Cytokines and Chemokines in Infectious Diseases Handbook

Infectious Disease

SERIES EDITOR: *Vassil St. Georgiev*

National Institute of Allergy and Infectious Diseases
National Institutes of Health

Cytokines and Chemokines in Infectious Diseases Handbook

Edited by

Malak Kotb, PhD

*Departments of Surgery and Molecular Sciences, University of Tennessee
VA Medical Center, Memphis, TN*

Thierry Calandra, MD, PhD

*Division of Infectious Diseases, Department of Internal Medicine,
Centre Hospital Universitaire Vaudois, Lausanne, Switzerland*

Humana Press ✳ Totowa, New Jersey

© 2003 Humana Press Inc.
999 Riverview Drive, Suite 208
Totowa, New Jersey 07512

www.humanapress.com

For additional copies, pricing for bulk purchases, and/or information about other Humana titles, contact Humana at the above address or at any of the following numbers: Tel.: 973-256-1699; Fax: 973-256-8341, E-mail: humana@humanapr.com; or visit our Website: http://humanapr.com

Production Editor: Robin B. Weisberg.
Cover illustration: Extracellular group A streptococci invading tissue and producing superantigens that elicit potent inflammatory cytokine responses. Norrby-Teglund A., et al. Unpublished data.
Cover design by Patricia F. Cleary.

This publication is printed on acid-free paper. ∞
ANSI Z39.48-1984 (American National Standards Institute) Permanence of Paper for Printed Library Materials.

Library of Congress Cataloging-in-Publication Data

Cytokines and chemokines in infectious diseases handbook / edited by Malak Kotb and Thierry Calandra.
        p. ; cm. -- (Infectious disease)
    Includes bibliographical references and index.
    ISBN 0-89603-908-0 (alk. paper); 1-59259-309-7 (e-ISBN)
      1. Cytokines—Physiological effect—Handbooks, manuals, etc. 2. Cytokines—Pathophsiology—Handbooks, manuals, etc. 3. Chemokines—Physiological effect—Handbooks, manuals, etc. 4. Chemokines—Pathophsiology—Handbooks, manuals, etc. 5. Infection—Handbooks, manuals, etc. 6. Communicable diseases—Immunological aspects—Handbooks, manuals, etc. I. Kotb, Malak. II. Calandra, Thierry. III. Infectious disease (Totowa, N.J.)
      [DNLM: 1. Chemokines—immunology. 2. Cytokines—immunology. 3. Communicable Diseases—immunology. QW 568 H2357 2003]
    QR185.8.C95 H355 2003
      616.9'0479—dc21   2002032871

This book is dedicated in loving memory to my mother whose love, friendship, beauty of the soul, and extraordinary strength have guided me throughout my life.

—*Malak Kotb*

Preface

Cytokines and chemokines are an important class of effector molecules that play a fundamental role in orchestrating the innate and acquired immune responses needed to eliminate or wall off invading pathogens. In vitro and in vivo studies have been instrumental in revealing the complexity of the cytokine network and the many facets of cytokine biology, such as pleiotropism (i.e., the capacity for a given cytokine to stimulate several cell types) and redundancy (i.e., the ability of different cytokines to exert similar effects). However, the development of sensitive reagents to detect and measure human cytokines and chemokines has provided opportunities to investigate the role of these important mediators in human inflammatory and infectious diseases. Despite many similarities, important differences in cytokine responses and mode of action between human and animal models became evident. A shift in focus from animal to clinical studies was, therefore, inevitable.

In recent years, we have witnessed an outpouring of information on the role of cytokines and chemokines in human infectious diseases. These studies have led to a deeper understanding of the pathogenesis of infectious diseases, an appreciation for differences of cytokine and chemokine production profiles in response to various pathogens, and a realization that genetic host factors influence the type and magnitude of cytokine and chemokine responses to a given microorganism. Our understanding of the immunopathogenesis of specific infections has become much more profound and thorough, and has thus contributed to the design of better and more effective therapeutic interventions for the management of patients with infectious diseases.

While playing a pivotal role in host defense against infection, cytokines also contribute to pathology when released in excessive amounts. Much work, both in academic institutions and in the biotechnology and pharmaceutical industries, has been devoted to the development of cytokine or anticytokine treatment strategies in infectious diseases. Although some strategies have failed, there have been numerous successes that have led to effective interventions for inflammatory and infectious diseases. One reason for the failure of cytokine-based therapies in infectious diseases may have stemmed from a lack of understanding of important differences in cytokine biology in infections caused by different pathogens.

Cytokines and Chemokines in Infectious Diseases Handbook is meant to provide a unique and up-to-date reference on the role of cytokines and chemokines in a variety of human infectious diseases. International leaders in the field present a comprehensive overview of cytokine and chemokine responses in bacterial, viral, fungal, and parasitic infections. Readers will gain a better appreciation for the differences in cytokine profiles in distinct infectious diseases and will see how this knowledge has led to a deeper understanding of host–pathogen interactions, as well as the pathogenetic basis of infectious diseases. In addition, *Handbook of Cytokines and Chemokines in Infectious Diseases* is intended to provide a critical evaluation of the use of cytokines and anticytokines in the treatment of infectious diseases and to demonstrate how knowledge of cytokine pleiotropic effects, redundancy, and the complexity of the cytokine network has impacted the use of cytokines as therapeutic tools.

Malak Kotb, PhD
Thierry Calandra, MD, PhD

vii

Contents

Contributors

LAURENCE ARBIBE, MD • *Unité de Biologie Moléculaire de l'Expression Génique, Institut Pasteur, Paris, France*

ANTONIO BERTOLETTI, MD • *Institute of Hepatology, Royal Free University College Medical School, University College London, UK*

PIERRE-YVES BOCHUD, MD • *Division of Infectious Diseases, Department of Internal Medicine, Centre Hospital Universitaire Vaudois, Lausanne, Switzerland*

THIERRY CALANDRA, MD, PhD • *Division of Infectious Diseases, Department of Internal Medicine, Centre Hospital Universitaire Vaudois, Lausanne, Switzerland*

JEAN-LAURENT CASANOVA, MD, PhD • *Laboratory of Human Genetics of Infectious Diseases, and Pediatric Immunology Hematology Unit, Necker Enfants Malades Medical School, Paris, France*

JEAN-MARC CAVAILLON, DSC • *Unit Cytokines and Inflammation, Institut Pasteur, Paris, France*

DAVID C. DALE, MD • *Department of Medicine, University of Washington, Seattle, WA*

CHARLES A. DINARELLO, MD • *University of Colorado Health Sciences Center, Division Infectious Diseases, Denver, Colorado*

STÉPHANIE DUPUIS, PhD • *Laboratory of Human Genetics of Infectious Diseases, Necker Enfants Malades Medical School, Paris, France*

STEFAN EHLERS, MD • *Division of Molecular Infection Biology, Center for Medicine and Biosciences, Borstel, Germany*

JERROLD J. ELLNER, MD • *University of Medicine and Dentistry of New Jersey, Newark, NJ*

CLAIRE FIESCHI, MD • *Laboratory of Human Genetics of Infectious Diseases, Necker Enfants Malades Medical School, Paris, France*

JOANNA FILIOTI, MD • *3rd Department of Pediatrics, Aristotle University of Thessaloniki, Hippokration Hospital, Thessaloniki, Greece*

CLAUDIO FORTIS, MD • *Laboratory of Clinical Immunology, San Raffaele Scientific Institute, Milano, Italy*

JOHN I. GALLIN, MD • *Laboratory of Host Defenses, National Institute of Allergy and Infectious Diseases, National Institutes of Health, Bethesda, MD*

CRISTINA GIL-LAMAIGNERE, PhD • *3rd Department of Pediatrics, Aristotle University of Thessaloniki, Hippokration Hospital, Thessaloniki, Greece*

MICHEL P. GLAUSER, MD • *Division of Infectious Diseases, Department of Internal Medicine, Centre Hospital Universitaire Vaudois, Lausanne, Switzerland*

KLAUS HEEG, MD • *Institute of Medical Microbiology and Hygiene, Philipps University of Marburg, Germany*

STEVEN M. HOLLAND, MD • *Clinical Pathophysiology Section, Laboratory of Host Defenses, National Institute of Allergy and Infectious Diseases, National Institutes of Health, Bethesda, MD*

HANS HOLMBERG, MD • *Department of Infectious Diseases, Örebro University Hospital, Örebro, Sweden*

KAI HÜBEL, MD • *Department of Medicine, University of Washington, Seattle, WA*

BRIGITTE T. HUBER, PhD • *Department of Pathology, Tufts University School of Medicine, Boston, MA*

CHRISTOPHER A. HUNTER, PhD • *Department of Pathobiology, University of Pennsylvania, Philadelphia, PA*

STEFAN H. E. KAUFMANN, PhD • *Department of Immunology, Max Planck Institute for Infection Biology, Berlin, Germany*

MALAK KOTB, PhD • *Departments of Surgery and Molecular Sciences, University of Tennessee VA Medical Center, Memphis, TN*

PETER KRAGSBJERG, MD • *Department of Internal Medicine, Division of Hematology, Örebro University Hospital, Örebro, Sweden*

ADRIANO LAZZARIN, MD • *Division of Infectious Diseases, San Raffaele Scientific Institute, Milano, Italy*

W. CONRAD LILES, MD • *Department of Medicine, University of Washington, Seattle, WA*

GRAHAM LORD, MD • *Department of Immunology, Division of Medicine, Faculty of Medicine, Imperial College of Science, Technology and Medicine, Hammersmith Hospital, London*

JACQUES A. LOUIS, MD • *Institute of Biochemistry, WHO-IRTC, Epalinges, Switzerland*

DONALD E. LOW, MD, PhD • *Department of Microbiology, Mount Sinai Hospital and the University of Toronto, Toronto, Canada*

PAOLO LUSSO, MD • *Unit of Human Virology, Department of Biological and Technological Research, San Raffaele Scientific Institute, Milan, Italy*

MALA K. MAINI, MRCP, PhD • *Departments of Sexually Transmitted Diseases and Immunology, Royal Free and University College Medical School, University College London, UK*

GRANT McFADDEN, MD • *Department of Microbiology and Immunology, University of Western Ontario and The John P. Robarts Research Institute, London, Ontario, Canada*

ABBIE L. MEYER, PhD • *Department of Pathology, Tufts University School of Medicine, Boston, MA*

GENEVIÈVE MILON, DVM • *Pasteur Institute, Paris France*

MILTON OZORIO MORAES, PhD • *Leprosy Laboratory, Oswaldo Cruz Institute, Rio de Janeiro, Brazil*

ANNA NORRBY-TEGLUND, PhD • *Center for Infectious Medicine, Department of Medicine, Karolinska Institute, Huddinge University Hospital, Stockholm, Sweden*

M. CRISTINA VIDAL PESSOLANI, PhD • *Leprosy Laboratory, Oswaldo Cruz Institute, Rio de Janeiro, Brazil*

CAPUCINE PICARD, MD • *Laboratory of Human Genetics of Infectious Diseases, and Pediatric Immunology Hematology Unit, Necker Enfants Malades Medical School, Paris, France*

GUIDO POLI, MD • *AIDS Immunopathogenesis Unit, San Raffaele Scientific Institute, Milan, Italy*

EMMANUEL ROILIDES, MD • *3rd Department of Pediatrics, Aristotle University of Thessaloniki, Hippokration Hospital, Thessaloniki, Greece*

MICHAEL S. ROLPH, PhD • *Garvan Institute of Medical Research, Darlinghurst, Sydney, NSW, Australia*

LUIGINA ROMANI, MD • *Microbiology Section, Department of Experimental Medicine and Biochemical Sciences, University of Perugia, Italy*

RICHARD K. ROOT, MD • *Department of Medicine, University of Washington, Seattle, WA*

ELIZABETH PEREIRA SAMPAIO, PhD • *Leprosy Laboratory, Oswaldo Cruz Institute, Rio de Janeiro, Brazil*

PHILIPPE SANSONETTI, MD • *Unité de Pathogénie Microbienne Moléculaire et Unité, Institut Pasteur, Paris, France*

EUZENIR NUNES SARNO, PhD • *Leprosy Laboratory, Oswaldo Cruz Institute, Rio de Janeiro, Brazil*

FRANK STÜBER, MD • *Molecular Research Lab, University Hospital Bonn, Friedrich-Wilhelms-Universität Bonn, Germany*

FABIENNE TACCHINI-COTTIER, PhD • *Institute of Biochemistry, WHO-IRTC, Epalinges, Switzerland*

GIUSEPPE TAMBUSSI, MD • *Division of Infectious Diseases, San Rafaelle Scientific Institute, Milano, Italy*

ZAHRA TOOSSI, MD • *Division of Infectious Diseases, Case Western Reserve University, Cleveland, OH*

ULRIKE WILLE, PhD • *Department of Pathobiology, University of Pennsylvania, Philadelphia, PA*

Introduction:
Cytokine Biology Relevant to Infectious Diseases

Charles A. Dinarello

1. INTRODUCTION

Cytokine- and anticytokine-based therapies have already entered the mainstream of medical practice. Regulatory agencies continue to approve anticytokine therapies for patients with rheumatoid arthritis, and it appears highly likely that more will be approved in the near future. Cytokines also play a role in the pathogenesis of sepsis and septic shock. Two cytokines are particularly important: interleukin-1 (IL-1) and tumor necrosis factor-α (TNF-α). However, these are not the only cytokines that are involved in sepsis, and many other cytokines are likely therapeutic targets. Whether blocking other cytokines, blocking more than one cytokine, or a combination of these will reduce mortality in the septic patient is unclear at the present time. As with many new areas in science and technology, spin-offs are anticipated. From the results of current trials examining the blocking of IL-1 and TNF-α in patients with rheumatoid arthritis, it is certain that more will be learned about the role of these cytokines in sepsis.

The proinflammatory and anti-inflammatory cytokines discussed in this book have been selected because of their association with the pathogenesis of infectious diseases. Hundreds of investigators have carried out extensive studies determining the type, location, and quantities of cytokines produced during infections in various body fluids of affected patients. The levels of circulating cytokines and the production of cytokines from peripheral blood cells of patients with active infections have also been reported. Often, the results from these studies have been contrasted with results from patients with noninfectious disease, such as generalized trauma. Sepsis and the entire septic syndrome have attracted the most interest in cytokine biology. This is understandable because of the high mortality in these patients. The septic patient has also been the target of many studies using specific anticytokine-based therapies. In fact, a meta-analysis of anticytokine trials in the septic patient have been examined and more than 10,000 patients have been entered in several placebo-controlled, double-blind, randomized trials *(1)*.

As a result, it can be readily observed that dysregulation of innate immunity (also called nonspecific immunity) to the detriment of the host is prominent in sepsis. Dysregulation of innate immunity, also to the detriment of the host, is prominent in rheumatoid arthritis. However, in the case of rheumatoid arthritis, the same anti-cytokine agents that failed to improve 28-d all-cause mortality in sepsis trials have been highly successful in reducing the signs and symptoms of rheumatoid arthritis and related autoimmune diseases. There are more than 250,000 patients currently receiving either anti-TNF-α or IL-1 receptor blockade for the treatment of rheumatoid arthritis. In several studies, the effects of anticytokine therapy has reduced the progression of the joint destructive nature of the disease *(2–4)*. In fact, the TNF-α-soluble receptor (p75) that resulted in a dose-dependent worsening of 28-d all-cause mortality *(5)* is highly effective in treating juvenile rheumatoid arthritis *(6)* as well as psoriatic arthritis and psoriasis. The success of these anticytokine therapies in patients with rheu-

From: *Cytokines and Chemokines in Infectious Diseases Handbook*
Edited by: M. Kotb and T. Calandra © Humana Press Inc., Totowa, NJ

matoid arthritis provides strong evidence that these cytokines (TNF-α and IL-1) are, in fact, causal in the pathogenesis of rheumatoid arthritis.

The true test of a causal relationship between any one cytokine and a specific disease, however, comes from the results of clinical trials that demonstrate a correlation between the blockade or neutralization of a specific cytokine and a reduction in disease severity or disease progression. A great deal has been learned from the sepsis clinical studies, and there have been some remarkably consistent findings. Of considerable importance, these clinical trials have not validated results obtained from animal models of sepsis or septic shock. No animal model completely recapitulates the local and systemic picture of human sepsis; nevertheless, these models have yielded vital preclinical information on the role of individual cytokines in the pathologic processes of sepsis. Not all animal models have shown a benefit for survival, particularly when anticytokines are used in live bacterial models compared to the endotoxemia models.

In view of the increasing use of anticytokine-based therapies in patients with rheumatoid arthritis and related autoimmune diseases, the role of cytokines in host defense against infection becomes an important issue. There is a growing body of clinical evidence that neutralization of TNF-α is associated with an increased risk of opportunistic infection. Moreover, because of physician underreporting, the true incidence of infections, both serious and nonserious, will remain unknown. Nevertheless, does the increase in infections associated with anticytokine-based therapies come as a surprise? From a wealth of rodent studies, the following conclusions can be drawn: (1) neutralization of TNF-α is frequently associated with the reduction of host defense in models of live Gram-positive or Gram-negative infections; (2) reduced IL-1 activity can also result in decreased resistance to these same infectious agents, although possibly to a lesser extent; (3) TNF-α, IL-1, IL-6, IL-12, or interferon (IFN)-γ is required for defense against infection caused by *Mycobacterium tuberculosis*. It must be stressed, however, that the effect of blockade or deficiency of any particular cytokine or combination of cytokines in animal models of live infection does not necessarily predict the human experience, particularly in patients cotreated with a disease-modifying antirheumatic drug.

Because homologs of proinflammatory cytokines have been found in primitive species, cytokines likely play some continuing role in the survival of the host. There are numerous animal studies showing that several proinflammatory cytokines are essential for natural resistance to specific infections, particularly intracellular organisms. The reduction in the production and/or activities of proinflammatory cytokines in rheumatoid arthritis remains a therapeutic objective for many patients. However, this raises the perennial issue of what is an acceptable risk in the use of these therapies. Rheumatoid arthritis is a chronic disease, and anticytokine-based therapies require chronic administration. Thus, the long-term effects of cytokine blockade may interfere with host defense functions. The two areas of host defense that may be affected by chronic anticytokine therapies are resistance to infection and immune surveillance for cancer. In this chapter, the mechanisms by which cytokines affect immune mechanisms of tumor surveillance are not discussed but, rather, the chapter focuses on their role in infections.

2. MODELS USING MICE WITH TARGETED GENE DELETIONS (KNOCKOUT MICE)

2.1. Advantages of Using Knockout Mice

The use of mice with specific cytokine or cytokine receptor gene deletion(s) (knockouts) offers several advantages over chronic pharmacologic administration, primarily because of an absolute absence of the gene product from conception to death. Compared to the use of cytokine inhibitors, when using knockout mice there are seldom questions concerning inadequate doses of neutralizing antibodies, low-affinity antibodies, poor antibody specificity, or similar issues for soluble receptors on binding proteins where ligand passing or a carrier function may exist. For example, some antibodies to IL-6 neutralize IL-6 in vitro but act as carriers of IL-6 in vivo and, in doing so, prolong the activity of IL-6 in models of disease. Therefore, IL-6 knockout mice are preferred to address the role of IL-6 in models of disease.

With the use of knockout mice, there is no question concerning drug penetration into tissues. In other models of rheumatoid arthritis or autoimmune encephalomyelitis, however, penetration of the affected joint by large molecules may be reduced, and dosing becomes an issue. Another advantage of the cytokine knockout models is the lack of an immune response to an antibody or a soluble receptor when either is exogenously administered over long periods of time. For example, when testing whether daily infusions of human IL-1 receptor antagonist (IL-1Ra) affect the development of a disease that evolves over several weeks, the animal will likely develop antibodies to the human IL-1Ra that reduce the effectiveness of the infusions.

2.2. Disadvantages of Using Knockout Mice

The primary disadvantage of using cytokine knockout mice is the lack of clinical relevance of absent cytokine activity in knockout mice compared to reduced cytokine activity when using anticytokine therapies. For example, the administration of any TNF inhibitor results in a peak of the inhibitor, followed by a nadir prior to the next injection. It is unlikely that complete and sustained neutralization of TNF-α occurs with current dosing. In the case of IL-1 inhibition, 24 h after an intravenous infusion of anakinra (a recombinant form of IL-1Ra) at 1 mg/kg in healthy volunteers, the blood levels of anakinra had fallen to levels less than 1.0 ng/mL *(7)*. Therefore, in order to predict a clinically relevant defect in host defense during anticytokine therapy using data derived from cytokine knockout mice, one would have to sustain a high level of the anticytokine in the relevant body compartment to match the situation in the knockout mouse for the same cytokine. It is questionable whether that could be accomplished in the clinical setting.

Another widely held view is that the absence of a particular cytokine or cytokine receptor from conception into adult life results in other cytokines being overexpressed and compensating for the deleted signaling pathways. In the IL-1β knockout mouse, the response to IL-1α is enhanced *(8)* suggesting that lacking receptor occupancy by IL-1β, the intracellular signaling by IL-1α by the same receptor has changed. These unusual responses have also been observed with other cytokine knockout models. When mice deficient in TNF-RII are challenged with bacterial endotoxin, TNF-α production is markedly enhanced *(9)*. Therefore, it is unclear whether the increased mortality in these TNF-RII knockout mice challenged with endotoxin is the result of the absence of TNF-RII signaling or is secondary to increased TNF-α and TNF-RI signaling.

When a cytokine knockout mouse fails to develop an inducible disease, one can conclude that such a cytokine likely plays a role in the development of that disease. For example, the IL-1β knockout mouse does not develop an inflammatory response to local tissue necrosis *(10)*. One can assume from these mouse studies that in the clinical setting, there may be a role for IL-1β in patients with local trauma injuries. On the other hand, when a cytokine knockout mouse fails to resist infection, one cannot conclude that a comparable clinical condition may exist in humans. The best example is the IFN-γ receptor knockout mouse. This mouse is unusually susceptible to *Mycobacterium bovis* BCG (Bacille–Calmette–Guérin) infection *(11)*. Humans lacking a functional IFN-γ receptor are also susceptible to mycobacterial infections *(12)*.

3. A COMPARISON OF MOUSE AND HUMAN RESPONSES TO BACTERIAL ENDOTOXINS

In critically ill patients with sepsis syndrome or septic shock, the transient overproduction of proinflammatory cytokines likely contributes to manifestation of the systemic inflammatory response, development of organ failure, and even death. In order to study the role of cytokines in sepsis, injection of purified endotoxins and exotoxins have been used to mimic Gram-negative and Gram-positive infections, respectively. In animal models of endotoxemia or exotoxemia, blocking the production and/or activity of proinflammatory cytokines such as IL-1, TNF-α, IL-12, or IFN-γ has reduced mortality, improved hemodynamic performance, and provided a comprehensive body of evidence showing the detrimental effects of overproduction of these cytokines. Indeed, this evidence provided the rationale for clinical trials blocking any one of these cytokines in high-risk patients with sepsis. Although this has been a logical strategy, the failure to reduce 28-d all-cause mortality at a statistically significant level using any one of several agents to neutralize TNF-α or to block the IL-1 receptor with anakinra has raised the issue of whether these animal models of endotoxemia were appropriate for humans at risk of death from sepsis *(1)*. Therefore, some investigators have compared models of live infection with those of noninfectious endotoxemia and have shown substantial differences between anticytokine interventions for the outcome of these models. For example, in rodent models of sepsis that result from a nidus of infection, blocking endogenous TNF-α has often been ineffective or has worsened disease and increased mortality compared to controls. This is in contrast to the beneficial effect of anti-TNF-α on survival in endotoxemia. In particular, in mice subjected to a nonlethal peritonitis resulting from cecal ligation and puncture, blocking TNF-α resulted in lethal peritonitis *(13)*. These studies showed that an endogenous TNF-α response was actually essential for the formation of an abscess to sequester the infectious agents. In subsequent studies, an endogenous TNF-α response and signaling through the TNF-RI was required for the formation of fibrin deposits and granulocyte function. The mast cell and mast-cell-derived TNF-α appeared to play a central role in this protective effect. Such studies have raised the issue that TNF blockade in septic humans may impair the natural host defense mechanisms to combat or prevent the downward spiral from infection to death. They also emphasize the subtle but critically important observation that the absence of any given cytokine may be as detrimental as its excess.

Purified LPS or killed suspensions of Gram-negative bacteria can be injected intraperitoneally, intravenously, or intratracheally. However, in general, rodents and primates are particularly insensitive to endotoxins when compared to humans. In fact, the lethal amount of disease-inducing endotoxin given to mice and rats ranges from 1 to 10 mg/kg, and mg/kg doses produce a systemic inflammatory response. In contrast, in humans, an intravenous bolus injection of only 3 or 4 ng/kg of *Escherichia coli* lipopolysaccharide (LPS) produces fever, reduces hemodynamic functions, is a cardiosuppressant, and results in increased procoagulant activities. Other indications of systemic inflammation in the endocrine and hematopoietic systems are manifested within 3–4 h in humans injected with endotoxin. There is little question that humans are exquisitely sensitive to the systemic effects of LPS, whereas rodents and primates are impressively resistant. To make rodents more vulnerable to endotoxemia, animals can be pretreated with transcriptional inhibitors, such as D-galactosamine or actinomycin D, which prevent the synthesis of "survival genes" that protect against endotoxemia. It should be noted, however, that although the use of these transcriptional inhibitors markedly increases the sensitivity to LPS, the mechanisms of lethality are profoundly different. Whereas high-dose LPS kills predominantly through vascular injury, hypotension, shock, and necrotic injury, D-galactosamine-sensitized mice treated with low-dose LPS die predominantly from apoptotic liver injury.

Nevertheless, models of endotoxemia overwhelmingly dominate the literature, especially in intervention experiments with anticytokines. Extensive literature exists on the beneficial effects of blocking TNF-α, IL-1, and other cytokines in these various models of endotoxemia. Furthermore, using cytokine and cytokine receptor knockout mice, similar data have been reported. Is the endotoxemia model relevant to the role of a cytokine in combating an indolent infection and preventing it from becoming life threatening? The appropriate models use live organisms.

4. POLYMICROBIAL SEPSIS AS A MODEL

Several studies have examined the role of cytokines using live infection, particularly cecal ligation and puncture. In this model, mice or rats undergo ligation of the cecum followed by a single or double puncture with a small or large needle. After the procedure, the peritoneal cavity is surgically closed. The rapidly evolving peritonitis varies in severity depending on the size and number of holes, but even with antibiotic treatment, death generally takes place in 2–10 d. Bacteria are found in the peritoneal cavity, in the liver, and, occasionally, in the lungs. The ability to form an abscess to contain the infection is critical for survival *(13)*. Neutrophils are also important in that attempts to decrease the numbers or the ability of neutrophils to emigrate and phagocytize bacteria worsen the infection.

Endotoxemia is part of the cecal ligation and puncture model, but death is usually the result of a large bacterial burden. Therefore, increasing neutrophil function often results in increased survival. For example, the administration of chemokines such as the CC chemokine C10 increases survival *(14)*. Consistent with this observation, blocking TNF-α decreases the survival response to a mixed flora bacterial infection, but this appears to be dependent on the severity of the infectious challenge. For example, reducing the size of the needle used to puncture the cecum can produce a model with a modest mortality (approx 10%). When endogenous TNF-α was neutralized in these mice using a monoclonal antibody, mortality was dramatically increased. Those studies revealed a requirement for TNF-α to form an abscess and sequester the infectious agents. When the severity of the model is increased to nearly 100% lethality by increasing the size and/or number of the punctures, passive immunization against TNF-α alone produces no improvement in survival.

In addition to suppressing TNF-a and IL-1, IL-10 can be immunosuppressive, in part through its ability to block Th1 and promote Th2-mediated immune response. This has been most evident in models where an endogenous IL-10 response to injury may contribute to the immunosuppression leading to secondary infections. For example, following a burn injury, mice are more susceptible to lethal cecal ligation and puncture. However, this increased susceptibility could be prevented by treating the mice with a monoclonal antibody against IL-10 in the interim between the burn injury and the cecal ligation and puncture. Similarly, an endogenous IL-10 response following cecal ligation and puncture was responsible for the decreased antimicrobial response and increased mortality resulting from lung exposure to *Pseudomonas aeruginosa*.

The administration of recombinant IL-1Ra either alone (15) or with polyethelyne glycol TNF-RI (16) remarkably increased survival in rodent models with lethal cecal ligation and puncture. The protective effect of IL-1Ra compared to the decreased survival in animals either deficient in TNF-a or given anti-TNF-a antibodies is a consistent finding. One possible mechanism for the survival benefit of IL-1Ra may be to reduce the inflammatory component of the disease while not impairing antimicrobial responses to the peritonitis.

REFERENCES

1. Zeni, F., Freeman, B., and Natanson, C. (1997) Anti-inflammatory therapies to treat sepsis and septic shock: a reassessment. *Crit. Care Med.* **25,** 1095–1100.
2. Bresnihan, B., Alvaro-Gracia, J.M., Cobby, M., Doherty, M., Domljan, Z., et al. (1998) Treatment of rheumatoid arthritis with recombinant human interleukin-1 receptor antagonist. *Arthritis Rheum.* **41,** 2196–2204.
3. Lipsky, P.E., van der Heijde, D.M., St Clair, E.W., Furst, D.E., Breedveld, F.C., et al. (2000) Infliximab and methotrexate in the treatment of rheumatoid arthritis. *N. Engl. J. Med.* **343,** 1594–1602.
4. Moreland, L.W., Baumgartner, S.W., Schiff, M.H., Tindall, E.A., Fleischmann, R.M., et al. (1997) Treatment of rheumatoid arthritis with a recombinant human tumor necrosis factor receptor (p75)-Fc fusion protein. *N. Engl. J. Med.* **337,** 141–147.
5. Fisher, C., Jr., Agosti, J.M., Opal, S.M., Lowry, S.F., Balk, R.A., et al. (1996) Treatment of septic shock with the tumor necrosis factor receptor:Fc fusion protein. *N. Engl. J. Med.* **334,** 1697–1702.
6. Takei, S., Groh, D., Bernstein, B., Shaham, B., Gallagher, K., and Reiff, A. (2001) Safety and efficacy of high dose etanercept in treatment of juvenile rheumatoid arthritis. *J. Rheumatol.* **28,** 1677–1680.
7. Granowitz, E.V., Porat, R., Mier, J.W., Pribble, J.P., Stiles, D.M., Bloedow, D.C., et al. (1992) Pharmacokinetics, saftey, and immunomodulatory effects of human recombinant interleukin-1 receptor antagonist in healthy humans. *Cytokine* **4,** 353–360.
8. Alhei, K., Chai, Z., Fantuzzi, G., Hasanvan, H., Malinowsky, D., Di Santo, E., et al. (1997) Hyperresponsive febrile reactions to interleukin (IL)-1alpha and IL-1beta, and altered brain cytokine mRNA and serum cytokine levels, in IL-1beta-deficient mice. *Proc. Natl. Acad. Sci. USA* **94,** 2681–2686.

9. Peschon, J.J., Torrance, D.S., Stocking, K.L., Glaccum, M.B., Otten, C., Willis, C.R., et al. (1998) TNF receptor-deficient mice reveal divergent roles for p55 and p75 in several models of inflammation. *J. Immunol.* **160,** 943–952.
10. Zheng, H., Fletcher, D., Kozak, W., Jiang, M., Hofmann, K., Conn, C.C., et al. (1995) Resistance to fever induction and impaired acute-phase response in interleukin-1β deficient mice. *Immunity* **3,** 9–19.
11. Kamijo, R., Le, J., Shapiro, D., Havell, E.A., Huang, S., Aguet, M., et al. (1993) Mice that lack the interferon-gamma receptor have profoundly altered responses to infection with Bacillus Calmette-Guerin and subsequent challenge with lipopolysaccharide. *J. Exp. Med.* **178,** 1435–1440.
12. Jouanguy E, Altare F, Lamhamedi S, Revy P, Emile JF, Newport M, et al. (1996) Interferon-gamma-receptor deficiency in an infant with fatal bacille Calmette–Guerin infection. *N. Engl. J. Med.* **335,** 1956–1961.
13. Echtenacher, B., Falk, W., Mannel, D.N., and Krammer, P.H. (1990) Requirement of endogenous tumor necrosis factor/cachectin for recovery from experimental peritonitis. *J. Immunol.* **145,** 3762–3766.
14. Steinhauser, M.L., Hogaboam, C.M., Matsukawa, A., Lukacs, N.W., Strieter, R.M., et al. (2000) Chemokine C10 promotes disease resolution and survival in an experimental model of bacterial sepsis. *Infect. Immun.* **68,** 6108–6114.
15. Alexander, H.R., Doherty, G.M., Venzon, D.J., Merino, M.J., Fraker, D.L., and Norton, J.A. (1992) Recombinant interleukin-1 receptor antagonist (IL-1ra): effective therapy against gram-negative sepsis in rats. *Surgery* **112,** 188–194.
16. Remick, D.G., Call, D.R., Ebong, S.J., Newcomb, D.E., Nybom, P., Nemzek, J.A., and Bolgos, G.E. (2001) Combination immunotherapy with soluble tumor necrosis factor receptors plus interleukin 1 receptor antagonist decreases sepsis mortality. *Crit. Care. Med.* **29,** 473–481.

I
Cytokines in Infectious Diseases

Leptin

Its Role in Immunomodulation and Susceptibility to Infection

Graham Lord

1. INTRODUCTION

The field of leptin and the immune system has expanded rapidly since the first article described the interrelationship of this cytokine, initially thought of as a weight-reducing hormone, with the optimal functioning of the immune system in vitro and in vivo *(1)*. There is still a great deal of work to be done in order to define precisely the role that leptin plays in the host response to infection and this chapter attempts to summarize the current thinking in this field. The chapter starts with an introduction to the biology of leptin, which is crucial in understanding how it compares with other cytokine systems. This section also highlights what is considered by many to be the main physiological role of leptin; namely that it acts as a signal of failing energy reserves. A brief discussion of the in vivo models of leptin deficiency follows, which leads in to the immune changes seen in starvation and malnutrition, a situation in which leptin may have its most profound effect on immunity and also susceptibility to infectious diseases.

The final section deals with the specific effects of leptin on the various cells of the immune system and how this relates to responses to pathogens.

The chapter attempts to address what may be the true physiological role for leptin as an immunomodulator. It is tempting to just write down a list of the known actions of a cytokine without trying to put the data into a biological context. Hopefully, I have gone some way toward putting the large amount of data into perspective.

2. THE BIOLOGY OF THE ACTION OF LEPTIN

2.1. The Obese Gene and its Protein Product Leptin

In 1994, the mouse obese (ob) gene and its human homolog were isolated by positional cloning *(2)*. In humans, the gene is positioned at 7q31. The mouse ob gene resides on chromosome 6 and consists of three exons and two introns and encodes a 4.5-kilobase (kb) mRNA. The coding sequence is contained within exons 2 and 3. The wild-type obese gene encodes a 167-amino-acid protein named leptin, expressed almost exclusively in white adipose tissue, although recently its expression has been found at lower levels in the placenta, stomach, and brain *(3–5)*. The homozygous mutant mouse ob/ob has a mutation in the obese gene, either as a result of a 5-kb ETn transposon inserted into the first intron of ob (ob^{2j} mice) or of a nonsense mutation causing protein truncation *(6)*. Leptin (leptos [Greek]: thin) is a 16-kDa class I cytokine, with structural similarity to interleukin (IL)-2, the para-

From: *Cytokines and Chemokines in Infectious Diseases Handbook*
Edited by: M. Kotb and T. Calandra © Humana Press Inc., Totowa, NJ

digm T-cell growth factor, although there is no sequence similarity *(7)*. It consists of 167 amino acids and is a helical cytokine, belonging to the family of hemopoietic cytokines, which includes IL-2, IL-3, IL-4, and granulocyte-macrophage colony-stimulating factor (GM-CSF). Leptin circulates in the bloodstream bound to plasma proteins and soluble leptin receptor (ObRe) *(8)*. The ratio of free:bound leptin in serum increases with increasing obesity *(9)*. Its serum levels are proportional to body fat mass *(10)* and are dynamically regulated, being increased by inflammatory mediators such as tumor necrosis factor (TNF)-a, IL-1, and lipopolysaccaride (LPS) *(11–13)* and being rapidly reduced by starvation *(14,15)*. The release of leptin is pulsatile *(16)* and is inversely related to ACTH and cortisol secretion *(17)*. The fact that obesity is associated with high leptin levels rather than vice versa, as would be predicted by the obese phenotype of the ob/ob mouse, has lead to the hypothesis that appetite suppression is not the main physiological role of leptin *(18)*. It is excreted via the kidneys and is, therefore, elevated in patients with end-stage renal failure (19). The regulation of leptin gene expression is highly complex, as it involves multiple mediators whose relative importance is, as yet, undetermined *(20)*. A high serum leptin level reduces leptin gene expression and changes in nutrient availability result in rapid alterations in gene expression *(21)*. Other important regulatory factors are glucocorticoids, insulin, and thyroid hormones. Corticosteroids enhance gene expression and protein secretion, whereas insulin causes release of leptin from an intracellular pool *(22)*. Thyroid hormones inhibit leptin gene expression *(23)* and sex steroids such as estrogen increase leptin mRNA levels *(24)*. This latter fact may underlie the sexual dimorphism observed in serum leptin concentration, such that for a given body mass index (BMI = weight [kg] / height^2 [m]), females have significantly higher leptin levels than males *(19,25)*.

2.2. Role of Leptin in the Regulation of Body Weight

Chronic administration of recombinant *ob* protein has been shown to produce a significant reduction in body weight in *ob/ob* and normal mice because of a reduction in food intake but also an increase in energy expenditure *(26–28)*. Centrally administered leptin (into the lateral or third cerebral ventricles) has been shown to be particularly effective in promoting anorexia and weight loss at doses which when administered peripherally were without effect on feeding behavior *(26)*. This suggests that leptin acts on receptors within the central nervous system, probably at the level of the hypothalamus and clearly implicate leptin as an important factor in the regulation of body weight in rodents *(29)*. Further evidence that implicates leptin as a regulator of body weight is the fact that total deficiency in leptin in mouse and man causes obesity, *(29,30)* which is reversed by leptin treatment *(27,31)*. However, as mentioned earlier, leptin levels are high in rodent and human models of obesity, *(10,32)* leading to the hypothesis that either there is resistance to the actions of leptin akin to insulin resistance in type 2 diabetes mellitus *(33)* or that the main function of leptin is a signal of starvation and not body weight regulation (*see* Section 2.3) *(14)*. There is some experimental evidence for the occurrence of leptin resistance because leptin induces the expression of SOCS-3 (suppressor of cytokine signaling), which subsequently prevents that cell from responding to further leptin *(34,35)*. The poor clinical results of leptin as a weight-reducing agent have cast further doubt on the assertion that its main role is as a body weight regulator *(36)*.

2.3. Role of Leptin as a Signal of Starvation

In 1996, Ahima et al. proposed a role for leptin as a signal of energy deficiency *(14)*. Circulating leptin levels fall rapidly in response to starvation when energy intake is limited and energy stores (fat) are declining. It was suggested that leptin may have evolved to signal the shift between sufficient and insufficient energy stores *(18)*. The hypothesis that reduced circulating leptin levels signal nutrient deprivation is supported by the demonstration that prevention of the starvation-induced fall in plasma leptin levels by exogenous replacement is able to prevent the starvation-induced delay in ovulation in female mice. In addition, such a regime of leptin replacement was also shown to partially prevent the fasting-induced rise in plasma corticosterone levels and the fall in plasma thyroid hormone (total T4) levels *(14)*. It is likely that leptin exerts these effects at the level of the central nervous system *(18)*.

2.4. Peripheral Effects of Leptin

In addition to the centrally mediated effects of leptin, many peripheral effects have been reported. Leptin receptor expression has been demonstrated in the pancreas *(37,38)*, hemopoietic stem cells *(39)*, endothelial cells, *(40)* and reproductive organs *(39)* where leptin has been shown to have direct effects in vitro. Thus, leptin can influence ovarian hormone synthesis, can induce proliferation and differentiation of bone marrow cells, *(41)* and can act as an angiogenic factor by its action on endothelial cells *(40)*. Leptin can also affect insulin secretion from pancreatic β-cells by inhibiting glucose-stimulated insulin release both in vitro and in vivo *(37,38)*. Metabolic effects of leptin are partially peripheral and partly central, via the sympathetic nervous system *(42)*. Leptin directly promotes glucose uptake and glycogen synthesis in skeletal muscle *(43,44)* and promotes lipolysis with no increase in free fatty acids *(45)*. The relative importance of these central and peripheral effects of leptin still remains to be determined. It will be difficult to dissect observed responses completely, however, because many effects are likely to be both peripherally and centrally mediated *(20)*.

2.5. Leptin Receptor Genetics and Structure

The receptor for leptin was identified by expression cloning in 1995. Sequencing of the original mouse cDNA demonstrated that it coded for a single membrane spanning protein of the class I cytokine receptor family residing on chromosome 4 (human: 1p31). It consists of 20 exons, of which the first 2 are noncoding *(46)*. This family includes gp130, G-CSF, interleukin-6, and leukemia inhibitory factor receptors among its members and is consistent with predictions that leptin itself was a helical cytokine structurally homologous to growth hormone and interleukin-2. There are several isoforms of the leptin receptor (ObRa–e) in both mice and humans arising from alternative RNA splicing at the most C-terminal coding exon of the leptin receptor gene. All isoforms have a common extracellular domain but differ in the length of their intracytoplasmic domain *(46–48)*. One isoform (OBRe) is predicted to be a soluble receptor, as it lacks the transmembrane domain *(48)*. The "long isoform" of the leptin receptor (ObRb) has a long intracellular domain of about 303 amino acids and contains sequence motifs enabling it to employ the JAK–STAT pathway for signal transduction *(49,50)*. Mice and humans that have mutant receptors with impaired or no signal transducing capacity have a phenotype of obesity and insulin resistance identical to that of *ob* gene mutations *(47,51)*.

2.6. Distribution of the Leptin Receptor

The short leptin receptor isoforms appear to be ubiquitously expressed, although their function remains to be established *(50)*. It has been suggested that the high levels of ObRa observed in the choroid plexus may play a role in transporting leptin from the bloodstream into the cerebrospinal fluid (CSF), from where it can access centers in the hypothalamus involved in energy homeostasis *(52)*. The long isoform of the leptin receptor, ObRb, is expressed at high levels in the hypothalamic nuclei known to be of importance in the regulation of body weight *(53,54)*. However, ObRb mRNA expression has also been detected in rodent peripheral tissues such as pancreatic β-cells *(38)* and lymph nodes, *(28,50)* suggesting that leptin may have a broader physiological role. We and others have shown that ObRb is expressed in T-cells *(1,55)* and there is good evidence to suggest that it is also expressed by macrophages *(53,56)*.

2.7. Signal Transduction via the Receptor

As with other class I cytokine receptors, ObRb has been shown to signal through the JAK–STAT pathway *(57)*. To date, only STAT-3 activation has been detected following exogenous leptin administration in vivo, although there are reports that as well as STAT-3, STAT-1, -5, and -6 are stimulated in COS cells transfected with ObRb *(49,50)*. No STAT protein activation has been observed following leptin administration to db/db mice *(50)*. ObRa has been shown to be capable of signal transduction and to weakly activate gene expression in vitro *(58,59)*. The physiological importance of this signaling capability of the short isoforms in vivo, however, remains unclear. Indeed, the db/db mouse displays a phenotype identical to the leptin-deficient ob/ob mouse despite expression of all but the long ObRb isoform of the leptin receptor, underscoring the prime importance of ObRb in leptin-mediated signaling. Leptin binding to ObRb causes tyrosyl phosphorylation of the cytoplasmic domain of the receptor. SHP-2 (SH2 domain containing protein tyrosine phosphatase-2) binds to these regions and serves to reduce JAK-2 phosphorylation. This would serve to reduce the signaling capacity of ObRb, providing a means of controlling signal transduction *(60)*. It has been postulated that the short receptor isoforms may act as a type of molecular sink for leptin *(52)*, thus flattening out the ultradian oscillations that typify leptin release *(16)*. It has also been suggested that the short isoform (ObRa) found in abundance in the choroid plexus may serve as a transport protein across the blood-brain barrier and that this mechanism is saturable, giving another mechanism for the proposed state of leptin resistance (*see* Section 2.2) *(61,62)*. In this vein, new molecules called Ob-binding protein 1 and 2 (OB-BP1/2) have recently been cloned. They are expressed on B-lymphocytes and their function is assumed to be similar to that of the short leptin receptor isoforms *(63)*.

Recently, it has also been shown that leptin can activate PI3-kinase and the signaling pathways distal to this *(64)*. Futhermore, leptin has also been shown to activate the mitogen-activated protein (MAP) kinase pathway of signal transduction *(65)*. Interestingly, both of these pathways are activated in macrophages. The significance of the activation of these different signaling pathways remains to be determined.

2.8. Dynamics and Kinetics of Ligand–Receptor Binding

As is the case for the class I cytokine receptors, ObRb probably dimerizes in order to signal optimally *(66)*. Unlike the other receptors of this class that form heterodimers with gp130 *(57)*, ObRb forms homodimers or homo-oligomers *(67)*. This homo-oligomerization is ligand independent and signaling via ObRb is not susceptible to dominant negative repression by the short isoforms, even when they are present in great excess *(66)*. The leptin receptor is able to homo-oligomerize in an isoform-specific manner, such that long isoforms specifically oligomerize even in the presence of an excess of short forms of the receptor. This probably occurs via the JAK-binding motif in the intracytoplasmic domain of ObRb *(68)*. This is an important finding, as it provides a mechanism whereby leptin can exert potent effects even in issues with a relatively low density of ObRb. Following ligand binding, the leptin receptor is internalized via clathrin-mediated endocytosis at different rates; ObRb is downregulated to the greatest extent and reaches the lysosome more rapidly than the other isoforms *(69,70)*.

Given that the extracellular domains of all the isoforms of the leptin receptor are identical, their binding kinetics are also equivalent. Using a soluble extracellular receptor domain, the apparent affinity constant (*Kd*) was 9.5 nM, as measured by surface plasmon resonance *(71)*. These data, along with measured association and dissociation rate constants, give a calculated ligand–receptor half-life of approximately 8 min. Furthermore, as the range of serum leptin levels in humans lies between 0.1 and 10 nM *(10)*, then at steady state, over 50% of leptin receptors will be occupied by ligand. This may be an important consideration when trying to understand the physiological role of leptin, because a reduction of receptor occupancy from a high initial level may be more biologically significant that an increase under the same circumstances.

3. IN VIVO MODELS OF LEPTIN DEFICIENCY

3.1. The ob/ob and db/db Mouse

Recessive mutations in the mouse *diabetes* (*db*) and *obese* (*ob*) genes have long been recognized to cause a syndrome of obesity and diabetes resembling morbid obesity in humans *(32,72)*. These mice are phenotypically identical, each weighing three times more than normal mice, with a fivefold increase in body fat content. In his pioneering parabiosis work, Coleman showed that the obesity in the *ob/ob* mouse was the result of the lack of a circulating satiety factor and that the phenotype of the *db/db* mouse was probablycaused by a receptor defect for that factor *(73,74)*. The *ob/ob* phenotype has since been found to result from two different mutations in two different strains of mice. The mutation in *ob²ʲ* mice prevents synthesis of leptin caused by a mutation that results in the insertion of a retrovirallike transposon in the first intron of the *ob* gene. This insertion contains several splice acceptor and polyadenylation sites, which leads to the production of chimaeric RNAs in which the first exon is spliced to sequences in the transposon. Thus, mature mRNA is not produced *(6)*. In the C57BL/6 *ob/ob* mutant, a nonsense mutation results in the production of a truncated inactive leptin *(2)*.

The *db/db* mouse has been shown to have a missense mutation (G-T transversion) within an exon encoding the extreme C-terminus and 3' untranslated region of ObRa, the predominant short isoform. This generates a new splice donor site that results in the truncation of the intracellular domain of what would have been the long isoform splice variant of the leptin receptor and instead generates a transcript encoding for a protein that is identical to the major short isoform, ObRa *(48)*. The demonstration that the defect in the *db/db* mouse is in the leptin receptor gene confirmed the importance of the ObRb receptor in body weight regulation *(47)*. In vivo, the *db/db* mouse is resistant to the actions of exogenous leptin administration *(27,28)*.

All of these mice strains are obese and have insulin resistance, which leads to frank diabetes later in life. The mice also exhibit the development of raised circulating corticosterone, which is partly responsible for the insulin resistance *(72)*. Male and female mice are sterile because of a variety of reproductive disturbances. This sterility can be reversed in *ob/ob* mice with recombinant exogenous leptin, but it is, of course, without effect on the *db/db* mouse *(75)*. An additional phenotypic feature of these mice is that they have impaired immunity, as will be discussed below.

3.2. Immunological Abnormalities of the ob/ob and db/db Mouse

Impaired cellular immune function was noted nearly 20 yr ago in both *ob/ob* and *db/db* mice, long before the discovery of leptin *(76–80)*. Leptin-deficient *ob/ob* mice and receptor-defective *db/db* mice have been found to exhibit defective cell-mediated immunity and lymphoid atrophy analogous to that observed in chronic human undernutrition, in which leptin levels are low. In one study, skin graft rejection from a fully allogeneic mouse strain was delayed when grafted onto *db/db* mice compared with wild-type controls *(77)*. These mutant mouse strains also show increased susceptibility to pathogens, most notably to coxsackie virus. In one study, infection of *db/db* mice with coxsackie virus caused 100% mortality, as opposed to less than 10% mortality in the wild-type control group *(80)*. Of note, there seemed to be a discrepancy between the in vivo and in vitro results in that cell-mediated immune responses were significantly impaired in vivo, but in vitro T-cell responses were less affected *(77)*. Further defects were found in thymic and splenic cellularity *(76,77)*. All of these defects were considered to be the result of some unidentified aspect of obesity *(76)*.

4. STARVATION AND IMMUNE RESPONSES

4.1. Models of Starvation in Normal Mice

Animal models have been set up to investigate the effects of food restriction on immune responses. It is important to define the terms of reference carefully when assessing the literature. Starvation is defined as withholding all food for a short defined period and allowing the animal free access to water. Following this short period of starvation, the animal is then allowed free access to food. A period of 48 h of food withdrawal is usually used in mice, because 24 h produces mild immunosuppression only and 72 h causes unacceptable mortality. Most studies using rat models have employed 72-h food deprivation for similar reasons *(14,81,82)*. Food restriction generally means reducing the calorific intake to approx 30–50% of normal.

Starvation causes significant immune impairment *(83)*. It has been shown that acute starvation in mice reduces the number of CD4$^+$ T-cells and suppresses the development of T-cell-mediated immunity *(84)*. Furthermore, starvation causes delayed repopulation of the lymphoid compartment following an insult, such as sublethal irradiation *(85)*. The timing of the acute starvation appears to be crucial in terms of influencing immune responses. Starvation around the time of priming to an antigen has the greatest effect on reducing the subsequent T-cell immune response to that antigen. Starvation around the time of rechallenge also reduces the immune response, although by not to as great an extent *(82)*. Food restriction can also impair immune responses such that it can prevent death from autoimmune nephritis in the NZB × NZW F$_1$ model of murine lupus *(86)*.

4.2. The ob/ob and db/db Mouse as a Model of Starvation

It has been suggested that the *ob/ob* and the *db/db* mice are models of "perceived" starvation, despite their obvious obesity. Given that a falling leptin concentration can be considered a signal of starvation, then mice deficient in leptin or its receptor become obese because they perceive that they are starving and thus become hyperphagic *(14)*. Furthermore, these strains of mice share many of the other physiological and behavioral features of chronic starvation such as infertility, reduced thermogenesis, reduced physical activity, and food-seeking behaviour *(18)*. Indeed, many authors consider these mice to be good animal models of chronic starvation in man *(20)*.

4.2. Malnutrition and Impaired Immune Responses

It has been well established that malnutrition and starvation cause significant impairment of the immune system *(87)*. The mechanism underlying this starvation-induced immunosuppression (SII) has never been elucidated *(88)*. This phenomenon is predominantly a selective impairment of the cell-mediated immune response, with T-lymphocytes being particularly affected *(89)*. Non-T-dependent antibody responses and innate immune responses seem to be much less affected *(90)*.

4.3. The Cell-Mediated Immune Response in Starvation

As mentioned earlier, the cellular immune system seems particularly sensitive to undernutrition and starvation. The reasons for this are unknown and it has been hypothesized that much immunosuppression is the result of specific micronutrient deficiency. However, these deficiencies occur relatively sporadically, yet the type of immune impairment seen is fairly consistent, casting some doubt on this hypothesis. The immune phenotype seen in SII includes reduced delayed-type hypersensitivity responses (DTH), which is a sensitive measure of T-cell-dependent in vivo immune responses. Furthermore, circulating peripheral T-cells are reduced, particularly naïve (CD45RA$^+$) T-Cells *(91)*. T cell antigen-specific responses are severely impaired and vaccination efficacy is poor *(92)*. Antibody responses are relatively preserved, but production of interferon (IFN)-γ is markedly reduced both in vitro and in vivo *(93)*. Children seem particularly affected by SII because of the immaturity of their immune systems with diseases that are dependent on CD4$^+$ T-cell responses being particularly devastating *(91,94)*. Worldwide, malnutrition is the commonest cause of immunodeficiency *(93)*.

Anorexia nervosa is a human disease associated with marked weight loss. The immunological changes observed in this condition mirror those seen in the SII discussed earlier. In particular, T-cell production of IFN-γ is impaired, *(95)* as are DTH responses *(96)*. Markers of T-cell activation are reduced, as are circulating numbers of naïve T-cells *(97)*. All of these situations are associated with markedly suppressed leptin levels *(14,15,98)*.

It has recently been shown that food restriction can alter immunity in such a way as to ameliorate autoimmune disease in humans. Food restriction reduced CD4$^+$ T-cell activation, increased IL-4 production, and improved clinical and laboratory indicators of disease *(99)*.

4.5. Epidemiology of Starvation and Infection

The association between malnutrition and infection has been recognized since the 12th century, when church records displayed an association between years of famine and epidemics of communicable disease *(91)*. More recently, similar conclusions have been reached in a more scientific epidemiological study relating times of famine to disease epidemics *(100,101)*. Malnutrition and infection are responsible for 70% of deaths of children under 5 yr of age worldwide *(91)*. Attempts to improve these figures by vaccination against communicable diseases have been hampered by the fact that the generation of immunological memory is impaired when the primary immune response is so poor *(92)*.

5. THE EFFECTS OF LEPTIN ON THE IMMUNE SYSTEM

5.1. The Innate Immune Reponse

As mentioned earlier, the pattern of leptin release during an acute-phase response mirrors other cytokine gene expression, particularly IL-6 *(11–13)*. It has been shown that LPS, IL-1, TNF-α, and other inflammatory stimuli increase gene expression and serum concentration of leptin as early as 6 h after the initial stimulus. The induction of gene expression makes leptin an ideal candidate to be a key player in an immune/inflammatory response. It is of particular interest that LPS binds to a Toll-like receptor (TLR-4) on adipocytes and induces adipocyte expression of TLR-2 and secretion of leptin and other proinflammatory cytokines *(102)*. TLR engagement provides an elegant mechanism whereby the production of leptin is induced at the start of an immune response before cognate recognition of a foreign antigen has occurred, which will, in turn, upregulate Th1 cognate immune responses if appropriate *(see* Section 5.2). This further illustrates the well-accepted concept of a critical interplay between noncognate and cognate immune responses, which serves to coordinate the host response to any foreign or "dangerous" antigen *(103)*. Leptin itself does not cause induction of other acute-phase proteins, which distinguishes it from other members of the IL-6 family *(104)*.

It was initially thought that the induction of leptin expression during an acute-phase response was responsible for the anorexia of infection *(11)*. However, it has since been shown that LPS-induced anorexia occurs in the absence of leptin *(105)*, indicating that other factors are responsible for this phenomenon.

Leptin induces proinflammatory or Th1-type cytokines from a variety of cell types, including T-cells *(see* Section 5.2). It has been clearly shown that macrophages express the leptin receptor and respond to added exogenous leptin by increasing the synthesis and release of TNF-α, IL-6, and IL-12 *(56,106)*. It is important to note that in most studies, the basal synthesis of these cytokines is not affected by leptin. It is only the stimulated production that is enhanced (e.g., after addition of LPS), indicating that leptin does not initiate immune responses *per se*, but rather influences their outcome. There is some in vitro and in vivo data to suggest that leptin enhances the phagocytic and bactericidal activity of neutrophils and macrophages *(107)*. One study showed that leptin-deficient mice were unable to clear *Escherichia coli* as efficiently as normal mice and that phagocytosis by peritoneal macrophages from these mice was significantly impaired *(56)*. Other experiments show that in vitro, leptin enhances the phagocytic activity of macrophages against *Leishmania major* and *Candida parapsilosis (108)*. In contrast with these data, there is evidence that leptin can induce IL-1Ra production from monocytes in vitro, which acts as an anti-inflammatory protein *(109)*.

There is a body of data relating the responses of leptin-deficient *ob/ob* mice to septic shock, which indicates that these mice are more sensitive to LPS-, or TNF-α- induced injury *(110,111)*. It has been suggested that *ob/ob* mice have increased numbers of circulating monocytes and that this may underlie their hypersensitivity to septic shock *(112)*. The cytokine responses in *ob/ob* mice in these models do show marked dysregulation, but, as yet, there is not a clear mechanism to explain these findings. It may well be that in the total absence of leptin, these mice have a chronic undiagnosed infection that renders them susceptible to LPS-induced shock, such as occurs in normal mice primed with *Propionibacterium acnes (113)*. Alternatively, alterations in lymphocyte apoptosis may underlie this phenomenon, as enhanced lymphocyte apoptosis is associated with impaired survival in LPS-induced shock and leptin has been shown to have antiapoptotic properties (*see* Section 5.3) *(114)*. Whatever the mechanism, it is clear that in the absence of leptin, either congenitally in the *ob/ob* mouse or acutely during starvation *(115)*, sensitivity to septic shock is markedly increased and that this hypersensitivity is reversed by exogenous leptin treatment.

5.2. The Cognate Immune Response

As mentioned earlier, the innate and cognate immune systems are interlinked, so that many of the effects of leptin discussed in Section 4 will have implications for the behavior of responding lymphocytes. It is also clear that an organism mounts a coordinated immune response to an infectious pathogen that initially comprises innate immunity and then evolves, if appropriate to involve the cognate immune system. An important point of communication between the innate and cognate arms of the immune systems lies with macrophages and dendritic cells. These cells produce cytokines that polarize and activate T-cell responses and act as professional antigen-presenting cells by presenting peptide bound to major histocompatibility complex (MHC) molecules to T-cells along with high levels of costimulation. As leptin can effect the production of proinflammatory cytokines from macrophages *(56)* and dendritic cells (GM Lord, unpublished data) and also increase expression of MHC molecules and costimulatory molecules *(106)*, it can be seen how this will affect T-cell immune responses.

As mentioned in Section 3 of this chapter, mice deficient in either leptin or its receptor were known to have marked defects in T-cell-mediated immunity long before leptin was cloned. Since the discovery of leptin, these findings have been extended in other T-cell-dependent in vivo models. It has also been possible to confirm that these defects are directly attributable to leptin, as it is possible to add back recombinant leptin to the system studied and see correction of the deficit. The only articles regarding specific pathogen responses in leptin-deficient hosts are the studies by Loffreda et al. *(56)* showing that *ob/ob* mice display impaired clearance of *E. coli* and the article by Webb *(80)* demonstrating the startling susceptibility of *db/db* mice to coxsackie virus infection. Further studies are currently ongoing and suggest that *ob/ob* mice have impaired cellular immune responses to BCG (Lord, unpublished data). Therefore, in terms of in vivo responses to other pathogens in animals, we have to extrapolate from the autoimmune models already studied, for the time being.

It has been shown that *ob/ob* mice are completely resistant to a concanavalin A (Con A)-induced T-cell-mediated hepatitis. This resistance was abrogated by exogenous leptin replacement *(112)*. It was also demonstrated that equally obese mice that had had their endogenous leptin levels raised by a hypothalamic lesion induced by an injection of gold thioglucose had worse hepatitis that lean wild-type mice *(116)*. This would suggest that the key cytokine in this T-cell-dependent model was leptin. Similar findings have been reported in a Th1-dependent model of colitis, which shows elevated leptin levels during the induction of colitis that correlate with the severity of the colonic inflammation *(117)*. Interestingly, human studies have reported that serum leptin levels do not necessarily correlate with the severity or the presence of colitis. This is entirely consistent with the animal model, whereby at later stages of the disease, leptin levels are not particularly raised. The *ob/ob* mice are protected from induction of this disease and this protection is reversed by administration of exogenous recombinant leptin. Furthermore, much lower levels of the proinflammatory cytokines IFN-γ, TNF-α, and IL-18 were found in the *ob/ob* mice in this model.

Probably the best studied model of T-cell-mediated autoimmune disease is experimental autoimmune encephalomyelitis (EAE), a murine model of multiple sclerosis in humans. This disease is critically dependent on antigen-specific CD4[+] Th1 cells that produce IFN-γ, because it can be adoptively transferred by these cells into a naïve host. Antigen-specific CD4[+] T-cells that have a Th2 phenotype and produce IL-4 do not cause disease and, under some circumstances, can be protective.

The *ob/ob* mice are totally resistant to induction of EAE but develop disease to the same extent as wild-type mice when given leptin exogenously *(118)*. This disease protection is caused by skewing of the immune response toward a Th2 phenotype. When leptin is given to *ob/ob* mice, Th1 CD4⁺ T-cells are generated normally and produce similar amounts of IFN-γ in vitro to wild-type mice. Associated with this is impaired antibody isotype switching. In untreated *ob/ob* mice, all of the antigen-specific antibody produced in IgG1 (Th2-dependent antibody). In wild-type and leptin-treated mice, the antigen-specific antibody is mainly IgG2a, which is a Th1-dependent isotype. These findings have been essentially replicated in a murine arthritis model *(119)*. To extend these findings further, we looked at EAE-prone and EAE-resistant normal mice strains. Male SJL mice, which have lower endogenous leptin levels, are resistant to EAE, whereas females are susceptible. Exogenous leptin rendered the male mice susceptible to EAE and worsened disease in females *(120)*. These data may well be informing us of an additional factor in the sexual dimorphism of autoimmune disease *(121)*.

Findings in vitro support the above in vivo data. Essentially, T-cells respond to exogenous leptin by increased proliferation and increased Th1-type cytokine production in the context of the mixed lymphocyte reaction in both humans and mice. This is associated with suppression of Th2 cytokine production *(1,55)*. In the case of polyclonal stimulation, memory T-cell (CD45RO⁺) proliferation is inhibited, IFN-γ production is increased, and naïve T-cell (CD45RA⁺) proliferation is increased *(122)*. Therefore, in two different in vitro systems, leptin seems to have differential proliferative effects on naïve and memory T-cell proliferation, but consistently upregulates Th1 cytokine production. These differential effects have been confirmed using naïve T-cells from cord blood as responder cells *(1,122)*.

5.3. Leptin and the Thymus

The thymus is known as the barometer of nutrition and its size and function are severely impaired in malnutrition *(91)*. It would appear that leptin is a key mediator of thymic atrophy in starvation because *ob/ob* mice have a hypocellular thymus as a result of enhanced apoptosis and this is reversed by leptin administration *(112,123)*. Furthermore, a model of acute starvation in mice induces profound thymic atrophy, which can be entirely prevented by leptin administration during the period of starvation *(123)*. Thymic output is more pronounced in the earlier years of life in humans and this may explain the greater susceptibility of children to infectious diseases, although it is clear that thymic output occurs throughout life and can be increased when the T-cell repertoire needs to be replenished.

In vitro, leptin prevents steroid-induced apoptosis of thymocytes *(123)*. This antiapoptotic phenomenon of leptin has also been observed in myeloid cells *(124)* and pancreatic β-cells and probably occurs as a result of leptin-induced maintenance of bcl-2 expression *(125)*.

5.4. Leptin and Infectious Diseases: The Immunosuppression of Starvation?

It has been suggested earlier that the main effects of leptin on immune responses may well be in relatively hypoleptinaemic states. These occur primarily during starvation and may be important in explaining starvation-induced immunosuppression that is responsible for a great deal of infectious disease worldwide. There are good animal data to suggest that in models of acute and chronic starvation or food restriction, cellular immune responses are particularly affected *(89–91,94)*. This immune dysfunction can, for the most part, be abrogated by the administration of leptin. This has been shown to be true in delayed-type hypersensitivity responses *(1,123)*, thymic atrophy and apoptosis *(123)*, and septic shock *(115)*.

In humans, the data seem to suggest that leptin may be important in protection from infectious disease. Most of these studies have looked at serum leptin levels and correlated them with survival from sepsis. As mentioned earlier, leptin levels usually correlate with severity of inflammation in rodent models and humans if early enough time-points are analyzed (*see* Section 5.4). Two independent studies have shown that there is a positive correlation between leptin levels and survival from sepsis in the setting of an intensive care unit *(126,127)*, although one other study found no change in serum levels of leptin during sepsis *(128)*. It has been suggested that leptin may be useful as adjunctive therapy in the treatment of infectious disease, but there is no animal or human data to support this view as yet *(129)*.

It is clear, however, that in the complete absence of leptin in humans, the propensity to infectious disease is markedly increased. In one consanguineous pedigree, 64% of individuals homozygous for a deletion of the *ob* gene died from infectious disease compared with none of the heterozygotes *(130)*.

CONCLUSION

Initially, leptin was implicated in the regulation of body weight and reproductive function *(29)*. However, recent reports of its effect on the immune system both in vitro and in vivo indicate that it has a role in modulation of a wide variety of immune responses. The light in which we see the biological role of leptin is changing to reflect its pleiotrophic functions, and the most satisfactory evolutionary explanation is that falling leptin concentrations signal impending energy/nutrient deficiency. This is supported by most of the experimental data to date and implies that falling leptin levels reduce the energy utilization of extraneous or nonimmediately vital systems such as the immune system and the reproductive system. This would serve to preserve limited energy for cardiac and cerebral metabolism, but at the expense of an increased risk of infection. Immune responses use up significant amounts of energy, which can be life threatening at times of energy scarcity. We propose that one of the functions of leptin is to prevent this from happening *(131)*. The data discussed here may help to explain the occurrence of immune dysfunction in humans with low body weight and the observation that caloric restriction is able to abrogate autoimmune disease in several animal models. Leptin may, therefore, be the key link between nutritional status and an optimal immune response and may provide the explanation for starvation-induced immunosuppression, which is responsible for millions of deaths per year worldwide. Furthermore, leptin represent a novel axis of control of immune responses, which may lead to the possibility of pharmacological intervention for the treatment of a variety of disease states.

REFERENCES

1. Lord, G.M., Matarese, G., Howard, J.K., Baker, R.J., Bloom, S.R., et al. (1998) Leptin modulates the T cell immune response and reverses starvation induced immunosuppression. *Nature* **394**, 897–901.
2. Zhang, Y., Proenca, R., Maffei, M., Barone, M., Leopold, L., and Friedman, J.M. (1994) Positional cloning of the mouse obese gene and its human homologue. *Nature* **372**, 425–432.
3. Bado, A., Levasseur, S., Attoub, S., Kermorgant, S., Laigneau, J.P., Bortoluzzi, M.N., et al. (1998) The stomach is a source of leptin. *Nature* **394**, 790–793.
4. Masuzaki, H., Ogawa, Y., Sagawa, N., Hosoda, K., Matsumoto, T., Mise, H., et al. (1997) Nonadipose tissue production of leptin: leptin as a novel placenta-derived hormone in humans. *Nat. Med.* **3**, 1029–1033.
5. Morash, B., Li, A., Murphy, P.R., Wilkinson, M., and Ur, E. (1999) Leptin gene expression in the brain and pituitary gland. *Endocrinology* **140**, 5995–5998.
6. Moon, B.C. and Friedman, J.M. (1997) The molecular basis of the obese mutation in ob2J mice. *Genomics* **42**, 152–156.
7. Zhang, F., Basinski, M.B., Beals, J.M., Briggs, S.L., Churgay, L.M., Clawson, D.K., et al. (1997b) Crystal structure of the obese protein leptin-E100. *Nature* **387**, 206–209.
8. Sinha, M.K., Opentanova, I., Ohannesian, J.P., Kolaczynski, J.W., Heiman, M.L., Hale, J., et al. (1996a) Evidence of free and bound leptin in human circulation. Studies in lean and obese subjects and during short-term fasting. *J. Clin. Invest.* **98**, 1277–1282.
9. Houseknecht, K.L., Mantzoros, C.S., Kuliawat, R., Hadro, E., Flier, J.S., and Kahn, B.B. (1996) Evidence for leptin binding to proteins in serum of rodents and humans: modulation with obesity. *Diabetes* **45**, 1638–1643.
10. Considine, R.V., Sinha, M.K., Heiman, M.L., Kriauciunas, A., Stephens, T.W., et al. (1996) Serum immunoreactive-leptin concentrations in normal-weight and obese humans. *N. Engl. J. Med.* **334**, 292–295.
11. Grunfeld, C., Zhao, C., Fuller, J., Pollack, A., Moser, A., Friedman, J., et al. (1996) Endotoxin and cytokines induce expression of leptin, the ob gene product, in hamsters. *J. Clin. Invest.* **97**, 2152–2157.
12. Janik, J.E., Curti, B.D., Considine, R.V., Rager, H.C., Powers, G.C., Alvord, W.G., et al. (1997) Interleukin 1 alpha increases serum leptin concentrations in humans. *J. Clin. Endocrinol. Metab.* **82**, 3084–3086.
13. Sarraf, P., Frederich, R.C., Turner, E.M., Ma, G., Jaskowiak, N.T., Rivet, D.J., et al. (1997) Multiple cytokines and acute inflammation raise mouse leptin levels: potential role in inflammatory anorexia. *J. Exp. Med.* **185**, 171–175.

14. Ahima, R.S., Prabakaran, D., Mantzoros, C., Qu, D., Lowell, B., Maratos Flier, E., et al. (1996) Role of leptin in the neuroendocrine response to fasting. *Nature* **382,** 250–252.
15. Boden, G., Chen, X., Mozzoli, M., and Ryan, I. (1996) Effect of fasting on serum leptin in normal human subjects. *J. Clin. Endocrinol. Metab.* **81,** 3419–3423.
16. Sinha, M.K., Sturis, J., Ohannesian, J., Magosin, S., Stephens, T., Heiman, M.L., et al. (1996b) Ultradian oscillations of leptin secretion in humans. *Biochem. Biophys. Res. Commun.* **228,** 733–738.
17. Licinio, J., Mantzoros, C., Negrao, A.B., Cizza, G., Wong, M.L., Bongiorno. P.B., et al. (1997) Human leptin levels are pulsatile and inversely related to pituitary-adrenal function. *Nat. Med.* **3,** 575–579.
18. Flier, J.S. (1998) What's in a name? In search of leptin's physiologic role. *J. Clin. Endocrinol. Metab.* **83,** 1407–1413.
19. Howard, J.K., Lord, G.M., Clutterbuck, E.J., Ghatei, M.A., Pusey, C.D., and Bloom, S.R. (1997) Plasma Immunoreactive Leptin Concentration in End Stage Renal Disease. *Clin. Sci.* **93,** 119–126.
20. Friedman, J.M. and Halaas, J.L. (1998) Leptin and the regulation of body weight in mammals. *Nature* **395,** 763–770.
21. Wang, J., Liu, R., Liu, L., Chowdhury, R., Barzilai, N., Tan, J., and Rossetti, L. (1999) The effect of leptin on Lep expression is tissue-specific and nutritionally regulated. *Nat. Med.* **5,** 895–899.
22. Bradley, R.L. and Cheatham, B. (1999) Regulation of ob gene expression and leptin secretion by insulin and dexamethasone in rat adipocytes. *Diabetes* **48,** 272–278.
23. Kristensen, K., Pedersen, S.B., Langdahl, B.L., and Richelsen, B. (1999) Regulation of leptin by thyroid hormone in humans: studies in vivo and in vitro. *Metabolism* **48,** 1603–1607.
24. Brann, D.W., De, Sevilla, L., Zamorano, P.L., and Mahesh, V.B. (1999) Regulation of leptin gene expression and secretion by steroid hormones. *Steroids* **64,** 659–663.
25. Saad, M.F., Damani, S., Gingerich, R.L., Riad Gabriel, M.G., Khan, A., Boyadjian, R., et al. (1997) Sexual dimorphism in plasma leptin concentration. *J. Clin. Endocrinol. Metab.* **82,** 579–584.
26. Campfield, L.A., Smith, F.J., Guisez, Y., Devos, R., and Burn, P. (1995) Recombinant mouse OB protein: evidence for a peripheral signal linking adiposity and central neural networks. *Science* **269,** 546–549.
27. Halaas, J.L., Gajiwala, K.S., Maffei, M., Cohen, S.L., Chait, B.T., Rabinowitz, D., et al. (1995) Weight-reducing effects of the plasma protein encoded by the obese gene. *Science* **269,** 543–546.
28. Pelleymounter, M.A., Cullen, M.J., Baker, M.B., Hecht, R., Winters, D., Boone, T., et al. (1995) Effects of the obese gene product on body weight regulation in ob/ob mice. *Science* **269,** 540–543.
29. Friedman, J.M. (1997) Leptin, leptin receptors and the control of body weight. *Eur. J. Med. Res.* **2,** 7–13.
30. Montague, C.T., Farooqi, I.S., Whitehead, J.P., Soos, M.A., Rau, H., Wareham, N.J., et al. (1997) Congenital leptin deficiency is associated with severe early- onset obesity in humans. *Nature* **387,** 903–908.
31. Farooqi, I.S., Jebb, S.A., Langmack, G., Lawrence, E., Cheetham, C.H., Prentice, A.M., et al. (1999) Effects of recombinant leptin therapy in a child with congenital leptin deficiency. *N. Engl. J. Med.* **341,** 879–884.
32. Friedman JM and Leibel RL. (1992) Tackling a weighty problem. *Cell* **69,** 217–220.
33. Friedman, J.M. (1997) The alphabet of weight control. *Nature* **385,** 119–120.
34. Bjorbaek, C., Elmquist, J.K., Frantz, J.D., Shoelson, S.E., and Flier, J.S. (1998) Identification of SOCS-3 as a potential mediator of central leptin resistance. *Mol. Cell.* **1,** 619–625.
35. Bjorbaek, C., El-Haschimi, K., Frantz, J.D., and Flier, J.S. (1999) The role of SOCS-3 in leptin signaling and leptin resistance. *J. Biol. Chem.* **274,** 30,059–30,065.
36. Gura, T. (1999) Obesity research. Leptin not impressive in clinical trial. *Science* **286,** 881–882.
37. Emilsson, V., Liu, Y.L., Cawthorne, M.A., Morton, N.M., and Davenport, M. (1997) Expression of the functional leptin receptor mRNA in pancreatic islets and direct inhibitory action of leptin on insulin secretion. *Diabetes* **46,** 313–316.
38. Kulkarni, R.N., Wang, Z.L., Wang, R.M., Hurley, J.D., Smith, D.M., Ghatei, M.A., et al. (1997) Leptin rapidly suppresses insulin release from insulinoma cells, rat and human islets and, in vivo, in mice. *J. Clin. Invest.* **100,** 2729–2736.
39. Cioffi, J.A., Shafer, A.W., Zupancic, T.J., Smith Gbur, J., Mikhail, A., Platika, D., et al. (1996) Novel B219/OB receptor isoforms: possible role of leptin in hematopoiesis and reproduction. *Nat. Med.* **2,** 585–589.
40. Sierra, H.M., Nath, A.K., Murakami, C., Garcia, C.G., Papapetropoulos, A., Sessa, W.C., et al. (1998) Biological action of leptin as an angiogenic factor. *Science* **281,** 1683–1686.
41. Bennett, B.D., Solar, G.P., Yuan, J.Q., Mathias, J., Thomas, G.R., and Matthews, W. (1996) A role for leptin and its cognate receptor in hematopoiesis. *Curr. Biol.* **6,** 1170–1180.
42. Haque, M.S., Minokoshi, Y., Hamai, M., Iwai, M., Horiuchi, M., and Shimazu, T. (1999) Role of the sympathetic nervous system and insulin in enhancing glucose uptake in peripheral tissues after intrahypothalamic injection of leptin in rats. *Diabetes* **48,** 1706–1712.
43. Berti, L. and Gammeltoft, S. (1999) Leptin stimulates glucose uptake in C2C12 muscle cells by activation of ERK2. *Mol. Cell. Endocrinol.* **157,** 121–130.
44. Kamohara, S., Burcelin, R., Halaas, J.L., Friedman, J.M., and Charron, M.J. (1997) Acute stimulation of glucose metabolism in mice by leptin treatment. *Nature* **389,** 374–377.
45. Wang, M.Y., Lee, Y., and Unger, R.H. (1999) Novel form of lipolysis induced by leptin. *J. Biol. Chem.* **274,** 17,541–17,544.
46. Tartaglia, L.A., Dembski, M., Weng, X., Deng, N., Culpepper, J., Devos, R., et al. (1995) Identification and expression cloning of a leptin receptor, OB-R. *Cell* **83,** 1263–1271.
47. Chen, H., Charlat, O., Tartaglia, L.A., Woolf, E.A., Weng, X., Ellis, S.J., et al. (1996) Evidence that the diabetes gene encodes the leptin receptor: identification of a mutation in the leptin receptor gene in db/db mice. *Cell* **84,** 491–495.

48. Lee, G.H., Proenca, R., Montez, J.M., Carroll, K.M., Darvishzadeh, J.G., Lee, J.I., et al. (1996) Abnormal splicing of the leptin receptor in diabetic mice. *Nature* **379**, 632–635.
49. Baumann, H., Morella, K.K., White, D.W., Dembski, M., Bailon, P.S., Kim, H., et al. (1996) The full-length leptin receptor has signaling capabilities of interleukin 6-type cytokine receptors. *Proc. Natl. Acad. Sci. USA* **93**, 8374–8378.
50. Ghilardi, N., Ziegler, S., Wiestner, A., Stoffel, R., Heim, M.H., and Skoda, R.C. (1996) Defective STAT signaling by the leptin receptor in diabetic mice. *Proc. Natl. Acad. Sci. USA* **93**, 6231–6235.
51. Clement, K., Vaisse, C., Lahlou, N., Cabrol, S., Pelloux, V., Cassuto, D., et al. (1998) A mutation in the human leptin receptor gene causes obesity and pituitary dysfunction. *Nature* **392**, 398–401.
52. Tartaglia, L.A. (1997) The leptin receptor. *J. Biol. Chem.* **272**, 6093–6096.
53. Fei, H., Okano, H.J., Li, C., Lee, G.H., Zhao, C., Darnell, R., et al. (1997) Anatomic localization of alternatively spliced leptin receptors (Ob-R) in mouse brain and other tissues. *Proc. Natl. Acad. Sci. USA* **94**, 7001–7005.
54. Mercer, J.G., Hoggard, N., Williams, L.M., Lawrence, C.B., Hannah, L.T., and Trayhurn, P. (1996) Localization of leptin receptor mRNA and the long form splice variant (Ob-Rb) in mouse hypothalamus and adjacent brain regions by in situ hybridization. *FEBS Lett.* **387**, 113–116.
55. Martin-Romero, C., Santos-Alvarez, J., Goberna, R., and Sanchez-Margalet, V. (2000) Human leptin enhances activation and proliferation of human circulating T lymphocytes. *Cell Immunol* **199**, 15–24.
56. Loffreda, S., Yang, S.Q., Lin, H.Z., Karp, C.L., Brengman, M.L., Wang, D.J., et al. (1998) Leptin regulates proinflammatory immune responses. *FASEB J.* **12**, 57–65.
57. Heldin, C.H. (1995) Dimerization of cell surface receptors in signal transduction. *Cell* **80**, 213–223.
58. Bjorbaek, C., Uotani, S., da Silva, B., and Flier, J.S. (1997) Divergent signaling capacities of the long and short isoforms of the leptin receptor. *J. Biol. Chem.* **272**, 32,686–32,695.
59. Murakami, T., Yamashita, T., Iida, M., Kuwajima, M., and Shima, K. (1997) A short form of leptin receptor performs signal transduction. *Biochem. Biophys. Res. Commun.* **231**, 26–29.
60. Li, C. and Friedman, J.M. (1999) Leptin receptor activation of SH2 domain containing protein tyrosine phosphatase 2 modulates Ob receptor signal transduction. *Proc. Natl. Acad. Sci. USA* **96**, 9677–9682.
61. Caro, J.F., Kolaczynski, J.W., Nyce, M.R., Ohannesian, J.P., Opentanova, I., Goldman, W.H., et al. (1996) Decreased cerebrospinal-fluid/serum leptin ratio in obesity: a possible mechanism for leptin resistance. *Lancet* **348**, 159–161.
62. Koistinen, H.A., Karonen, S.L., Iivanainen, M., and Koivisto, V.A. (1998) Circulating leptin has saturable transport into intrathecal space in humans. *Eur. J. Clin. Invest.* **28**, 894–897.
63. Patel, N., Brinkman-Van der Linden, E.C., Altmann, S.W., Gish, K., Balasubramanian, S., Timans, J.C., et al. (1999) OB-BP1/Siglec-6. a leptin- and sialic acid-binding protein of the immunoglobulin superfamily. *J. Biol. Chem.* **274**, 22,729–22,738.
64. O'Rouke, L., Yeaman, S.J., and Shepherd, P.R. (2001) Insulin and leptin acutely regulate cholesterol ester metabolism in macrophages by novel signaling pathways. *Diabetes* **50**, 955–961.
65. Martin-Romero, C. and Sanchez-Margalet, V. (2001) Human leptin activates PI3K and MAPK pathways in human peripheral blood mononuclear cells: possible role of Sam68. *Cell Immunol.* **212**, 83–91.
66. White, D.W., Kuropatwinski, K.K., Devos, R., Baumann, H., and Tartaglia, L.A. (1997) Leptin receptor (OB-R) signaling. Cytoplasmic domain mutational analysis and evidence for receptor homo-oligomerization. *J. Biol. Chem.* **272**, 4065–4071.
67. Nakashima, K., Narazaki, M., and Taga, T. (1997) Leptin receptor (OB-R) oligomerizes with itself but not with its closely related cytokine signal transducer gp130. *FEBS Lett.* **403**, 79–82.
68. White, D.W. and Tartaglia, L.A. (1999) Evidence for ligand-independent homo-oligomerization of leptin receptor (OB-R) isoforms: a proposed mechanism permitting productive long-form signaling in the presence of excess short-form expression. *J. Cell. Biochem.* **73**, 278–288.
69. Barr, V.A., Lane, K., and Taylor, S.I. (1999) Subcellular localization and internalization of the four human leptin receptor isoforms. *J. Biol. Chem.* **274**, 21,416–21,424.
70. Uotani S, Bjorbaek C, Tornoe J, and Flier JS. (1999) Functional properties of leptin receptor isoforms: internalization and degradation of leptin and ligand-induced receptor downregulation. *Diabetes* **48**, 279–286.
71. Rock, F.L., Peterson, D., Weig, B.C., Kastelein, R.A., and Bazan, J.F. (1996) Binding of leptin to the soluble ectodomain of recombinant leptin receptor: a kinetic analysis by surface plasmon resonance. *Horm. Metab. Res.* **28**, 748–750.
72. Coleman, D.L. (1978) Obese and diabetes: two mutant genes causing diabetes–obesity syndromes in mice. *Diabetologia* **14**, 141–148.
73. Coleman, D.L. and Hummel, K.P. (1967) Effects of parabiosis of normal with genetically diabetic mice Studies with the mutation, diabetes, in the mouse. *Am. J. Physiol.* **3**, 238–248.
74. Coleman, D.L. and Hummel, K.P. (1969) Effects of parabiosis of normal with genetically diabetic mice. *Am. J. Physiol.* **217**, 1298–1304.
75. Mounzih, K., Lu, R., and Chehab, F.F. (1997) Leptin treatment rescues the sterility of genetically obese ob/ob males. *Endocrinology* **138**, 1190–1193.
76. Chandra, R.K. (1980) Cell-mediated immunity in genetically obese C57BL/6J ob/ob) mice. *Am. J. Clin. Nutr.* **33**, 13–16.
77. Fernandes, G., Handwerger, B.S., Yunis, E.J., and Brown, D.M. (1978) Immune response in the mutant diabetic C57BL/Ks-dt⁺ mouse. Discrepancies between in vitro and in vivo immunological assays. *J. Clin. Invest.* **61**, 243–250.
78. Mandel MA and Mahmoud AA. (1978) Impairment of cell-mediated immunity in mutation diabetic mice (db/db). *J. Immunol.* **120**, 1375–1377.

79. Meade, C.J., Sheena, J., and Mertin, J. (1979) Effects of the obese (ob/ob) genotype on spleen cell immune function. *Int. Arch. Allergy. Appl. Immunol.* **58**, 121–127.
80. Webb, S.R., Loria, R.M., Madge, G.E., and Kibrick, S. (1976) Susceptibility of mice to group B coxsackie virus is influenced by the diabetic gene. *J. Exp. Med.* **143**, 1239–1248.
81. Legradi, G., Emerson, C.H., Ahima, R.S., Flier, J.S., and Lechan, R.M. (1997) Leptin prevents fasting-induced suppression of prothyrotropin- releasing hormone messenger ribonucleic acid in neurons of the hypothalamic paraventricular nucleus. *Endocrinology* **138**, 2569–2576.
82. Martinez, D., Cox, S., Lukassewycz, O.A., and Murphy, W.H. (1975) Immune mechanisms in leukemia: suppression of cellular immunity by starvation. *J. Natl. Cancer. Inst.* **55**, 935–939.
83. Chandra, R.K. (1991) Immunocompetence is a sensitive and functional barometer of nutritional status. *Acta. Paediatr. Scand.* **374(Suppl.)**, 129–132.
84. Wing, E.J., Magee, D.M., and Barczynski, L.K. (1988) Acute starvation in mice reduces the number of T cells and suppresses the development of T-cell-mediated immunity. *Immunology* **63**, 677–682.
85. Wing, E.J. and Barczynski, L.K. (1984) Effect of acute nutritional deprivation on immune function in mice. II. Response to sublethal radiation. *Clin. Immunol. Immunopathol.* **30**, 479–487.
86. Fernandes, G., Yunis, E.J., and Good, R.A. (1976) Influence of diet on survival of mice. *Proc. Natl. Acad. Sci. USA* **78**, 1279–1283.
87. Neumann, C.G., Lawlor, G.J., Jr., Stiehm, E.R., Swenseid, M.E., Newton, C., Herbert, J., et al. (1975) Immunologic responses in malnourished children. *Am. J. Clin. Nutr.* **28**, 89–104.
88. McMurray, D.N., Loomis, S.A., Casazza, L.J., Rey, H., and Miranda, R. (1981) Development of impaired cell-mediated immunity in mild and moderate malnutrition. *Am. J. Clin. Nutr.* **34**, 68–77.
89. Chandra, R.K. and Kumari, S. (1994) Effects of nutrition on the immune system. *Nutrition* **10**, 207–210.
90. Chandra, R.K. and Kumari, S. (1994) Nutrition and immunity: an overview. *J Nutr* **124**, 1433S–1435S.
91. Chandra, R.K. (1992) Protein-energy malnutrition and immunological responses. *J. Nutr.* **122**, 597–600.
92. Saha, K., Mehta, R., Misra, R.C., Chaudhury, D.S., and Ray, S.N. (1977) Undernutrition and immunity: smallpox vaccination in chronically starved, undernourished subjects and its immunologic evaluation. *Scand. J. Immunol.* **6**, 581–589.
93. Beisel, W.R. (1992) History of nutritional immunology: introduction and overview. *J. Nutr.* **122**, 591–596.
94. Beisel, W.R. (1996) Nutrition in pediatric HIV infection: setting the research agenda. Nutrition and immune function: overview. *J. Nutr.* **126**, 2611S–2615S.
95. Polack, E., Nahmod, V.E., Emeric Sauval, E., Bello, M., Costas, M., Finkielman, S., et al. (1993) Low lymphocyte interferon-gamma production and variable proliferative response in anorexia nervosa patients. *J. Clin. Immunol.* **13**, 445–451.
96. Cason, J., Ainley, C.C., Wolstencroft, R.A., Norton, K.R., and Thompson, R.P. (1986) Cell-mediated immunity in anorexia nervosa. *Clin. Exp. Immunol.* **64**, 370–375.
97. Allende, L.M., Corell, A., Manzanares, J., Madruga, D., Marcos, A., Madrono, A., et al. (1998) Immunodeficiency associated with anorexia nervosa is secondary and improves after refeeding. *Immunology* **94**, 543–551.
98. Grinspoon, S., Gulick, T., Askari, H., Landt, M., Lee, K., Anderson, E., et al. (1996) Serum leptin levels in women with anorexia nervosa. *J. Clin. Endocrinol. Metab.* **81**, 3861–3863.
99. Fraser, D.A., Thoen, J., Reseland, J.E., Forre, O., and Kjeldsen-Kragh, J. (1999) Decreased CD4⁺ lymphocyte activation and increased interleukin-4 production in peripheral blood of rheumatoid arthritis patients after acute starvation. *Clin. Rheumatol.* **18**, 394–401.
100. Moore, S.E., Cole, T.J., Poskitt, E.M.E., Sonko, B.J., Whitehead, R.G., McGregor, I.A., et al. (1997) Season of birth predicts mortality in rural Gambia. *Nature* **388**, 434–434.
101. Scrimshaw, N.S. (1987) The phenomenon of famine. *Annu. Rev. Nutr.* **7**, 1–21.
102. Lin, Y., Lee, H., Berg, A.H., Lisanti, M.P., Shapiro, L. and Scherer, P.E. (2000) The lipopolysaccharide-activated Toll-like receptor (TLR)-4 induces synthesis of the closely related TLR-2 in adipocytes. *J. Biol. Chem.* **275**, 24,255–24,263.
103. Janeway, C.A.J. and Medzhitov, R. (1998) Introduction: the role of innate immunity in the adaptive immune response. *Semin. Immunol.* **10**, 349–350.
104. Agnello, D., Meazza, C., Rowan, C.G., Villa, P., Ghezzi, P. and Senaldi, G. (1998) Leptin causes bodyweight loss in the absence of in vivo activities typical of cytokines of the IL-6 family. *Am. J. Physiol.* **275**, R1518–R1525.
105. Faggioni, R., Fuller, J., Moser, A., Feingold, K.R. and Grunfeld, C. (1997) LPS-induced anorexia in leptin-deficient (ob/ob) and leptin-receptor deficient (db/db) mice. *Am. J. Physiol.* **273**, R181–R186.
106. Santos-Alvarez, J., Goberna, R., and Sanchez-Margalet, V. (1999) Human leptin stimulates proliferation and activation of human circulating monocytes. *Cell Immunol.* **194**, 6–11.
107. Caldefie-Chezet, F., Poulin, A., Tridon, A., Sion, B. and Vasson, M.P. (2001) Leptin: a potential regulator of polymorphonuclear neutrophil bactericidal action? *J. Leukocyte Biol.* **69**, 414–418.
108. Gainsford, T., Willson, T.A., Metcalf, D., Handman, E., McFarlane, C., Ng, A., et al. (1996) Leptin can induce proliferation, differentiation and functional activation of hemopoietic cells. *Proc. Natl. Acad. Sci. USA* **93**, 14,564–14,568.
109. Gabay, C., Dreyer, M., Pellegrinelli, N., Chicheportiche, R. and Meier, C.A. (2001) Leptin directly induces the secretion of interleukin 1 receptor antagonist in human monocytes. *J. Clin. Endocrinol. Metab.* **86** 783–791.
110. Faggioni, R., Fantuzzi, G., Gabay, C., Moser, A., Dinarello, C.A., Feingold, K.R., et al. (1999) Leptin deficiency enhances sensitivity to endotoxin-induced lethality. *Am. J. Physiol.* **276**, R136–R142.
111. Takahashi, N., Waelput, W. and Guisez, Y. (1999) Leptin is an endogenous protective protein against the toxicity exerted by tumor necrosis factor. *J. Exp. Med.* **189**, 207–212.

112. Faggioni, R., Jones-Carson, J., Reed, D.A., Dinarello, C.A., Feingold, K.R., Grunfeld, C., et al. (2000a) Leptin-deficient (ob/ob) mice are protected from T cell-mediated hepatotoxicity: role of tumor necrosis factor alpha and IL-18. *Proc. Natl. Acad. Sci. USA* **97**, 2367–2372.

113. Guebre-Xabier, M., Yang, E.K., Lin, H.Z., Schwenk, R., Krzych, U. and Diehl, A.M. (2000) Altered hepatocyte lymphocyte subpopulations in obesity-related murine fatty livers: potential mechanisms for sensitization to liver damage. *Hepatology* **31**, 633–640.

114. Hotchkiss, R.S., Tinsley, K.W., Swanson, P.E., Chang, K.C., Cobb, J.P., Buchman, T.G., et al. (1999) Prevention of lymphocyte cell death in sepsis improves survival in mice. *Proc. Natl. Acad. Sci. USA* **96**, 14,541–14,546.

115. Faggioni, R., Moser, A., Feingold, K.R. and Grunfeld, C. (2000b) Reduced leptin levels in starvation increase susceptibility to septic shock. *Am. J. Pathol.* **156**, 1781–1787.

116. Siegmund, B., Lear-Kaul, K.C., Faggioni, R., Fantuzzi, G. (2002) Leptin deficiency, not obesity, protects mice from Con A-induced hepatitis. *Eur. J. Immunol.* **32**, 552–560.

117. Fantuzzi, G., Lehr, H.A., Dinarello, C.A., and Siegmund, B. (2001) Leptin deficient (*ob/ob*) mice are resistant to experimental colitis: role of Th1 cytokines. *FASEB J.* 15: A1067 (abstract).

118. Matarese, G., Di Giacomo, A., Sanna, V., Lord, G.M., Howard, J.K., Di Tuoro, A., et al. (2001) Requirement for leptin in the induction and progression of autoimmune encephalomyelitis. *J. Immunol.* **166**, 5909–5916.

119. Busso, N., So, A., Chobaz-Peclat, V., Morard, C., Martinez-Soria, E., Talabot-Ayer, D. et al. (2002) Leptin signaling deficiency impairs humoral and cellular immune responses and attenuates experimental arthritis. *J. Immunol.* **168**, 875–882.

120. Matarese, G., Sanna, V., Di Giacomo, A., Lord, G.M., Howard, J.K, Bloom, S.R., et al. (2001) Leptin potentiates experimental autoimmune encephalomyelitis in SJL female mice and confers susceptibility to males. *Eur. J. Immunol.* **31**, 1324–1332.

121. Matarese, G., La Cava, A., Sanna, V., Lord, G.M., Lechler, R.I., Fontana, S., et al. (2002) Balancing susceptibility to infection and autoimmunity: a role for leptin? *Trends Immunol.* **23**, 182–187.

122. Lord, G.M., Matarese, G., Howard, J.K., Bloom, S.R., Lechler, R.I. (2002) Leptin inhibits the anti-CD3 driven proliferation of peripheral blood T cells but enhances the production of pro-inflammatory cytokines. *J. Leukocyte Biol.*, in press.

123. Howard, J.K., Lord, G.M., Matarese, G., Vendetti, S., Ghatei, M.A., Ritter, M.A., et al. (1999) Leptin protects mice from starvation-induced lymphoid atrophy and increases thymic cellularity in ob/ob mice. *J. Clin. Invest.* **104**, 1051–1059.

124. Konopleva, M., Mikhail, A., Estrov, Z., Zhao, S., Harris, D., Sanchez-Williams, G., et al. (1999) Expression and function of leptin receptor isoforms in myeloid leukemia and myelodysplastic syndromes: proliferative and anti-apoptotic activities. *Blood* **93**, 1668–1676.

125. Shimabukuro, M., Wang, M.Y., Zhou, Y.T., Newgard, C.B., and Unger, R.H. (1998) Protection against lipoapoptosis of beta cells through leptin-dependent maintenance of Bcl-2 expression. *Proc. Natl. Acad. Sci. USA* **95**, 9558–9561.

126. Bornstein, S.R., Licinio, J., Tauchnitz, R., Engelmann, L., Negrao, A.B., Gold, P., et al. (1998) Plasma leptin levels are increased in survivors of acute sepsis: associated loss of diurnal rhythm, in cortisol and leptin secretion. *J. Clin. Endocrinol. Metab.* **83**, 280–283.

127. Arnalich, F., Lopez, J., Codoceo, R., Jimemnz, M., Madero, R. and Montiel, C. (1999) Relationship of plasma leptin to plasma cytokines and human survival in sepsis and septic shock. *J. Infect. Dis.* **180**, 908–911.

128. Carlson, G.L., Saeed, M., Little, R.A. and Irving, M.H. (1999) Serum leptin concentrations and their relation to metabolic abnormalities I human sepsis. *Am. J. Physiol.* **276**, E658–E662.

129. De Fanti, B.A., Lamas, O., Milagro, F.I., Martínez-Ansó, E. and Martínez, J.A. (2002) Immunoneutralization and anti-idiotype production: two-sided applications of leptin. *Trends Immunol.* **23**, 180–181.

130. Ozata, M., Ozdemir, I.C., and Licinio, J. (1999) Human leptin deficiency caused by a missense mutation: multiple endocrine defects, decreased sympathetic tone, and immune system dysfunction indicate new targets for leptin action, greater central than peripheral resistance to the effects of leptin, and spontaneous correction of leptin-mediated defects. *J. Clin. Endocrinol. Metab.* **84**, 3686–3695.

131. Lord, G.M., Matarese, G., Howard, J.K., and Lechler, R.I. (2001) The bioenergetics of the immune system. *Science* **292**, 855–856.

2
Cytokine Gene Polymorphism and Host Susceptibility to Infection

Frank Stüber

1. INTRODUCTION

The individual susceptibility to infection of any organism is determined by a variety of factors such as environmental conditions of the host, pathogenicity of infecting microbes, and the effectiveness of the host's defense systems. The induction of specific immune responses such as antibodies released by β-cells and effector T-cells directed against antigens of invading microbes rely on antigen-presenting cells such as macrophages and dendritic cells. These "smart weapons" guarantee the elimination and clearance of antigens and invaders from the body without harming the host's own cellular and organ structure and function. In contrast, molecules as part of the evolutionary older innate immune system like defensins or cytokines may prove to be harmful for the host if released in excessive amounts into systemic circulation. On the other hand, low levels of these molecules locally released at the site of infection may result in insufficient clearance of invading microbes.

The host's inflammatory response to infection contributes as a main factor to morbidity and mortality in today's intensive care units, and it displays a high interindividual variation *(1)* that is not sufficiently explained by single factors such as gender *(2)*. Comparable amounts of infectious units of microbial organisms induce a wide range of severity of infectious diseases. The role of an individual's genetic background and predisposition to the extent of inflammatory responses is also determined by genetic variants of endogenous mediators that constitute the pathways of endogenous mediators of host responses to infection. Important candidate genes for host susceptibility to infection are cytokine genes.

Primary responses in inflammation are mediated by pro-inflammatory cytokines such as tumor necrosis factor (TNF) and interleukin 1 (IL-1) *(3)*. Recent evidence suggests that anti-inflammatory mediators have important effects on the host's immune system *(4)*. Anti-inflammatory mediators induce a state of immunosuppression in sepsis that has also been named "immunoparalysis" *(5)*. Pro-inflammatory and anti-inflammatory responses contribute to the outcome of patients with systemic inflammation and sepsis in humans. The genetically determined capacity of cytokine production and release may contribute to a wide range of clinical manifestations of inflammatory disease: a patient with peritonitis, for example, may present without symptoms of sepsis and recover within days or may suffer from fulminant septic shock, resulting in death within hours.

From: *Cytokines and Chemokines in Infectious Diseases Handbook*
Edited by: M. Kotb and T. Calandra © Humana Press Inc., Totowa, NJ

2. CYTOKINE GENE POLYMORPHISM: CANDIDATE GENES

2.1. *Tumor Necrosis Factor*

Primary proinflammatory cytokines like TNF and IL-1 induce secondary proinflammatory and anti-inflammatory mediators like IL-6 and IL-10. They have been shown to contribute substantially to the host's primary response to infection. Both TNF and IL-1 are capable of inducing the same symptoms and the same severity of septic shock and organ dysfunction as endotoxin in experimental settings as well as in humans *(6)*. Genetic variations in the TNF and IL-1 genes are of major interest concerning genetically determined differences in the susceptibility and response to infection.

Tumor necrosis factor is considered one of the most important mediators of endotoxin induced effects. Interindividual differences of TNF release have been described *(7,8)*.

The TNF locus consists of three functional genes. TNF is positioned between lymphotoxin β (LTβ) in the upstream direction and lymphotoxin α (LTα) in the downstream direction. Genomic polymorphisms within in the TNF locus have been under intense investigation.

Genetic variation within the TNF locus is rare, as the TNF gene is well conserved throughout evolution *(9)*. Especially, the coding region is highly conserved.

The main interest has been focused on the genomic variations of the TNF locus: Biallelic polymorphisms defined by restriction enzymes (NcoI, AspHI) or other single base-changes (−308, −238) as well as multiallelic microsatellites (TNFa–e) have been investigated in experimental in vitro studies and also in various diseases in which TNF is considered as an important or possible pathogen. Functional importance for regulation of the TNF gene has been suggested for two polymorphisms within the TNF promoter region. Single-base changes have been detected at positions −850, −376, −308, and −238 *(10–13)*. A G to A transition at position −308 has been associated with susceptibility to cerebral malaria *(14)*. These results could not be confirmed by another malaria study that showed fewer fever episodes in heterozygous carriers of the allele TNF2 *(15)*. In contrast, more recent findings link altered OCT-1 binding in the TNF promoter with susceptibility to severe malaria *(11)*. Further evidence for the association of quantitative cytokine responses with susceptibility to parasitemia has been reported very recently *(16)*. Even susceptibility to *Helicobacter pylori* infection has been examined and shows a correlation of the rare allele TNF2 of the −308 polymorphism with infection with the cagA subtype in Korean patients with gastric disease *(17)*. Studies linking TNF genomic variability to the incidence or severity of viral hepatitis C infection or response to antiviral therapy could not be confirmed by Rosen et al. *(18)*, whereas allele TNF2 might display protective effects in cytomegalovirus infection *(19)*.

The rare allele TNF2 (A at position −308) was suggested to be linked to high TNF promoter activity *(14)*. Autoimmune diseases like diabetes mellitus or lupus erythematosus did not show differences of allele frequencies or genotype distribution between patients and controls *(20,21)*. In addition, patients with severe sepsis and a high proportion of Gram-negative infection also did not display altered allele frequencies concerning both biallelic promoter polymorphisms (positions −238 and −308) *(22)*. Analysis of the TNF promoter by means of reporter gene constructs revealed contradictory results. A first report supposed a functional importance of the −308 G to A transition *(14)*. Two articles could not confirm differences of the TNF promoter activity in relation to the −308 polymorphism *(22,23)*. A recent article reported a possible influence on TNF promoter activity by the −308 G to A transition in a B-cell line *(214)*. Data demonstrating an impact of this genomic polymorphism on transcription are rather weak, as reports predominantly derive from one group *(25)* *(see* Table 1), findings seem to be restricted to few cell lines, and impaired or enhanced binding of transcription factors has not been shown. In addition, the difference in transcription rates in the responsive cell line seems to require a specific stimulus (PMA plus retinoic acid) *(26)*.

Table 1
Actual Evidence that Association of TNF Polymorphisms with Gene Function is Weak

TNF promoter polymorphisms	Promoter activity	Association with Protein expression	Susceptibility to infection
–238	Uncertain	Uncertain	Uncertain
–308	In B-Lymphocytes	In septic shock	Uncertain
TNF locus polymorphisms			
NcoI	Unknown	In peritonitis	In trauma
TNFa–e microsatellites	Unknown	Uncertain	Unknown

Studies trying to associate incidence or severity of infectious disease with TNF polymorphisms have been published on a variety of pathogens. Positive associations of the biallelic TNF –308 as well as LTα polymorphisms with susceptibility to mucocutaneous leishmaniasis and leprosy have been reported *(27,28)*.

Genotyping of this polymorphism in patients with severe sepsis or septic shock still shows controversial results. In contrast to the negative findings in sepsis are the results of two recent studies that suggest an association of the rare allele TNF2 with nonsurvivors of septic shock *(29,30)*. These publications again open the discussion about functionality of the –308 TNF promoter polymorphism and its possible relevance for routine clinical use. In addition to the discussion about the relevance of association, formal standards of genotyping techniques have to be established. Are there typing techniques like allele-specific amplification that imply overestimation or underestimation of certain alleles and genotypes?

In contrast to genomic variations located in the promoter region, intronic polymorphisms are more difficult to associate with a possible functional relevance. Two biallelic polymorphisms located within intron 1 of LTα have been studied in autoimmune disease *(31,32)*. One polymorphism is characterized by the absence or presence of a NcoI restriction site. First reports demonstrated genomic blots revealing characteristic 5.5- or 10.5-kb bands after genomic NcoI digest, which hybridize to TNF-specific probes *(33)*. These bands correspond to presence and absence, respectively, of a NcoI restriction site within intron 1 of lymphotoxin α.

The allele TNFB2 of this NcoI polymorphism (10.5-kb band) has been shown to be associated with high TNF release ex vivo *(34)*. Other studies showed no differences between genotypes in other models of ex vivo TNF induction, whereas another study suggests an increased LTα response in TNFB2 homozygotes *(8)*. The question of which genotype is clearly associated with a high proinflammatory response in the clinical situation of severe Gram-negative infection and severe sepsis cannot yet be answered by ex vivo studies. Different conditions of cell culture and cytokine induction contribute to differing results. In addition, the genomic NcoI polymorphism within intron 1 of the LTα gene may represent a genomic marker without evidence for own functional importance in gene regulation. This genomic marker may coincide with so far undetected genomic variations that are responsible for genetic determination of a high proinflammatory responses to infection. Results from studies in patients with severe intra-abdominal sepsis suggest TNFB2 homozygotes to be associated with a high TNF response. In contrast, genotyping for another biallelic polymorphism within intron 1 of LTα (AspHI) did not show significant association to TNF plasma levels (data not shown).

Several studies in chronic inflammatory autoimmune diseases suggest an association between TNFB2 and incidence or severity and outcome of the disease *(31,32,35)*. Studies in acute inflammatory diseases like severe sepsis in patients in surgical intensive care units showed a correlation between

TNFB2 homozygosity and mortality *(22)* or incidence of septic states in traumatized patients *(36)*. TNFB2 homozygotes displayed a relative risk of 2.9 of dying from severe sepsis when compared to corresponding genotypes.

2.2. Interleukin-1

In addition to TNF, IL-1 is another potent proinflammatory cytokine released by macrophages in the systemic inflammatory response. IL-1 is capable of inducing the symptoms of septic shock and organ failure in animal models and is regarded as a primary mediator of the systemic inflammatory response. Antagonizing IL-1 in endotoxin challenged animals including primates abrogates the lethal effects of endotoxin *(37)*. A biallelic TaqI polymorphism has been described within the coding region (exon 5) of IL-1β *(38,39)* Despite the finding that a homozygous TaqI genotype correlates with high IL-β secretion *(38)*, genotyping of patients with severe sepsis did not reveal any association with incidence or outcome of the disease. In contrast, the allele T of the IL-1BC-31T polymorphisms has been linked to susceptibility to persistent *H. pylori* infection in Japanese patients following an eradication program *(40)*.

2.3. Interleukin-1 Receptor Antagonist

Proinflammatory mediators comprise the hyperinflammatory side of the host's response to infection. At the same time, anti-inflammatory mediators are induced by proinflammatory cytokines and try to counterbalance the increased inflammatory activity. This physiologic process of limiting the extent of inflammation by release of anti-inflammatory proteins may escape physiologic boundaries of local and systemic concentrations of these mediators. Proteins like IL-4, IL-10, IL-11 or IL-13, or IL-1ra contribute to a very powerful downregulation of cellular and humoral proinflammatory activities. This downregulation results in decreased expression of class II molecules in antigen presenting cells as well as in low ex vivo responses of immuncompetent cells to inflammatory stimuli. This state of imunosuppression has also been termed "immunoparalysis" *(5)*. It results in a situation of anergy and diminished capabilities of fighting infectious pathogens. A new term for this status, which is a consequence of the systemic inflammatory response, is "compensatory anti-inflammatory response syndrome" (CARS) *(41)*. The outcome of patients with, for example, severe sepsis is not only influenced by hyperinflammation in fulminant situations of progressing organ dysfunction but may also be limited by immunosuppression and lack of restoration of immune function. In this view, an overwhelming anti-inflammatory response with a possible genetic background of interindividual differences in the release of anti-inflammatory mediators following infection contributes to the human systemic inflammatory reaction to a similar extent as proinflammatory responses.

A genomic polymorphism of the anti-inflammatory cytokine IL-1ra is located within intron 2 and consists of variable numbers of a tandem repeat (VNTR) of a 86-bp motif. This 86-bp motif contains at least three known binding sites for DNA-binding proteins *(42)*. Ex vivo experiments suggest that higher IL-1ra responses combined with alleles containing low numbers of the 86-bp repeat. Ex vivo studies also demonstrate a higher level of IL-1ra protein expression and protein release of A2 homozygous individuals compared to heterozygotes following stimulation with lipopolysaccharide *(43)*.

The allele A2 has been associated with the incidence of autoimmune diseases like lupus erythematosus and insulin-dependent diabetes mellitus *(44,45)*. In acute systemic inflammation, there is no difference between surviving or nonsurviving patients with severe sepsis. This finding is in contrast to the results concerning the biallelic NcoI polymorphism within intron 1 of LTα: Homozygotes for the TNFB2 genotype revealed a high mortality when compared to heterozygotes and TNFB1 homozygotes. The overall group of patients with severe sepsis did not show an increase in the TNFB2 allele frequency. For the IL-1ra polymorphism, however, an increase of the allele A2 in the patients with severe sepsis was detected. Patients carrying the haplotype TNFB2 homozygous and A2 homozygous did not survive in this study.

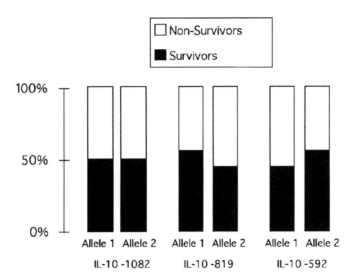

Fig. 1. Comparison of allele frequencies of IL-10 promoter polymorphisms in nonsurvivors ($n = 67$) and survivors ($n = 63$) with severe abdominal sepsis ($p > 0.05$).

Negative associations between IL-1ra polymorphisms and susceptibility to infection have been suggested for vaginal mycoplasma colonization, cytomegalovirus and Epstein–Barr virus infection as well as human immunodeficiency virus (HIV) reproductivity and hemorrhagic fever caused by a hantavirus (*see* reviews in refs. *46,47*).

3. FINDINGS IN OTHER CYTOKINE CANDIDATE GENES

Interleukin-10 shows well-defined haplotypic promoter variation. High IL-10 secretors presenting with fever of unknown origin display an increased mortality rate *(48)*, whereas susceptibility to severe meningococcal disease as well as poor outcome seem to be linked to inherited high IL-10 secretion and low TNF release in a family study testing ex vivo cytokine inducibility *(49)*. IL-10 promoter genotypes could not be associated with incidence or outcome of severe abdominal sepsis (Fig. 1).

In viral infections, IL10-1082 promoter polymorphism has been associated with susceptibility to chronic hepatitis C infection and resistance to antiviral therapy *(50)*. Another publication suggests that high IL-10 secretion indicated by the –1082 polymorphism or the promoter haplotype defined by single nucleotide polymorphisms at positions –1082, –819, and –592 protects against Epstein–Barr virus infection *(51,52)*.

Interestingly, another cytokine promoter polymorphism, interleukin-8-251A, has been associated with high IL-8 release and, possibly because of the IL-8 proinflammatory profile, also associated with the incidence of virus bronchiolitis in an excellent family-based study *(53)*.

Other results show that lipopolysaccharide (LPS)-binding protein may contribute to susceptibility to severe sepsis *(54)*, as suggested in a study also investigating the effects of gender. Genomic variability in chemokine genes have been demonstrated to influence the course of HIV infection *(55–57)*.

4. SIGNAL TRANSDUCTION PATHWAYS IN INFECTION INDUCING CYTOKINES

Transduction of the LPS signal into the cell has been an unknown mechanism until recently. An analogon of the so-called Toll-like receptor in *Drosophila* species that transduces signals for the elaboration of innate immune responses in flies directed against bacteria and fungi has been identified in mice and other species *(58)*. A single-basepair change resulting in an amino acid change of the murine Toll-like receptor 4 (TLR4) renders the extensively studied mouse strain CH3/HeJ highly resistant to LPS challenge *(59)*. Ten Toll-like receptors (TLR1–10) *(60)* have been identified in mammals so far. TLR2 has been identified to transduce peptidoglycan stimulation by Gram-positive organisms *(61–63)*. In contrast, TLR4 seems to play a key role in the LPS-induced signaling pathway. TLR9 transduces inflammatory effects of bacterial DNA.

The presence of a functional TLR4 gene and gene product appears to be one of several determinants of outcome in Gram-negative infection. A first preliminary report suggests that a rare Arg753Gln mutation might render patients with sepsis susceptible to staphylococcal infection *(64)*. Another rare Arg677Trp variation of TLR2 has been linked to susceptibility to lepromatous leprosy *(65)*. Studies to test the association of the rare TLR4 variations with incidence and course of infectious disease are ongoing *(66,67)*.

5. CONCLUSION

Uncovering and understanding the genetic determination of the susceptibility to infection offers the chance of developing valuable diagnostic tools and new therapeutic approaches in severe sepsis. Evaluation of candidate genomic markers for risk stratification of individuals at high risk of developing infectious disease has just begun. Many candidate genes still have to be studied and clinical significance of genomic markers will be tested. In addition, this new approach may prove to be a valuable inclusion criterion for studies testing the prevention of infectious diseases in subpopulations known to be at high risk because of genomic predisposition. Most studies so far include rather small numbers of individuals and are in danger of being statistically underpowered and lack quality control of genotyping. New study designs will provide the scientific community with adequately powered studies, well-established concepts of genetic epidemiology, and quality control criteria of genotyping. These designs will include the determination of the genomic background variability in a given population to control for false-positive association (concept of genomic controls). Technical progress will allow researchers to step beyond candidate gene approaches and scan the genome to discover previously unnoticed loci of interest. Extension of single genomic marker analysis to haplotype analyses including functionally relevant alleles may reveal the highest informativity and diagnostic relevance even before the era of widely available genomic scans.

REFERENCES

1. Sasse, K.C., Nauenberg, E., Long, A., Anton, B., Tucker, H. J., and Hu, T.W. (1995) Long-term survival after intensive care unit admission with sepsis. *Crit. Care. Med.* **23,** 1040–1047.
2. Schlegel, R.J. and Bellanti, J.A. (1969) Increased susceptibility of males to infection. *Lancet* **2,** 826–827.
3. Blackwell, T.S. and Christman, J.W. (1996) Sepsis and cytokines: current status. *Br. J. Anaesth.* **77,** 110–117.
4. van der Poll, T., de Waal Malefyt, R., Coyle, S.M., and Lowry, S.F. (1997) Anti-inflammatory cytokine responses during clinical sepsis and experimental endotoxemia: sequential measurements of plasma soluble interleukin (IL)-1 receptor type II, IL-10, and IL-13. *J. Infect. Dis.* **175,** 118–122.
5. Volk, H. D., Reinke, P., Krausch, D., Zuckermann, H., Asadullah, K., Muller, J. M., et al. (1996) Monocyte deactivation—rationale for a new therapeutic strategy in sepsis. *Intens Care Med.* **22 (Suppl 4),** S474–481.
6. Weinberg, J.R., Boyle, P., Meager, A., and Guz, A. (1992) Lipopolysaccharide, tumor necrosis factor, and interleukin-1 interact to cause hypotension. [see comments]. *J. Lab. Clin. Med.* **120,** 205–211.
7. Westendorp, R.G., Langermans, J.A., Huizinga, T.W., Elouali, A.H., Verweij, C.L., Boomsma, D.I., et al. (1997) Genetic influence on cytokine production and fatal meningococcal disease. [see comments]. *Lancet* **349,** 170–173.
8. Whichelow, C.E., Hitman, G.A., Raafat, I., Bottazzo, G. F., and Sachs, J.A. (1996) The effect of TNF*B gene polymorphism on TNF-alpha and -beta secretion levels in patients with insulin-dependent diabetes mellitus and healthy controls. *Eur. J. Immunogenet.* **23,** 425–435.
9. Gray, P.W., Aggarwal, B.B., Benton, C.V., Bringman, T.S., Henzel, W.J., Jarrett, J.A., et al. (1984) Cloning and expression of cDNA for human lymphotoxin, a lymphokine with tumour necrosis activity. *Nature* **312,** 721–724.
10. Kato, T., Honda, M., Kuwata, S., Juji, T., Kunugi, H., Nanko, S., et al. (1999) Novel polymorphism in the promoter region of the tumor necrosis factor alpha gene: No association with narcolepsy. *Am J. Med. Genet.* **88,** 301–304.
11. Knight, J.C., Udalova, I., Hill, A.V., Greenwood, B.M., Peshu, N., Marsh, K., et al. (1999) A polymorphism that affects OCT-1 binding to the TNF promoter region is associated with severe malaria. [see comments]. *Nat. Genet.* **22,** 145–150.
12. Wilson, A.G., di Giovine, F.S., Blakemore, A.I., and Duff, G.W. (1992) Single base polymorphism in the human tumour necrosis factor alpha (TNF alpha) gene detectable by NcoI restriction of PCR product. *Hum. Mol. Genet.* **1,** 353.

13. Brinkman, B.M., Huizinga, T.W., Kurban, S.S., van der Velde, E.A., Schreuder, G.M., Hazes, J.M., et al. (1997) Tumour necrosis factor alpha gene polymorphisms in rheumatoid arthritis: association with susceptibility to, or severity of, disease? *Br. J. Rheumatol.* **36,** 516–521.
14. McGuire, W., Hill, A. V., Allsopp, C.E., Greenwood, B.M., and Kwiatkowski, D. (1994) Variation in the TNF-alpha promoter region associated with susceptibility to cerebral malaria. *Nature* **371,** 508–510.
15. Stirnadel, H.A., Stockle, M., Felger, I., Smith, T., Tanner, M., and Beck, H.P. (1999) Malaria infection and morbidity in infants in relation to genetic polymorphisms in Tanzania. Trop. Med. Int. *Health* **4,** 187–193.
16. Dodoo, D., Omer, F.M., Todd, J., Akanmori, B.D., Koram, K.A., and Riley, E.M. (2002) Absolute levels and ratios of pro-inflammatory and anti-inflammatory cytokine production in vitro predict clinical immunity to plasmodium falciparum malaria. *J. Infect. Dis.* **185,** 971–979.
17. Yea, S.S., Yang, Y.I., Jang, W.H., Lee, Y.J., Bae, H.S., and Paik, K.H. (2001) Association between TNF-alpha promoter polymorphism and Helicobacter pylori cagA subtype infection. *J. Clin. Pathol.* **54,** 703–706.
18. Rosen, H.R., McHutchison, J.G., Conrad, A.J., Lentz, J.J., Marousek, G., Rose, S.L., et al. (2002) Tumor necrosis factor genetic polymorphisms and response to antiviral therapy in patients with chronic hepatitis C. *Am. J. Gastroenterol.* **97,** 714–720.
19. Hurme, M. and Helminen, M. (1998) Resistance to human cytomegalovirus infection may be influenced by genetic polymorphisms of the tumour necrosis factor-alpha and interleukin-1 receptor antagonist genes. *Scand. J. Infect. Dis.* **30,** 447–449.
20. Pociot, F., Wilson, A.G., Nerup, J., and Duff, G.W. (1993) No independent association between a tumor necrosis factor-alpha promotor region polymorphism and insulin-dependent diabetes mellitus. *Eur. J. Immunol.* **23,** 3050–3053.
21. Wilson, A.G., Gordon, C., di Giovine, F.S., de Vries, N., van de Putte, L.B., Emery, P., et al. (1994) A genetic association between systemic lupus erythematosus and tumor necrosis factor alpha. *Eur. J. Immunol.* **24,** 191–195.
22. Stuber, F., Udalova, I.A., Book, M., Drutskaya, L.N., Kuprash, D.V., Turetskaya, R. L., et al. (1995) –308 tumor necrosis factor (TNF) polymorphism is not associated with survival in severe sepsis and is unrelated to lipopolysaccharide inducibility of the human TNF promoter. [see comments]. *J. Inflamm.* **46,** 42–50.
23. Brinkman, B.M., Zuijdeest, D., Kaijzel, E.L., Breedveld, F.C., and Verweij, C.L. (1995) Relevance of the tumor necrosis factor alpha (TNF alpha) –308 promoter polymorphism in TNF alpha gene regulation. [see comments]. *J. Inflamm.* **46,** 32–41.
24. Wilson, A.G., Symons, J.A., McDowell, T.L., McDevitt, H.O., and Duff, G.W. (1997) Effects of a polymorphism in the human tumor necrosis factor alpha promoter on transcriptional activation. *Proc. Natl. Acad. Sci. USA* **94,** 3195–3199.
25. Abraham, L.J. and Kroeger, K.M. (1999) Impact of the –308 TNF promoter polymorphism on the transcriptional regulation of the TNF gene: relevance to disease. *J. Leukoc. Biol.* **66,** 562–566.
26. Kroeger, K.M., Steer, J.H., Joyce, D.A., and Abraham, L.J. (2000) Effects of stimulus and cell type on the expression of the –308 tumour necrosis factor promoter polymorphism. *Cytokine* **12,** 110–119.
27. Cabrera, M., Shaw, M.A., Sharples, C., Williams, H., Castes, M., Convit, J., et al. (1995) Polymorphism in tumor necrosis factor genes associated with mucocutaneous leishmaniasis. *J. Exp. Med.* **182,**1259–1264.
28. Knight, J.C. and Kwiatkowski, D. (1999) Inherited variability of tumor necrosis factor production and susceptibility to infectious disease. *Proc Assoc Am Physicians.* **111,** 290–298.
29. Mira, J.P., Cariou, A., Grall, F., Delclaux, C., Losser, M.R., Heshmati, F., et al. (1999) Association of TNF2, a TNF-alpha promoter polymorphism, with septic shock susceptibility and mortality: a multicenter study. [see comments]. *JAMA* **282,** 561–568.
30. Tang, G.J., Huang, S.L., Yien, H.W., Chen, W.S., Chi, C.W., Wu, C.W., et al. (2000) Tumor necrosis factor gene polymorphism and septic shock in surgical infection. [in process citation]. *Crit. Care Med.* **28,** 2733–2736.
31. Pociot, F., Molvig, J., Wogensen, L., Worsaae, H., Dalboge, H., Baek, L., et al. (1991) A tumour necrosis factor beta gene polymorphism in relation to monokine secretion and insulin-dependent diabetes mellitus. *Scand. J. Immunol.* **33,** 37–49.
32. Bettinotti, M.P., Hartung, K., Deicher, H., Messer, G., Keller, E., Weiss, E.H., et al. (1993) Polymorphism of the tumor necrosis factor beta gene in systemic lupus erythematosus: TNFB-MHC haplotypes. *Immunogenetics* **37,** 449–454.
33. Badenhoop, K., Schwarz, G., Trowsdale, J., Lewis,V., Usadel, K.H., Gale, E.A., et al. (1989) TNF-alpha gene polymorphisms in type 1 (insulin-dependent) diabetes mellitus. *Diabetologia* **32,** 445–448.
34. Pociot, F., Briant, L., Jongeneel, C.V., Molvig, J., Worsaae, H., Abbal, M., et al. (1993) Association of tumor necrosis factor (TNF) and class II major histocompatibility complex alleles with the secretion of TNF- alpha and TNF-beta by human mononuclear cells: a possible link to insulin- dependent diabetes mellitus. *Eur. J. Immunol.* **23,** 224–231.
35. Vinasco, J., Beraun, Y., Nieto, A., Fraile, A., Mataran, L., Pareja, E., et al. (1997) Polymorphism at the TNF loci in rheumatoid arthritis. *Tissue Antigens* **49,** 74–78.
36. Majetschak, M., Flohe, S., Obertacke, U., Schroder, J., Staubach, K., Nast, Kolb D., et al. (1999) Relation of a TNF gene polymorphism to severe sepsis in trauma patients. *Ann Surg* **230,** 207–214.
37. Boermeester, M.A., Van Leeuwen, P.A., Coyle, S.M., Wolbink, G.J., Hack, C.E., and Lowry, S.F. (1995) Interleukin-1 blockade attenuates mediator release and dysregulation of the hemostatic mechanism during human sepsis. *Arch. Surg.* **130,** 739–748.
38. Pociot, F., Molvig, J., Wogensen, L., Worsaae, H., and Nerup, J. (1992) A TaqI polymorphism in the human interleukin-1 beta (IL-1 beta) gene correlates with IL-1 beta secretion in vitro. *Eur. J. Clin. Invest.* **22,** 396–402.

39. Guasch, J.F., Bertina, R.M., and Reitsma, P.H. (1996). Five novel intragenic dimorphisms in the human interleukin-1 genes combine to high informativity. *Cytokine* **8**, 598–602.
40. Hamajima, N., Matsuo, K., Saito, T., Tajima, K., Okuma, K., Yamao, K., et al. (2001) Interleukin 1 polymorphisms, lifestyle factors, and Helicobacter pylori infection. *Jpn. J. Cancer Res.* **92**, 383–389.
41. Bone, R.C. (1996) Sir Isaac Newton, sepsis, SIRS, and CARS. *Crit. Care. Med.* **24**, 1125–1128.
42. Tarlow, J.K., Blakemore, A.I., Lennard, A., Solari, R., Hughes, H.N., Steinkasserer, A., et al. (1993) Polymorphism in human IL-1 receptor antagonist gene intron 2 is caused by variable numbers of an 86-bp tandem repeat. *Hum. Genet.* **91**, 403–404.
43. Danis, V.A., Millington, M., Hyland, V.J., and Grennan, D. (1995) Cytokine production by normal human monocytes: inter-subject variation and relationship to an IL-1 receptor antagonist (IL- 1Ra) gene polymorphism. *Clin. Exp. Immunol.* **99**, 303–310.
44. Blakemore, A.I., Tarlow, J.K., Cork, M.J., Gordon, C., Emery, P., and Duff, G.W. (1994) Interleukin-1 receptor antagonist gene polymorphism as a disease severity factor in systemic lupus erythematosus. *Arthritis. Rheum.* **37**, 1380–1385.
45. Metcalfe, K.A., Hitman, G.A., Pociot, F., Bergholdt, R., Tuomilehto-Wolf, E., Tuomilehto, J., et al. (1996) An association between type 1 diabetes and the interleukin-1 receptor type 1 gene. The DiMe Study Group. Childhood Diabetes in Finland. *Hum. Immunol.* **51**, 41–48.
46. Witkin, S.S., Gerber, S., and Ledger, W.J. (2002) Influence of interleukin-1 receptor antagonist gene polymorphism on disease. *Clin. Infect. Dis.* **34** 204–209.
47. Makela, S., Hurme, M., Ala-Houhala, I., Mustonen, J., Koivisto, A.M., Partanen, J., et al. (2001) Polymorphism of the cytokine genes in hospitalized patients with *Puumala hantavirus* infection. *Nephrol. Dial. Transplant.* **16**, 1368–1373.
48. van-Dissel, J.T., van-Langevelde, P., Westendorp, R.G., Kwappenberg, K., and Frolich, M. (1998) Anti-inflammatory cytokine profile and mortality in febrile patients. [see comments]. *Lancet* **351**, 950–953.
49. Westendorp, R.G., Langermans, J.A., Huizinga, T.W., Elouali, A.H., Verweij, C.L., Boomsma, D.I., et al. (1997) Genetic influence on cytokine production and fatal meningococcal disease [published erratum appears in *Lancet* 1997, **349(9052)** :656]. [see comments]. *Lancet* **349**, 170–173.
50. Vidigal, P.G., Germer, J.J., and Zein, N.N. (2002) Polymorphisms in the interleukin-10, tumor necrosis factor-alpha, and transforming growth factor-beta1 genes in chronic hepatitis C patients treated with interferon and ribavirin. *J. Hepatol.* **36**, 271–277.
51. Helminen, M., Lahdenpohja, N., and Hurme, M. (1999) Polymorphism of the interleukin-10 gene is associated with susceptibility to Epstein–Barr virus infection. *J. Infect. Dis.* **180**, 496–499.
52. Helminen, M.E., Kilpinen, S., Virta, M., and Hurme, M. (2001) Susceptibility to primary Epstein-Barr virus infection is associated with interleukin-10 gene promoter polymorphism. *J. Infect. Dis.* **184**, 777–780.
53. Hull, J., Thomson, A., and Kwiatkowski, D. (2000) Association of respiratory syncytial virus bronchiolitis with the interleukin 8 gene region in UK families. *Thorax* **55**, 1023–1027.
54. Hubacek, J. A., Stuber, F., Frohlich, D., Book, M., Wetegrove, S., Ritter, M., et al. (2001) Gene variants of the bactericidal/permeability increasing protein and lipopolysaccharide binding protein in sepsis patients: gender-specific genetic predisposition to sepsis. *Crit Care Med.* **29**, 557–561.
55. Alvarez, V., Lopez-Larrea, C., and Coto, E. (1998) Mutational analysis of the CCR5 and CXCR4 genes (HIV-1 co-receptors) in resistance to HIV-1 infection and AIDS development among intravenous drug users. *Hum. Genet.* **102**, 483–486.
56. McDermott, D.H., Beecroft, M.J., Kleeberger, C.A., Al Sharif, F.M., Ollier, W.E., Zimmerman, P.A., et al. (2000) Chemokine RANTES promoter polymorphism affects risk of both HIV infection and disease progression in the Multicenter AIDS Cohort Study. *AIDS* **14**, 2671–2678.
57. Gonzalez, E., Dhanda, R., Bamshad, M., Mummidi, S., Geevarghese, R., Catano, G., et al. (2001) Global survey of genetic variation in CCR5, RANTES, and MIP-1alpha: impact on the epidemiology of the HIV-1 pandemic. *Proc. Natl. Acad. Sci. USA* **98**, 5199–5204.
58. Janeway-CA, Jr and Medzhitov, R. (1999) Lipoproteins take their toll on the host. *Curr. Biol.* **9**, R879–R882.
59. Poltorak, A., He, X., Smirnova, I., Liu, M.Y., Huffel, C.V., Du, X., et al. (1998) Defective LPS signaling in C3H/HeJ and C57BL/10ScCr mice: mutations in Tlr4 gene. *Science* **282**, 2085–2088.
60. Takeuchi, O., Kawai, T., Sanjo, H., Copeland, N.G., Gilbert, D.J., Jenkins, N.A., et al. (1999) TLR6: A novel member of an expanding toll-like receptor family. *Gene* **231**, 59–65.
61. Schwandner, R., Dziarski, R., Wesche, H., Rothe, M., and Kirschning, C.J. (1999) Peptidoglycan- and lipoteichoic acid-induced cell activation is mediated by toll-like receptor 2. *J. Biol. Chem.* **274**, 17,406–17,409.
62. Yoshimura, A., Lien, E., Ingalls, R.R., Tuomanen, E., Dziarski, R., and Golenbock, D., et al. (1999) Cutting edge: recognition of Gram-positive bacterial cell wall components by the innate immune system occurs via Toll-like receptor 2. *J. Immunol.* **163**, 1–5.
63. Takeuchi, O., Kaufmann, A., Grote, K., Kawai, T., Hoshino, K., Morr, M., et al. (2000) Cutting edge: preferentially the R-stereoisomer of the mycoplasmal lipopeptide macrophage-activating lipopeptide-2 activates immune cells through a toll-like receptor 2- and MyD88-dependent signaling pathway. *J. Immunol.* **164**, 554–557.
64. Lorenz, E., Mira, J.P., Cornish, K.L., Arbour, N.C., and Schwartz, D.A. (2000) A novel polymorphism in the toll-like receptor 2 gene and its potential association with staphylococcal infection. *Infect. Immun.* **68**, 6398–6401.
65. Kang, T.J. and Chae, G.T. (2001) Detection of Toll-like receptor 2 (TLR2) mutation in the lepromatous leprosy patients. *FEMS Immunol. Med. Microbiol.* **31**, 53–58.
66. Smirnova, I., Hamblin, M.T., McBride, C., Beutler, B., and Di Rienzo, A. (2001) Excess of rare amino acid polymorphisms in the Toll-like receptor 4 in humans. *Genetics* **158**, 1657–1664.
67. Read, R.C., Pullin, J., Gregory, S., Borrow, R., Kaczmarski, E.B., di Giovine, F.S., et al. (2001) A functional polymorphism of toll-like receptor 4 is not associated with likelihood or severity of meningococcal disease. *J. Infect. Dis.* **184**, 640–642.

II
Cytokines in Gram-Negative Infections

3

Proinflammatory and Anti-Inflammatory Cytokines as Mediators of Gram-Negative Sepsis

Jean-Marc Cavaillon

1. INTRODUCTION

Severe sepsis represents 2.26 cases per 100 hospital discharges in the United States *(1)*. With an estimate of 751,000 cases a year in the United States and a 28.6% mortality, severe sepsis is responsible for 9.3% of the deaths in this country (i.e., as many deaths annually as those from acute myocardial infarction). Although in the past, Gram-negative sepsis cases were most frequent, recent surveys suggest that around 35% of the sepsis cases are the result of Gram-negative infections *(2,3)*. Gram-negative bacteria possess the capacity to elicit the production of numerous cytokines by host cells, particularly monocytes/macrophages. Endotoxin (lipopolysaccharide [LPS]), a major component of the cell wall of Gram-negative bacteria, is one of the most potent inducers of inflammatory cytokines. It is worth noting that endotoxins activate complement and coagulation, of which derived factors further act synergistically with LPS to generate higher release of cytokines. LPS binds to CD14, and CD14 knockout (KO) mice are resistant to a lethal injection of LPS, whereas lethal administration of *Escherichia coli* produces little or no response *(4)*. However, in the cecal ligature and puncture model of sepsis, no significant differences in mortality between CD14 KO and control mice were reported, although CD14 KO mice consistently showed lower levels of cytokines *(5)*. In human volunteers receiving an injection of LPS, anti-CD14 attenuated LPS-induced clinical symptoms and strongly inhibited LPS-induced proinflammatory cytokines, but only delaying the enhancement of circulating soluble tumor necrosis factor (TNF) receptors and interleukin (IL)-1 receptor antagonists *(6)*. CD14 is anchored to the membrane by a phosphatidyl-inositol group and is associated with heterotrimeric G-proteins that regulate p38 mitogen-activated protein kinase (MAPK) and cytokine production *(7)*. The recent discovery of the Toll-like receptors (TLRs) has allowed the identification of an important component of the LPS-receptor, which signals the cells and leads to cell activation: Signaling by LPS is mediated by a molecular complex including the TLR4, and MD2 molecules express on the cell surface *(8,9)*. However, in a model of Gram-negative sepsis, TLR4-deficient mice (C3H/HeJ) displayed sensitivity to iv injection of *E. coli* equal to that of normal mice and had a similar interferon-γ (IFN-γ) plasma levels despite an attenuated TNF response *(10)*. It is worth recalling that, in vitro, whole bacteria lead to higher levels of TNF by human monocytes than isolated LPS *(11)*. This is also true for IL-1α and IL-6, whereas interleukin-12 production by dendritic cell requires the lipopolysaccharide expression in intact *Neisseria meningitidis* bacteria *(12)*. Indeed, many other bacterial components possess the property to generate cytokine production. Recently, the contribution of various members of the TLR family was established: fimbriae activate cells via TLR4 *(13)*, flagelin via TLR5 *(14)*, lipoprotein and peptidoglycan via TLR2 *(8)*, and fragment of bacterial DNA containing CpG sequence via TLR9 *(15)*. Because of

From: *Cytokines and Chemokines in Infectious Diseases Handbook*
Edited by: M. Kotb and T. Calandra © Humana Press Inc., Totowa, NJ

their exacerbated productions, proinflammatory cytokines can be detected in many biological fluids and particularly in the bloodstream. Their production is essential to fight the infectious process, and their neutralization by antibodies or their absence in knockout mice has always been shown to be deleterious. In contrast, their excessive production is accompanied by numerous side effects that can result in organ damage and death (Fig. 1). Anti-inflammatory cytokines are also produced in great excess in sepsis and, in most cases, their high concentrations correlate with a poor outcome. Although the anti-inflammatory actors are required to limit the excessive inflammatory process, most probably the immune depression observed in sepsis patients is, in part, a consequence of their excessive production.

2. DETECTION OF CYTOKINES IN THE BLOOD COMPARTMENT

2.1. Circulating Cytokines and Soluble Receptors

2.1.1. Tumor Necrosis Factor and Lymphotoxin-α

In 1986, TNF was the first cytokine identified in the sera of patients with septicemia *(16)* and later in patients with meningococcal sepsis *(17,18)*. Although a correlation between poor outcome and high levels of circulating TNF exists in the case of meningococcal sepsis *(17,18)*, in other forms of sepsis, some authors also observe such a correlation *(19,20)*, whereas others did not *(21,22)*. Kinetics of plasma TNF have been reported *(20,22)*: The persistence of detectable TNF rather than the peak level is associated with fatal outcome *(21,23)*, and high TNF levels are correlated with severity of illness and elevated APACHE II scores. In contrast, during intraperitoneal sepsis, high levels of circulating TNF are associated with a favorable prognosis, whereas low levels are correlated with fatal outcome *(24,25)*. Some authors reported that the TNF levels were higher in Gram-negative than in Gram-positive sepsis, although this was not observed in all studies. In meningococcal sepsis, levels of TNF are higher in cerebrospinal fluids (CSFs) than in plasma *(26)* and not detected in CSFs of nonbacterial meningitis *(27)*. Injection of LPS in human volunteers and in animal models leads to a plasma peak of TNF at 90 min, and its level may be upregulated by administration of ibuprofen *(28)* or G-CSF *(29)* and downregulated by epinephrine *(30)*.

Lymphotoxin-α (Ltα) is a cytokine essentially produced by activated T-lymphocytes. It shares with TNF the same receptors and, thus, most of its activities. Essentially, Ltα should be expected in Gram-positive sepsis because Gram-positive bacteria release various T-cell activators known as superantigens *(31)*. To our knowledge, Ltα has never been reported in human Gram-negative sepsis *(32)*. On the contrary, in patients with streptococcal toxic shock syndrome, circulating Ltα was found to parallel the levels of the circulating superantigen *(33)*.

2.1.2. Interleukin-1

Interleukin-1β has been regularly reported in plasma of sepsis patients, whereas IL-1α has rarely been observed when investigated. IL-1β was found in 0–90% of septic patients, depending on the studies, the nature of the sepsis, and the nature of the technique used to assess its presence. The highest frequency of detectable levels of IL-1β was observed among patients with meningococcal sepsis *(34)* and high levels of IL-1β correlate with the severity of meningococcaemia, the presence of shock, high APACHE II scores, and rapid fatal outcome *(18,32,34)*. Such correlations were not observed in other forms of sepsis *(22)*. In some studies, an IL-1β survey was performed and either high levels at admission followed by a decrease or sustained levels were reported *(20,22)*.

2.1.3. Interleukin-6

The presence of IL-6 in plasma of sepsis patients was first reported in 1989 *(32,35)*. Plasma IL-6 has been observed in 64–100% of the studied patients. Most investigators have demonstrated that levels of circulating IL-6 correlate with severity of sepsis and may predict outcome *(22,32,35,36)*, as illustrated by the correlation between IL-6 levels and APACHE II scores[*(37)*]. Numerous correlations between IL-6 levels and other markers have been reported including C3a, lactate *(35)*, circulat-

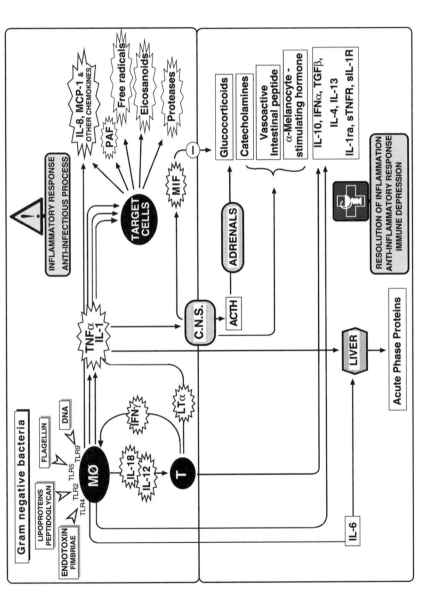

Fig. 1. Gram-negative bacteria and Gram-negative bacteria-derived products interact with macrophages (MØ) via various receptors, including the Toll-like receptors (TLR), and induce numerous proinflammatory cytokines that, in turn, induce a cascade of cytokines and other proinflammatory mediators. The inflammatory response is essential for the anti-infectious process (upper part of the schema). Bacteria and bacterial derived products also induce the release of anti-inflammatory cytokines and anti-inflammatory mediators targeting interleukin-1 (IL-1 receptor antagonist, IL-1ra; soluble IL-1 receptors, sIL-1R) and tumor necrosis factor (soluble TNF receptors, sTNFR). The central nervous system (CNS) is the source of numerous neuromediators that also counteract the inflammatory response. The anti-inflammatory response is required to induce the resolution of the inflammation but may be associated with an induction of an immune depression (lower part of the scheme).

ing endotoxin *(34,38)*, C-Reactive protein (CRP) *(37)*, and TNF *(32,34,36)*. IL-6 levels are similar in Gram-positive or Gram-negative sepsis *(22)*. Injection of endotoxin in human volunteers revealed that the peak level was reached 2 h after injection *(39,40)*.

2.1.4. Members of the gp130 Superfamily

Numerous cytokines share with IL-6 the gp130 chain of the receptor. This defines a cytokine superfamily that includes IL-11, leukemia inhibitory factor (LIF), ciliary neurotrophic factor (CNTF), and oncostatin M (OSM). Divergent reports concern IL-11, which was detected in 67% of patients with disseminated intravascular coagulation complicated by sepsis *(41)* but not in patients suffering from septic shock *(42)*. First reported in 1992 *(43)*, detectable levels of LIF were found in plasma of 9–40% septic patients *(42,44)*. Levels of circulating LIF correlate with shock, temperature, creatinine, and IL-6 *(44)*. The correlation between LIF and IL-6 has been confirmed in a baboon model of sepsis *(45)*. Elevated levels of plasma CNTF and OSM have been observed in 60% and 100% septic patients, respectively *(42)*.

2.1.5. Chemokines

Interleukin-8 was detected in plasma of baboons following injection of LPS, live *E. coli*, or IL-1 *(46)*. Indeed, a great amount of IL-8 is detectable within the blood compartment during human sepsis *(47,48)* and in broncho-alveolar lavage (BAL) and edema fluids of patients with acute respiratory distress syndrome (ARDS) associated with sepsis *(49)*. In this study, ARDS patients with high levels of IL-8 in BAL had a high mortality rate. Similarly, high levels of plasma IL-8 correlate with the occurrence of shock *(50)*, with the presence of infectious multiple-organ failure *(51)*, and with poor outcome *(47,48,51)*. No difference in IL-8 plasma levels were found between Gram-negative and Gram-positive infection *(48)*, whereas in bacteremic pneumonia, the type of pathogen influenced the measurable levels of IL-8 *(52)*. IL-8 levels also correlate with various markers, including IL-6 *(34,48,51)*, C3a, α_1-antitrypsin, lactate *(48)*, IL-10, IL-1ra, and soluble TNF receptors (sTNFRs) *(34)*. Correlation with plasma TNF led to controversial results *(34,53)*. More interestingly, local levels of IL-8 often correlate with the number of recruited neutrophils *(49)*, and plasma levels are associated with granulocyte activation as evidenced by massive release of elastase detectable in the circulation of bacteremic baboons *(54)* and by a correlation between elastase and IL-8 in human sepsis *(50)*.

The presence of other circulating chemokines has been reported in mice following LPS injection. MIP-1α and MIP-2 were rapidly elevated in serum within 1 h of LPS administration and the magnitude of monocyte-chemoattractant protein-1 (MCP-1) production was the greatest and remained substantially elevated 48 h after LPS *(55)*. Sustained levels of MCP-1 were also reported following a lethal injection of *E. coli* in baboons *(56)*. In a murine sepsis model induced by cecal ligation and puncture (CLP), levels of KC, a murine IL-8 homolog, and MIP-2 correlated with the severity of sepsis *(57)*. Increased levels of different chemokines have been found in plasma of septic patients or following LPS injection in human volunteers. This is the case for MCP-1 and MCP-2 *(58)*, MIP-1α and MIP-1β *(59)*, and IP-10 *(60)*. MCP-1 levels being higher in patients with the more severe forms of sepsis (i.e., those with shock or a lethal outcome). In contrast, in a preliminary study, we found that plasma levels of RANTES were inversely correlated with APACHE II score, and lower levels of this chemokine were found in nonsurviving sepsis patients (Cavaillon and Payen, unpublished observation).

2.1.6. Interleukin-2 and Interleukin-15

Interleukin-2 is a cytokine that reflects T-cell activation. Although rarely reported in human sepsis *(23,32)*, IL-2 was found in the circulation within 2 h following injection of bacterial superantigens in mice *(61)* and baboons *(62)*.

Interleukin-15 shares many functions with IL-2. The specific IL-15 receptor α-chain is associated with the IL-2 receptor β- and γ-chains. Interleukin-15 is produced by endothelial cells and by monocytes/macrophages in response to exogenous stimuli such as bacteria and LPS and, importantly, is expressed on the cell surface as an active molecule *(63)*. Although its presence has been reported in the plasma of septic patients *(64)*, its role during sepsis remains to be fully characterized .

2.1.7. Interleukin-12

Interleukin-12 is a heterodimeric cytokine constituted of p40 and p35 subunits. IL-12 is a potent inducer of IFN-γ. The measurement of p70 heterodimer is correlated with IL-12 bioactivity. Bioactive IL-12 was detected in mouse serum at 2–4 h after LPS injection *(65)*. In baboons, surprisingly, higher levels of IL-12 were detectable in plasma of animals injected with sublethal doses of *E. coli* than in animals challenged with lethal doses *(66)*. In humans, an intravenous bolus injection of *E. coli* LPS in volunteers did not lead to changes in the plasma levels of IL-12 *(67)*, and IL-12 could not be measured in most of septic patients *(68)*. Although levels of IL-12p40 were found higher in patients with severe melioidosis (infection with *Burkholderia pseudomallei*) than in healthy controls, IL-12p70, not detectable in controls, was only found in 10% of the patients *(64)*.

2.1.8. Interleukin-18

Interleukin-18 is structurally related to the IL-1 family and its maturation is under the control of caspase-1. Produced by activated macrophages and Kupffer cells, IL-18 is a potent inducer of IFN-γ *(69)*. Plasma IL-18 is found in healthy controls and its level was enhanced in patients with melioidosis, was higher in bacteremic patients, and correlated with APACHE II score, and there was a weak correlation with IFN-γ levels *(64)*. Levels of IL-18 were also enhanced in human sepsis, whereas, surprisingly, injection of LPS did not modify the levels of circulating IL-18 in human healthy volunteers *(70)*. Enhanced levels of IL-18 were also reported in the BAL of septic patients *(71)*.

2.1.9. Interferon-γ

Interferon-γ is an efficient amplifying cytokine produced by superantigen-activated or virus-activated T-lymphocytes. IFN-γ is also produced in response to IL-12 and/or IL-18 released by monocytes/macrophages activated by microbial products. The study of circulating IFN-γ in human sepsis led to contradictory results. In sepsis and purpura fulminans, IFN-γ was found in patients with the most severe disease *(18)*, but no correlation was reported with outcome in other studies on sepsis and septic shock *(20,23)*. No detectable IFN-γ was reported in meningococcal septic shock *(32)* and in human volunteers receiving systemic endotoxin *(67)*, although it was detected in 71% of patients with melioidosis *(64)*. In a baboon model of septic shock, the IFN-γ level was threefold higher in lethally challenged animals than in those receiving sublethal doses *(66)*. LPS injection also leads to detectable circulating IFN-γ in mice. It is noteworthy that in mice rendered tolerant to endotoxin, no further IFN-γ could be measured in plasma, whereas levels of IL-12 and IL-18 remained elevated *(72)*

2.1.10. Colony-Stimulating Factors

In human, macrophage-colony-stimulating factor (M-CSF) is present at homeostasis in the circulation and its level is increased in patients with sepsis and to a greater degree in patients with hemophagocytosis associated with sepsis *(73)*. Granulocyte-CSF (G-CSF) is also increased in sepsis and reaches higher levels in severe sepsis as compared to sepsis or bacteremia *(74)*. Enhanced levels of circulating G-CSFs have been particularly associated with infection and sepsis in neonates *(75)*. In meningococcemia, plasma GM-CSF concentrations were briefly present in subjects with life-threatening septic shock and were strongly associated with fulminant disease *(74)*. GM-CSF was also markedly elevated in septic preterm infants *(76)*.

2.1.11 Interleukin-1 Receptor Antagonist (IL-1ra)

Interleukin-1 receptor antigen (IL-1ra) is present in plasma at homeostasis. Enhanced levels of IL-1ra have been regularly reported in critically ill patients, septic adults and newborn patients *(77–79)*. It may correlate with the APACHE II score *(79)*. As an antagonist, its concentration must be at least 100-fold higher than that of IL-1 to efficiently block the effects of this cytokine. In a patient who died within 8 h after admission with a *N. meningitides* septicemia, we found a 61,000-fold higher concentration of plasma IL-1ra than IL-1β *(80)*. This observation suggests that the balance between proinflammatory and anti-inflammatory cytokines seems adequate to limit the effects of proinflammatory cytokines.

2.1.12. Soluble IL-1 Receptors

Both IL-1 receptors can be shed by the cells and bind to IL-1β. However, soluble form of IL-1R (sIL-1R) type I has no discernable anti-inflammatory property following endotoxin administration in human volunteers *(81)*. This may reflect the fact that sIL-1RI has a similar affinity for IL-1α and IL-1β than for IL-1ra *(82)*. In contrast, the soluble form of the type II receptor, also known as the decoy receptor, binds IL-1β with higher affinity than IL-1ra and inhibits IL-1 activity. Plasma levels of sIL-1RII in patients with sepsis syndrome were in higher concentrations than those of sIL-1RI *(83)*.

2.1.13. Soluble TNF Receptors

The soluble forms of the TNF receptors (sTNFRI and sTNFRII) are natural inhibitors capable of limiting TNF bioactivity. Injection into animal models of sepsis has also shown to be essentially protective *(84,85)*. Sepsis is associated with an enhanced plasma level of soluble TNF receptors. In children with severe meningococcemia, high levels of sTNFRI and II correlate with a poor clinical outcome *(86)*. In meningococcemia and in sepsis, high levels of sTNFRI and sTNFRII correlate with TNF-α levels *(87,88)*. Increased levels of sTNFR can be induced by an injection of LPS *(87,88)* or following injections of IL-1 *(89)* or TNF *(90)*. Although the ratio sTNFR/TNF has been proposed to illustrate the clinical status of patients, this readout is meaningless: Indeed, the measurement of sTNFR in the circulation reflects most (if not all) of the available molecules, whereas the measurement of plasma TNF only corresponds to the accessible circulating part of the molecules when most of the active TNF is linked to its receptors on leukocytes and on the endothelium.

2.1.14. Interleukin-10

Significant amounts of IL-10 are detected in the circulation of septic patients *(91,92)*. The highest plasma levels of this regulatory molecule are detected in the most severe cases (with shock, with poor prognosis) *(93,94)*. A high ratio of IL-10 to TNF is also associated with poor outcome *(94)*. These observations further illustrate that sepsis is not associated with a deficient anti-inflammatory response. In contrast, the exacerbated production of anti-inflammatory cytokines in sepsis cautions against a widespread use of therapeutical approaches only targeting the proinflammatory mediators. Indeed, the overproduction of anti-inflammatory cytokines and mediators led to the concept of "compensatory anti-inflammatory response syndrome" (CARS) *(95)*. This is further suggested by the work of Brantzaeg *(96)*, who showed that plasma IL-10 was, in part, responsible of the monocyte deactivation noticed in sepsis *(see* Section 5).

2.1.15. Transforming Growth Factor-β

Measurements of circulating transforming growth factor-β (TGF-β) led to controversial results, most probably because of technical difficulties (latent and active forms exist, platelets are an important source). Karres et al. *(97)* and Astiz et al. *(98)* reported reduced TGF-β levels in sera from septic patients. On the other hand, we found enhanced TGF-β levels in plasma and platelet-poor plasma in patients with sepsis *(99)*. In a rat model of sepsis, circulating levels of TGF-β were found to be increased *(100)*, and in a baboon model of sepsis, active TGF-β levels were increased, whereas total TGF-β were decreased *(101)*.

2.2. Cell-Associated Cytokines

Circulating cytokines represent the tip of the iceberg *(102)*. Once produced, cytokines can been detected within the producing cells and/or on the cell surface for some cytokines such as IL-1α, TNF, IL-10, IL-15, or IFN-γ which exist as membrane forms. Once released, cytokines are present within a cellular environment and, consequently, can be efficiently trapped by surrounding cells that possess specific receptors. Accordingly, detection of cell-associated cytokines should not only be interpreted as an indication of the cellular source of a given cytokine because internalization of receptor-bound environmental cytokine can also take place. If one considers the human blood compartment, circulating leukocytes may be considered as useful examples. Indeed, we showed that IL-1α, IL-1β, and, particularly, TNF could be found associated to human monocytes *(22)*. Interestingly, at the end of the survey (around d 14), although most survivors did not have any more detectable circulating TNF, a majority had still detectable cell-associated TNF. The membrane form of TNF may be part of this observation, as recently suggested by studies on monocytes from patients with fracture and soft tissue hematomas *(103)* and on alveolar macrophages from patients with ARDS *(104)*. Using flow-cytometric analysis in intensive care unit (ICU) patients, Yentis et al. *(105)* confirmed the presence of IL-1β-positive cells among circulating leukocytes. We also investigated cell-associated IL-8 in septic patients *(106)*. A tremendous amount of cell-associated IL-8 has been detected in lysates of mononuclear cells and of neutrophils, whereas levels of IL-8 trapped by red blood cells via their Duffy antigen were lower. Such measurements may offer more precise informations in terms of follow-up and possible association with infection. This was recently confirmed in human volunteers receiving iv injection of LPS. Interestingly, although IL-8 was found associated to red blood cells and leukocytes, GROα and MCP-1 were only found to be associated to red blood cells and MIP-1β was never recovered from any cell fractions *(107)*. In ARDS patients, the presence of numerous IL-8-positive alveolar macrophages has confirmed the putative detrimental role of IL-8 in the development of that syndrome *(108)*. The presence of cell-associated IL-10 has also been reported in monocytes of trauma patients *(109)*.

2.3. Sources of Cytokines

2.3.1. Immunohistochemical Analysis

Different approaches have helped to identify the sites of production of cytokines during endotoxic shock or bacterial sepsis. Immunohistochemical analysis of tissues have revealed the presence of IL-1β and TNF in the spleen, liver, lung, heart, pituitary gland, and kidney following injection of LPS or bacteria in mice *(110–113)*. In the CLP model of peritonitis and sepsis, the presence of IL-1β and TNF in mice liver has been demonstrated by immunohistochemical analysis, whereas IL-1β was not detected in plasma *(114)*. Mast cells, Paneth cells, and one type of crypt endocrine cell of the intestinal mucosa possess granules, which contain preformed-TNF. It has been shown that after endotoxin treatment, the two types of intestinal cell had degranulated, whereas the appearance of TNF in the secretory granules of all eosinophils, neutrophils, and monocytes in the bone marrow, spleen, lung, and the proximal intestine was noticed *(115)*. Using mast-cell-deficient mice, it was elegantly demonstrated that during CLP-induced peritonitis or following ip injection of *Klebsiella pneumoniae*, mast cells were the main source of the protective TNF *(116,117)*. Transgenic mice in which the TNF coding sequence and introns were replaced by a chloramphenicol acetyltransferase (CAT) reporter gene were studied following LPS ip injection. CAT activity was observed in the kidney, heart, islet of Langherans, fallopian tubes, and uterus, and to a lesser extent in the spleen and lung, but absent in brain, muscle, liver, and small bowel *(118)*. In human sepsis, TNF and IL-1β were found in skin, muscle fat, arteries and the site of infection, and inflamed and putrescent areas *(119)*.

2.3.2. Cytokine Genes Expression

Investigation of cytokine mRNA is another means of identifying the source of cytokines during sepsis. Of course, gene transcription can occur without protein translation. In contrast with the results reported with the CAT reporter gene, other reports noticed the detection of TNF mRNA in the diaphragm muscle and liver following endotoxin administration, as well as in the spleen and lungs *(120–122)*. Injection of endotoxin also induces IL-1β mRNA in the brain *(123)*, gene expression of

IL-1α, IL-1β, and IL-1ra in the lung, liver, spleen and bowel *(124)*, and interleukin-6 mRNA expression in small intestinal mucosa *(125)*, peritoneal macrophages, liver, spleen, lungs, and kidney *(121)*. Most interestingly, Baumgarten et al. *(126)* showed that the heart expression of IL-1β and TNF-α mRNA in mice injected with LPS was dependent on the myocardial TLR4 expression. This observation was confirmed by a direct measurement of IL-1β and TNF-α in hearts. The CLP model of peritonitis does not seem to activate the same sources of cytokines as does an injection of LPS. CLP is associated with the expression of TNF and IL-6 mRNA in the liver and lung *(122,127)* but not in the spleen and gut *(122,128)*. After ip injection of LPS, the mouse liver expresses mRNA for numerous chemokines, including IP10, KC, MIP-2 MIP-1α, MIP-1β, RANTES, MCP-1, and MCP-5 *(55)*. RANTES mRNA was also detected in lung after LPS ip treatment, whereas minimal quantities of RANTES mRNA were detected in the blood buffy coat

2.3.3. Blood Leukocytes

Despite the fact that blood leukocytes studied in vitro, either in whole-blood samples or after isolation, have been shown to be a source of most cytokines after activation, their contribution during sepsis remains unclear. Nevertheless, one can hypothesize that cytokine-producing cells within the bloodstream might be difficult to identify because of the rapid and specific adherence of activated cells to the endothelium and their rapid margination toward inflamed tissues. Accordingly, endotoxin infusion in sheep is associated with an intrapulmonary sequestration of leukocytes that immunohistochemically express tumor necrosis factor *(129)*. Indeed, no or minimal mRNA expression could be detected for either TNF or IL-6 in circulating leukocytes of patients with sepsis *(47,121)*. In contrast, IL-8 and IL-18 mRNA content were raised in peripheral blood mononuclear cells (PBMCs) of septic patients *(47,71)*.

2.3.4. Compartmentalization

Differential levels of cytokines in different blood compartments may suggest the involvement of certain tissues in the local production of circulating cytokines. Accordingly, we showed that following abdominal aortic surgery, levels of TNF were higher in portal vein than in systemic blood *(130)*, suggesting that the gut, which may suffer of hypoperfusion during sepsis, may be a source of cytokine. Similarly, Douzinas et al. *(131)* showed in multiple-organ failure (MOF) patients with hepatic involvement that IL-6 levels were higher in hepatic sinusoidal blood than in peripheral vein blood; in MOF patients with ARDS, the authors reported higher IL-1β levels in pulmonary capillary blood than in peripheral vein blood. These results strongly suggest the production of the aforementioned cytokines within tissue and their subsequent release into the downstream vein. On the other hand, we found a strong correlation ($r = 0.87$, $p = 0.01$) between levels of TGF-β in pleural effusion and in bronchoalveolar lavages of septic patients, whereas there was no correlation with plasma levels *(132)*. This suggested that either there was an active exchange of this specific cytokine between pleura and the alveolar space and not with plasma or that a similar response occurred in both compartments. In an elegant study, Kurahashi et al. *(133)* demonstrated in *Pseudomonas aeruginosa* pneumonia that instillated, radiolabeled TNF in the lung leaked into the circulation as a consequence of the epithelial injury caused by the cytotoxic bacteria. The production of cytokines at the site of infection has been suggested by the measurement of the chemokines IL-8, GRO-α, and ENA-78 in the urine of patients with usosepsis *(134)*: The concentrations of all three chemokines were strongly elevated in urine; IL-8 levels were also enhanced in patients' plasma as compared to healthy controls, whereas plasma levels of GRO-α and ENA-78 were not increased. In contrast, in volunteers challenged with LPS, very high levels of all three chemokines were found in plasma and very little elevation was observed in urine. In peritonitis-associated sepsis, peritoneal levels of cytokines has been shown to be elevated as compared to plasma levels *(135)*. In the CLP model of sepsis in mice, it was reported that relative levels between both systemic and local compartment were dependent upon the studied cytokines *(5)*. Most interestingly, the neutralization of TNF by a pretreatment with an adenovirus-mediated TNF receptor fusion protein did not similarly affect the cytokine expression in plasma and in the heart *(136)*; whereas plasma levels of IL-1β, IL-6, MCP-1, and IL-12 were reduced after LPS injection in mice, and heart expression of IL-6, MCP-1, and IL-12 were unaffected. This illustrates that any treatment targeting proinflammatory cytokines may not equally affect their expression in different compartments.

2.3.5. Tissue Removal

Removal of organs may also help to identify the source of cytokines. However, the analysis may be complex, as illustrated by the analysis after splenectomy: Splenectomy in dogs significantly decreased the levels of plasma IL-6, whereas it did not affect the levels of circulating TNF after LPS challenge *(137,138)*. However, it was demonstrated that the reduced levels of circulating IL-6 was not caused by the absence of splenic production but by a decrease in nonsplenic IL-6 production *(138)*. Partial hepatectomy did reduce the plasma level of TNF *(139)*. In addition, gadolinium chloride treatment that reduces the number of Kupffer cells was associated with a reduced levels of plasma IL-1β and IL-6 in CLP performed in rats *(140)*. Finally, unilateral nephrectomy improved the resistance to LPS injection or to CLP *(141)*. All of these studies further confirm that most tissues contribute to cytokine production during sepsis.

3. DO PROINFLAMMATORY CYTOKINES ALWAYS CONTRIBUTE TO ADVERSE EFFECTS ASSOCIATED WITH SEPSIS?

3.1. Tumor Necrosis Factor

Tumor necrosis factor toxicity includes hemodynamic instability, fever, diarrhea, metabolic acidosis, capillary leak syndrome, activation of coagulation, late hypoglycemia, induction of a catabolic state, neurotoxicity, cachexia, and renal and hematological disorders, all phenomena associated with sepsis syndrome *(142)*. In addition, together with IL-1, TNF induces on the endothelial cell the expression of adhesion molecules involved in organ infiltration by leukocytes. The lethal effect of TNF was synergistically enhanced by IL-1 *(143)*, interferon-γ *(144)*, and LPS itself *(145)*. Anti-TNF treatments have been shown to be highly efficient in protecting animals against endotoxic shock *(146)* and lethal bacteremia *(147)*. Such treatments also protected against pulmonary microvascular injury after intestinal ischemia injury, which is associated with endotoxin translocation *(148)*. Studies with mice rendered deficient for TNF or its receptors led to controversial results, which reflected the different experimental models: use of galactosamine; injection of bacteria; cecal ligation and puncture; injection of high dose of LPS. It is worth noting that in the absence of the hepatotoxic galactosamine, TNF KO mice die after injection of similar amounts of LPS than normal mice *(149)*. Finally, as recently suggested by van der Meer's group in Nijmegen, the bacterial origin of the LPS itself contribute to the heterogeneity of the results *(150)*.

3.2. Interleukin-1

The cascade of inflammatory events is mainly orchestrated by IL-1 and TNF. Injection of IL-1 into animals results in hypotension, increased cardiac output and heart rate, leukopenia, thrombocytopenia, hemorrhage, and pulmonary edema *(143)*. Cyclo-oxygenase inhibitors greatly prevent these different effects. Interleukin-1 receptor antagonist (IL-1ra), a natural IL-1 inhibitor, reduces mortality from endotoxic shock *(151)*. IL-1β- converting enzyme (ICE) or caspase-1 is the enzyme required for the maturation of the 30-kDa biologically inactive IL-1β precursor to the mature 17-kDa active form of IL-1β. Survival to a lethal dose of endotoxin reaches 70% among ICE-deficient animals *(152)*, whereas IL-1β-deficient mice are normally sensitive to the lethal effect of LPS *(153)*. These results most probably reflect that caspase-1 is also involved in the maturation of IL-18.

3.3. LIF and OSM

Whereas IL-6 and IL-11 possess certain anti-inflammatory properties (*see* Subheading 4.1.), two other members of the gp130 superfamily, LIF and OSM, can be considered as proinflammatory cytokines. Indeed, LIF is involved in the pathogenesis of inflammation and sepsis syndrome *(43)*. Induced by LPS and TNF, LIF can induce the release of other cytokines, including IL-1, IL-6, and IL-8, by various cell types. Passive immunization against LIF in mice challenged with intraperitoneal administration of endotoxin protected them from lethality and blocked increases in serum levels of IL-1 and IL-6 *(154)*. Subcutaneous injection of OSM in mice caused an acute inflammation reaction *(155)*. OSM favors Polymorphonuclear (PMN) adhesion to endothelial cells and transmigration via its capacity to enhance the expression of P- and E-selectin, Intracellular Adhesion molecule-1 (ICAM-1), and Vascual Cell Adhesion molecule-1 (VCAM-1). Furthermore, OSM induces the release of IL-6 and ENA-78 (an a-chemokine) but not that of IL-8.

3.4. Chemokines

Sepsis and Systemic Inflammatory Response Syndrome (SIRS) are often associated with organ dysfunction, which reflects the inflammatory process occurring in the tissues. One of the major features of this phenomenon is the recruitment of inflammatory leukocytes. This involves the adherence of circulating cells to the endothelium and their margination toward the tissues in response to the locally produced chemokines. Chemokines represent a family of more than 40 members. These chemokines contribute to the inflammatory cell infiltrate that participates in the damaging of tissue integrity. For example, neutralization of IL-8 profoundly inhibited neutrophil recruitment in an endotoxin-induced rabbit model of pleurisy, indicating that IL-8 is a major chemotactic factor in this model of acute inflammation *(156)*. During sepsis, a great amount of IL-8 was detectable within the blood compartment, not only as a free cytokine *(51)* but also in cell-associated form *(106)*. This first encounter of neutrophils with IL-8 lead to their desensitization to further signals delivered locally by IL-8 or by other chemokines sharing the same receptors. Accordingly, the presence of IL-8 in the vascular space may well be a mechanism that limits neutrophil accumulation at extracellular sites, as illustrated by the defect in neutrophil migration capacity during sepsis or endotoxemia *(157,158)*. Similarly, although monocyte-chemoattractant protein-1 (MCP-1) contributes to the recruitment of inflammatory macrophages within the tissues, neutralization of MCP-1 by specific antibodies before LPS administration resulted in a striking increase in mortality, and the injection of MCP-1 confirmed that MCP-1 was protective *(159)*. Likewise, murine chemokine C10, which enhances bacterial phagocytic activity of peritoneal macrophages, was shown to promote disease resolution and to favor survival in the CLP model of murine sepsis *(160)*. In contrast, mice rendered deficient for the receptor of MCP-1 (CCR4–/–), which also binds MIP-1α, RANTES, macrophage-derived chemokine (MDC), and TARC, exhibited significantly decreased mortality upon administration of LPS *(161)*. These controversial results illustrate, once again, the influence of the experimental models. Furthermore, one should keep in mind that the recruitment of leukocytes by chemokines is a prerequisite for addressing the infectious process, as elegantly shown by the deleterious effect of blocking MDC in the CLP model of peritonitis in mice *(162)*.

3.5. Interleukin-12

The injection of IL-12 in chimpanzees induces an increase in plasma concentrations of IFN-γ as well as IL-15, IL-18, α- and β-chemokines, and anti-inflammatory mediators *(163)*. Among the adverse effects of IL-12, hepatomegaly and splenomegaly, leukopenia, anemia, and myelodepression have been reported *(164)*. These phenomena were largely IFN-γ-dependent because they were not reported to occur in IFN-γ-receptor-deficient mice. Hepatomegaly is associated with infiltration of activated macrophages and natural killer (NK) cells and single-cell necrosis. In contrast, pulmonary edema and interstitial macrophage infiltration generated by IL-12 injection were shown to be IFN-γ independent. In a Bacillus Calmette–Guerin (BCG)-primed model of LPS-induced shock and lethality, anti-IL-12 antibodies were associated with decreased IFN-γ and were shown to protect mice if injected before endotoxin *(165)*. In contrast, in a CLP model, IL-12 neutralization was deleterious *(166)*. The later observation is in agreement with other reports that demonstrated the beneficial effects of IL-12 to address the infectious process *(167,168)*. In this context, it is worth remembering that in contrast to all other cytokines, plasma IL-12 levels were higher in baboons injected with sublethal doses of *E. coli* than in animals challenged with lethal doses *(66)*. The association of enhanced levels of IL-12 and protection has also been observed in signal transducer and activator of transcription (Stat)6-deficient mice, which display an enhanced survival to the CLP model of sepsis *(169)*: the bacterial clearance from the peritoneum and survival were increased and, in parallel, peritoneal levels of IL-12, TNF, and chemokines MDC and C10 were higher in these mice as compared to control animals.

3.6. Interleukin-18

Although IL-18 promotes resolution of bacterial infection in mice *(170)*, it accounts for both TNF and Fas-ligand-mediated hepatotoxic pathways in endotoxin-induced liver injury in this model *(171)*. Neutralization of IL-18 protects mice against lethal *E. coli* and *S. typhimurium* endotoxemia *(172)*, and IL-18-deficient mice showed decreased sensitivity toward LPS-induced shock *(173)*, although this might depend on the model because *Propionibacterium acnes*-primed IL-18–/– mice were highly susceptible to LPS *(174)*. It is worth noting that in contrast, IL-18–/– mice and normal mice were similarly responsive to bacterial superantigen *(173)*.

3.7. Interferon-γ

The synergy of IFN-γ with the detrimental activities of LPS has been clearly established: IFN-γ enhanced LPS-induced circulating TNF as well as LPS- and TNF-induced mortality *(144,175)* and anti-IFN-γ antibodies protected against LPS- and *E. coli*-induced mortality *(175,176)*. As a consequence, a clinically silent viral infection may induce hypersensitivity to Gram-negative bacterial endotoxin through T-cell activation and subsequent IFN-γ production, leading to a hyperproduction of TNF *(177)*. Mice lacking IFN-γ receptor have been shown to be resistant to LPS challenge after priming with BCG *(178)* or treatment with GalNH2 *(179)*. A mouse model of endotoxinemia revealed that IFN-γ was not involved in pulmonary edema *(180)*, although side effects of IFN-γ include tachychardia, myalgia, malaise, leukopenia, and weakness.

3.8. Interleukin-16 and Interleukin-17

Interleukin-16 and IL-17 are recently described cytokines with ill-defined physiologic properties. Both were discovered as a T-cell product. IL-16 can also be produced by eosinophils, mast cells, and epithelial cells. It is worth mentioning that both can stimulate the production of proinflammatory cytokines. IL-16 induces the secretion of IL-1β, IL-6, IL-15, and TNF *(181)*, and IL-17 upregulates the expression of IL-1β, TNF, IL-6, IL-12, and prostaglandin E_2 (PGE_2) as well as IL-1ra and IL-10 *(182)*. However, their involvement during sepsis has not been addressed so far.

3.9. Colony-Stimulating Factors

In addition to their well-known action on hematopoiesis, CSFs favor the anti-infectious process and may reduce the natural apoptosis of neutrophils. However, among these cytokines, IL-3, previously called "multi-CSF," and granulocyte–macrophage-CSF (GM-CSF) can amplify the production of IL-1 and TNF and thus behave as proinflammatory cytokines *(183)*. The deleterious effect of GM-CSF is exemplified by the response of GM-CSF-deficient mice to endotoxin: Following LPS injection, hypothermia, and loss in body weight, levels of circulating IFNg, IL-1β, and IL-6 were markedly reduced as compared to normal mice. Furthermore, the survival to one LD_{100} of LPS was 42% among

GM-CSF–/– mice *(184)*. In contrast, numerous studies have reported that granulocyte-CSF (G-CSF) possesses many beneficial properties. It has been demonstrated that G-CSF reduces endotoxemia and improves survival during E. coli pneumonia *(185)*, reduces bacterial translocation resulting from burn wound sepsis *(186)*, and enhances the phagocytic function of neutrophils of sepsis animals *(187)*. Furthermore, in combination with antibiotics, G-CSF can prevent severe infectious complication in a peritonitis model *(188)*, and in combination with IL-11, it prevents the occurrence of lethality to a bacterial challenge in neutropenic animals *(189)*.

3.10. Fas Ligand

Fas (CD95) is a member of the TNF receptor superfamily that contains a cytoplasmic death domain. Binding of FasL to Fas induces apoptosis. Fas ligand (FasL) exists as a membrane form of a soluble molecule. Sepsis is associated with a delayed apoptosis of neutrophils, but with an increased apoptosis in hematopoietic tissues such as thymus, Peyer's patch, spleen, and bone marrow. Using FasL-deficient mice, it was established that the sepsis-associated apoptosis of lymphoid cells was a FasL-dependent process *(190)*. During the acute phase of human ARDS following sepsis, mRNA for Fas and FasL were highly upregulated in cells of BALs and enhanced levels of soluble FasL have been measured in the BAL of these patients, whereas soluble FasL was absent from BAL of healthy controls *(191)*. Because it has been shown that preventing apoptosis may protect mice against CLP-induced lethality *(192)*, one can suggest that Fas-induced apoptosis could have deleterious effects in human sepsis.

3.11. Macrophage Migration Inhibitory Factor

Macrophage inhibitory factor (MIF) was first discovered in 1966 as a T-cell product released during delayed-type hypersensitivity *(193)* and rediscovered in 1993 as a pituitary-derived cytokine that potentiates lethal endotoxemia *(194)* as well as a macrophage product *(195)* induced by the action of glucocorticoids *(196)*. MIF is expressed constitutively in many tissues, including lung, liver, kidney, spleen, adrenal gland, and skin. MIF exists as a preformed cytokine that is rapidly released following LPS injection *(197)*. Bernhagen et al. *(194)* reported that injection of MIF together with one LD_{40} of LPS greatly potentiated lethality and that anti-MIF antibodies fully protected against one LD_{50} of LPS. Accordingly, MIF-deficient mice were more resistant to LPS-induced lethality *(198)*. This phenomenon was associated with a reduced level of circulating TNF, an enhanced level of nitric oxide (NO) and no effect on IL-6, IL-10, and IL-12 levels. Anti-MIF antibodies also protected mice from lethal experimental peritonitis, even when treatment was started up to 8 h after induction of peritonitis *(199)*. MIF is present at homeostasis in the plasma of healthy controls and its levels are significantly enhanced during sepsis *(199)* (*see* Chapter 5).

3.12. High-Mobility Group-1 Protein

High mobility group-1 is a highly conserved nuclear protein that binds cruciform DNA. It exists as a membrane form and as an extracellular form that interacts with plasminogen and tissue-type plasminogen activator. It is produced by macrophages in response to LPS and by the pituitary cell stimulated by IL-1 or TNF *(200)*. HMG-1 was reported to be a late mediator of endotoxin lethality in mice and found in plasma of septic patients, with significantly higher levels in nonsurvivors than in survivors *(200)*.

3.13. Interleukin-15

In vivo, IL-15 is induced by IL-12 *(163)*. In concert with other monokines (e.g., IL-12), IL-15 stimulates IFN-γ production by NK cells and is involved in the LPS-induced general Shwartzman reaction *(201)*. However, inhibition by specific antibodies of endogenous IL-15 production during in vitro LPS activation of murine macrophages further amplify the TNF-α production *(202)*. The role of IL-15 in human sepsis remains to be fully established.

4. ANTI-INFLAMMATORY CYTOKINES: FROM PROTECTION TO IMMUNODEPRESSION

4.1. Interleukin-6 and Interleukin-11

Although IL-6 is often considered as an inflammatory cytokine, most of its activities are probably associated with a negative control of inflammation as a result of its potent capacity to induce the production of acute-phase proteins by the liver (Fig. 1). Acute-phase proteins are essentially protective and limit the inflammatory process via their antiprotease and scavenger activities. It was also mentioned that IL-6 inhibits the release of IL-1 and TNF *(203)* and favors that of soluble TNF receptor *(204)*. Accordingly, intraperitoneal injection of LPS in IL-6 knockout mice led to higher levels of circulating TNF, MIP-2, GM-CSF, and IFN-γ than in control mice and administration of IL-6 abolished these differences *(205)*. Furthermore, numerous experimental models, including systemic or local endotoxemia, demonstrated the protective activity of IL-6 either by studying the direct effect of exogenous IL-6 injection *(206)* or by demonstrating the enhanced sensitivity of IL-6 KO mice to LPS *(205)*. However, in contrast, IL-6 can induce bone resorption *(207)*, muscle atrophy *(208)*, and anemia *(209)* and can prime neutrophils for the production of platelet activating factor (PAF) and superoxide anion *(210,211)*. Although IL-6 does not activate endothelial cells, it induces MCP-1, MCP-3, and IL-8 production, STAT-3 activation, and ICAM-1 expression, in the presence of its soluble receptor gp80, which is naturally found in plasma *(212)*. Deleterious activities of IL-6 in vivo have been suggested by experimental models of ischemia reperfusion and of lung injury performed in IL-6 knockout mice, which were shown to exhibit lower inflammatory responses *(213,214)*.

Although IL-11 stimulated the production of several major acute-phase proteins by hepatoma cells, circulating IL-11 did not significantly participate in the production of acute-phase proteins by the liver *(215)*. One of the major beneficial effects of IL-11, which has been described, is related to its healing activity on the intestinal tract. For example, chemotherapy and radiation both damage the small-intestine mucosal barrier and lead to the entry of gastrointestinal flora into the blood. In this lethal model, IL-11 was able to protect 80% of the animals *(216)*. Beneficial properties of IL-11 have also been demonstrated in a rat neonatal infectious model with group B streptococci. Prophylactic use of IL-11 enhanced the survival in this model in association with an increased number of platelets *(217)*.

4.2. Interleukin-1 Receptor Antagonist

Interleukin-1 receptor antagonist (IL-1ra) is a natural IL-1 inhibitor. Produced by many cell types, including monocytes/macrophages, IL-1ra is also produced by the liver as an acute-phase protein *(218)*. Early treatment with IL-1ra reduced mortality from endotoxic shock *(151)*, improved survival and hemodynamic performance in *E. coli* septic shock *(219)*, and, depending on the dosage either reduced or enhanced lethality in a model of *K. pneumoniae* infection of newborn rats *(220)*. In agreement with these observations, IL-1ra-deficient mice were more susceptible than controls to lethal endotoxemia *(221)*.

4.3. Interleukin-10

Interleukin-10 is a well-known cytokine that exerts its anti-inflammatory properties particularly on monocytes/macrophages, neutrophils, and T-lymphocytes. IL-10 is capable of preventing lethality in experimental endotoxemia *(222)*, and IL-10-deficient mice were far more sensitive to LPS-induced lethality than wild-type animals *(223)*. In addition, neutralization of IL-10 in endotoxemia and during experimental septic peritonitis illustrated that endogenously produced IL-10 was instrumental in downregulating the abundant production of proinflammatory cytokines *(224,225)*. In the CLP model of sepsis, it was reported that IL-10 was a major mediator involved in the impairment of lung antibacterial response *(226)*, whereas in humans, Donnelly et al. *(93)* reported that the lowest levels of IL-10 in the lung fluids were significantly associated with a poor prognosis in patients with adult respiratory distress syndrome. In contrast, in patients resuscitated after cardiac arrest, high levels of systemic IL-10 were associated with poor outcome *(226a)*. Indeed, it appears that, depending on the experimental models or the clinical status, IL-10 may be beneficial or deleterious. Some authors have suggested *(227)* and demonstrated *(96)* that IL-10 was responsible of the monocyte deactivation observed in sepsis; however, this has not been confirmed by other studies *(228)*.

4.4. Interleukin-4 and Interleukin-13

In addition to IL-10, IL-4 and IL-13 also possess strong anti-inflammatory activities and a potent capacity to inhibit the synthesis of the proinflammatory cytokines. Each individual anti-inflammatory cytokine has been demonstrated to be capable of reducing mortality in various endotoxic or septic shock models. IL-4 prevented mortality from acute but not from chronic murine peritonitis *(229)*. All mice pretreated with IL-4 survived an ip injection of 10^7 live *E. coli* and 10^9 *Bacteroides fragilis*, which kill 90% of untreated animals. Using IL-4-deficient mice, it was established that IL-4 can protect against TNF-mediated cachexia and death during parasitic infection *(230)*. However, the fact that a pretreatment with IL-4 administration before the induction of sepsis was protective while an increased mortality was reported when IL-4 was given at the time of infection *(231)*, illustrates the importance of the timing and reinforces the idea that one should be very cautious when referring to a too simplistic dichotomy between proinflammatory and anti-inflammatory cytokines *(232)*. IL-13, which shares many activities with IL-4, fully protected mice from an LD_{90} ip injection of LPS *(233,234)*. IL-13 blockade with anti-IL-13 antibodies significantly decreased the survival rate of mice after experimental peritonitis and enhanced tissue injury that was associated with an increased expression of many chemokines *(235)*. This latter result suggests that, despite the absence of detectable circulating IL-4 or IL-13 in human sepsis *(67,236)*, these cytokines may well be involved in the control of the exacerbated release of proinflammatory cytokines.

4.5. Transforming Growth Factor-β

Injection of TGF-β in mice before or even together with high doses of LPS was associated with a reduced mortality *(237)*. In a rat model of endotoxemia, TGF-β markedly reduced inducible NO synthase mRNA and protein levels in organs, arrested LPS-induced hypotension, and decreased mortality *(238)*. In murine and rat models of sepsis, circulating levels of TGF-β were found to be increased and it was demonstrated that TGF-β contributed to the depressed T-cell functions *(100,239)*.

4.6. Interferon-α

Interferon-α also prevented LPS-induced mortality in mice and reduced TNF mRNA expression in the spleen and liver *(240)*. The most fascinating observation with IFN-α was its capacity to be effective even when administrated few hours after LPS. This contrasts with many reports in which the protective cytokine or drug had to be administrated before or simultaneously with LPS. Surprisingly, very few further studies have addressed the role of IFN-α in sepsis.

4.7. Interleukin-9

Interleukin-9 is a T-cell-derived cytokine, originally described as a growth factor for T-cells and mast cells. Prophylactic injections of IL-9 conferred resistance of mice challenged with a lethal concentration of *Pseudomonas aeruginosa (241)*. This protective effect correlated with a marked decrease of serum levels of TNF, IL-12, and IFN-γ, as well as an increase of circulating IL-10 and IL-10 mRNA expression in the spleen. Interestingly, a shorter and lower expression of IL-9 mRNA was observed in the spleen of mice after a lethal challenge than in mice after a sublethal bacterial challenge. To our knowledge, the role of IL-9 has not yet been investigated in human sepsis.

5. EX VIVO CYTOKINE PRODUCTION IN SEPSIS

5.1. Ex Vivo Cytokine Production by Lymphocytes

Sepsis syndrome is associated with an exacerbated in vivo production of proinflammatory and anti-inflammatory cytokines as assessed by their increased levels in the blood stream. Paradoxically, a reduced capacity of circulating leukocytes from septic patients to produce cytokines has been regularly reported as compared to cells from healthy controls. The very first observation on the hyporeactivity of circulating cells in septic patients was demonstrated in peripheral blood lymphocytes: Wood et al. *(242)* reported a decreased IL-2 production upon phytohemaglutinin (PHA) stimulation. More recently, interferon-γ production was also reported to be affected in sepsis as well as in patients with severe injury *(243)*. It is often suggested that the depressed response mainly affects the production of the Th1 cytokines (IL-2, IFN-γ), whereas production of Th2 cytokines would be upregulated. In human volunteers receiving an injection of LPS, T-cell-derived cytokine productions were assessed in vitro *(244)*: 3–6 h after LPS injection, (anti-CD3 + anti-CD28)-induced IFN-γ production was reduced, whereas IL-2 and IL-4 production were unchanged; staphylococcal enterotoxin B-induced production of IFN-γ and IL-2 were reduced and IL-5 production was enhanced. The authors conclude that endotoxemia favors a shift in the Th1/Th2 balance toward a Th2-type immune response. However, we demonstrated in sepsis and in SIRS patients that the production of Th2 cytokines (IL-5, IL-10) could also be altered and that the nature of the triggering agent itself influences the observation *(245)*.

5.2. Ex Vivo Cytokine Production by Neutrophils

Similar hyporeactivity has been reported for the production of IL-1β, IL-1ra, and IL-8 by LPS-activated neutrophils from septic patients *(246–248)*. We showed that, in contrast to monocytes, PMNs could not be rendered tolerant to endotoxin in vitro by previous contact with LPS and even released enhanced levels of IL-8 after reexposure to LPS *(247)*. Most interestingly, van der Poll's group *(249)* demonstrated that in vivo treatment of normal humans with endotoxin led to hyporeactive blood-derived PMN when further challenged in vitro with either LPS, heat-killed *S. pneumoniae* or heat-killed *P. aeruginosa:* The PMN production of the chemokines IL-8, GRO-α and ENA-78 were reduced.

5.3. Ex Vivo Cytokine Production by Monocytes

Monocyte reactivity to LPS stimulation has been particularly studied in isolated monocytes and in whole-blood assays. Monocytes from septic patients have a diminished capacity to release TNFα, IL-1α, IL-1β, IL-6, IL-10, and IL-12 *(227,228,243,250,251)*, whereas this is not the case for IL-1ra *(251)* and G-CSF *(252)*. Reduced cytokine production has also been observed with other stimuli such as silica, staphylococcal enterotoxin B, and killed *Streptococcus* and *Staphylococcus (98,243, 253,254)*. In human volunteers, intravenous endotoxin suppresses the cytokine response of PBMCs when activated in vitro by LPS *(255)*. The anergy of leukocytes observed in septic patients has been associated with endotoxin tolerance *(246,256)*. We have shown that upon LPS activation, PBMC of systemic inflammatory response syndrome patients show patterns of necrosis factor (NF)-κB expression that resemble those reported during LPS tolerance [i.e., a global downregulation of NF-κB in survivors of sepsis and trauma patients, and the presence of large amounts of the inactive homodimer in the nonsurvivors of sepsis *(257)*]. In many stressful conditions, including trauma, thermal injury, hemorrhage, and severe surgery, hyporesponsiveness of circulating leukocytes and low cytokine production have been well documented and associated with immune depression observed in these patients. However, the cellular hyporeactivity is not a global phenomenon and some signaling pathways are unaltered and allow the cells to normally respond to certain stimuli *(258)*. During sepsis and SIRS, cells derived from tissues are either fully responsive to ex vivo stimuli or even primed, in contrast to cells derived from hematopoietic compartments (blood, spleen), which are hyporeactive. This dichotomy illustrates the concept of compartmentalization that occurs within the body during sepsis *(259)*. Indeed, immune depression reported in sepsis and SIRS patients, often revealed by a diminished capacity of leukocytes to respond to lipopolysaccharide, is not a generalized phenomenon. Thus, during systemic inflammation, SIRS and the compensatory anti-inflammatory response syndrome (CARS) *(95)* seem to be present concomitantly, SIRS predominating within the inflamed tissues, whereas in the blood, the leukocytes show hyporeactivity.

REFERENCES

1. Angus, D.C., Linde-Zwirble, W.T., Lidicker, J., Clermont, G., Carcillo, J., and Pinsky, M.R. (2002) The epidemiology of severe sepsis in the United States: analysis of incidence, outcome, and associated costs of care. *Crit. Care Med.* **29,** 1303–1310.
2. Brun-Buisson, C., Doyon, F., Carlet, J., et al. (1996) Bacteremia and severe sepsis in adults: a multicenter prospective survey in ICUs and wards of 24 hospitals. *Am. J Respir. Crit. Care Med.* **154,** 617–624.
3. Sands, K.E., Bates, D.W., Lanken, P.N., Grasman, P.S., Hibberd, P.L., Kahn, K.L., et al. (1997) Epidemiology of sepsis syndrome in 8 academic medical centers. *JAMA* **278,** 234–240.
4. Haziot, A., Ferrero, E., Köntgen, F., Hijiya, N., Yamamoto, S., Silver, J., et al. (1996) Resistance to endotoxin shock and reduced dissemination of Gram negative bacteria in CD14-deficient mice. *Immunity* **4,** 407–414.
5. Ebong, S.J., Goyert, S.M., Nemzek, J.A., Kim, J., Bolgos, G.L., and Remick, D.G. (2001) Critical role of CD14 for production of inflammatory cytokines and cytokines inhibitors during sepsis with failure to alter morbidity or mortality. *Infect Immun.* **69,** 2099–2106.
6. Verbon, A., Dekkers, P.E.P., ten Hove, T., Hack, E., Pribble, J. P., Turner, T., et al. (2001) IC14, an anti-CD14 antibody, inhibits endotoxin-mediated symptoms and inflammatory responses in humans. *J. Immunol.* **166,** 3599–3605.
7. Solomon, K.R., Kurt-Jones, E.A., Saladino, R.A., Stack, A.M., Dunn, I.F., Ferretti, M., et al. (1998) Heterotrimeric G proteins physically associated with the lipopolysaccharide receptor CD14 modulate both in vivo and in vitro responses to lipopolysaccharide. *.J Clin. Invest.* **102,** 2019–2027.
8. Takeuchi, O., Hoshin, K., Kawai, T., Sanjo, H., Takada, H., Ogawa, T., et al. (1999) Differential roles of TLR2 and TLR4 in recognition of Gram-negative and Gram-positive bacterial cell wall components. *Immunity* **11,** 443–451.
9. Shimazu, R., Akashi, S., Ogata, H., Nagai, Y., Fukudome, K., Miyake, K., et al. (1999) MD-2, a molecule that confers LPS responsiveness on Toll-like receptor 4. *J. Exp. Med.* **189,** 1777–1782.
10. Evans, T.J., Strivens, E., Carpenter, A., and Cohen, J. (1993) Differences in cytokine response and induction of nitric oxide synthase in endotoxin-resistant and endotoxin-sensitive mice after intravenous Gram-negative. *J. Immunol.* **150,** 5033–5040.
11. Cavaillon, J.-M. (1994) Cytokines and macrophages. *Biomed. Pharmacother.* **48,** 445–453.
12. Dixon, G.L.J., Newton, P.J., Chain, B.M., Katz, D., Andersen, S.R., Wong, S., et al. (2001) Dendritic cell activation and cytokine production induced by group B *Neisseria meningitidis:* interleukin-12 production depends on lipopolysaccharide expression in intact bacteria. *Infect. Immun.* **69,** 4351–4357.
13. Frendéus, B., Wachtler, C., Hedlund, M., Fischer, H., Samuelsson, P., Svensson, M., et al. (2001) *Escherichia coli* P fimbriae utilize the Toll-like receptor 4 pathway for cell activation. *Mol. Microbiol.* **40,** 37–51.
14. Hayashi, F., Smith, K.D., Ozynsky, A., Hawn, T.R., Yi, E.C., Goodlett, D.R., Eng, J.K., Akira, S., Underhill, D.M., and Aderem, A. (2001) The innate immune response to bacterial flagellin is mediated by Toll-like receptor 5. *Nature* **410,** 1099–1103.
15. Hemmi, H., Takeuchi, O., Kawai, T., Kalsho, T., Sato, S., Sanjo, H., et al. (2000) A Toll-like receptor recognizes bacterial DNA. *Nature* **408,** 740–745.
16. Waage, A., Espevik, T., and Lamvik, J. (1986) Detection of TNF-like cytotoxicity in serum from patients with septicemia but not from untreated cancer patients. *Scand. J. Immunol.* **24,** 739–743.
17. Waage, A., Halstensen, A., and Espevik, T. (1987) Association between tumor necrosis factor in serum and fatal outome in patients with meningococal disease. *Lancet* **i,** 355–357.
18. Girardin, E., Grau, G., Dayer, J., Roux-Lombard, P., and Lambert, P. (1988) Tumor necrosis factor and IL-1 in the serum of children with severe infectious purpura. *N. Engl. J. Med.* **319,** 397–400.
19. Offner, F., Philippé, J., Vogelaers, D., Colardyn, F., Baele, G., Baudrihaye, M., et al. (1990) Serum tumor necrosis factor levels in patients with infectious diseases and septic shock. *J. Lab. Clin. Med.* **116,** 100–105.
20. Calandra, T., Baumgartner, J.D., Grau, G.E., Wu, M.M., Lambert, P.H., Schellekens, J., et al. (1990) Prognostic values of tumor necrosis factor, interleukin-1, interferon-α, and interferon-γ in the serum of patients with septic shock. *J. Infect. Dis.* **161,** 982–987.
21. Baud, L., Cadranel, J., Offenstadt, G., Luquel, L., Guidet, B., and Amstutz, P. (1990) Tumor necrosis factor and septic shock. *Crit. Care Med.* **18,** 349–350.
22. Muñoz, C., Misset, B., Fitting, C., Bleriot, J.P., Carlet, J., and Cavaillon, J.-M. (1991) Dissociation between plasma and monocyte-associated cytokines during sepsis. *Eur. J. Immunol.* **21,** 2177–2184.
23. Pinsky, M.R., Vincent, J.L., Deviere, J., Alegre, M., Kahn, R.J., and Dupont, E. (1993) Serum cytokine levels in human septic shock. Relation to multiple-system organ failure and mortality. *Chest* **103,** 565–575.

24. Hamilton, G.H., Hofbauer, S., and Hamilton, B. (1992) Endotoxin, TNF-alpha, IL-6 and parameters of the cellular immune system in patients with intraabdominal sepsis. *Scand. J. Infect. Dis.* **24**, 361–368.
25. Riche, F., Panis, Y., Laisne, M.J., Briard, C., Cholley, B., Bernard-Poenaru, O., et al. (1996) High TNF serum level is associated with increased survival in patients with abdominal septic shock: a prospective study in 59 patients. *Surgery* **120**, 801–807.
26. Arditi, M., Manogue, K.R., Caplan, M., and Yogev, R. (1990) Cerebrospinal fluid tumor necrosis factor-alpha and PAF concentrations and severity of bacterial meningitis in children. *J. Infect. Dis.* **162**, 139–147.
27. Dulkerian, S.J., Kilpatrick, L., Costarino, A.T., McCawley, L., Fein, J., Corcoran, L., et al. (1995) Cytokine elevations in infants with bacterial and aseptic meningitis. *J. Pediatr.* **126**, 872–876.
28. Engelhardt, R., Mackensen, A., Galanos, C., and Andreesen, R. (1990) Biological response to intravenously administered endotoxin in patients with advanced cancer. *J. Biol. Respir. Models* **9**, 480–491.
29. Pollmächer, T., Korth, C., Mullington, J., Schreiber, W., Sauer, J., Vedder, H., et al. (1996) Effects of G-CSF on plasma cytokine and cytokine receptor levels and on the in vivo host response to endotoxin in healthy men. *Blood* **87**, 900–905.
30. van der Poll, T., Coyle, S.M., Barbosa, K., Braxton, C.C., and Lowry, S.F. (1996) Epinephrine inhibits tumor necrosis factor-alpha and potentiates interleukin-10 production during human endotoxemia. *J. Clin. Invest.* **97**, 713–719.
31. Müller-Alouf, H., Alouf, J., Gerlach, D., Ozegowski, J., Fitting, C., and Cavaillon, J.-M. (1994) Comparative study of cytokine release by human peripheral blood mononuclear cells stimulated with *Streptococcus pyogenes* superantigen erythrogenic toxins, heat-killed streptococci and lipopolysaccharide. *Infect. Immun.* **62**, 4915–4921.
32. Waage, A., Brandtzaeg, P., Halstensen, A., Kierulf, P., and Espevik, T. (1989) The complex pattern of cytokines in serum from patients with meningococcal septic shock. Association between interleukin-6, interleukin-1, and fatal outcome. *J. Exp. Med.* **169**, 333–338.
33. Sriskandan, S., Moyes, D., and Cohen, J. (1996) Detection of circulating bacterial superantigen and lymphotoxin-alpha in patients with streptococcal toxic-shock syndrome. *Lancet* **348**, 1315–1316.
34. Van Deuren, M., Van Der Ven-Jongekrijg, H., Baterlink, A.K.N., Van Dalen, R., Sauerwein, R.W., and van Der Meer, J.W.M. (1995) Correlation between proinflammatory cytokines and antiinflammatory mediators and the severity of disease in meningococcal infections. *J. Infect. Dis.* **172**, 433–439.
35. Hack, C., de Groot, E., Felt-Bersma, R., Nuijens, J., Strack Van Schijndel, R., Eerenberg-Belmer, A., et al. (1989) Increased plasma levels of interleukin-6 in sepsis. *Blood* **74**, 1704–1710.
36. Calandra, T., Gerain, J., Heumann, D., Baumgartner, J.D., and Glauser, M.P. (1991) High circulating levels of interleukin-6 in patients with septic shock: evolution during sepsis, prognostic value, and interplay with other cytokines. The Swiss-Dutch J5 Immunoglobulin Study Group. *Am. J. Med.* **91**, 23–29.
37. Damas, P., Ledoux, D., Nys, M., Vrindts, Y., De Groote, D., Franchimont, P., et al. (1992) Cytokine serum level during severe sepsis in human IL-6 as a marker of severity. *Ann Surg.* **215**, 356–362.
38. Yoshimoto, T., Nakanishi, K., Hirose, S., Hiroishi, K., Okamura, H., Takemoto, Y., et al. (1992) High serum IL-6 level reflects susceptible status of the host to endotoxin and IL-1 / TNF. *J. Immunol.* **148**, 3596–3603.
39. Fong, Y., Moldawer, L.L., Marano, M., Wei, H., Tatter, S.B., Clarick, R.H., et al. (1989) Endotoxemia elicits increased circulating beta 2-IFN/IL-6 in man. *J. Immunol.* **142**, 2321–2324.
40. van Deventer, S.J.H., Büller, H.R., ten Cate, J.W., Aarden, L.A., Hack, C.E., and Sturk, A. (1990) Experimental endotoxemia in humans: analysis of cytokine release and coagulation, fibrinolytic and complement pathways. *Blood* **76**, 2520–2526.
41. Endo, S., Inada, K., Arakawa, N., Yamada, Y., et al. (1996) IL-11 in patients with disseminated intravascular coagulation. Res Com *Mol. Pathol. Pharmac.* **91**, 253–256.
42. Guillet, C., Fourcin, M., Chevalier, S., Pouplard, A., and Gascan, H. (1995) ELISA detection of circulating levels of LIF, OSM and CNTF in septic shock. *Ann. NY Acad. Sci.* **762**, 407–412.
43. Waring, P., Wycherley, K., Cary, D., Nicola, N., and Metcalf, D. (1992) Leukemia inhibitory factor levels are elevated in septic shock and various inflammatory body fluids. *J. Clin. Invest.* **90**, 2031–2037.
44. Villers, D., Dao, T., Nguyen, J.M., Bironneau, E., Godard, A., Moreau, M., et al. (1995) Increased plasma levels of human interleukin for DA1a cells / leukemia inhibitory factor in sepsis correlate with shock and poor prognosis. *J. Infect. Dis.* **171**, 232–236.
45. Jansen, P.M., de Jong, I.W., Hart, M., Kim, K.J., Aarden, L.A., Hinshaw, L.B., et al. (1996) Release of leukemia inhibitory factor in primate sepsis. Analysis of the role of TNFα. *J. Immunol.* **156**, 4401–4407.
46. Van Zee, K.J., De Forge, L.E., Fischer, E., Marano, M.A., Kenney, J.S., Remick, D.G., et al. (1991) IL-8 in septic shock, endotoxemia, and after IL-1 administration. *J. Immunol.* **146**, 3478–3482.
47. Friedland, J., Suputtamongkol, Y., Remick, D., Chaowagul, W., Strieter, R., Kunkel, S., et al. (1992) Prolonged elevation of interleukin-8 and interleukin-6 concentrations in plasma and of leukocyte interleukin-8 m-RNA levels during septicemic and localized *Pseudomonas pseudomallei* infection. *Infect .Immun.* **60**, 2402–2408.
48. Hack, C., Hart, M., Strack van Schijndel, R., Eerenberg, A., Nuijens, J., Thijs, L., et al. (1992) IL-8 in sepsis: relation to shock and inflammatory mediators. *Infect. Immun.* **60**, 2835–2842.
49. Miller, E.J., Cohen, A.B., Nagao, S., Griffith, D., Maunder, R.J., Martin, T.R., et al. (1992) Elevated levels of NAP-1/Interleukin-8 are present in the airspaces of patients with the adult respiratory distress syndrome and are associated with increased mortality. *Am. J. Respir. Dis.* **148**, 427–432.
50. Endo, S., Inada, K., Ceska, M., Takakuwa, T., Yamada, Y., Nakae, H., et al. (1995) Plasma interleukin 8 and polymorphonuclear leukocyte elastase concentrations in patients with septic shock. *J. Inflamm.* **45**, 136–142.
51. Marty, C., Misset, B., Tamion, F., Fitting, C., Carlet, J., and Cavaillon, J.-M. (1994) Circulating interleukin-8 concentrations in patients with multiple organ failure of septic and nonseptic origin. *Crit. Care Med.* **22**, 673–679.

52. Kragsbjerg, P., Holmberg, H., and Vikerfors, T. (1996) Dynamics of blood cytokine concentrations in patients with bacteremic infections. *Scand .J. Infect. Dis.* **28**, 391–398.
53. Friedland, J. S., Porter, J. C., Daryanani, S., Bland, J. M., Screaton, N. J., Vesely, M. J. J., et al. (1996) Plasma proinflammatory cytokine concentrations, acute physiology and chronic health evaluation (APACHE) III scores and survival in patients in an intensive care unit. *Crit. Care Med.* **24**, 1775–1781.
54. Redl, H., Schlag, G., Bahrami, S., Schade, U., Ceska, M., and Stutz, P. (1991) Plasma neutrophil-activating peptide-1/ interleukin-8 and neutrophil elastase in a primate bacteremia model. *J. Infect. Dis.* **164**, 383–388.
55. Kopydlowski, K.M., Salkowski, C.A., Cody, M.L., van Rooijen, N., Major, J., Hamilton, T.A., et al. (1999) Regulation of macrophage chemokine expression by lipopolysaccharide in vitro and in vivo. *J. Immunol.* **163**, 1537–1544.
56. Jansen, P.M., van Damme, J., Put, W., de Jong, I.W., Taylor, F., Jr., and Hack, C.E. (1995) Monocyte chemotactic protein 1 is released during lethal and sublethal bacteremia in baboons. *J. Infect. Dis.* **171**, 1640–1642.
57. Ebong, S., Call, D., Nemzek, J., Bolgos, G., Newcomb, D., and Remick, D. (1999) Immunopathologic alteration in murine models of sepsis of increasing severity. *Infect. Immun.* **67**, 6603–6610.
58. Bossink, A.W., Paemen, L., Jansen, P.M., Hack, C.E., Thijs, L.G., and Van Damme, J. (1995) Plasma levels of the chemokines monocyte chemotactic proteins-1 and -2 are elevated in human sepsis. *Blood* **86**, 3841–3847.
59. O'Grady, N.P., Tropea, M., Preas, H.L., Reda, D., Vandiveir, R.W., Banks, S.M., et al. (1999) Detection of macrophage inflammatory protein (MIP)-1α and MIP-1β during experimental endotoxemia and human sepsis. *J. Infect. Dis.* **179**.
60. Olszyna, D.P., Prins, J.M., Dekkers, P.E.P., De Jonge, E., Speelman, P., van Deventer, S.J.H., et al. (1999) Sequential measurements of chemokines in urosepsis and experimental endotoxemia. *J. Clin. Immunol.* **19**.
61. Wagner, H., Heeg, K., and Miethke, T. (1992) T cell mediated lethal shock induced by bacterial superantigens. *Behring. Inst. Mitt.* **91**, 46–53.
62. Tokman, M.G., Carey, K.D., and Quimby, F.W. (1995) The pathogenesis of experimental toxic shock syndrome: the role of interleukin-2 in the induction of hypotension and release of cytokines. *Shock* **3**, 145–151.
63. Musso, T., Calosso, L., Zucca, M., Millesimo, M., Ravarino, D., Giovarelli, M., et al. (1999) Human monocytes constitutively express membrane-bound, biologically active, and interferon-γ upregulated IL-15. *Blood* **93**, 3531–3539.
64. Lauw, F.N., Simpson, A.J.H., Prins, J.M., Smith, M.D., Kurimoto, M., van Deventer, S.J.H., et al. (1999) Elevated plasma concentrations of interferon (IFN) and the IFN-inducing cytokines interleukin (IL)18, IL-12, and IL-15 in severe melioidosis. *J. Infect. Dis.* **180**, 1878–1885.
65. Heinzel, F.P., Rerko, R.M., Ling, P., Hakimi, J., and Schoenhaut, D.S. (1994) IL-12 is produced in vivo during endotoxemia and stimulates synthesis of γ-interferon. *Infect. Immun.* **62**, 4244–4251.
66. Jansen, P.M., van der Pouw Kraan, T.C.T.M., de Jong, I.W., van Mierlo, G., Wijdenes, J., Chang, A.A., et al. (1996) Release of IL-12 in experimental *Escherichia coli* septic shock in baboons : relation to plasma levels to IL-10 and IFN-gamma. *Blood* **87**, 5144–5151.
67. Zimmer, S., Pollard, V., Marshall, G.D., Garofalo, R.P., Traber, D., Prough, D., et al. (1996) The 1996 Moyer Award. Effects of endotoxin on the Th1/Th2 response in humans. *J. Burn Care Rehabil.* **17**, 491–496.
68. Presterl, E., Staudinger, T., Pettermann, M., Lassnigg, A., Burgmann, H., Winkler, S., et al. (1997) Cytokine Profile and Correlation to the APACHE III and MPM II Scores in Patients with Sepsis. *Am. J. Respir. Crit. Care Med.* **156**, 825–832.
69. Puren, A.J., Razeghi, P., Fantuzzi, G., and Dinarello, C.A. (1998) Interleukin-18 enhances LPS-induced interferon-γ production in human whole blood cultures. *J. Infect. Dis.* **178**, 1830–1834.
70. Grobmyer, S.R., Lin, E., Lowry, S.F., Rivadeneira, D.E., Potter, S., Barie, P.S., and Nathan, C.F. (2000) Elevation of IL-18 in human sepsis. *J. Clin. Immunol.* **20**, 212–215.
71. Mathiak, G., Neville, L.F., Grass, G., Boehm, S.A., Luebke, T., Herzmann, T., et al. (2001) Chemokines and interleukin-18 are up-regulated in bronchoalveolar lavage fluid but not in serum of septic surgical ICU patients. *Shock* **15**, 176–180.
72. Rayhane, N., Fitting, C., and Cavaillon, J.-M. (1999) Dissociation of INFγ from IL-12 and IL-18 during endotoxin tolerance. *J. Endotoxin Res.* **5**, 319–324.
73. Francois, B., Trimoreau, F., Vignon, P., Fixe, P., Praloran, V., and Gastinne, H. (1997) Thrombocytopenia in the sepsis syndrome: role of hemophagocytosis and macrophage colony-stimulating factor. *Am. J. Med.* **103**, 114–120.
74. Waring, P.M., Presneill, J., Maher, D.W., Layton, J.E., Cebon, J., Waring, L.J., et al. (1995) Differential alterations in plasma colony-stimulating factor concentrations in meningococcaemia. *Clin. Exper. Immunol.* **102**, 501–506.
75. Cairo, M.S., Suen, Y., Knoppel, E., Dana, R., Park, L., Clark, S., et al. (1992) Decreased G-CSF and IL-3 production and gene expression from mononuclear cells of newborn infants. *Pediatr. Res.* **31**, 574–578.
76. Kantar, M., Kultursay, N., Kutukculer, N., Akisu, M., Cetingul, N., and Caglayan, S. (2000) Plasma concentration of granulocyte-macrophage colony stimulating factor and interleukin-6 in septic and healthy preterms. *Eur. J. Pediat.* **159**, 156–157.
77. Fischer, E., Van Zee, K.J., Marano, M.A., Rock, C.S., Kenney, J.S., Poutsiaka, D.D., et al. (1992) Interleukin-1 receptor antagonist circulates in experimental inflammation and in human disease. *Blood* **79**, 2196–2200.
78. Rogy, M.A., Coyle, S.M., Oldenburg, H.S., Rock, C.S., Barie, P.S., Van Zee, K.J., et al. (1994) Persistently elevated soluble TNF receptor and interleukin-1 receptor antagonist levels in critically ill patients. *J. Am. Coll. Surg.* **178**, 132–138.
79. Gardlund, B., Sjölin, J., Nilsson, A., Roll, M., Wickerts, C.J., and Wretlind, B. (1995) Plasma levels of cytokines in primary septic shock in humans: correlation with disease severity. *J. Infect. Dis.* **172**, 296–301.
80. Cavaillon, J.-M. (1998) Pathophysiological role of pro- and anti-inflamatory cytokines in sepsis. *Sepsis* **2**, 127–140.
81. Preas, H.L., Reda, D., Tropea, M., Vandivier, R.W., Banks, S.M., Agosti, J.M., et al. (1996) Effects of recombinant soluble type I interleukin-1 receptor on human inflammatory responses to endotoxin. *Blood* **88**, 2465–2472.

82. Giri, J.G., Wells, J., Dower, S.K., McCall, C.E., Guzman, R.N., Slack, J., et al. (1994) Elevated levels of shed type II IL-1 receptor in sepsis. Potential role for type II receptor in regulation of IL-1 responses. *J. Immunol.* **153,** 5802–5809.

83. Pruitt, J.H.,B,W.M., Edwards, P.D., Harward, R.R.S., Seeger, J.W., Martin, T.D., et al. (1996) Increased soluble interleukin-1 type II receptor concentrations in postoperative patients and in patients with sepsis syndrome. *Blood* **87,** 3282–3288.

84. Lesslauer, W., Tabuchi, H., Gentz, R., Brockhaus, M., Schlaeger, E., Grau, G., et al. (1991) Recombinant soluble tumor necrosis factor receptor proteins protect mice from LPS-induced lethality. *Eur. J. Immunol.* **21,** 2883–2886.

85. Ashkenazi, A., Marsters, S., Capon, D., Chamow, S., Figari, I., Pennica, D., et al. (1991) Protection against endotoxic shock by a tumor necrosis factor receptor immunoadhesin. *Proc. Natl. Acad. Sci. USA* **88,** 10,535–10,539.

86. Girardin, E., Roux-Lombard, P., Grau, G.E., Suter, P., Gallati, H., and Dayer, J.M. (1992) Imbalance between tumour necrosis factor-alpha and soluble TNF receptor concentrations in severe meningococcaemia. *Immunology* **76,** 20–23.

87. Van Zee, K.J., Kohno, T., Fischer, E., Rock, C.S., Moldawer, L.L., and Lowry, S.F. (1992) Tumor necrosis factor soluble receptors circulate during experimental and clinical inflammation and can protect against excessive TNFα in vitro and in vivo. *Proc. Natl. Acad. Sci. USA* **89,** 4845–4849.

88. van der Poll, T., Jansen, J., van Leenen, D., von der Mohlen, M., Levi, M., ten Cate, H., et al. (1993) Release of soluble receptors for tumor necrosis factor in clinical sepsis and experimental endotoxemia. *J. Infect. Dis.* **168,** 955–960.

89. van der Poll, T., Fischer, E., Coyle, S.M., Van Zee, K.J., Pribble, J.P., Stiles, D.M., et al. (1995) Interleukin-1 contributes to increased concentrations of soluble tumor necrosis factor receptor type I in sepsis. *J. Infect. Dis.* **172,** 577–580.

90. Lantz, M., Malik, S., Slevin, M.L., and Olsson, I. (1990) Infusion of tumor necrosis factor (TNF) causes an increase in circulating TNF-binding protein in humans. *Cytokine* **2,** 402–406.

91. Marchant, A., Devière, J., Byl, B., De Groote, D., Vincent, J., and Goldman, M. (1994) Interleukin-10 production during septicaemia. *Lancet* **343,** 707–708.

92. Derkx, B., Marchant, A., Goldman, M., Bijlmer, R., and van Deventer, S. (1995) High levels of IL-10 during the initial phase of fulminant meningococcal septic shock. *J. Infect. Dis.* **171,** 229–232.

93. Donnelly, S.C., Strieter, R.M., Reid, P.T., Kunkel, S.L., Burdick, M.D., Armstrong, I., et al. (1996) The association between mortality rates and decreased concentrations of interleukin-10 and interleukin-1 receptor antagonist in the lung fluids of patients with the adult respiratory distress syndrome. *Ann. Intern. Med.* **125,** 191–196.

94. van Dissel, J.T., van Langevelde, P., Westendorp, R.G.J., Kwappenberg, K., and Frolich, M. (1998) Anti-inflammatory cytokine profile and mortality in febrile patients. *Lancet* **351,** 950–953.

95. Bone, R.C., Grodzin, C.J., and Balk, R.A. (1997) Sepsis: a new hypothesis for pathogenesis of the disease process. *Chest* **121,** 235–243.

96. Brandtzaeg, P., Osnes, L., Øvstebø, R., Joø, G. B., Westwik, A. B., and Kierulf, P. (1996) Net inflammatory capacity of human septic shock plasma evaluated by a monocyte-based target cell assay : identification of IL-10 as a major functional deactivator of human monocytes. *J. Exp. Med.* **184,** 51–60.

97. Karres, I., Kremer, J.P., Sterckholzer, U., Kenney, J.S., and Ertel, W. (1996) TGF-β1 inhibits synthesis of cytokines in endotoxin-stimulated human whole blood. *Arch. Surg.* **131,** 1310–1317.

98. Astiz, M., Saha, D., Lustbader, D., Lin, R., and Rackow, E. (1996) Monocyte response to bacterial toxins, expression of cell surface receptors, and release of anti-inflammatory cytokines during sepsis. *J. Lab. Clin. Med.* **128,** 597–600.

99. Marie, C., Cavaillon, J.-M., and Losser, M.-R. (1996) Elevated levels of circulating transforming growth factor-β1 in patients with the sepsis syndrome. *Ann. Intern. Med.* **125,** 520–521.

100. Ahmad, S., Choudhry, M.A., Shankar, R., and Sayeed, M.M. (1997) Transforming growth factor-β negatively modulates T-cell responses in sepsis. *FEBS Lett.* **402,** 213–218.

101. Junger, W.G., Hoyt, D.B., Redl, H., Liu, F.C., Loomis, W.H., Davies, J., et al. (1995) Tumor necrosis factor antibody treatment of septic baboons reduces the production of sustained T-cell suppressive factors. *Shock* **3,** 173–178.

102. Cavaillon, J.M., Muñoz, C., Fitting, C., Misset, B., and Carlet, J. (1992) Circulating cytokines: the tip of the iceberg? *Circ. Shock* **38,** 145–152.

103. Hauser, C.J., Zhou, X., Joshi, P., Cuchens, M.A., Kregor, P., Devidas, M., et al. (1997) The immune microenvironment of human fracture/soft-tissue hematomas and its relationship to systemic immunity. *J. Trauma Injury Infect Crit. Care.* **42,** 895–903.

104. Armstrong, L., Thickett, D.R., Christie, S.J., Kendall, H., and Millar, A.B. (2000) Increased expression of functionally active membrane-associated tumor necrosis factor in acute respiratory distress syndrome. *Am. J. Respir. Cell Mol. Biol.* **22,** 68–74.

105. Yentis, S.M., Rowbottom, A.W., and Riches, P.G. (1995) Detection of cytoplasmic IL-1β in peripheral blood mononuclear cells from intensive care unit patients. *Clin. Exp. Immunol.* **100,** 330–335.

106. Marie, C., Fitting, C., Cheval, C., Losser, M.R., Carlet, J., Payen, D., et al. (1997) Presence of high levels of leukocyte-associated interleukin-8 upon cell activation and in patients with sepsis syndrome. *Infect. Immun.* **65,** 865–871.

107. Olszyna, D.P., De Jonge, E., Dekkers, P.E.P., van Deventer, S. J.H., and van der Poll, T. (2001) Induction of cell-associated chemokines after endotoxin administration to healthy humans. *Infect. Immun.* **69,** 2736–2738.

108. Donnelly, S., Strieter, R., Kunkel, S., Walz, A., Robertson, C., Carter, D., et al. (1993) Interleukin-8 and development of adult respiratory distress syndrom in at-risk patients groups. *Lancet* **341,** 643–647.

109. Shimonkevitz, R., Bar-Or, D., Harris, L., Dole, K., McLaughlin, L., and Yukl, R. (1999) Transient monocyte release of interleukin-10 in response to traumatic brian injury. *Shock* **12,** 10–16.

110. Koenig, J.I., Snow, K., Clark, B.D., Toni, R., Cannon, J.G., Shaw, A. R., et al. (1990) Intrinsic pituitary interleukin-1β is induced by bacterial lipopolysaccharide. *Endocrinol.* **126,** 3053–3058.

111. Kita, T., Tanaka, N., and Nagano, T. (1993) The immunocytochemical localization of TNF and leukotriene in the rat kidney aftert treatment with lipopolysaccharide. *Int. J. Exp. Path.* **74,** 471–479.
112. Ge, Y., Ezzel, R.M., Clarck, B.D., Loiselle, P.M., Amato, S.F., and Warren, H.S. (1997) Relationship of tissue and cellular interleukin-1 and lipopolysaccharide after endotoxemia and bacteremia. *J. Infect. Dis.* **176,** 1313–1321.
113. Yao, L., Berman, J.W., Factor, S.M., and Lowy, F.D. (1997) Correlation of histopathologic and bacteriologic changes with cytokine expression in an experimental murine model of bacteremic *Staphylococcus aureus* infection. *Infect. Immun.* **65,** 3889–3895.
114. Chen, J., Raj, N., Kim, P., Andrejko, K.M., and Deutschman, C.S. (2001) Intrahepatic nuclear factor-κB activity and α1-acid glycoprotein transcription do not predict outcome after cecal ligation and puncture in the rat. *Crit. Care. Med.* **29,** 589–596.
115. Schmauder-Chock, E.A., Chock, S.P., and Patchen, M.L. (1994) Ultrastructural localization of tumour necrosis factor-alpha. *Histochem. J.* **26,** 142–151.
116. Malavija, R., Ikeda, T., Ross, E., and Abraham, S. (1996) Mast cell modulation of neutrophil influx and bacterial clearance at sites of infection through TNFα. *Nature* **381,** 77–80.
117. Echtenacher, B., Männel, D., and Hültner, L. (1996) Critical protective role of mast cells in a model of acute septic peritonitis. *Nature* **381,** 75–77.
118. Giroir, B.P., Johnson, J.H., Brown, T., Allen, G.L., and Beutler, B. (1992) The tissue distribution of tumor necrosis factor biosynthesis during endotoxemia. *J. Clin. Invest.* **90,** 693–698.
119. Annane, D., Sanquer, S., Sébille, V., Faye, A., Djuranovic, D., Raphaël, J.-C., et al. (2000) Compartmentalised inducible nitric-oxide synthase activity in septic shock. *Lancet* **355,** 1143–1148.
120. Shindoh, C., Hida, W., Ohkawara, Y., Yamauchi, K., Ohno, I., Takishima, T., et al. (1995) TNF-α mRNA expression in diaphragm muscle after endotoxin administration. *Am. J. Respir. Crit. Care Med.* **152,** 1696–1696.
121. Chapoval, A.I., Kamdar, S.J., Kremlev, S.G., and Evans, R. (1998) CSF-1 differentially sensitizes mononuclear phagocyte subpopulations to endotoxin in vivo: a potential pathway that regulates the severity of Gram-negative infections. *J. Leukocyte Biol.* **63,** 245–252.
122. Tannahill, C.L., Fukuzuka, K., Marum, T., Abouhamze, Z., MacKay, S.L.D., Copeland, E.M., et al. (1999) Discordant tumor necrosis factor-α superfamily gene expression in bacterial peritonitis and endotoxemic shock. *Surgery* **126,** 349–357.
123. Buttini, M., and Boddeke, H. (1995) Peripheral lipopolysaccharide stimulation induces interleukin-1β mRNA in rat brain microglial cells. *Neuroscience* **65,** 523–530.
124. Ulich, T. R., Guo, K., Yin, S., del Castillo, J., Yi, E. S., Thompson, R. C., et al. (1992) Endotoxin-induced cytokine gene expression in vivo. IV. Expression of interleukin-1 alpha/beta and interleukin-1 receptor antagonist mRNA during endotoxemia and during endotoxin-initiated local acute inflammation. *Am. J. Pathol.* **141,** 61–68.
125. Meyer, T.A., Wang, J., Tiao, G.M., Ogle, C.K., Fischer, J.E., and Hasselgren, P.O. (1995) Sepsis and endotoxemia stimulate intestinal interleukin-6 production. *Surgery* **118,** 336–342.
126. Baumgarten, G., Knuefermann, P., Nozaki, N., Sivasubramanian, N., Mann, D.L., and Vallejo, J.G. (2001) In vivo expression of proinflammatory mediators in the adult heart after endotoxin administration: the role of toll-like receptor 4. *J. Infect. Dis.* **183,** 1617–1624.
127. Wang, P., Ba, Z.F., and Chaudry, I.H. (1997) Mechanism of hepatocellular dysfunction during early sepsis. Key role of increased gene expression and release of proinflammatory cytokines tumor necrosis factor and interleukin-6. *Arch. Surg.* **132,** 364–370.
128. Koo, D.J., Zhou, M., Jackman, D., Cioffi, W.G., Bland, K.I., Chaudry, I.H., et al. (1999) Is gut the major source of proinflammatory cytokine release during polymicrobial sepsis? *Biochem. Biophys. Acta.* **1454,** 289–295.
129. Cirelli, R.A., Carey, L.A., Fisher, J.K., Rosolia, D.L., Elsasser, T.H., Caperna, T.J., et al. (1995) Endotoxin infusion in anesthetized sheep is associated with intrapulmonary sequestration of leukocytes that immunohistochemically express tumor necrosis factor-α. *J. Leukocyte Biol.* **57,** 820–826.
130. Cabié, A., Farkas, J.-C., Fitting, C., Laurian, C., Cormier, J.-M., Carlet, J., et al. (1993) High levels of portal TNF-α during abdominal aortic surgery in man. *Cytokine* **5,** 448–453.
131. Douzinas, E. E., Tsidemiadou, P. D., Pitaridis, M. T., Andrianakis, I., Bobotachloraki, A., Katsouyanni, K., et al. (1997) The regional production of cytokines and lactate in sepsis-related multiple organ failure. *Am. J. Respir.Crit. Care Med.* **155,** 53–59.
132. Marie, C., Losser, M.R., Fitting, C., Kermarrec, N., Payen, D., and Cavaillon, J.-M. (1997) Cytokines and soluble cytokines receptors in pleural effusions from septic and nonseptic patients. *Am. J. Respir. Crit. Care Med.* **156,** 1515–1522.
133. Kurahashi, K., Kajikawa, O., Sawa, T., Ohara, M., Gropper, M.A., Frank, D.W., et al. (1999) Pathogenesis of septic shock in *Pseudomonas aeruginosa* pneumonia. *J. Clin. Invest.* **104,** 743–750.
134. Olszyna, D. P., Opal, S. M., Prins, J. M., Horn, D. L., Speelman, P., van Deventer, S. J. H., et al. (2000) Chemotactic activity of CXC chemokines interleukin-8, growth-related oncogen-α and epithelial cell-derived neutrophil-activating protein-78 in urine of patients with urosepsis. *J. Infect Dis.* **182,** 1731–1737.
135. Holzheimer, R.G., Schein, M., and Wittmann, D.H. (1995) Inflammatory response in peritoneal exudate and plasma of patients undergoing planned relaparotomy for severe secondary peritonitis. *Arch. Surg.* **130,** 1314–1319.
136. Kadokami, T., McTiernan, C.F., Kubota, T., Frye, C.S., Bounoutas, G.S., Robbins, P.D., et al. (2001) Effects of soluble TNF receptor treatment on lipopolysaccharide-induced myocardial cytokine expression. *Am. J. Physiol.* **280,** H2281–H2291.
137. Kohno, H., Yamamoto, M., Iimuro, Y., Fujii, H., and Matsumoto, Y. (1995) The role of splenic macrophages in plasma tumor necrosis factor levels in endotoxemia. *Eur. Surg. Res.* **29,** 176–186.
138. Moeniralam, H.S., Bemelman, W.A., Endert, E., Koopmans, R., Sauerwein, H.P., and Romijn, J.A. (1997) The decrease in nonsplenic interleukin-6 production after splenectomy indicates the existence of a positive feedback loop of IL-6 production during endotoxemia in dogs. *Infect. Immun.* **65,** 2299–2305

139. Kumins, N.H., Hunt, J., Gamelli, R.L., and Filkins, J.P. (1996) Partial hepatectomy reduces the endotoxin induced peak of circulating level of TNF in rats. *Shock* **5,** 385–388.
140. Koo, D.J., Chaudry, I.H., and Wang, P. (1999) Kupffer cells are responsible for producing inflammatory cytokines and hepatocellular dysfunction during early sepsis. *J. Surg.Res.* **83,** 151–157.
141. Zurovsky, Y. and Eligal, Z. (1996) Reduction of risk following endotoxin injection in unilaterally nephrectomized rats. *Exp. Toxic Pathol.* **48,** 41–46.
142. Van der Poll, T., Romijn, J.A., Endert, E., Borm, J.J., Buller, H.R., and Sauerwein, H.P. (1991) Tumor necrosis factor mimics the metabolic response to acute infection in healthy humans. *Am. J. Physiol.* **261,** E457–E465.
143. Okusawa, S., Gelfand, J., Ikejima, T., Connolly, R., and Dinarello, C. (1988) Interleukin-1 induces a shock like state in rabbit. Synergism with tumor necrosis factor and the effect of cyclooxygenase inhibition. *J. Clin. Invest.* **81,** 1162–1172.
144. Doherty, G.M., Lange, J.R., Langstein, H.N., Alexander, H.R., Buresh, C.M., and Norton, J.A. (1992) Evidence for IFN-gamma as a mediator of the lethality of endotoxin and tumor necrosis factor-alpha. *J. Immunol.* **149,** 1666–1670.
145. Rothstein, J.L., and Schreiber, H. (1988) Synergy between TNF and bacterial products causes hemorrhagic necrosis and lethal shock in normal mice. *Proc. Natl. Acad. Sci. USA* **85,** 607–611.
146. Beutler, B., Milsark, I.W., and Cerami, A.C. (1985) Passive immunization against cachectin/tumor necrosis factor protects mice from lethal effect of endotoxin. *Science* **229,** 869–871.
147. Tracey, K.J., Fong, Y., Hesse, D.G., Manogue, K.R., Lee, A. T., Kuo, G.C., et al. (1987) Anti-cachectin/TNF monoclonal antibodies prevent septic shock during lethal bacteraemia. *Nature* **330,** 662–664.
148. Caty, M.G., Guice, K.S., Oldham, K.T., Remick, D.G., and Kunkel, S.I. (1990) Evidence for tumor necrosis factor-induced pulmonary microvascular injury after intestinal ischemia-reperfusion injury. *Ann. Surg.* **212,** 694–700.
149. Amiot, F., Fitting, C., Tracey, K. J., Cavaillon, J.-M., and Dautry, F. (1997) LPS-induced cytokine cascade and lethality in Ltα/TNFα deficient mice. *Mol. Med.* **3,** 864–875.
150. Netea, M.G., Kullberg, B.J., Verschueren, I., and Van der Meer, J.W.M. (2000) Differential susceptibility of cytokine knock-out mice for lipopolysaccharides derived from different Gram negative bacteria. *J. Endotoxin Res.* **6,** 188.
151. Ohlsson, K., Bjökk, P., Bergenfield, M., Hageman, R., and Thompson, R. (1990) Interleukin-1 receptor antagonist reduces mortality from endotoxin shock. *Nature* **348,** 550–552.
152. Li, P., Allen, H., Banerjee, S., Francklin, S., Herzog, L., Johnston, C., et al. (1995) Mice defeficient in IL-1β converting enzyme are defective in production of mature IL-1β and resistant to endotoxic shock. *Cell* **80,** 401–411.
153. Fantuzzi, G., Hui, Z., Faggioni, R., Benigni, F., Ghezzi, P., Sipe, J. D., et al. (1996) Effect of endotoxin in IL-1β deficient mice. *J. Immunol.* **157,** 291–296.
154. Block, M.I., Berg, M., McNamara, M.J., Norton, J.A., Fraker, D.L., and Alexander, H.R. (1993) Passive immunization of mice against D factor blocks lethality and cytokine release during endotoxemia. *J. Exp. Med.* **178,** 1085–1090.
155. Modur, V., Feldhaus, M.J., Weyrich, A.S., Jicha, D.L., Prescotte, S.M., Zimmerman, G.A., et al. (1997) Oncostanin M is a proinflammatory mediator. In vivo effects correlates with endothelial cell expression of inflammatory cytokines and adhesion molecules. *J. Clin. Invest.* **100,** 158–168.
156. Broaddus, V.C., Boylan, A.M., Hoeffel, J.M., Kim, K.J., Sadick, M., and Chuntharapai, A. (1994) Neutralization of IL-8 inhibits neutrophils influx in a rabbit model of endotoxin-induced pleurisy. *J. Immunol.* **152,** 2960–2967.
157. Gimbrone, M.A., Obin, M.S., Brock, A.F., Luis, E.A., Hass, P.E., Hébert, C.A., et al. (1989) Endothelial IL-8: a novel inhibitor of leukocyte–endothelial interactions. *Science* **246,** 1601–1603.
158. Cunha, F.Q. and Cunha Tamashiro, W.M.S. (1992) Tumour necrosis factor-alpha and interleukin-8 inhibit neutrophil migration in vitro and in vivo. *Mediators Inflam.* **1,** 397–401.
159. Zisman, D.A., Kunkel, S.L., Strieter, R.M., Tsai, W.C., Bucknell, K., Wilkowski, J., et al. (1997) MCP-1 protects mice in lethal endotoxemia. *J. Clin. Invest.* **99,** 2832–2836.
160. Steinhauser, M.L., Hogaboam, C.M., Matsukawa, A., Lukacs, N.W., Strieter, R.M., and Kunkel, S.L. (2000) Chemokine C10 promotes disease resolution and survival in an experimental model of bacterial sepsis. *Infect. Immun.* **68,** 6108–6114.
161. Chvatchko, Y., Hoogewerf, A. J., Meyer, A., Alouani, S., Jullard, P., Buser, R., et al. (2000) A key role for CC chemokine receptor 4 in lipopolysaccharide-induced endotoxic shock. *J. Exp. Med.* **191,** 1755–1763.
162. Matsukawa, A., Hogaboam, C.M., Lukacs, N.W., Lincoln, P.M., Evanoff, J.L., and Kunkel, S.L. (2000) Pivotal role of the CC chemokine, macrophage derived chemokine, in the innate immune response. *J. Immunol.* **164,** 5362–5368.
163. Lauw, F. N., Dekkers, P. E., te Velde, A. A., Speelman, P., Levi, M., Kurimoto, M., et al. (1999) Interleukin-12 induces sustained activation of multiple host inflammatory mediators systems in chimpanzees. *J. Infect. Dis.* **179,** 646–652.
164. Ryffel, B. (1997) Interleukin-12: role of interferon-γ in IL-12 adverse effects. *Clin. Immunol. Immunopath.* **83,** 18–20.
165. Wysocka, M., Kubin, M., Vieira, L. Q., Ozmen, L., Garotta, G., Scott, P., et al. (1995) Interleukin-12 is required for interferon-gamma production and lethality in lipopolysaccharide-induced shock in mice. *Eur. J. Immunol.* **25,** 672–676.
166. Steinhauser, M.L., Hogaboam, C.M., Lukacs, N.W., Strieter, R.M., and Kunkel, S.L. (1999) Multiples roles for IL-12 in a model of acute septic peritonitis. *J. Immunol.* **162,** 5437–5443.
167. Mancuso, G., Cusumano, V., Genovese, E., Gambuzza, M., Beninati, C., and Teti, G. (1997) Role of IL-12 in experimental neonatal sepsis caused by group B streptococci. *Infect. Immun.* **65,** 3731–3735.
168. Yamaguchi, T., Hirakata, Y., Izumikawa, K., Miyazaki, Y., Maesaki, S., Tomono, K., et al. (2000) Prolonged survival of mice with *Pseudomonas aeruginosa*-induced sepsis with rIL-12 modulation of IL-10 and IFN-γ. *J. Med. Microbiol.* **49,** 701–707.
169. Matsukawa, A., Kaplan, M.H., Hogaboam, C.M., Lukacs, N.W., and Kunkel, S.L. (2001) Pivotal role of signal transducer and activator of transcription (Stat)4 and Stat6 in the innate immune response during sepsis. *J. Exp. Med.* **193,** 679–688.

170. Bohn, E., Sing, A., Zumbihl, R., Biefeldt, C., Okamura, H., Kurimoto, M., et al. (1998) IL-18 regulates early cytokine production in, and promotes resolution of, bacterial infection in mice. *J. Immunol.* **160**, 299–307.

171. Tsutsui, H., Matsui, K., Kawada, N., Hyodo, Y., Nahashi, N., Okamura, H., et al. (1997) IL-18 accounts for both TNFα and Fas Ligand-mediated hepatotoxic pathways in endotoxin-induced liver injury in mice. *J. Immunol.* **159**, 3961–3967.

172. Netea, M.G., Fantuzzi, G., Kullberg, B.J., Stuyt, R.J.L., Pulido, E.J., McIntyre, R.C., et al. (2000) Neutralization of IL-18 reduces neutrophil tissue accumulation and protects mice against lethal *Escherichia coli* and *Salmonella typhimurium* endotoxemia. *J. Immunol.* **164**, 2644–2649.

173. Hochholzer, P., Lipford, G.B., Wagner, H., Pfeffer, K., and Heeg, K. (2000) Role of interleukin-18 during lethal shock: decreased lipopolysaccharide sensitivity but normal surperantigen reaction in IL-18-deficient mice. *Infect. Immun.* **68**, 3502–3508.

174. Sakao, Y., Takeda, K., Tsutsui, H., Kaisho, T., Nomura, F., Okamura, H., et al. (1999) IL-18-deficient mice are resistant to endotoxin-induced liver injury but highly susceptible to endotoxic shock. *Intern. Immunol.* **11**, 471–480.

175. Heinzel, F.P. (1990) The role of interferon-gamma in the pathology of experimental endotoxemia. *J. Immunol.* **145**, 2920–2924.

176. Silva, A.T. and Cohen, J. (1992) Role of interferon-gamma in experimental Gram-negative sepsis. *J. Infect. Dis.* **166**, 331–335.

177. Nansen, A., Pravsgaard Christensen, J., Marker, O., and Randrup Thomsen, A. (1997) Sensitization to lipopolysaccharide in mice with asymptomatic viral infection: role of T-cell-dependent production of interferon-γ. *J. Infect. Dis.* **176**, 151–157.

178. Kamijo, R., Le, J., Shapiro, D., Havell, E.A., Huang, S., Aguet, M., et al. (1993) Mice that lack the interferon-gamma receptor have profoundly altered responses to infection with Bacillus Calmette-Guerin and subsequent challenge with lipopolysaccharide. *J. Exp. Med.* **178**, 1435–1440.

179. Car, B.D., Eng, V.M., Schnyder, B., Ozmen, L., Huang, S., Gallay, P., et al. (1994) Interferon-gamma receptor deficient mice are resistant to endotoxic shock. *J. Exp. Med.* **179**, 1437–1444.

180. Heremans, H., Dillen, C., Groenen, M., Matthys, P., and Billiau, A. (2000) Role of interferon-γ and nitric oxide in pulmonary edema and death induced by lipopolysaccharide. *Am. J. Respir. Crit. Care Med.* **161**, 110–117.

181. Mathy, N.L., Scheuer, W., Lanzendörrfer, M., Honold, K., Ambrosius, D., and Norley, S. (2000) Interleukin-16 stimulates the expression and production of proinflammatory cytokines by human monocytes. *Immunology* **100**, 63–69.

182. Jovanovic, D.V., Di Battista, J.A., Martel-Pelletier, J., Jolicoeur, F.C., He, Y., Zhang, M., et al. (1998) IL-17 stimulates the production and expression of proinflammatory cytokines, IL-1β and TNFα by human macrophages. *J. Immunol.* **160**, 3513–3521.

183. Cohen, L., David, B., and Cavaillon, J.M. (1991) Interleukin-3 enhances cytokine production by LPS-stimulated macrophages. *Immunol. Lett.* **28**, 121–126.

184. Basu, S., Dunn, A.R., Marino, M.W., Savoia, H., Hodgson, G., Lieschke, G.J., et al. (1997) Increased tolerance to endotoxin by granulocyte-macrophage colony stimulating factor deficient mice. *J. Immunol.* **159**, 1412–1417.

185. Freeman, B.D., Ouezado, Z., Zeni, F., Natanson, C., Danner, R. L., Banks, S., et al. (1997) G-CSF reduces endotoxemia and improves survival during E. coli pneumonia. *J. Appl. Physiol.* **83**, 1467–1475.

186. Yalcin, O., Soybir, G., Koksoy, F., Kose, H., Ozturk, R., and Cokneseli, B. (1997) Effects of granulocyte colony-stimulating factor on bacterial translocation due to burn wound sepsis. *Surg. Today* **27**, 154–158.

187. Zhang, P., Bagby, G.J., Stoltz, D.A., Summer, W.R., and Nelson, S. (1998) Enhancement of peritoneal leukocyte function by granulocyte colony-stimulating factor in rats with abdominal sepsis. *Crit. Care Med.* **26**, 315–321.

188. Villa, P., Shakle, C.L., Meazza, C., Agnello, D., Ghezzi, P., and Senaldi, G. (1998) Granulocyte colony stimulating factor and antibiotics in the prophylaxis of a murine model of polymicrobial peritonitis and sepsis. *J. Infect. Dis.* **178**, 471–477.

189. Opal, S.M., Jhung, J.W., Keith, J.C., Goldman, S.J., Palardy, J.E., and Parejo, N.A. (1999) Additive effects of human recombinant interleukin-11 and granulocyte colony stimulating factor in experimental gram negative sepsis. *Blood* **93**, 3467–3472.

190. Ayala, A., Chung, C.S., Xu, Y.X., Evans, T.A., Redmond, K.M., and Chaudry, I.H. (1999) Increased inducible apoptosis in CD4+ T lymphocytes during polymicrobial sepsis is mediated by Fas ligand and not endotoxin. *Immunology* **97**, 45–55.

191. Hashimoto, S., Kobayashi, A., Kooguchi, K., Kitamura, Y., Onodera, H., and Nakajima, H. (2000) Upregulation of two death pathways of perforin/granzyme and FasL/Fas in septic acute respiratory distress syndrome. *Am. J. Respir. Crit. Care Med.* **161**, 237–243.

192. Hotchkiss, R.S., Tinsley, K.W., Swanson, P.E., Chang, K.C., Cobb, J.P., Buchman, T.G., et al. (1999) Prevention of lymphocyte cell death in sepsis improves survival in mice. *Proc. Natl. Acad. Sci. USA* **96**, 14,541–14,546.

193. David, J.R. (1966) Delayed hypersensitivity in vitro. Its mediation by cell free substances formed by lymphoid cell-antigen interaction. *Proc. Natl. Acad. Sci. USA* **65**, 72–77.

194. Bernhagen, J., Calandra, T., Mitchell, R.A., Martin, S.B., Tracey, K.J., Voelter, W., et al. (1993) MIF is a pituitary-derived cytokine that potentiates lethal endotoxaemia. *Nature* **365**, 756–759.

195. Calandra, T., Bernhagen, J., Mitchell, R.A., and Bucala, R. (1994) The macrophage is an important and previously unrecognized source of macrophage migration inhibitory factor. *J. Exp. Med.* **179**, 1895–1902.

196. Calandra, T., Bernhagen, J., Metz, C.N., Spiegel, L.A., Bacher, M., Donnelly, T., et al. (1995) MIF as a glucocorticoid-induced modulator of cytokine production. *Nature* **376**, 68–71.

197. Bacher, M., Meinhardt, A., Lan, H.Y., Mu, W., Metz, C.N., Chesney, J.A., et al. (1997) Migration inhibitory factor expression in experimentally induced endotoxemia. *Am. J. Pathol.* **150**, 235–246.

198. Bozza, M., Satoskar, A.R., Lin, G., Lu, B., Humbles, A.A., Gerard, C., et al. (1999) Targeted disruption of migration inhibitory factor gene reveals its critical role in sepsis. *J. Exp. Med.* **189**, 341–346.

199. Calandra, T., Echtenacher, B., Le Roy, D., Pugin, J., Metz, C.N., Hültner, L., et al. (2000) Protection from septic shock by neutralization of macrophage migration inhibitory factor. *Nat. Med.* **6,** 164–170.
200. Wang, H., Bloom, O., Zhang, M., Vishnubhakat, J.M., Ombrellino, M., Che, J., et al. (1999) HMG-1 as a late mediator of endotoxin lethality in mice. *Science* **285,** 248–251.
201. Fehniger, T.A., Yu, H., Cooper, M.A., Suzuki, K., Shah, M.H., and Caligiuri, M.A. (2000) IL-15 costimulates the general Shwartzman reaction and innate immune IFNγ production in vivo. *J. Immunol.* **164,** 1643–1647.
202. Alleva, D.G., Kaser, S.B., Monroy, M.A., Fenton, M.J., and Beller, D.I. (1997) IL-15 functions as a potent autocrine regulator of macrophage proinflammatory cytokine production. Evidence for differential receptor subunit utilization associated with stimulation or inhibition. *J. Immunol.* **159,** 2941–2951.
203. Schindler, R., Mancilla, J., Endres, S., Ghorbani, R., Clark, S.C., and Dinarello, C.A. (1990) Correlations and interactions in the production of interleukin-6 (IL-6), IL-1, and tumor necrosis factor (TNF) in human blood mononuclear cells: IL-6 suppresses IL-1 and TNF. *Blood* **75,** 40–47.
204. Tilg, H., Trehu, E., Atkins, M.B., Dinarello, C.A., and Mier, J.W. (1994) Interleukin-6 (IL-6) as an anti-inflammatory cytokine: induction of circulating IL-1 receptor antagonist and soluble tumor necrosis factor receptor p55. *Blood* **83,** 113–118.
205. Xing, Z., Gauldie, J., Cox, G., Baumann, H., Jordana, M., Lei, X.F., et al. (1998) IL-6 is an antiinflammatory cytokine required for controlling local or systemic acute inflammatory responses. *J. Clin. Invest.* **101,** 311–320.
206. Yoshizawa, K.I., Naruto, M., and Ida, N. (1996) Injection time of interleukin-6 determines fatal outcome in experimental endotoxin shock. *J. Interferon Cytokine Res.* **16,** 995–1000.
207. Ishimi, Y., Miyaura, C., Jin, C. H., Akatsu, T., Abe, E., Nakamura, Y., et al. (1990) IL-6 is produced by osteoblasts and induces bone resorption. *J. Immunol.* **145,** 3297–3303.
208. Tsujinaka, T., Fujita, J., Ebisui, C., Yano, M., Kominami, E., Suzuki, K., et al. (1996) Interleukin-6 receptor antibody inhibits muscle atrophy and modulates proteolytic systems in interleukin-6 transgenic mice. *J. Clin. Invest.* **97,** 244–249.
209. Jongen-Lavrencic, M., Peeters, H.R.M., Rozemuller, H., Rombouts, W.J.C., Martens, A.C.M., Vreugdenhil, G., et al. (1996) IL-6 induced anaemia in rats: possible pathogenic implications for anaemia observed in chronic inflammations. *Clin. Exp. Immunol.* **103,** 328–334.
210. Biffl, W.L., Moore, E.E., Moore, F.A., Barnett, C.C., Silliman, C.C., and Peterson, V.M. (1996) Interleukin-6 stimulates neutrophil production of platelet activating factor. *J. Leukocyte Biol.* **59,** 569–574.
211. Borish, L., Rosenbaum, R., Albury, L., and Clark, S. (1989) Activation of neutrophils by recombinant interleukin-6. *Cell Immunol.* **121,** 280–289.
212. Romano, M., Sironi, M., Toniatti, C., Polentarutti, N., Fruscella, P., Ghezzi, P., et al. (1997) Role of IL-6 and its soluble receptor in induction of chemokines and leukocyte recruitment. *Immunity* **6,** 315–325.
213. Cuzzocrea, S., Sautebin, L., De Sarro, G., Costantino, G., Rombola, L., Mazzon, E., et al. (1999) Role of IL-6 in the pleurisy and lung injury caused by carrageeenan. *J. Imunol.* **163,** 5094–5104
214. Cuzzocrea, S., De Sarro, G., Costantino, G., Ciliberto, G., Mazzon, E., De Sarro, A., et al. (1999) IL-6 knock-out mice exhibit resistance to splanchnic artery occlusion shock. *J. Leukocyte Biol.* **66,** 471–480.
215. Gabay, C., Singwe, M., Genin, B., Meyer, O., Mentha, G., Lecoultre, C., et al. (1996) Circulating levels of IL-11 and leukaemia inhibitory factor (LIF) do not significantly participate in the production of acute-phase proteins by the liver. *Clin. Exp. Immunol.* **105,** 260–265.
216. Du, X.X., Doerschuk, C.M., Orazi, A., and Williams, D.A. (1994) A bone marrow stromal-derived growth factor, interleukin-11, stimulates recovery of small intestinal mucosal cells after cytoablative therapy. *Blood* **83,** 33–37.
217. Chang, M., Williams, A., Ishizawa, L., Knoppel, A., van de Ven, C., and Cairo, M. S. (1996) Endogenous interleukin-11 (IL-11) expression is increased and prophylactic use of exogenous IL-11 enhances platelet recovery and improves survival during thrombocytopenia associated with experimental group B streptococcal sepsis in neonatal rats. *Blood Cells Mol. Dis.* **22,** 57–67.
218. Gabay, C., Smith, M.F., Eidlen, D., and Arend, W.P. (1997) Interleukin-1 receptor antagonist is an acute phase protein. *J. Clin. Invest.* **99,** 2930–2940.
219. Fischer, E., Marano, M.A., Van Zee, K.J., Rock, C.S., Hawes, A.S., Thompson, W.A., et al. (1992) Interleukin-1 receptor blockade improves survival and hemodynamic performance in *Escherichia coli* septic shock, but fails to alter host responses to sublethal endotoxemia. *J. Clin. Invest.* **89,** 1551–1557.
220. Mancilla, J., Garcia, P., and Dinarello, C.A. (1993) The IL-1 receptor antagonist can either reduce or enhance the lethality of *Klebsiella pneumoniae* sepsis in newborn rats. *Infect Immun.* **61,** 926–932.
221. Hirsch, E., Irikura, V.M., Paul, S.M., and Hirsh, D. (1996) Functions of interleukin-1 receptor antagonist in gene knockout and overproducing mice. *Proc. Natl. Acad. Sci. USA* **93,** 11,008–11,013.
222. Gérard, C., Bruyns, C., Marchant, A., Abramowicz, D., Vandenabeele, P., Delvaux, A., et al. (1993) Interleukin-10 reduces the release of tumor necrosis factor and prevents lethality in experimental endotoxemia. *J. Exp. Med.* **177,** 547–550.
223. Berg, D., Kühn, R., Rajewsky, K., Müller, W., Menon, S., Davidson, N., et al. (1995) IL-10 is a central regulator of the response to LPS in murine models of endotoxin shock and the Shwartzman reaction but not endotoxin tolerance. *J. Clin. Invest.* **96,** 2339–2347.
224. Standiford, T.J., Strieter, R.M., Lukacs, N.W., and Kunkel, S.L. (1995) Neutralization of IL-10 increases lethality in endotoxemia. *J. Immunol.* **155,** 2222–2229.
225. van der Poll, T., Marchant, A., Buurman, W.A., Berman, L., Keogh, C.V., Lazarus, D.D., et al. (1995) Endogenous Il-10 protects mice from death during septic peritonitis. *J. Immunol.* **155,** 5397–5401.
226. Steinhauser, M.L., Hogaboam, C.M., Kunkel, S.L., Lukacs, N.W., Strieter, R.M., and Standiford, T.J. (1999) Il-10 is a major mediator of sepsis-induced impairment in lung antibacterial host defense. *J. Immunol.* **162,** 392–399.

226a. Adrie, C., Adib-Conquy, M., Laurent, I., Munchi, M., Vinsonneau, C., Fitting, C., et al. (2002) Successful Cardiopulmonary resuscitation after cardiac arrest as a "sepsis-like" syndrome. *Circulation* **106**, 562–568.

227. Randow, F., Syrbe, U., Meisel, C., Krausch, D., Zuckermann, H., Platzer, C., et al. (1995) Mechanism of endotoxin desensitization: involvement of interleukin-10 and transforming growth factor β. *J. Exp. Med.* **181**, 1887–1892.

228. Marchant, A., Alegre, M., Hakim, A., Piérard, G., Marécaux, G., Friedman, G., et al. (1995) Clinical and biological significance of interleukin-10 plasma levels in patients with septic shock. *J. Clin. Immunol.* **15**, 265–272.

229. Sawyer, R.G., Rosenlof, L.K., and Pruett, T.L. (1996) IL-4 prevents mortality from acute but not chronic murine peritonitis and induces an accelerated TNF response. *Eur. Surg. Res.* **28**, 119–123.

230. Brunet, L.R., Finkelman, F.D., Cheever, A.W., Kopf, M.A., and Pearce, E.J. (1997) IL-4 protects against TNF-α-mediated cachexia and death during acute shistosomiasis. *J. Immunol.* **159**, 777–785.

231. Giampietri, A., Grohmann, U., Vacca, C., Fioretti, M. C., Puccetti, P., and Campanile, F. (2000) Dual effect of IL-4 on resistance to systemic Gram-negative infection and production of TNFα. *Cytokine* **12**, 417–421.

232. Cavaillon, J.-M. and Adib-Conquy, M. (2000) The proinflammatory cytokine cascade, in *Immune Response in the Critically Ill* (Marshal, J.C. and Vincent J.L., eds). Update in Intensive Care and Emergency Medicine Vol. 31. Verlag, New York, pp. 37–66.

233. Muchamuel, T., Menon, S., Pisacane, P., Howard, M.C., and Cockayne, D.A. (1997) IL-13 protects mice from lipopolysaccharide-induced lethal endotoxemia —Correlation with down-modulation of TNFα, IFN-γ, and IL-12 production. *J. Immunol.* **158**, 2898–2903.

234. Nicoletti, F., Mancuso, G., Cusumano, V., Di Marco, R., Zaccone, P., Bendtzen, K., et al. (1997) Prevention of endotoxin-induced lethality in neonatal mice by interleukin-13. *Eur. J. Immunol.* **27**, 1580–1583.

235. Matsukawa, A., Hogaboam, C.M., Lukacs, N.W., Lincoln, P.M., Evanoff, H.L., Strieter, R.M., et al. (2000) Expression and contribution of endogenous IL-13 in an experimental model of sepsis. *J. Immunol.* **164**, 2738–2744.

236. van der Poll, T., de Waal Malefyt, R., Coyle, S.M., and Lowry, S.F. (1997) Antiinflammatory cytokine responses during clinical sepsis and experimental endotoxemia: sequential measurements of plasma soluble interleukin (IL)-1 receptor type II, IL-10, and IL-13. *J. Infect. Dis.* **175**, 118–122.

237. Urbaschek, R. and Urbaschek, B. (1990) *Induction of Endotoxin Tolerance by Endotoxin, its Mediators and by Monophosphoryl Lipid* A, in Endotoxin research Series (Nowotny, A. Spitzer, J.J., and Ziegler, E.J., eds). Elsevier Science, Amsterdam, pp. 455–463.

238. Perrella, M. A., Hsieh, C. M., Lee, W. S., Shieh, S., Tsai, J. C., Patterson, C., et al. (1996) Arrest of endotoxin induced hypotension by transforming growth factor-β1. *Proc. Natl. Acad. Sci. USA* **93**, 2054–2059.

239. Ayala, A., Knotts, J.B., Ertel, W., Perrin, M.M., Morrison, M.H., and Chaudry, I.H. (1993) Role of interleukin 6 and transforming growth factor-beta in the induction of depressed splenocyte responses following sepsis. *Arch. Surg.* **128**, 89–94.

240. Tzung, S.P., Mahl, T.C., Lance, P., Andersen, V., and Cohen, S.A. (1992) Interferon-alpha prevents endotoxin-induced mortality in mice. *Eur. J. Immunol.* **22**, 3097–3101.

241. Grohmann, U., Van Snick, J., Campanile, F., Silla, S., Giampietri, A., Vacca, C., et al. (2000) IL-9 protects mice from Gram-negative bacterial shock : suppression of TNFα, Il-12 and IFNg and induction of IL-10. *J. Immunol.* **164**, 4197–4203.

242. Wood, J., Rodrick, M., O'Mahony, J., Palder, S., Saporoschetz, I., D'Eon, P., et al. (1984) Inadequate interleukin 2 production. A fundamental immunological deficiency in patients with major burns. *Ann. Surg.* **200**, 311–320.

243. Ertel, W., Keel, M., Neidhardt, R., Steckholzer, U., Kremer, J. P., Ungethuem, U., et al. (1997) Inhibition of the defense system stimulating interleukin-12 interferon-γ pathway during critical illness. *Blood* **89**, 1612–1620.

244. Lauw, F.N., Ten Hove, T., Dekkers, P.E.P., de Jonge, E., van Deventer, S.J.H., and van der Poll, T. (2000) Reduced Th1, but not Th2, cytokines production by lymphocytes after in vivo exposure of healthy subjects to endotoxin. *Infect Immun.* **68**, 1014–1018.

245. Muret, J., Marie, C., Fitting, C., Payen, D., and Cavaillon, J.-M. (2000) Ex vivo T-lymphocyte derived cytokine production in SIRS patients is influenced by experimental procedures. *Shock* **13**, 169–174.

246. McCall, C.E., Grosso-Wilmoth, L.M., LaRue, K., Guzman, R.N., and Cousart, S.L. (1993) Tolerance to endotoxin-induced expression of the interleukin-1β gene in blood neutrophils of humans with the sepsis syndrome. *J. Clin. Invest.* **91**, 853–861.

247. Marie, C., Muret, J., Fitting, C., Losser, M.-R., Payen, D., and Cavaillon, J.-M. (1998) Reduced ex vivo interleukin-8 production by neutrophils in septic and non-septic systemic inflammatory response syndrome. *Blood* **91**, 3439–3446.

248. Marie, C., Muret, J., Fitting, C., Payen, D., and Cavaillon, J.-M. (2000) IL-1 receptor antagonist production during infectious and noninfectious systemic inflammatory response syndrome. *Crit. Care Med.* **28**, 2277–2283.

249. Schultz, M.J., Olszyna, D.P., de Jonge, E., Verbon, A., van Deventer, S.J.H., and van der Poll, T. (2000) Reduced ex vivo chemokine production by polymorphonuclear cells after in vivo exposure of normal humans to endotoxin. *J. Infect. Dis.* **182**, 1264–1267.

250. Muñoz, C., Carlet, J., Fitting, C., Misset, B., Bleriot, J.P., and Cavaillon, J.M. (1991) Dysregulation of in vitro cytokine production by monocytes during sepsis. *J. Clin. Invest.* **88**, 1747–1754.

251. Van Deuren, M., Van Der Ven-Jongekrijg, H., Demacker, P.N.M., Baterlink, A.K.N., Van Dalen, R., Sauerwein, R.W., et al. (1994) Differential expression of proinflammatory cytokines and their inhibitors during the course of meningococcal infections. *J. Infect. Dis.* **169**, 157–161.

252. Weiss, M., Fisher, G., Barth, E., Boneberg, E., Schneider, E.-M., Georgieff, M., et al. (2000) Dissociation of LPS-induced monocytic ex vivo production of granulocyte colony stimulating factor and TNFα in patients with septic shock. *Cytokine* **13**, 51–54.

253. Luger, A., Graf, H., Schwarz, H.P., Stummvoll, H.K., and Luger, T.A. (1986) Decreased serum interleukin-1 activity and monocytes interleukin-1 production in patients with fatal sepsis. *Crit. Care Med.* **14**, 458–461.

254. Cavaillon, J.-M., Muñoz, C., Marty, C., Cabié, A., Tamion, F., Misset, B., et al. (1993) Cytokine production by monocytes from patients with sepsis syndrome and by endotoxin-tolerant monocytes, in *Bacterial Endotoxin: Recognition and Effector Mechanisms* (Levin, J., Alving, C.R., Munford, R.S., and Stütz, P.L., eds.) Elsevier Science, Amsterdam.
255. Granowitz, E.V., Porat, R., Mier, J.W., Orencole, S.F., Kaplanski, G., Lynch, E.A., et al. (1993) Intravenous endotoxin suppresses the cytokine response of peripheral blood mononuclear cells of healthy humans. *J. Immunol.* **151,** 1637–1645.
256. Cavaillon, J.M. (1995) The nonspecific nature of endotoxin tolerance. *Trends Microbiol.* **3,** 320–324.
257. Adib-Conquy, M., Adrie, C., Moine, P., Asehnoune, K., Fitting, C., Pinsky, M. R., et al. (2000) NF-κB expression in mononuclear cells of septic patients resembles that observed in LPS-tolerance. *Am. J. Respir. Crit. Care Med.* **162,** 1877–1883.
258. Cavaillon, J.-M., Adib-Conquy, M., Cloëz-Tayarani, I., and Fitting, C. (2001) Immunodepression in sepsis and SIRS assessed by ex vivo cytokine production is not a generalized phenomenon: a review. *J. Endotoxin Res.* **7,** 85–93.
259. Munford, R.S. and Pugin, J. (2001) Normal response to injury prevent systemic inflammation and can be immunosuppressive. *Am. J. Respir. Crit. Care Med.* **163,** 316–321.

4

Host Response to Pathogenic Bacteria at Mucosal Sites

Laurence Arbibe and Philippe Sansonetti

1. INTRODUCTION

Epithelial cells at mucosal surfaces constitute the first line of defense against pathogens. Intestinal epithelial cells (IECs) form a single layer of cells that isolate the host's internal milieu from gut luminal environment. IECs from the distal ileum and colon are in constant contact with a rich microbial flora, and yet, under normal conditions, no pathological inflammation is present. However, IECs possess the ability to discriminate between pathogenic and nonpathogenic bacteria because infection of these cells by pathogenic bacteria induces an inflammatory response. Because of the repertoire of proinflammatory molecules they produce when activated by microbial agents or proinflammatory cytokines, IECs can function as sensors of mucosal injury and actively participate in the innate immune mucosal response. Therefore, these cells play an essential role in the maintenance of a delicate balance between the defensive immune response and tolerance to local microflora. This chapter outlines some of the mechanisms by which IEC acts as sensor for microbial pathogens and how the proinflammatory response mediated by IEC plays a role in the pathogenesis of inflammatory bowel disease (IBD).

2. IMPORTANCE OF IEC IN THE MUCOSAL IMMUNE RESPONSE

Bacterial products such as lipopolysaccharide (LPS) of Gram-negative organisms and peptidoglycan (PG) from the cell walls of Gram-positive organisms are found in high concentration in the colon. To avoid overreaction to normal microbial flora while remaining adequately responsive to pathogens, IECs must have developed a bacterial recognition system able to discriminate pathogens from commensals. Innate immune system recognition in cells of the myeloid lineage involves a family of protein known as Toll-like receptors (TLRs). Ten TLRs have been cloned and are characterized by a leucin-rich extracellular domain and a cytoplasmic domain that is similar to the interleukin (IL)-1 receptor (1). Innate recognition of LPS proceeds through TLR4, and PG through TLR2. Downstream signaling through TLR leads to necrosis factor (NF)-κB activation, a transcriptional factor that is central to the immune and inflammatory responses, leading to cytokine production. LPS-dependent TLR4 signaling requires the presence of LPS-binding protein, which acts as an opsonin, and soluble or membrane-associated CD14, which acts as an opsonin receptor (2). Another critical component of the TLR4 signaling complex is MD2, a secreted protein that binds to the extracellular domain of TLR4, where it facilitates LPS-mediated NF-κB activation and is essential for LPS-mediated mitogen-activated protein kinase (MAPk) kinase activation (3,4). TLR expression was investigated in several epithelial cell lines. TLR4 was constitutively expressed at a low level by the human cell lines HT29, Caco-2, and T84 (5,6), compared to endothelial cells. CD14, the LPS coreceptor necessary to mediate LPS signaling through TLR4, was not detected (5). These cells respond to a high concentration of LPS(10 μg range) and only in the presence of serum, which might provide soluble proteins like soluble CD14. These serum proteins may be released from the vascular space when the intestinal epithelial monolayer is disrupted and invaded by pathogens. However, using a purified LPS preparation, Abreu et al. found that these intestinal cell lines were completely unresponsive to LPS, even when TLR4 was overexpressed (6). Importantly, the coreceptor molecule MD2 was not constitutively expressed, and its coexpression with TLR4 confers LPS-responsiveness to IEC at a concentration of LPS as low as the nanogram range. Taken together, these results show that LPS is an effective inducer of NF-κB in IEC in vitro and suggest that careful regulation of TLR4 and MD2 expression may be a central point of regulation of the mucosal immune response.

One in vivo study was performed on 16 patients with inflammatory bowel disease, Crohn's disease (CD), and ulcerative colitis (UC) (7). Primary IECs in normal tissue appear to express very little TLR4. However, TLR4 expression is strongly upregulated throughout the lower gastrointestinal tract regardless of whether assessed in active or inactive disease in both CD and UC patients. Because luminal LPS is usually well tolerated in large quantities within the healthy intestine, this tolerance may result from TLR4 downregulation minimizing LPS recognition. In IBD, host tolerance toward luminal bacterial toxins may be broken, thereby reflecting aberrant TLR4 expression. Finally, the fact that activation of NF-κB in IEC can be triggered by bacterial adhesion without the direct uptake of the micro-organism into the cell, which suggests that pathogenic organisms are able to stimulate a receptor(s) on the surface of the cells (8). Interestingly, increased apical distribution of TLR4 in CD has been observed (7). However, it is unknown whether this overexpression confers hyperresponsiveness to luminal LPS or reflects loss of response. Interestingly, the C3H/HeJ mice and the substrain C3H/HeJBir show a high susceptibility phenotype for spontaneous colitis (9). Both strains harbor the LPS response mutation (LPSd), a single-point mutation of TLR4, which renders them resistant to the effect of bacterial endotoxin. The disease onset coincides with bacterial colonization of the gut, and these animals have a high frequency of serum antibodies to antigens of the normal enteric flora. However, the role that endotoxin resistance and/or TLR4 mutation might play in colitis susceptibility is totally unknown.

The ability of epithelial cells to discriminate between pathogens and nonpathogens might be based also on the subcellular localization of the recognition system. The expression of pathogen-detection molecules may be localized such that they will be engaged if a bacterium is able to gain access to the basolateral compartment of the epithelium. Interestingly, TLR5 is expressed on the basolateral side of the intestinal epithelium, where it can sense flagellin, a conserved protein from both Gram-positive and Gram-negative bacteria (10,11). Flagellin is a potent activator of intestinal epithelial proinflammatory gene expression via Ca^{2+}-mediated activation of the NF-κB pathway (12). Although secreted by both pathogenic and commensal bacteria, flagellin must be translocated from the luminal domain, to the basolateral domain where it activates epithelial chemokine secretion through TLR5. Such translocation can be mediated by a pathogen such as *Salmonella typhimurium* but not by commensal *Escherichia coli* strains, which cannot cross the epithelial barrier. Although the mechanism of flagellin translocation remains undefined, the ability to translocate flagellin across the mucosa appears to be an important determinant of virulence in certain bacteria that elicit IL-8 in the absence of physical break in the mucosa.

The importance of TLR5 in mucosal immunity is also supported by the recent finding that various mutations in TLR5 have been identified in susceptible MOLF/Ei mice to *Salmonella* infection (13). In human intestinal biopsy specimens, TLR5 was found to be expressed on epithelial cells throughout the normal lower gastrointestinal tract and selectively by the surface epithelium because it was not present in either crypt epithelium or cell population from the lamina propria or submucosa. No difference between normal control and IBD patients have been detected (7).

Another means by which epithelial cells can discriminate between pathogens and nonpathogens may be related to the expression of intracellular pathogen-detection molecules, which are only engaged once the bacterium invade the cells. It was indeed shown that some pathogens like *S.*

typhimurium can release LPS once it is located in the intracellular environment of epithelial cells *(14)*. LPS is liberated from vacuolar compartments where intracellular bacteria reside, to vesicles present in the host cell cytosol. Because a release of cytokine mediators has been found in epithelial cells infected by *S. typhimurium*, it was tempting to speculate that a cytoplasmic pathogen-detection molecules may exist. To address this question, it was recently shown that microinjection of a bacterial culture supernatant or purified LPS activates NF-κB and JNK in HeLa and Caco-2 epithelial cells *(15,16)*. A protein called caspase-activating and recruitment domain 4 (CARD4, also known as Nod1), first shown to activate NF-κB following its overexpression *(17)*, is implicated in this response *(16,18)*. Nod1 is a cytoplasmic protein with a carboxy-terminal leucin-rich repeat (LRR) domain and an amino-terminal CARD domain similar to the apoptosis proteins CED-4 and APAF-1. Interestingly, dominant negative versions of CARD4 block activation of NF-κB and JNK by *Shigella flexneri*, as well as microinjected LPS *(16)*. Further studies are required to investigate whether Nod1 binds LPS directly or through an intrinsic cytosolic factor. Nod1 is expressed in intestinal, lung, and nasal epithelial surfaces in the late mouse embryo *(19)*. The recently identified Nod2 protein is homologous to Nod1 (34% amino acid identity), contains an additional N-terminal CARD domain, and is mainly expressed in monocyte *(20)*. Both LPS and peptidoglycan (PGN) preparations from *S. aureus* stimulate NF-κB in cells overexpressing Nod2 *(18)*. Recently, two independent groups have linked human Nod2 to the development of Crohn's disease *(21,22)*. Three independent mutations (one frame-shift and two missense variants) that alter the carboxy-terminal leucin-rich repeat domain or the adjacent region were found in up to 15% of sufferers. The frame-shift mutation leads to a truncation in the 10 leucin-rich repeats in Nod2 and, surprisingly, the truncated Nod2 was unable to respond to LPS. One might predict a resultant constitutive or enhanced responsiveness that would have been proinflammatory. However, these authors speculate that a deficit in sensing bacteria in monocyte might result in an exaggerated inflammatory response by the immune system. A second possibility is that wild-type Nod2 might mediate the production of anti-inflammatory cytokines such as interleukin-10. Although the functional connection between Nod2 mutation and Crohn's disease remains to be examined, these studies confirm suspicions of a link between the immune response to bacteria and IBD.

3. THE IEC: A UNIQUE CYTOKINE SIGNAL TRANSDUCTION AND NF-κB ACTIVATION

Cytokines are well recognized as key mediators in the inflammatory cascade causing IBD. Importantly, several line of evidence indicate that cytokines and chemokines are central mediators of tissue damage. For example, in shigellosis, severe disease was observed in patients with an increase in the number of interleukin (IL)-1β-, IL-6-, tumor necrosis factor (TNF)-α- and interferon (IFN)-γ producing cells *(23)*. Monocytes expressed IL-1, TNF-α, and IFN-γ whereas epithelial cells accounted for the production of IL-6 and IL-8. In the rabbit ligated-loop model of shigellosis, intravenous infusion of receptor antagonist IL1-ra controls the inflammatory symptoms *(24)*, thus emphasizing the role of IL-1 in the generation of the lesions. Furthermore, the key role played by IL-8 during *S. flexneri* infection was recently demonstrated in the rabbit model of shigellosis *(25)*. This proinflammatory cytokine is a potent chemoattractant for polymorphonuclear cells to the subepithelial area and pretreatment of rabbits with antibodies to IL-8 before bacterial challenge dramatically reduced both fluid accumulation within the infected ileal loop and the level of inflammation in the infected tissue. Immunohistochemistry analysis indicate that infected IEC are a major cellular source of IL-8. This result is in line with an in vitro study showing that the colonic epithelial cell line (T84, HT-29, and Caco-2) stimulated by invasive Gram-negative bacteria produces a large amount of IL-8 and other proinflammatory cytokines such as monocyte-chemoattractant protein (MCP-1), granulocyte–macrophage colony-stimulating factor (GM-CSF) and TNF-α *(26)*. Therefore, in a situation of intestinal infection, IECs, which are the first cellular barrier against the pathogen, act as sentinels by orchestrating early nonspecific immune responses by the secretion of cytokines and chemokines.

An important transcriptional regulator of cytokine/chemokine gene expression is NF-κB. The active form of NF-κB consists of heterogenous dimers, where the p50 heterodimer is the predominant form of active NF-κB. It is stored in an inactive state in the cytoplasm bound to inhibitory proteins of the IkB family that mask the nuclear localization signal of NF-κB and thus prevent its nuclear translocation. Following stimulation by a wide variety of agents such as LPS or proinflammatory cytokines, the inhibitor of NF-κB (IκB) protein becomes phosphorylated by a kinase complex that consists of the two kinases IKK1 and IKK2 and the regulatory subunit *(27)*, which is then ubiquitinated and targeted for degradation by the proteasome pathway. Free NF-κB translocates to the nucleus and induces transcription of multiple kB-dependent genes.

The intestinal mucosa is composed of a dynamic cell population in perpetual change from a proliferative and undifferentiated stage (crypt base) to mature surface villus epithelial cells. NF-κB expression and activity change as colonic cells mature: Active p65–p50 complexes predominate in proliferating cells, whereas the p50–p50 dimer is prevalent in mature cells at the luminal surface *(28)*. Interestingly, the inhibitor IκBβ is highly expressed in mature surface epithelial cells *(29)*. Therefore, colonic epithelial cells appear to be designed to have a low NF-κB response at the surface. Studies of transgenic chimeric mice that disrupt the epithelial-cell-adhesion molecule E-cadherin along the entire crypt–villus axis, but not in the villus epithelium alone, produced an inflammatory bowel disease resembling Crohn's disease *(30)*. Interestingly, the IL-1β signaling pathway leading to IKK and NF-κB activation is downregulated in differentiated HT-29 cells *(31)*. Taken together, these studies indicate that a physiological gradient of NF-κB activation may exist along the crypt–surface axis in response to stimulation and suggest that attenuation of the normal immune response in the differentiated epithelial compartment may be one of the mechanisms used to prevent immune activation in the normal state.

The unique tolerance of the gastrointestinal mucosa to proinflammatory stimuli is also maintained by the ability of the luminal microflora to regulate the epithelial response. Indeed, nonpathogenic bacteria are able to downregulate IL-8 response induced by pathogenic strain or proinflammatory cytokines such as TNF-α *(32)*.

The immunosuppressive effect on nonpathogenic *Salmonella* involved inhibition of IκBα degradation by abrogation of the polyubiquinization step that occurs following phosphorylation. Therefore, prokaryotic determinants potentially can mediate an immunosuppressive effect that may participate to the unique tolerance of the gastrointestinal mucosa to proinflammatory stimuli.

Necrosis factor-κB regulated the transcription of a number of proinflammatory molecules involved in acute response to injury, as mentioned earlier, including IL-1, TNF-α, IL-6, and IL-12. NF-κB activation and p65 nuclear translocation have been extensively documented in IBD *(33,34)*. Their critical role in intestinal inflammation is illustrated by the profound inhibition of the inflammatory response following administration of p65 antisense oligonucleotide or proteasome inhibitor in experimental model of colitis *(33,35)* and by the efficiency of anticytokine strategy such as anti-TNF-α in Crohn's disease *(36)*. However, an inflammatory response is also essential in host defense because it has been shown in an experimental model of *Shigellosis* that anti-IL-8 neutralization led to a dramatic effect on mucosal invasion by *Shigella*, which expands into the lamina propria instead of remaining restricted to the epithelium *(25)*. The key role of IL-8 in polymorphonuclear leukocytes (PMN) infiltration is essential to control the translocation of bacteria such *S. flexneri*. Finally, another example of the importance of NF-κB in the regulation of mucosal immunity in response to pathogenic organisms may also be illustrated by the strong association between the Nod2 mutation and Crohn's disease, a lack of NF-κB response leading to unregulated bacterial invasion.

4. CONCLUSION

Because of their unique position as sentinels of host defense, IEC must be able to discriminate between pathogens and nonpathogens and to initiate an adapted defensive response. Continued research in this area will undoubtedly impact on our understanding on intestinal inflammatory processes like those seen in IBD. Progress in the understanding of how the immune response generated by IEC participate in bacterial clearance at the stage of primary infection should help to identify new therapeutic strategy to combat pathogen-associated diseases.

REFERENCES

1. Medzhitov, R. (2001) Toll-like receptors and innate immunity. *Nat. Rev.* **1**, 135–145.
2. Akashi, S., Ogata, H., Kirikae, F., Kirikae, K., Kawasaki, K., Nishijima, M, et al. (2000) Regulatory roles of CD14 and phosphatidyl inositol in the signaling via Toll-like receptor 4-MD-2. *Biochem. Biophys. Res. Commun.* **268**, 172–177.
3. Shimazu, R., Akashi, S., Ogata, H., Nagai, Y., Fukudome, K., Miyake, K., et al. (1999) MD2, a molecule that confers lipopolysaccharide responsiveness on Toll-like receptor 4. *J. Exp. Med.* **189**, 1777–1782.
4. Yang, H., Youg, F., Gusovsky, F., and Chow, J.C. (2000) Cellular events mediated by lipopolysaccharide-stimulated Toll-like receptor 4: MD-2 is required for activation of mitogen-activated protein kinases and Elk-1. *J. Biol. Chem.* **275**, 20,861.
5. Cario, E., Rosenberg, I.M., Brandwein, S.L., Beck, P.L ., Reinecker, H.C., and Podolsky, D.K. (2000) Lipopolysaccharide activates distinct signaling pathways in intestinal epithelial cell lines expressing Toll-like receptors. *J. Immunol.* **164**, 966–972.
6. Abreu, M.T., Vora, P., Faure, E., Thomas, L.S., Arnold, A.T., and Arditi, M. (2001) Decreased expression of Toll-like receptor 4 and MD-2 correlates with intestinal epithelial cell protection against dysregulated proinflammatory gene expression in response to bacterial lipopolysccharide. *J. Immunol.* **167**, 1609–1617.
7. Cario, E. and Podolsky, D. (2000) Differential alteration in intestinal epithelial cell expression of Toll-like receptor 3 (TLR3) and TLR4 in inflammatory bowel disease. *Infect. Immun.* **68**, 7010–7017.
8. Eaves-Pyles, T., Szabo, C., and Salsman, A.L. (1999) Bacterial invasion is not required for activation of NF-κB in enterocytes. *Infect. Immun.* **67**, 800–804.
9. Elso, C.O., Cong, Y., and Sundberg, J. (2000) The C3H/HeJBir mouse model: a high susceptibility phenotype for colitis. *Intern. Rev. Immunol.* **19**, 63–75.
10. Hayashi, F., Smith, K.D., Ozinsky, A., Hawn, T.R., Yi, E.C., Goodlett, D.R., et al. (2001) The innate immune response to bacterial flagellin is mediated by Toll-like receptor 5. *Nature* **410**, 1099–1103.
11. Gewirtz, A.T., Simon, P.O., Schmitt, C.K., Taylor, L.J., Hagedorn, C.T., O'Brien, A.D., et al. (2001) Salmonella typhimurium translocates flagellin across intestinal epithelia, inducing a proinflammatory response. *J. Clin. Invest.* **107**, 99–109.
12. Gewirtz, A.T., Navas, T.A., Lyons, S., Godowski, P.J. and Madara, J.L. (2001) Cutting edge: bacterial flagellin activates basolaterally expressed TLR5 to induce epithelial proinflammatory gene expression. *J. Immunol.* **167**,1882–1885.
13. Sebastiani, G., Leveque, G., Lariviere, L., Laroche, L., Skamene, E., Gros, P. et al. (2000) Cloning and characterization of the murine Toll-like receptor 5 (TLR5) gene: sequence and mRNA expression studies in Salmonella-susceptible MOLF/Ei mice. *Genomics* **64**, 230–240.
14. Garcia del Portillo, G., Stein, M.A., and Finlay, B.B. (1997) Release of lipopolysaccharide from intracellular compartments containing salmonella typhimurium to vesicles of the host epithelial cell. *Infect. Immun.* **65**, 24–34.
15. Philpott, D.J., Yamaoka, S., Israel, A., and Sansonetti, P.J. (2000) Invasive Shigella flexneri activates NF-κB through a lipopolysaccharide-dependent innate intracellular response and leads to IL-8 expression in epithelial cells. *J. Immunol.* **165**, 903–914.
16. Girardin, S.E., Tournebize, R., Mavris, M., Page, A.L., Li, X., Stark, G.R., et al. (2001) CARD/Nod1 mediates NF-κB and JNK activation by invasive Shigella flexneri. *EMBO Rep.* **21**, 736–742.
17. Bertin, J., Nir, W.J., Fischer, C.M., Tayber, O.V., Errada, P.R., Grant, J.R., et al. (1999) Human CARD4 protein is a novel CED/Apaf-1 cell death family cell death that activates NF-κB. *J. Biol. Chem.* **274**, 12,955–12,958.
18. Inoharan, N., Oguran, Y., Chenn, F.F., Muton, A. and Nunezn, G. (2001) Human nod1 confers responsiveness to bacterial lipopolysaccharides. *J. Biol. Chem.* **4**, 2551–2554.
19. Inohara, N., Koseki, T., Peso, L.D., Hu, Y., Yee, C., Chen, S., et al. (1999) Nod1, an apaf-like activator of caspase-9 and nuclear factor-κB. *J. Biol. Chem.* **21**, 14,560–14,567.
20. Ogura, Y., Inohara, N., Benito, A., Chen, F.F., Yamaoka, S. and Nunez, G. (2001). Nod 2, a nod1/Apaf-1 family member that is restricted to monocytes and activates NF-κB. *J. Biol. Chem.* **276**, 4812–4818.
21. Hugot, J.P., Chamaillard, M., Zouali, H., Lesaage, S., Cezard, J.P., Belaiche, J., et al. (2001) Association of NOD2 leucine-rich repeat variants with susceptibility to Crohn's disease. *Nature* **411**, 599–603.
22. Ogura, Y., Bonen, D.K., Inohara, N., Nicolae, D.L., Chen, F.F., Ramos, P., et al. (2001) A frameshift mutation in NOD2 associated with susceptibility to Crohn's disease. *Nature* **411**, 603–606.
23. Raqib, R., Lindberg, A., Wrething, B., Bardhan, P.K., Andersson, U., and Anderson, J. (1995) Persistence of local cytokine production in shigellosis in acute and convalescent stages. *Infect. Immun.* **63**, 289–296.
24. Sansonetti, P.J., Arondel, J., Cavaillon, J.M., and Huerre, M. (1995) Role of IL-1 in the pathogenesis of experimental shigellosis. *J. Clin. Invest.* **96**, 884–892.
25. Sansonetti, P.J., Arondel, J., Huerre, M., Hararada, A., and Matsuda, K. (1999) Interleukin-8 controls bacterial transepithelial translocation at the cost of epithelial destruction in experimental Shigellosis. *Infect. Immun.* **67**, 1471–1480.
26. Jung, H.C., Eckmann, L., Yang, S.K., Panja, A., Fierer, J., Morzycka-Wroblewska, E., et al. (1995) A distinct array of proinflammatory cytokines is expressed in human colonic epithelial cells in response to bacterial invasion. *J. Clin. Invest.* **95**, 55–65.

27. Yamaoka, S., Courtois, G., Bessia, C., Whiteside, S.T., Weil, R., Agou, F., et al. (1998) Complementation cloning of NEMO, a component of the IkB kinase complex essential for NF-κB activation. *Cell* **93,** 1231.

28. Inan, M.I., Tolmacheva, V., Qiang-Shu, W., Rosenberg, D.W., and Giardana, C. (2000) Transcription factor NF-(B participates in regulation of epithelial cell turnover in the colon. *Am. J. Physiol. Gastrointest. Liver Physiol.* **279,** G1282–G1291.

29. Wu, G.D., Huang, N., Wen, X., Keilbaugh, S.A., and Yang, H. (1999) High level expression of IkB-b in the surface epithelium of the colon: in vitro evidence for an immunomodulatory role. *J. Leucocyte Biol.* **66,** 1049–1056.

30. Hermiston, M.L., and Gordon, J.I. (1995) Inflammatory bowel disease and adenomas in mice expressing a dominant negative N-cadherin. *Science* **270,** 1203–1207.

31. Bocker, U, Schottelius, A, Watson, J, Holt, L, Licato, L.L, Brenner, D.A, et al. (2000) Cellular differentiation causes a selective down regulation of IL-1b-mediated NF-κB activation and IL-8 gene expression in intestinal epithelial cells. *J. Biol. Chem.* **275,** 12,207–12,213.

32. Neish, A.S., Gewirtz, A.T., Zeng, H., Young, A.N., Hobert, M.E., Karmali, V., et al. (2000) Prokaryotic regulation responses by inhibition of IkB-a ubiquinisation. *Science* **1,** 1560–1563.

33. Neurath, M., Pettersson, S., Meyer, K.H., Zum, Buschenfelde, K.H., and Strober, W. (1996). Local administration of antisense phophothioate oligonucleotides to the p65 subunit of NF-κB abrogates established experimental colitis in mice. *Nat. Med.* **2,** 998–1004.

34. Rogler, G. and Andus, T. (1998) Cytokines in inflammatory bowel disease. *World. J. Surg.* **22,** 382–389.

35. Conner, E.M., Brand, S., Davis, J.M., Larous, F.S., Palombella, V.J., Fuseler, J.W., et al. (1997) Proteasome inhibition attenuates nitric oxide synthase expression, VCAM-1 transcription and the development of chronic colitis. *J. Pharmacol. Exp. Ther.* **283,** 1–8.

36. Van Dullemen, H.M., Vandevnter, S.J.H, Hommes, D.W., Bijl, H.A., Jansen, J., Tytgat, G.N.J. and Woody, J. (1995) Treatment of Crohn's disease with anti-tumor necrosis factor chimeric monoclonal antibody (cA2). *Gastroenterology* **109,** 129–135.

5

Macrophage Migration Inhibitory Factor as a Cytokine of Innate Immunity

Thierry Calandra

1. INTRODUCTION

The innate immune system is the first line of host defenses against infection and is activated as soon as a pathogen crosses the host's natural defense barriers *(1–3)*. Recognition of invasive microbial pathogens is mediated by soluble factors (such as the lipopolysaccharide [LPS]-binding protein [LBP]) and by pattern recognition receptors (CD14 and Toll-like receptors [TLR]) expressed on myeloid cells (i.e., granulocytes, monocytes, macrophages, and dendritic cells). LBP, CD14, and TLR4 play an essential role in the recognition of endotoxin (LPS) of Gram-negative bacteria. CD14, TLR2, TLR4, and TLR6 are members of the receptor complex implicated in the recognition of peptidoglycan (PGN) and the lipoteichoic acids (LTA) of Gram-positive bacteria. In addition, Gram-positive exotoxins activate both the innate and acquired components of the immune system, acting as superantigens to stimulate T-lymphocytes, after crosslinking the major histocompatibility complex (MHC) class II molecules of antigen-presenting cells to specific chains of the T-cell receptor.

The binding of pathogens or of microbial toxins to pattern recognition receptors on immune cells activates intracellular signaling pathways, resulting in the release of numerous effector molecules, including cytokines. Cytokines play an essential role in establishing an inflammatory response. Inflammation is an integral component of the host response to infection and comprises coordinated cellular and hormonal reactions to ensure that the microbial infection is localized or eradicated. However, the inflammation must be tightly controlled, because an excessive inflammatory reaction may result in septic shock, whereas an insufficient response may result in overwhelming infection.

2. DISCOVERY OF MIF

Nearly 40 years ago, during a study of delayed-type hypersensitivity reactions in guinea pigs, a soluble nondialyzable factor was identified that inhibited the migration of peritoneal exudate cells *(4,5)*. Termed macrophage migration inhibitory factor (MIF) to reflect its activity, this factor was thought to be released by activated lymphocytes and was, therefore, one of the first cytokines to be identified. Subsequently, MIF was found to stimulate several macrophage functions, such as cell adhesion, phagocytosis, and killing of intracellular parasites (reviewed in ref. *6*). However, the biological activities of MIF remained undefined until the cloning of a human MIF complementary deoxyribonucleic acid (cDNA) in 1989 *(7)*. Soon after its cloning, MIF was rediscovered as a protein released in a hormonelike fashion by anterior pituitary cells stimulated with LPS *(8)*. Cloning of the mouse and human *Mif* genes, expression of recombinant proteins, and production of antibodies stimulated further studies to define the biological activities of MIF *(7,9–11)*.

From: *Cytokines and Chemokines in Infectious Diseases Handbook*
Edited by: M. Kotb and T. Calandra © Humana Press Inc., Totowa, NJ

3. THE MIF GENE

The human *Mif* gene, a single functional gene located on chromosome 22 (22q11.2), contains three exons that are separated by small introns *(9)*. The coding sequence of the human *Mif* gene is identical to the sequences of *Mif* cDNA of the human eye lens *(12)* and the Jurkat human T-cell line *(7,13)*. By Northern blotting, a single MIF messenger ribonucleic acid (mRNA) has been identified in all tissues examined, with high baseline levels of mRNA in organs such as kidneys, liver, and brain. The mouse *Mif* gene is located on chromosome 10 *(10,11)*, and more than 9 *Mif* pseudogenes exist in the mouse genome *(11,14)*. The sequences of the three exons of the mouse and human *Mif* genes are highly homologous (70–86%). The only noteworthy homology with MIF is shown by the DNA sequences coding for D-*dopachrome tautomerase*, which shares an approx 30% homology with *Mif (15)*, indicating that MIF does not belong to any of the recognized cytokine superfamilies.

4. STRUCTURE AND BIOCHEMICAL ACTIVITY OF THE MIF PROTEIN

The amino acid sequences of the mouse and human MIF are 90% identical. Similarly, the MIF proteins of mouse, rat, gerbil, chicken, calf, and man display more than 80% homology. MIF is identical to the protein known as glycosylation-inhibiting factor (GIF). GIF has been shown to inhibit the N-glycosylation of IgE-binding factors, resulting in suppression of IgE synthesis, and to be associated with antigen-specific suppressor activity *(16)*. Further search for MIF homologs has revealed the existence of MIF-like molecules in *Caenorhabditis elegans* and *Arabidopsis thaliana* and in filarial parasites (*Wuchereria bancrofti*, *Brugia malayi*, and *Onchocerca volvulus*). MIF also shares a 33% amino acid sequence homology with D-dopachrome tautomerase *(17)*.

Analysis of the crystal structure of human and rat MIF indicates that MIF is a trimer *(18–20)*. MIF has a three-dimensional structural similarity, but not sequence homology, with two microbial enzymes, 4-oxalocrotonate tautomerase and 5-carboxymethyl-2-hydroxymuconate isomerase *(21)*. MIF was found to exert tautomerase activity catalyzing the conversion of 2-carboxy-2,3-dihydroindole-5,6-quinone (dopachrome) into 5,6-dihydroxyindole-2-carboxylic acid *(22,23)*. Moreover, MIF has been shown to exhibit other enzymatic activities, including the enolization of phenylpyruvate and the ketonization of *p*-hydroxyphenylpyruvate, and to act as a thiol-protein oxidoreductase *(24)*. Deletions or replacement of the N-terminal proline of MIF abolish the tautomerase activity *(25)*, but not its ability to inhibit monocyte migration *(26)*. The physiological relevance of these enzymatic activities for the biological role of MIF remains unclear at the present time. Interestingly, mapping of the chromosomal positions of the *Mif* and dopachrome tautomerase genes has indicated that they are located close together. Therefore, it is tempting to speculate, because of the sequence homology, that both genes are duplications of a common ancestral gene that has evolved to exert different biological functions.

5. CELLULAR EXPRESSION OF MIF

5.1. T-Lymphocytes

For years, it was thought that MIF was secreted only by activated T-cells. However, recent studies have shown that MIF protein and MIF mRNA are normal constituents not only of T-cells but also of many other cell types (reviewed in ref. *27*). Unlike other cytokines, which are synthesized and secreted in response to exogenous stimuli, MIF is a preformed protein stored in cytoplasmic granules. MIF mRNA and MIF protein have been detected in T-cells derived from mouse spleen and from human peripheral blood. MIF is released from T-cells stimulated by mitogens such as phorbol myristate acetate and ionomycin or by tetanus toxoid, anti-CD3 antibody, superantigenic exotoxin toxic shock syndrome toxin-1 (TSST-1), and glucocorticoids *(28–30)*. TSST-1 was a very potent stimulator of MIF secretion from mouse splenocytes. Indeed, very low concentrations of TSST-1 (10 pg/mL) induced MIF release from splenocytes, whereas 1 ng/mL of TSST-1 was required to stimulate interleukin-2 (IL-2) or interferon-γ (IFN-γ) secretion. Similar to the observation made with macrophages *(31)*, glucocorticoids induce MIF secretion by T-cells in a concentration-dependent manner *(28)*. MIF production was initially attributed to the Th2 subset of CD4+ T-helper cells *(28)*, but, subsequently, mouse Th0 and Th1 cells were also found to express MIF (Calandra, unpublished). MIF stimulates T-cell activation in vivo and in vitro, indicating that MIF exerts autocrine effects on T-cells.

Anti-MIF antibodies inhibit antigen-driven T-cell activation, proliferation, and antibody production *(28)*. Moreover, anti-MIF antibodies inhibit T-cell proliferation and IL-2 production in vitro. Administration of neutralizing anti-MIF antibody before injection of TSST-1 prevents splenic enlargement in mice and reduces the ex vivo proliferation of splenocytes by 50% *(29)*. MIF also modulates the activity of cytotoxic CD8+ T-cells. Blocking MIF activity with anti-MIF monoclonal antibodies results in an increased expression of IFN-γ and a significant increase in cytotoxic T-cell responses *(30)*.

5.2. Monocytes and Macrophages

Macrophage migration inhibitory factor has also been found in large amounts in unstimulated macrophages and monocytes *(31,32)* and can be released by these cells during inflammatory and immune reactions. Factors that elicit the release of MIF from macrophages include microbial products, such as endotoxin (LPS), TSST-1, streptococcal pyrogenic exotoxin A (SPEA), and malaria pigment, but also Gram-negative and Gram-positive bacteria, mycobacteria, as well as the cytokines tumor necrosis factor-α (TNF-α) and IFN-γ *(29,32,33)*. MIF secretion from macrophages is evoked by very low concentrations of LPS, TSST-1, or SPEA. On the other hand, stimulation with high concentrations of these toxins decreases the production of MIF from the activated macrophages, resulting in a "bell-shaped" dose-response curve.

Surprisingly, glucocorticoid hormones do not inhibit MIF secretion, as they do for other cytokines, but induce MIF release by macrophages *(31)*. The dose-response curve of dexamethasone- or cortisol-induced MIF production by macrophages is also bell shaped, with a peak of MIF release at a glucocorticoid concentration of 10^{-12} to 10^{-14} *M*. Similar observations have been made with synoviocytes *(34)*.

5.3. B Lymphocytes, Neutrophils, Eosinophils, and Basophils

An Epstein–Barr-virus-transformed human B-cell line was reported to release MIF in large amounts *(35)*. MIF protein was also detected in the WEHI 231 B-cell line *(36)*. Several studies have suggested a role for MIF in antibody production by B-cells *(28)* and in the control of B-cell cycle progression and apoptosis *(36)*. MIF is also expressed in neutrophils *(20)*, albeit in much lower amounts than in other immune cells, such as macrophages or T-cells. Superoxide production by neutrophils stimulated with formyl methionyl-leucyl-phenylalanine (fMLP) was augmented after priming with recombinant MIF *(20)*. By contrast, recombinant MIF exerted inhibitory effects on chemoattractant-induced neutrophil chemotaxis or luminol- and lucigenin-amplified chemiluminescence (Markert and Calandra, unpublished). Neutralization of MIF activity decreases the migration of neutrophils into the lungs, as well as the pulmonary myeloperoxidase activity of rats injected with LPS *(37)*. In agreement with these results, neutrophil counts were lower in the broncho-alveolar lavage of MIF knockout mice than wild-type mice after tracheal instillation of *Pseudomonas aeruginosa* *(38)*. However, these results do not confirm a direct effect of MIF on neutrophils, because the observed effects may have been caused by another mediator. As with other leukocytes (i.e., monocytes, macrophages, and T- and B-lymphocytes), eosinophils are an abundant source of MIF *(39)*, which is released after stimulation with C5a, IL-5, and phorbol myristate acetate. In addition, constitutive expression of MIF mRNA and MIF protein were identified in the human HMC-1 immature mast cell line, in primary rat peritoneal mast cells, and in the KU812 basophil cell line *(40)*.

5.4. Endocrine Cells

In addition to leucocytes, preformed MIF protein is widely expressed in most tissues throughout the body *(32,41)*. Special mention, because of possible functional importance, will be made of the role of MIF in the endocrine system. Considerable quantities of MIF have been found in the pituitary gland *(8)*, in amounts similar to adrenocorticotrophic hormone (ACTH) and prolactin. In pituitary cells, MIF is found alone in granules or is associated with ACTH or thyroid-stimulating hormone (TSH) *(42)*. MIF is secreted from the pituitary gland in response to LPS and also following stimulation with corticotrophin-releasing factor, but in doses smaller than those which elicit release of ACTH *(8,42)*. Decrease in the pituitary content of MIF is associated with increased levels of circulating MIF. Analysis of tissue distribution of MIF in the rat demonstrates the colocalization of MIF and glucocorticoid hormones in the adrenal cortex *(41)*.

Macrophage migration inhibitory factor is found in the beta cells of the islets of Langerhans of the pancreas, where MIF production is regulated in a time- and concentration-dependent fashion by glucose *(43)*. MIF potentiates the glucose-stimulated secretion of insulin, indicating that it participates in the regulation of insulin secretion. MIF has also been detected in the testis (Leydig cells), ovary (granulosa cells of follicles), and prostate (epithelial cells).

6. ROLE OF MIF IN SEPSIS

During the past decade, MIF has emerged as a critical messenger of the innate immune system. The discovery in the early 1990s that MIF was released by the pituitary gland into the bloodstream suggested the possibility that MIF might play an important role in the regulation of inflammatory reactions and of host defenses against infection. This concept was rapidly supported by a series of intriguing observations. MIF was first shown to be constitutively expressed by pivotal cells of the innate immune system, such as monocytes and macrophages, and to be released from these cells after exposure to microbial products and proinflammatory cytokines *(32)*. Similarly, MIF is constitutively expressed in many organs (including the brain, pituitary gland, kidneys, lungs, liver, spleen, adrenal glands, and skin) *(41)*. Administration of LPS to experimental animals results in the release of preformed MIF from these tissues, followed by the induction of mRNA and reconstitution of the intracellular pool of MIF protein.

Macrophage migration inhibitory factor has been shown to be an important factor influencing the outcome of experimental toxic and septic shock. Although large doses of MIF, by themselves, are not lethal, MIF was found to aggravate lethal endotoxemia when injected together with LPS into mice, increasing mortality from 35% to 85% ($p = 0.003$) *(8)*. Moreover, anti-MIF antibodies reduce blood levels of TNFα (Fig. 1) and fully protect mice against endotoxic shock, reducing mortality from 50 to 0% ($p = 0.004$) (Fig. 2A). Similarly, mice with deletion of the *Mif* gene are more resistant than wild-type mice to endotoxic shock *(38)*. Protection from lethal endotoxemia is associated with reduced blood levels of TNF-α, but not of IL- and IL-10, and also with delayed increase of IL-12.

Macrophage migration inhibitory factor is also involved in the immune reactions to staphylococcal and streptococcal exotoxins. Macrophage MIF is released after exposure to low concentrations of TSST-1 or SPEA, and neutralization of MIF bioactivity with anti-MIF antibodies prevents death from toxic shock syndrome caused by the injection of TSST-1 into mice sensitized with D-galactosamine *(29)* (Fig. 2B). Similarly, compared with wild-type mice, MIF knockout mice were resistant to injection of lethal amounts of staphylococcal enterotoxin B *(38)*. These results show that Gram-negative and Gram-positive endotoxins are powerful inducers of MIF secretion from immune cells and that MIF is an important mediator of the pathogenesis of these toxic shock syndromes.

Macrophage migration inhibitory factor also contributes to the pathophysiology of experimental septic shock caused by live bacteria. Bacterial peritonitis elicited by the intraperitoneal injection of *Escherichia coli* or by cecal ligation and puncture (CLP) in mice results in increased concentrations of MIF in peritoneal fluid and in the circulation. Polyclonal and monoclonal anti-MIF antibodies

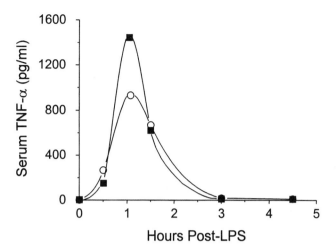

Fig. 1. Anti-MIF antibody reduces the serum concentrations of TNF-α in mice with lethal endotoxemia. BALB/c mice were injected intraperitoneally (ip) with 200 μL of anti-MIF or nonimmune rabbit serum 2 h before ip injection of a lethal dose of LPS (17.5 mg/kg). Serum was obtained before and 0.5, 1, 1.5, 3, and 4.5 h after LPS. Concentrations of TNF-α were measured using the L929 bioassay.

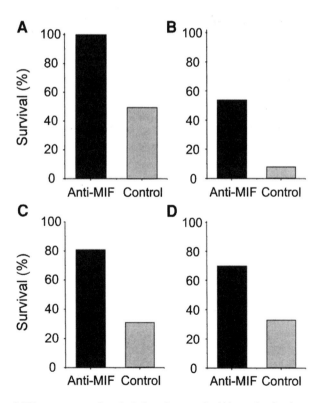

Fig. 2. Antibody against MIF protects against lethal endotoxemia (**A**), toxic shock syndrome induced by TSST-1 (**B**), and peritonitis induced by cecal ligation and puncture (CLP) (**C**) or injection of *E. coli* (**D**). (**A,B**) BALB/c mice were injected intraperitoneally (ip) with anti-MIF or nonimmune rabbit serum 2 h before ip injection of a lethal dose of LPS (**A**) or of TSST-1 and D-galactosamine (**B**) *(29)*. (**C,D**) NMRI mice were injected ip either with anti-MIF monoclonal antibody or control antibody (**C**), or with anti-MIF or control IgG (**D**), given immediately after CLP (**C**) or 2 h before the ip injection of *E. coli* (**D**) *(44)*.

protect mice from both types of lethal peritonitis *(44)*. Of note, in the CLP model of peritonitis, mice are protected even when treatment is started 8 h after the onset of bacterial peritonitis (Fig. 2C,D). The fact that protection is still provided by the delayed administration of anti-MIF therapy is clinically very important, as, under clinical conditions, antisepsis therapy is almost always given some hours after the onset of infection in septic patients. It has been shown previously that mice whose innate immune response is compromised by the deletion of the TNF-α gene or of type 1 TNF receptors are highly susceptible to otherwise nonlethal bacterial peritonitis. In agreement with this fact, TNF-α knockout mice were observed to be very sensitive to CLP. However, administration of a single dose of anti-MIF monoclonal antibodies immediately after CLP spectacularly increased survival from 0 to 62%, demonstrating that inhibition of MIF activity was capable of saving these immunocompromised animals from otherwise uniformly lethal septic shock. In the *E. coli* peritonitis model, the protection afforded by polyclonal anti-MIF antibodies was linked to a reduction of plasma TNF-α concentrations and circulating counts of *E. coli.* However, neither TNF-α nor *E. coli* are likely to be the primary targets of anti-MIF therapy in this model. Indeed, anti-MIF therapy protects TNF-α knockout mice from death, indicating that blocking MIF also prevents death in the absence of TNF-α evidence was found to support a direct causal relationship between neutralization of MIF activity and reduction of circulating bacteria *(44)*. Therefore, it is very likely that improved bacterial clearance is an early indicator of improved outcome after anti-MIF therapy.

The findings of a recent study indicate that the activation of the arachidonic acid–prostaglandins–leukotrienes pathway may account for some of the MIF-mediated effects during septic shock *(45)*. Studies conducted with antisense MIF macrophages and macrophages from MIF knockout mice have revealed an important role for MIF in the host responses to LPS and Gram-negative bacteria (Roger et al., unpublished). As observed in the endotoxemic mouse model, excessive MIF is also associated with poor outcome in bacterial septic shock. Mortality was 62% (15 of 24) in mice coinjected with recombinant MIF and *E. coli*, whereas it was only 21% (5 of 24) in mice exposed to *E. coli* alone ($p = 0.008$), supporting the conclusion that high tissue or systemic concentrations of MIF are damaging.

Elevated concentrations of MIF have been detected in the circulation of patients with severe sepsis or septic shock caused by Gram-negative or by Gram-positive bacteria. In agreement with the concept that high levels of MIF might be harmful in the context of an acute infection, plasma concentrations of MIF were higher in patients with septic shock (median: 17.8 ng/mL; range: 6.6–154.4 ng/mL) than in patients with severe sepsis (median: 12.2 ng/mL; range: 6.2–141.8 ng/mL) or healthy individuals (median: 3 ng/mL; range: 1.9–5.4 ng/mL) ($p = 0.001$) *(44)*. Similarly, on admission to an ICU, serum MIF levels were higher in patients with septic shock (mean ± SD: 14.3 ± 4.5 ng/mL) than in trauma patients (mean ± SD: 3.1 ± 1.7 ng/mL) or control patients (mean ± SD: 2.5 ± 2.1 ng/mL) ($p < 0.01$) *(46)*. In the subset of patients with septic shock, levels of MIF were higher in non-survivors than in survivors (mean ± SD: 18.4 ± 4.8 ng/mL vs 10.2 ± 4.2 ng/mL; $p = 0.001$) and higher in patients with, than in those without, the adult respiratory distress syndrome (ARDS) (mean ± SD: 19.4 ± 4.7 ng/mL vs 9.2 ± 4.2 ng/mL; $p = 0.115$). In a multiple logistic regression analysis, MIF levels were a better predictor of outcome than the presence of ARDS. In septic patients, concentrations of MIF were correlated with that of cortisol and IL-6.

7. MIF AND OTHER INFLAMMATORY DISEASES

In addition to sepsis, MIF has been shown to play an important role in the pathophysiology of several inflammatory diseases, including ARDS, arthritis, atopic dermatitis, glomerulonephritis, and allograft rejection. Increased concentrations of MIF have been detected in the broncho-alveolar lavage of patients with ARDS *(47)*. Stimulation of alveolar cells of ARDS patients ex vivo with recombinant MIF resulted in increased production of IL-8 and TNF-α, whereas treatment of these cells with anti-MIF antibodies reduced the release of these proinflammatory cytokines. In patients with rheumatoid arthritis (RA), synovial expression of MIF mRNA and protein are upregulated. Macrophages, T-cells, and fibroblastlike synoviocytes were reported to be the main sources of MIF in the synovium *(34,48)*. Levels of MIF in synovial fluid were found to be higher in patients with RA than in patients with osteoarthritis *(49)*. Interestingly, MIF production by synoviocytes was not increased by stimulation with IL-β, TNF-α, or IFN-γ possibly because synoviocyte MIF production was already maximal in these patients *(34)*. Circulating levels of MIF and expression of MIF in keratinocytes also were raised in patients with atopic dermatitis *(50)*. Anti-MIF therapy in animal models of glomerulonephritis and allograft rejection decreased inflammatory responses and improved pathological manifestations of these conditions.

8. MIF AND GLUCOCORTICOIDS AS PHYSIOLOGICAL MODULATORS OF INFLAMMATION

The secretion of ACTH and MIF by pituitary cells and the colocalization of MIF and glucocorticoid hormones in the adrenal cortex have called attention to the close relationship between the hypothalamo–pituitary–adrenal axis and MIF in the response to inflammation and infection. Circulating concentrations of MIF and glucocorticoids increase during inflammation, infection, or stress *(31,44)* and have been shown to be correlated in patients with septic shock *(46)*. However, unlike the classical inhibitory effects of glucocorticoids on the production of cytokines, MIF secretion is stimulated by physiological amounts of glucocorticoids *(28,31)*. This observation was at first difficult to reconcile with the proinflammatory activities of MIF. However, it has since been shown that secreted MIF antagonizes the anti-inflammatory effects of the glucocorticoids, so that MIF exerts proinflammatory effects on cytokine release and cellular function by reversing the glucocorticoid-induced inhibition of TNF-α, IL-1, IL-6, and IL-8 synthesis of peripheral blood mononuclear cells *(31)*. Indeed, although glucocorticoids can protect against the lethal effects of endotoxemia, by inhibiting the production of cytokines, administration of recombinant MIF to glucocorticoid-treated mice with endotoxemia reversed the protective effects of the glucocorticoids *(31)*. MIF also prevented dexamethasone-induced suppression of T-cell proliferation and cytokine production (IL-2 and IFN-γ) evoked by anti-CD3 antibodies *(28)*. Furthermore, although glucocorticoids inhibit cytosolic phospholipase A2 activity and arachidonic acid release from fibroblasts, MIF is capable of reversing these inhibitory effects *(45)*. In the macrophage, MIF has also be shown to reverse the transcriptional and posttranscriptional glucocorticoid-mediated suppression of proinflammatory gene expression (Roger et al., unpublished). Thus, MIF acts as a physiological antagonist of glucocorticoid activity, and MIF and glucocorticoids operate in concert to maintain some degree of proinflammatory and anti-inflammatory balance. The precise functional role of the interaction between MIF and glucocorticoids remains to be defined.

9. CONCLUSIONS

Macrophage migration inhibitory factor has emerged recently as an essential effector molecule of the innate immune system. The MIF protein is constitutively expressed in considerable amounts in the cells of many tissues of the body, including immune cells (monocytes, macrophages, and T- and B-lymphocytes), endocrine cells (pituitary and adrenal glands), and epithelial cells. During the course of inflammatory and infectious diseases, exposure of these cells to microbial products and proinflammatory cytokines induces the release of preformed MIF as well as *de novo* protein synthesis. When secreted into tissues or into the systemic circulation, MIF plays an important role in promoting inflammatory reactions and innate and adaptive immune responses and acts as a physiological antagonist of the anti-inflammatory and immunosuppressive effects of glucocorticoids. High blood levels of MIF are found in patients with inflammatory and infectious diseases, including severe sepsis and septic shock. Immunoneutralization of MIF or deletion of the *Mif* gene protects mice against lethal endotoxemia, Gram-positive toxic shock syndromes, and experimental bacterial peritonitis. Conversely, administration of recombinant MIF increases the lethality of endotoxemia and bacterial sepsis. It seems, therefore, that MIF has the potential to endanger life when expressed in excess during sepsis. Development of strategies that interfere with MIF production and function may have a role in the treatment of severe sepsis and inflammatory diseases.

ACKNOWLEDGMENTS

I am grateful to the colleagues who participated in these studies: M. Bacher, J. Bernhagen, R. Bucala, B. Echtenacher, M.P. Glauser, D. Heumann, L. Hültner, M. Knaup, S. Lengacher, D. Le Roy, D. Männel, C.N. Metz, R. Mitchell, J. Pugin, T. Roger, S. Rossier, and L. Spiegel. This work was supported by grants from the Swiss National Science Foundation (32-49129.96, 32-48916.96, 32-055829.98) and by a career award from the Leenards Foundation.

REFERENCES

1. Medzhitov, R. and Janeway, C.A., Jr. (1997) Innate immunity: the virtues of a nonclonal system of recognition. *Cell* **91,** 295–298.
2. Hoffmann, J.A., Kafatos, F.C., Janeway, C.A., and Ezekowitz, R.A. (1999) Phylogenetic perspectives in innate immunity. *Science* **284,** 1313–1318.
3. Kimbrell, D.A. and Beutler, B. (2001) The evolution and genetics of innate immunity. *Nat. Rev. Genet.* **2,** 256–267.
4. Bloom, B.R. and Bennett, B. (1966) Mechanism of a reaction in vitro associated with delayed-type hypersensitivity. *Science* **153,** 80–82.
5. David, J. (1966) Delayed hypersensitivity in vitro: its mediation by cell-free substances formed by lymphoid cell-antigen interaction. *Proc. Natl. Acad. Sci. USA* **56,** 72–77.
6. Calandra, T. and Bucala R. (1997) Macrophage migration inhibitory factor (MIF): a glucocorticoid counter-regulator within the immune system. *Crit. Rev. Immunol.* **17,** 77–88.
7. Weiser, W.Y., Temple, P.A., Witek-Gianotti, J.S., Remold, H.G., Clark, S.C., and David, J.R. (1989) Molecular cloning of a cDNA encoding a human macrophage migration inhibitory factor. *Proc. Natl. Acad. Sci. USA* **86,** 7522–7526.
8. Bernhagen, J., Calandra, T., Mitchell, R.A., Martin, S.B., Tracey, K.J., Voelter, W. et al. (1993) MIF is a pituitary-derived cytokine that potentiates lethal endotoxaemia. *Nature* **365,** 756–759.
9. Paralkar, V. and Wistow, G. (1994) Cloning the human gene for macrophage migration inhibitory factor (MIF). *Genomics* **19,** 48–51.
10. Mitchell, R., Bacher, M., Bernhagen, J., Pushkarskaya, T., Seldin, M., and Bucala, R. (1995) Cloning and characterization of the gene for mouse macrophage migration inhibitory factor (MIF). *J. Immunol.* **154,** 3863–3870.
11. Kozak, C.A., Adamson, M.C., Buckler, C.E., Segovia, L., Paralkar, V., and Wistow, G. (1995) Genomic cloning of mouse MIF (macrophage inhibitory factor) and genetic mapping of the human and mouse expressed gene and nine mouse pseudogenes. *Genomics* **27,** 405–411.
12. Wistow, G.J., Shaughnessy, M.P., Lee, D.C., Hodin, J., and Zelenka, P.S. (1993) A macrophage migration inhibitory factor is expressed in the differentiating cells of the eye lens. *Proc. Natl. Acad. Sci. USA* **90,** 1272–1275.
13. Bernhagen, J., Mitchell, R.A., Calandra, T., Voelter, W., Cerami, A., and Bucala, R. (1994) Purification, bioactivity, and secondary structure analysis of mouse and human macrophage migration inhibitory factor (MIF). *Biochemistry* **33,** 14,144–14,155.
14. Bozza, M., Kolakowski, L.F., Jenkins, N.A., Gilbert, D.J., Copeland, N.G., David, J.R., et al. (1996) Structural characterization and chromosomal location of the mouse macrophage migration inhibitory factor gene and pseudogenes. *Genomics* **27,** 412–419.
15. Esumi, N., Budarf, M., Ciccarelli, L., Sellinger, B., Kozak, C.A., and Wistow, G. (1998) Conserved gene structure and genomic linkage for D-dopachrome tautomerase (DDT) and MIF. *Mamm. Genome* **9,** 753–757.
16. Ishizaka, K., Ishii, Y., Nakano, T., and Sugie, K. (2000) Biochemical basis of antigen-specific suppressor T cell factors: controversies and possible answers. *Adv. Immunol.* **74,** 1–60.
17. Sugimoto, H., Taniguchi, M., Nakagawa, A., Tanaka, I., Suzuki, M., and Nishihira, J. (1999) Crystal structure of human D-dopachrome tautomerase, a homologue of macrophage migration inhibitory factor, at 1.54 Å resolution. *Biochemistry* **38,** 3268–3279.
18. Sun, H.W., Bernhagen, J., Bucala, R., and Lolis, E. (1996) Crystal structure at 2.6Å resolution of human macrophage migration inhibitory factor. *Proc. Natl. Acad. Sci. USA* **93,** 5191–5196.
19. Suzuki, M., Sugimoto, H., Nakagawa, A., Tanaka, I., Nishihira, J., and Sakai, M. (1996) Crystal structure of the macrophage migration inhibitory factor from rat liver. *Nat. Struct. Biol.* **3,** 259–266.
20. Swope, M.D. and Lolis, E. (1999) Macrophage migration inhibitory factor: cytokine, hormone, or enzyme? *Rev. Physiol. Biochem. Pharmacol.* **139,** 1–32.
21. Subramanya, H.S., Roper, D.I., Dauter, Z., Dodson, E.J., Davies, G.J., Wilson, K.S., et al. (1996) Enzymatic ketonization of 2-hydroxymuconate: specificity and mechanism investigated by the crystal structures of two isomerases. *Biochemistry* **95,** 792–802.
22. Rosengren, E., Bucala, R., Aman, P., Jacobsson, L., Odh, G., Metz, C.N., et al. (1996) The immunoregulatory mediator macrophage migration inhibitory factor (MIF) catalyzes a tautomerization reaction. *Mol. Med.* **2,** 143–149.

23. Rosengren, E., Aman, P., Thelin, S., Hansson, C., Ahlfors, S., Björk, P., et al. (1997) The macrophage migration inhibitory factor MIF is a phenylpyruvate tautomerase. *FEBS Lett.* **417,** 85–88.
24. Kleemann, R., Kapurniotu, A., Frank, R.W., Gessner, A., Mischke, R., Flieger, O., et al. (1998) Disulfide analysis reveals a role for macrophage migration inhibitory factor (MIF) as thiol-protein oxidoreductase. *J. Mol. Biol.* **280,** 85–102.
25. Bendrat, K., Al-Abed, Y., Callaway, D.J.E., Peng, T., Calandra, T., Metz, C.N., et al. (1997) Biochemical and mutational investigations of the enzymatic activity of macrophage migration inhibitory factor. *Biochemistry* **36,** 15,356–15,362.
26. Hermanowski-Vosatka, A., Mundt, S.S., Ayala, J.M., Goyal, S., Hanlon, W.A., Czerwinski, R.M., et al. (1999) Enzymatically inactive macrophage migration inhibitory factor inhibits monocyte chemotaxis and random migration. *Biochemistry* **38,** 12,841–12,849.
27. Martin, C., Roger, T., and Calandra, T. (2001) Macrophage migration inhibitory factor (MIF): a pro-inflammatory mediator of sepsis, in: (Eichacker, P.Q. and Pugin, J., eds.) *Evolving Concepts in Sepsis and Septic Shock* Kluwer Academic, Boston pp. 45–67.
28. Bacher, M., Metz, C.N., Calandra, T., Mayer, K., Chesney, J., Lohoff, M., et al. (1996) An essential regulatory role for macrophage migration inhibitory factor in T-cell activation. *Proc. Natl. Acad. Sci. USA* **93,** 7849–7854.
29. Calandra, T., Spiegel, L.A., Metz, C.N., and Bucala, R. (1998) Macrophage migration inhibitory factor is a critical mediator of the activation of immune cells by exotoxins of Gram-positive bacteria. *Proc. Natl. Acad. Sci. USA* **95,** 11,383–11,388.
30. Abe, R., Peng, T., Sailors, J., Bucala, R., and Metz, C.N. (2001) Regulation of the CTL response by macrophage migration inhibitory factor. *J. Immunol.* **166,** 747–753.
31. Calandra, T., Bernhagen, J., Metz, C.N., Spiegel, L.A., Bacher, M., Donnelly, T., et al. (1995) MIF as a glucocorticoid-induced modulator of cytokine production. *Nature* **377,** 68–71.
32. Calandra, T., Bernhagen, J., Mitchell, R.A., and Bucala, R. (1994) The macrophage is an important and previously unrecognized source of macrophage migration inhibitory factor. *J. Exp. Med.* **179,** 1895–1902.
33. Martiney, J.A., Sherry, B., Metz, C.N., Espinoza, M., Ferrer, A.S., Calandra, T., et al. (2000) Macrophage migration inhibitory factor release by macrophages after ingestion of plasmodium chabaudi-infected erythrocytes: possible role in the pathogenesis of malarial anemia. *Infect. Immun.* **68,** 2259–2267.
34. Leech, M., Metz, C., Hall, P., Hutchinson, P., Gianis, K., Smith, M., et al. (199) Macrophage migration inhibitory factor in rheumatoid arthritis: evidence of proinflammatory function and regulation by glucocorticoids. *Arthritis Rheum.* **42,** 1601–1608.
35. Wymann, D., Bluggel, M., Kalbacher, H., Blesken, T., Akdis, C.A., Meyer, H.E., et al. (1999) Human B cells secrete migration inhibition factor (MIF) and present a naturally processed MIF peptide on HLA-DRB1*0405 by a FXXL motif. *Immunology* **96,** 1–9.
36. Takahashi, A., Iwabuchi, K., Suzuki, M., Ogasawara, K., Nishihira, J., and Onoé, K. (1999) Antisense macrophage migration inhibitory factor (MIF) prevents anti-IgM mediated growth arrest and apoptosis of a murine B cell line by regulating cell cycle progression. *Microbiol. Immunol.* **43,** 61–67.
37. Makita, H., Nishimura, M., Miyamoto, K., Nakano, T., Tanino, Y., Hirokawa, J., et al. (1998) Effect of anti-macrophage migration inhibitory factor antibody on lipopolysaccharide-induced pulmonary neutrophil accumulation. *Am. J. Respir. Crit. Care Med.* **158,** 573–579.
38. Bozza, M., Satoskar, A.R., Lin, G., Lu, B., Humbles, A.A., Gerard, C., et al. (1997) Targeted disruption of migration inhibitory factor gene reveals its critical role in sepsis. *J. Exp. Med.* **189,** 341–346.
39. Rossi, A.G., Haslett, C., Hirani, N., Greening, A.P., Rahman, I., Metz, C.N., et al. (1999) Human circulating eosinophils secrete macrophage migration inhibitory factor (MIF). Potential role in asthma. *J. Clin. Invest.* **101,** 2869–2874.
40. Chen, H., Centola, M., Altschul, S.F., and Metzger, H. (1998) Characterization of gene expression in resting and activated mast cells. *J. Exp. Med.* **188,** 1657–1668.
41. Bacher, M., Meinhardt, A., Lan, H.Y., Metz, C.N., Chesney, J.A., Calandra, T., et al. (1997) MIF expression in experimentally-induced endotoxemia. *Am. J. Pathol.* **150,** 235–246.
42. Nishino, T., Bernhagen, J., Shiiki, H., Calandra, T., Dohi, K., and Bucala, R. (1995) Localization of macrophage migration inhibitory factor (MIF) to secretory granules within the corticotrophic and thyrotrophic cells of the pituitary gland. *Mol. Med.* **1,** 781–788.
43. Waeber, G., Calandra, T., Roduit, R., Haefliger, J-A., Bonny, C., Thompson, N., et al. (1997) Insulin secretion is regulated by the glucose-dependent production of islet b-cell macrophage migration inhibitory factor. *Proc. Natl. Acad. Sci. USA* **94,** 4783–4787.
44. Calandra, T., Echtenacher, B., Roy, D.L., Pugin, J., Metz, C.N., Hultner, L., et al. (2000) Protection from septic shock by neutralization of macrophage migration inhibitory factor. *Nat. Med.* **6,** 164–170.
45. Mitchell, R.A., Metz, C.N., Peng, T., and Bucala, R. (1999) Sustained mitogen-activated protein kinase (MAPK) and cytoplasmic phopholipase A2 activation by macrophage migration inhibitory factor (MIF). *J. Biol. Chem.* **274,** 18,100–18,106.
46. Beishuizen, A., Thijs, L.G., Haanen, C., and Vermes, I. (2001) Macrophage migration inhibitory factor and hypothalamo–pituitary–adrenal function during critical illness. *J. Clin. Endocrinol. Metab.* **86,** 2811–2816.
47. Donnelly, S.C., Haslett, C., Reid, P.T., Grant, I.S., Wallace, W.A.H., Metz, C.N., et al. (1997) Regulatory role for macrophage migration inhibitory factor in acute respiratory distress syndrome. *Nat. Med.* **3,** 320–323.
48. Onodera, S., Tanji, H., Suzuki, K., Kaneda, K., Mizue, Y., Sagawa, A., et al. (1999) High expression of macrophage migration inhibitory factor in the synovial tissues of rheumatoid joints. *Cytokine* **11,** 163–167.

49. Metz, C.N. and Bucala, R. (1997) Role of macrophage migration inhibitory factor in the regulation of the immune response. *Adv. Immunol.* **66,** 197–223.
50. Shimizu, T., Abe, R., Ohkawara, A., Mizue, Y., and Nishihira, J. (1997) Macrophage migration inhibitory factor is an essential immunoregulatory cytokine in atopic dermatitis. *Biochem. Biophys. Res. Commun.* **240,** 173–178.

III

Cytokines in Gram-Positive Infections

6
Cytokine Patterns in Severe Invasive Group A Streptococcal Infections

Anna Norrby-Teglund and Malak Kotb

1. INTRODUCTION

Group A streptococcus (GAS), *Streptococcus pyogenes*, is an important human pathogen that can cause a variety of diseases, ranging from superficial infections of the skin and mucous membranes to severe invasive infections. During the last two decades, a marked increase in the frequency of highly aggressive invasive GAS infections associated with high morbidity and mortality rates, including streptococcal toxic shock syndrome and necrotizing fasciitis, was noted world-wide. This resurgence prompted intense research in the field of GAS pathogenesis and revealed a complex host–pathogen interplay involving several different virulence factors and host defense systems. In this chapter, we focus on the immunopathogenesis of severe invasive GAS infections, with particular emphasis on GAS virulence factors triggering cytokine responses, and we highlight the importance of specific cytokine patterns in determining the severity of invasive disease.

2. PATHOGENESIS OF SEVERE INVASIVE GROUP A STREPTOCOCCAL INFECTIONS

Group A streptococcus expresses numerous factors, both cell associated and secreted, that interact with immune cells and other factors of the host to enhance the virulence of the bacteria. There are several cell surface molecules, such as hyaluronic acid capsule, M- and M-like proteins, C5a-peptidase, α_2-macroglobulin-binding protein, that are important for bacterial adherence and colonization, as well as for immune escape mechanisms (1–3). These proteins interact with a variety of human plasma proteins, including, among others, immunoglobulins, fibronectin, fibrinogen, albumin, plasminogen, kininogen, complement factor C5a, and inhibitors of the complement system, thereby promoting the attachment of the bacteria to host cells and the invasion into tissues, as well as evasion of immune attack and phagocytosis (2,3). The antiphagocytic M-protein is of special importance because type-specific antibodies against the M-protein confer protection against infection, and patients with invasive GAS disease generally have low levels of opsonic antibodies to the specific M-protein expressed by the infecting strain (4,5). In addition to these factors, GAS produces proteases that can modify host proteins and receptors expressed on host cells, thereby exerting tissue damage and inflammation. Interestingly, the same proteases can also act on bacterial virulence proteins to modulate their function and potentiate their biological activity.

Despite the involvement of many GAS virulence factors in pathogenesis, studies in patients with invasive infections have shown that the systemic effects seen in patients with streptococcal toxic

From: *Cytokines and Chemokines in Infectious Diseases Handbook*
Edited by: M. Kotb and T. Calandra © Humana Press Inc., Totowa, NJ

shock syndrome and necrotizing fasciitis are largely triggered by inflammatory mediators induced in response to the bacterial virulence factors, particularly the streptococcal pyrogenic exotoxins, which belong to the superantigen family of toxins and that are, by far, the most potent inducers of inflammatory responses in GAS infections.

3. PROINFLAMMATORY CELL WALL CONSTITUENTS

The role of bacterial cell wall components in Gram-negative bacteremia and sepsis has been studied in detail, and it is well established that the outer-membrane lipopolysaccharide (LPS) is the principal stimulus of inflammatory responses. Similarly, the Gram-positive cell wall is composed of several molecules—in particular peptidoglycan and lipoteichoic acid (LTA)—that exhibit proinflammatory activity (reviewed in ref. 6). Peptidoglycan is an essential bacterial cell wall component and is the major constituent of the Gram-positive cell wall. A study of *Streptococcus pneumoniae* peptidoglycan showed that the proinflammatory activity was attributed to highly active crosslinked stem peptides, with tripeptides demonstrating a >100-fold higher proinflammatory activity than intact peptidoglycan (7).

Lipoteichoic acids are sugar phosphate polymers that extend through the cell wall onto the surface of the Gram-positive cell. Both peptidoglycan and LTA have been shown to activate leukocytes and trigger production of proinflammatory cytokines, including interleukin (IL)-1β, IL-6, IL-8, IL-12, tumor necrosis factor (TNF)-α, and chemokines, as well as other inflammatory mediators, such as inducible nitric oxide synthetase (8–20). Most of these studies have focused on monocyte responses, but it was recently shown that circulating human T-cells also contribute to cytokine production in response to the *Staphylococcus aureus* cell wall (18).

Like the Gram-negative bacterial LPS, the Gram-positive bacterial LTA and peptidoglycan display pathogen-associated molecular patterns, which activate the innate immunity by interacting with cognate pattern recognition receptors, such as CD14 and Toll-like receptors (TLR) 2 and 4 (21) (Fig. 1). Engagement of the TLRs with microbial products triggers several intracellular signal transduction pathways, resulting in the activation of the transcription factor nuclear factor (NF)-κβ, and the subsequent induction of the expression of proinflammatory cytokines genes (21) (Fig. 1). The secreted small molecule MD2 functions as a helper molecule for both TLR2 and TLR4 in these responses (22–24).

The ability of purified peptidoglycan and LTA to trigger pathologic inflammatory conditions has been demonstrated in various animal models including experimental meningitis and septic shock (25–29). In a rat model of septic shock, it was shown that although administration of LTA resulted in moderate hypotension, it did not trigger multiorgan failure and death (26,27). However, when LTA was administered together with peptidoglycan, a synergistic effect was achieved and the anesthetized rats experienced shock and multiorgan failure (26–28).

4. SECRETED PROINFLAMMATORY VIRULENCE FACTORS

4.1. Superantigens

The most potent virulence factors of GAS are the superantigens, which are proteins that elicit excessive inflammatory responses in the host. They do so by circumventing the normal rules for antigen processing and presentation. Superantigens interact with the relatively invariable Vβ regions of the αβ heterodimeric T-cell receptor that are located outside the antigen-binding groove, and they also bind directly to major histocompatibility complex (MHC) class II molecules on antigen-presenting cells without prior cellular processing and outside of the conventional antigen-binding cleft (30). Each superantigen has a characteristic Vβ specificity, and activates preferentially T cells expressing certain Vβ elements. In humans, there are roughly 25 major Vβ families and most superantigens interact with 3–6 Vβ families, which may lead to the activation of 5–20% of the naive resting T-cell population. The fraction of stimulated T-cells may depend on the number of Vβ families engaged by

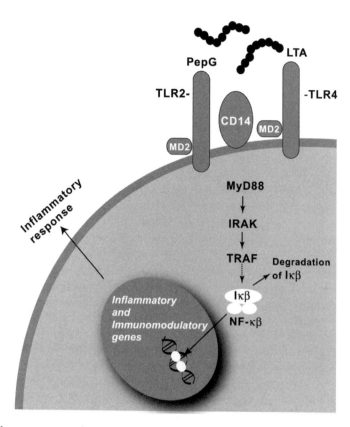

Fig. 1. Cell wall components activate macrophages through Toll-like receptors (TLRs). Gram-positive peptidoglycan (PepG, PGN) and lipoteichoic acid (LTA) interact with CD14 and activate TLR. MD2 enhances the responsiveness of TLR to microbial products. Upon TLR engagement, the adaptor protein MyD88 is recruited and associates with interleukin-1 receptor accessory protein kinase (IRAK), which results in phosphorylation of IRAK. Phosphorylated IRAK interacts with tumor necrosis-factor-receptor-associated factor 6 (TRAF6) adapter protein, leading to activation of MAP protein kinases that phosphorylate IκB leading to the release of NF-κB, which then translocates to the nucleus and activates genes involved in inflammatory and immune responses.

the secreted superantigens during an infection as well as on the relative expression of these cognate Vβ elements in the patient's repertoire. Furthermore, the interaction between superantigens and MHC class II molecules may differ depending on both the superantigen and the MHC class II allotype. The preferential binding of specific superantigens to certain class II alleles can influence the level of inflammatory response (reviewed in ref. *31*). Interestingly, although there is significant difference in the primary sequence of the superantigens, most share a common three-dimensional structure, which includes a folding of the superantigen into different domains, one amino-terminal hydrophobic β-barrel domain and a carboxy-terminal β-grasp domain (reviewed in *32*). It is believed that this structural fold plays an important role in allowing superantigens to exert their biological effects, but evidence is accumulating that this effect is modulated by host factors.

4.1.1. Cytokine-Induction Profile of Superantigens

The simultaneous binding of a superantigen to T-cells and antigen presenting cells results in potent activation of these cells and subsequent massive cytokine production (Fig 2). The superantigen-induction profile exhibits a wide array of cytokines and includes IL-1α, IL-1β, IL-1 receptor antagonist (IL-1ra), IL-6, IL-8, IL-12, macrophage migration inhibitory factor (MIF), TNF-α, IL-2,

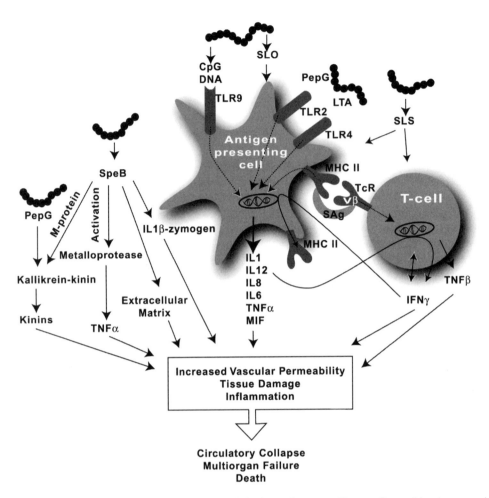

Fig. 2. Interactions between group A streptococcal virulence factors and host cells resulting in severe invasive infection. Lipoteichoic acid (LTA), peptidoglycan (PepG, PGN), and CpG DNA activate antigen-presenting cells through Toll-like receptors (TLRs). Activation results in the production of various cytokines, among others IL-12 which promoted interferon (IFN)-γ production by T-cells. Superantigens (SAg) interact with MHC class II molecules (MHC II) and the T-cell receptor (TcR) to activate both cell types, resulting in a high production of cytokines. The cysteine protease, streptococcal pyrogenic exotoxin (SpeB), also promotes a proinflammatory response. Streptolysin O and S (SLO, SLS) are cytotoxic and proinflammatory.

TNF-β, and interferon (IFN)-γ *(33–45)*. A much lower production of the Th2 cytokines IL-4, IL-5, and IL-10 is seen following stimulation with purified GAS superantigens *(35,43)*. A typical superantigen-induced cytokine production profile in human peripheral blood mononuclear cells is characterized by the rapid induction of IL-1α, IL-1β, and I-L8 production, which generally peaks between 24 and 48 h (Fig. 3). IL-1ra is also induced early, and its production persists over a prolonged period and usually reaches peak levels after 72 h of stimulation. Lower levels and a more gradual release without a distinct peak of production are seen for IL-2-, IL-6- and TNF-α-producing cells. However, the most pronounced and distinctive superantigen-induced production is seen for the Th1 cytokines TNF-β and IFN-γ, which can be detected in up to 20% of peripheral blood mononuclear cells following 72–96 h of superantigen stimulation in vitro *(35,43)* (Fig. 3). This potent cytokine response requires the participation of both T-cells and antigen-presenting cells and is perpetuated by the cytokines from these cells (Fig. 3). Superantigen-induced monokine production is

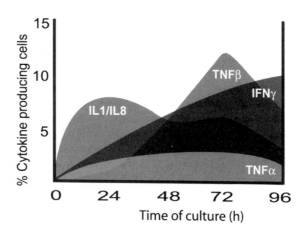

Fig. 3. Characteristic cytokine-induction profile of streptococcal superantigens. The figure shows cytokine production assessed after stimulation with the streptococcal pyrogenic exotoxin A by intracellular immunostaining technique. (Based on data from ref. *43.*)

dependent on the presence of T-cell-derived cytokines *(46,47)*. Production of IFN-γ is promoted by IL-12 *(48)*, and TNF-β production is dependent on IFN-γ *(47,48)*. Furthermore, the temporal production of cytokines has been shown to affect the overall cytokine cascade, and elevated IFN-γ causes a prolonged production of IL-1, IL-6, and TNF-α *(47)*.

A high degree of interindividual variation in mitogenic and cytokine responses induced by superantigens has been reported in several studies *(35,43,49)*. Some individuals responded consistently high to superantigens with the production of high levels of IL-1, TNF-β, and IFN-γ, and low levels of IL-4, whereas the reverse was true for a "low responder" *(49)*. This interindividual variation between the high and low responders seems to be attributed to host immunogenetic factors and significantly affects disease severity. This point is discussed further in Section 6.2 and is illustrated in ref. *50.*

4.1.2. Group A Streptococcal Superantigens

There are, to date, 11 distinct exotoxins produced by GAS, including the streptococcal pyrogenic exotoxins (Spe) A, B, C, F, G, H, J, streptococcal mitogenic exotoxin (Sme) Z, SmeZ-2, SmeZ-3, and streptococcal superantigen (SSA) (*see* Table 1; reviewed in ref. *61)*. The distribution of these superantigens among streptococcal strains varies significantly because some superantigens are chromosomally encoded and found in virtually all GAS strains, whereas others are associated with mobile genetic elements, such as bacteriophages or insertion sequences *(62)* (*see* Table 1). Several studies have attempted to identify the causative superantigen in the recent GAS outbreaks; however, the varying results of these studies indicate that the disease is not caused by any particular superantigen, but that rather several of the GAS superantigens have the potential of causing severe systemic inflammation and most likely these superantigens synergize with each other as well as with other streptococcal virulence factors in inducing severe disease *(65)* (*see* Table 2).

4.1.3. Superantigens and Disease

A critical role for superantigens has been shown in numerous experimental models of toxic shock syndrome using either superantigens from *Staphylococcus aureus* or from GAS (reviewed in refs. *31* and *66*). These studies showed the importance of the synergistic activity of superantigen-induced cytokines in the development of toxic shock, by demonstrating that protection against superantigen-induced toxic shock could be achieved by cyclosporine A, anticytokine antibodies, or the use of physically or functionally T-cell-deficient mice, including SCID and CD28-deficient mice *(33,45,67–69)*.

Table 1
Group A Streptococcal Superantigens

Superantigen	Distribution of genes[a]	Human Vβ-specificity	Ref.
SpeA	Variable	2, 12, 14, 15	*51*
SpeB	Universal	8	*51*
SpeC	Variable	1, 2, 5.1, 10	*51*
SpeF[b]	Universal	2, 4, 8, 15, 19	*52,53*
SpeG	Universal	2, 4, 6, 12	*54*
SpeH	Variable	2, 7, 9	*54*
Spe J	ND	2, 3, 12, 14, 17	*55*
SmeZ/Z2/Z3[c]	Universal	2, 4, 7, 8 / 14, 8 / 8[d]	*54,56–58*
SSA	Variable	1, 3, 5.2, 15	*59,60*

Note: Spe, streptococcal pyrogenic exotoxin; Sme, streptococcal mitogenic exotoxin; ND, not determined.
[a]Distribution of superantigen genes differ depending on whether or not they are genetically linked to mobile elements.
[b]Previously referred to as mitogenic factor (MF).
[c]Three distinct alleles of SmeZ have been identified with distinct Vβ usage.
[d]Determined by use of Vβ8-transfected cell lines.

Table 2
Synergistic Effects of Group A Streptococcal Virulence Factors

GAS virulence factor	Synergistic factor[a]	Consequence	Ref.
LTA	PepG	Shock	*26,28*
Superantigens	LPS	Shock	*61*
SpeA	SLO	Increased IL-1, TNF-α	*39*
CpG DNA	LPS	Increased TNF-α	*63*
Cystein protease (SpeB)	SLO	Lung injury	*64*
Cystein protease (SpeB)	GAS cell wall	Lung injury	*64*

Note: GAS, group A streptococcal; LTA, lipoteichoic acid; PepG (PGN), peptidoglycan; LPS, lipopolysaccharide; Spe, streptococcal pyrogenic exotoxin; SLO, streptolysin O.
[a]Include virulence factors of both group A streptococci and Gram-negative bacteria.

Another property of most pyrogenic superantigens is their augmentation of endotoxin-induced cytokine responses and their ability to enhance host-sensitivity to endotoxin-shock (reviewed in ref. *61*). It was recently shown that this enhancement was dependent on T-cells and most likely mediated by IFN-γ *(70,71)*. It is likely that this synergistic action of the Gram-positive superantigens and the Gram-negative endotoxins affects the pathogenesis and clinical outcome of infection, particularly in cases of polymicrobial sepsis.

Direct evidence of in vivo involvement of superantigens in fulminant GAS diseases was provided by studies of T-cell-receptor Vβ repertoires in patients with streptococcal toxic shock syndrome *(72,73)*. Watanabe-Ohnishi demonstrated that acute-phase blood from these patients showed a selective depletion of T-cells expressing certain Vβ elements that corresponded to the specificity of particular superantigens *(73)*. Furthermore, superantigens have been identified in the plasma of patients with streptococcal toxic shock syndrome *(74)*, as well as at the local site of infection in patients with deep tissue infections *(75)*. A critical role of superantigens in fulminant GAS infections was also demonstrated by the finding that patients with severe invasive GAS infections had significantly lower levels of protective antibodies against certain superantigens than did patients with uncomplicated tonsillitis or healthy individuals *(4,76)*. Administration of neutralizing antisuperantigen antibodies to patients by administration of intravenous polyspecific immunoglobulin G (IVIG) has been shown to reduce mortality in patients with streptococcal toxic shock syndrome *(77)*. Interestingly, comparison of humoral immunity in patients with varying severity of invasive GAS disease revealed that they all had equally low levels of protective antisuperantigen antibodies regardless of severity of invasive disease *(4,76)*. Thus, low levels of antisuperantigen antibodies renders the individuals susceptible to invasive disease, but it does not determine the severity of disease progression. As is seen in Section 6.2, severity is determined by the individual's propensity to mount high or low levels of cytokine responses to GAS superantigens.

4.2. Unmethylated CpG DNA

Specific motifs of prokaryotic DNA (i.e., unmethylated oligonucleotides containing cytidine–phosphate–guanosine [CpG]), have been reported to be immunostimulatory *(78,79)*. Unmethylated CpG DNA is abundant in prokaryotes, and when flanked by certain sequences these CpG motifs have been shown to activate macrophages, dendritic cells, and B-cells in a T-cell-independent manner, thereby triggering the production of IL-1, IL-6, TNF-α, IL-12, IL-10, and Th1-type cytokines (reviewed in ref. *80*). Activation of cellular responses by CpG DNA was recently shown to be mediated by Toll-like receptor 9 *(81)* *(see* Fig. 2). Although streptococcal DNA generally have a low GC-content, certain important virulence genes, such as the gene encoding the M1 protein, has been shown to have relatively high frequencies of immunostimulatory CpG motifs with a preferential specificity for human cells *(82)*. An enhanced proinflammatory response was achieved by the synergistic activity of CpG DNA and LPS, a property that may also be clinically relevant in cases of polymicrobial sepsis *(63)*.

4.3. Streptococcal Cysteine Proteinase

Aside from its superantigenic activity, SpeB exhibits protease activity and is also referred to as streptococcal cysteine protease. By virtue of its proteolytic activity, SpeB modulates several host defense systems, including the cytokine network system, kallikrein–kinin, coagulation, and complement system, and has, therefore, been suggested to cause tissue destruction and hypotension and contribute to the systemic effects seen in fulminant GAS infections *(83)* (Fig. 2). Numerous physiologically important host proteins, including IL-1β precursor *(84)*, metalloproteases *(85)*, the extracellular matrix proteins vitronectin and fibronectin *(86)*, immunoglobulins *(84)*, and kininogens *(87)*, are substrates for SpeB. Cleavage of human IL-1β precursor and activation of metalloproteases that cleaves the precursor form of TNF-α, results in the generation of bioactive IL-1β and TNF-α *(84,85)*. The proinflammatory response can be further augmented by the ability of SpeB to cleave kininogen, resulting in the release of the proinflammatory kinins, which increase vascular permeability, hypotension, and inflammation *(87)*. This effect can be further exacerbated by other streptococcal products, including the M-protein *(89)* and peptidoglycan *(90)*, which have been shown to also interact and activate the kallikrein–kinin system. A clinical relevance of these interactions was demonstrated in a recent study, which reported that the kallikrein–kinin system is activated during the acute phase of streptococcal toxic shock *(91)*.

Analyses of humoral immunity in patients with GAS infections supported an important role for SpeB in the pathogenesis of GAS infections, inasmuch as patients with invasive disease had significantly lower anti-SpeB antibodies during the acute phase of infections compared to patients with uncomplicated GAS infections or to healthy individuals *(4,76)*. Furthermore, experimental in vivo studies revealed reduced morbidity and mortality of invasive GAS infections by immunization against SpeB *(92)*, or by the administration of a protease-inhibiting synthetic peptide *(93)*. An excessive proinflammatory cytokine response and pronounced lung injury was induced in rats by the synergistic actions of SpeB and other streptococcal virulence factors, including streptolysin O and cell wall fragments *(64)*, *(see* Table 2). However, although several experimental models suggest an important role of SpeB in the dissemination of the bacteria and in destructive tissue inflammation, there have been other reports suggesting the opposite. For example, an association between SpeB expression and decreased virulence has been observed by several groups *(94–96)*. One potential explanation for this could be that several important cell-associated virulence factors of GAS, including M-protein, protein H, and C5a peptidase, can be cleaved by SpeB, resulting in either loss of or altered properties of essential virulence factors for the bacteria *(97,98)*. Thus, the role of SpeB in GAS pathogenesis is highly complex and remains to be better defined in the context of the route of infection as well as host–pathogen interactions.

4.4. The Streptolysins

Group A streptococcus produces two antigenically and functionally distinct haemolysins: streptolysin O (SLO) and S (SLS) *(99)*. SLS is a nonimmunogenic oxygen-stable cytolysin, which has a direct cytotoxic effect on several human cell types. The mechanism by which SLS mediates its cytotoxic activity is not well defined. However, SLS-deficient GAS strains were reported to be significantly less virulent in mice than their isogenic wild-type strains, as evident by the loss of the ability to induce inflammatory responses, weight loss, and necrotic lesions *(100)*.

Streptolysin O is a pore-forming cytolysin with well-established cell and tissue-destructive capacity *(99)*. SLO has been shown to be a potent inducer of IL-1β and TNF-α production in human monocytes *(39)*. This response was significantly enhanced by the synergistic effect of the superantigen SpeA *(39)*. As mentioned earlier, SLO also acts in synergy with the cysteine protease SpeB, which results in augmented lung injury in an experimental rat model *(64)*. Previous reports have shown that keratinocytes and Hep-2 cells express high levels of proinflammatory cytokines in response to adherent, but not to nonadherent, streptococci *(101–103)*, and, furthermore, that this phenomenon was coupled to the activities of SLO *(102)*. In an experimental murine skin model, SLO-deficient GAS strains were attenuated in virulence, and although the bacteria disseminated in these animals, they were less likely to cause lethal infection when compared to wild-type strains *(104)*.

5. CYTOKINES IN SEPSIS

One of the initial events in sepsis is the induction of proinflammatory cytokines, which trigger cytokine cascades, causes the activation of the complement and coagulation systems, induces endothelium and vessel injury, and elicits the release of proteases, arachidonic acid metabolites, and nitric oxide *(105,106)*. The cytokines that are most commonly associated with sepsis include IL-1, TNF-α, IL-6, IL-8, IL-12, IFN-γ, MIF, and high mobility group-1 (HMG-1) *(106–108)*. However, there are several additional cytokines being released during sepsis, and together with the above-mentioned ones, they interact in a complex network involving several crossover points and feedback loops. IL-1 and TNF-α induce potent pyrogenic and hypotensive responses, and the administration of either cytokine reproduces the clinical symptoms of sepsis (reviewed in ref. *106*). One of the best markers for sepsis outcome is IL-6. However, IL-6 *per se* does not induce a proinflammatory response, or hypotension, and does not cause shock in animal models. MIF is a pituitary- and macrophage-derived factor *(107)* that behaves as a proinflammatory cytokine and was recently shown to be a critical mediator of septic shock *(33,109)*. Gram-positive superantigens were identified as the most potent inducers of MIF *(33)*. HMG-1 is another recently identified critical mediator of septic shock *(108)*. HMG-1 is a potent proinflammatory cytokine that appears late in the cytokine cascade and is produced over a prolonged period *(108,110)*.

Because of the central role of cytokines in sepsis, immunotherapy directed against these inflammatory mediators has been a major area of investigations in this field. However, so far, anticytokine therapy, although very promising in experimental models, have failed to improve the survival rate in humans *(111)*. This failure may be attributed to compensatory mechanisms characteristic of cytokine networks and/or to the need to achieve a delicate balance in cytokine concentrations during infection. A better appreciation of the cytokine network and concentration-dependent variable effects of certain cytokines is needed for the design of more effective drugs that can halt the harmful effects of inflammatory cytokines without blocking the beneficial effects of these mediators in fighting the infection.

Another important factor to consider, in this regard, is the noted difference in the cytokine induction profile between Gram-negative and Gram-positive sepsis *(35)*. As mentioned earlier, Gram-positive superantigens induce powerful production of monokines as well as lymphokines, whereas Gram-negative bacteria and LPS predominantly induce monokine production, at least in the initial phases of infection *(35)*. The kinetic of the cytokine response also differs significantly, with a more rapid burst of monokine release noted for LPS as compared to superantigens *(35)*. Hence, the specificity of the pathogenic agent is likely to influence the profile of the cytokine response in vivo and, consequently, specific immunotherapies may have varying efficacies depending on the type of inciting pathogen and the timing of the therapeutic intervention. Novel cytokine targets include the recently identified late mediators of sepsis, including HMG-1 and MIF.

6. CYTOKINES IN GROUP A STREPTOCOCCAL INFECTIONS

6.1. In Vivo Cytokine Patterns in Experimental Group A Streptococcal Sepsis and Shock

In a baboon model, intravenous infusion of GAS resulted in a clinical picture that closely resembled that seen in streptococcal toxic shock syndrome, including profound hypotension, leukopenia, renal impairment, thrombocytopenia, disseminated coagulopathy, and high mortality rates *(112)*. A critical role for TNF-α was evident by the rapid rise in serum TNF levels as well as by the significantly improved survival rate following the administration of anti-TNF-α antibodies to these animals *(112)*. There have been several clinical trials of various anti-TNF-α therapies in sepsis; however, neither agent has been able to significantly lower the mortality rates *(113)*, and one trial, which assessed the efficacy and safety of a soluble TNF receptor, even showed a dose-dependent increased mortality in the active group *(114)*.

The need for a delicate balance between protective and detrimental effects of a given cytokine was underscored in a murine model of GAS skin infection *(115)*. In this model, the administration of IL-12, either prophylactically or therapeutically, protected mice against GAS infection, as shown by increased survival. The effect of IL-12 seemed to be attributed to its ability to induce IFN-γ, inasmuch as neutralization of IFN-γ, by use of antibodies or IFN-γ knockout mice, increased susceptibility to lethal infection and abrogated the protective effects of IL-12. Importantly, IL-12 was only protective at low doses; at high doses, it triggered detrimental effects that were associated with increased systemic levels of IFN-γ.

6.2. In Vivo Cytokine Responses in Patients with Invasive Group A Streptococcal Infections

In agreement with what has been reported for sepsis in general, patients with severe GAS sepsis were found to have elevated plasma levels of TNF-α and IL-6 compared to bacteremia or pharyngotonsillitis patients *(116)*. Furthermore, analysis of cytokine production by enumerating the percentage of cells producing specific cytokines using a single-cell immunostaining technique revealed very high frequencies of IL-2-, IL-6-, and TNF-α-producing cells *(117)*. In certain patients, 20% of the circulating peripheral blood mononuclear cells were producing TNF-α during the acute phase of invasive GAS infections. These frequencies corresponded well to the frequencies expected of a typical superantigen response, which usually stimulates 5–20% of resting mononuclear cells. Severe invasive cases suffering from toxic shock and/or necrotizing fasciitis had significantly higher frequencies of IL-2-, IL-6-, and TNF-α-producing cells in their circulation compared to nonsevere invasive cases (e.g., cases of bacteremia, erysipelas, or cellulitis). Importantly, this difference between severe and nonsevere cases could be reproduced in vitro during the convalescent phase (at least 1 mo after discharge and recovery). Paired age- and gender-matched severe and nonsevere cases infected with a clonal M1 GAS strain were tested in vitro during their convalescent phase for immune response to superantigens produced by their infecting isolates. The severe cases responded consistently higher to the streptococcal superantigens they had been exposed to during their infection than the nonsevere cases *(117)*. This reproducible difference between the high and low responders, who respectively had severe versus nonsevere disease, suggested a strong influence of host immunogenetic factors in modulating the outcome and severity in invasive GAS infections. The finding is in complete agreement with the recent discovery of a strong association between the human leukocyte antigen (HLA) class II haplotype of infected patients and disease progression, and the demonstration that the class II allotype strongly influenced the in vitro immune response induced by streptococcal superantigens *(50)*.

Similar to the predicted value of the number of proinflammatory cytokine-producing cells in the circulation of patients with severe GAS infections, a significant correlation between in vivo inflammatory responses and severity of infection was noted at the local site of infection in patients with soft tissue infection *(75)*. Increasing levels of IL-1 and significantly higher frequencies of Th1 cytokine-producing cells were found in more severely affected tissue biopsies *(see* Fig. 4). The finding of high frequencies of cells producing Th1 cytokines at the local site of infection was of special interest because neither TNF-β- nor IFN-γ-producing cells could not be detected at significant numbers in the peripheral circulation of patients with invasive GAS infection *(116–118)*. This is not unusual inasmuch as other studies have shown that cells producing these cells tend to leave the peripheral circulation and home to the infected tissue site *(119)*. Hence, the cytokine profile at the local site of infection mimicked that of a typical superantigen cytokine response and provided evidence for the direct actions of superantigens in GAS tissue infections *(75)*. Further experiments assessing the expression of homing receptors revealed a strong correlation between the magnitude of Th1 cytokines and certain homing receptors—in particular CCR5, CD44, and cutaneous lymphocyte antigen *(75)* *(see* Fig. 5). These data taken together with previous reports on superantigens and homing receptors *(120–127)*, suggest that superantigen activation of peripheral T-cells may induce upregulation of these homing receptors and thereby promote the migration of these activated T-cells to the skin and, subsequently, exacerbated inflammation at the local site of infection.

Further support for a critical role of superantigen-induced cytokine responses in the pathogenesis of invasive GAS infections was provided by studies of the use of IVIG *(77,128)* or superantigen peptide antagonists in severe invasive GAS infections *(129,130)*. Several in vitro studies have shown a complete abrogation of superantigen-induced cytokine production by IVIG (reviewed in ref. *131)*. In a case control study of IVIG in streptococcal toxic shock syndrome patients, it was shown that IVIG therapy significantly reduced TNF-α and IL-6 levels and correlated to improved survival *(77)*. The use and mechanism of IVIG is further discussed in Chapter 26, and it appears to involve both the action of antisuperantigen neutralizing antibodies and the immunodulatory effects of IVIG. Another promising therapeutic approach is to inhibit superantigens by peptides. Peptides representing common regions shared between both streptococcal and staphylococcal superantigens have been identified *(129–132)*, and peptides specific for these regions were able to inhibit the induction of cytokines and protect against lethal shock in experimental models of superantigen-induced toxic shock *(129,130,132)*.

7. CONCLUSIONS

Group A streptococci express several molecules with proinflammatory activity, including both cell wall components and secreted factors, of which the superantigens are the most potent inducers of inflammatory cytokine cascades. Cell wall virulence factors activate mainly innate immunity and interact with antigen-presenting cells to elicit the induction of chemokines and monokines. Superantigens, on the other hand, are powerful inducers of cytokines from the innate as well as the acquired arm of the immune system involving the activation of both antigen-presenting cells and T-cells. The proinflammatory and tissue-damaging effects caused by superantigen-induced responses is further exacerbated by the synergistic effect of several other GAS virulence factors. There is ample in vitro and in vivo evidence that superantigens and their induction of cytokines are critical in the

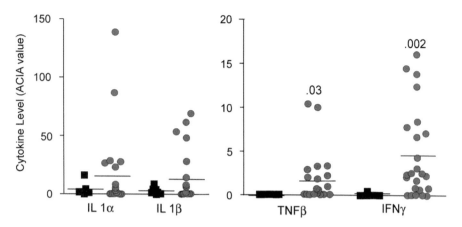

Fig. 4. Correlation between severity of tissue infection and increased expression of proinflammatory cytokines. Tissue biopsies were obtained from patients with tissue infections caused by group A streptococci and immunostained for IL-1α, IL-1β, TNF-β, and IFN-γ. The biopsies were classified according to clinical grade, defined as 1 = normal tissue, no signs of inflammation (squares), and 2 = cellulitis, fasciitis, and necrotizing fasciitis (circles). The stainings were evaluated by acquired computerized image analysis (ACIA) and the results are presented as ACIA values, which correspond to the area and intensity of positive stain (brown) in relation to the total cell area (hematoxylin counterstain). The horizontal bars indicate mean values. Statistical differences between biopsies of clinical grades 1 and 2 were analyzed by the Mann–Whitney U-test, and p-values are indicated above the bars. (Based on data from ref. *75.*)

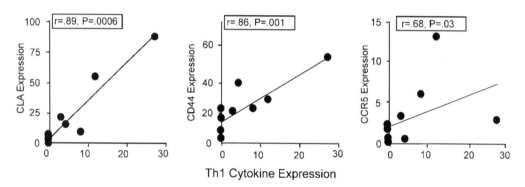

Fig. 5. Upregulation of CCR5, CD44, and CLA correlate with higher Th1 response. Tissue biopsies were obtained from patients with tissue infections caused by group A streptococci. Snap-frozen biopsies were immunostained for CCR5, CD44, CLA, TNF-β, and IFN-γ, and the stainings were evaluated by acquired computerized image analysis (ACIA). A significant correlation between Th1 cytokine levels (TNF-β + IFN-γ) and receptor expression was determined by Spearman's correlation test. Spearman R values and P-values are indicated in the figure. (Based on data from ref. *75*).

development of toxic shock and in destructive tissue infections caused by GAS. However, individuals vary considerably in their susceptibility to the superantigens, and this variability affects both the magnitude and type of cytokine response during the invasive infection. It has been shown that patients with a propensity to produce higher levels of inflammatory cytokines in response to streptococcal superantigens develop significantly more severe systemic manifestations than patients with a propensity to produce lower levels of inflammatory cytokines to the same superantigens. This difference in propensity to be a high or a low responder was attributed to differences in immunogenetic elements of the host, primarily the HLA class II genes, which encode molecules that regulate the magnitude of cytokine responses to superantigens. Thus, host factors clearly influence the magnitude of cytokine responses to superantigens and, consequently, the clinical outcome of the infection. The finding that superantigens are pivotal players in severe invasive GAS disease suggests that therapy directed toward superantigens, or against the excessive cytokines induced by these toxins, may afford an effective therapeutic strategy in these diseases.

REFERENCES

1. Rasmussen, M., Muller, H.P., and Bjorck, L. (1999) Protein GRAB of streptococcus pyogenes regulates proteolysis at the bacterial surface by binding alpha2-macroglobulin. *J. Biol. Chem.* **28,** 15,336–15,344.
2. Fischetti, V.A. (1989) Streptococcal M protein: molecular design and biological behavior. *Clin. Microbiol. Rev.* **2,** 285–314.
3. Boyle, M.D. (1995) Variation of multifunctional surface binding proteins—a virulence strategy for group A streptococci? *J. Theor. Biol.* **21,** 415–426.
4. Basma, H., Norrby-Teglund, A., Guedez, Y., McGeer, A., Low, D.E., El-Ahmedy, O., et al. (1999) Risk factors in the pathogenesis of invasive group A streptococcal infections: Role of protective humoral immunity. *Infect. Immun.* **67,** 1871–1877.
5. Holm, S.E., Norrby, A., Bergholm, A.-M., and Norgren, M. (1992) Aspects of the pathogenesis in serious group A streptococcal infections in Sweden 1988–1989. *J. Infect. Dis.* **166,** 31–37.
6. Sriskandan, S. and Cohen, J. (1999) Gram-positive sepsis. Mechanisms and differences from gram-negative sepsis. *Infect. Dis. Clin. North Am.* **13,** 397–412.
7. Majcherczyk, P.A., Langen, H., Heumann, D., Fountoulakis, M., Glauser, M.P., and Moreillon, P. (1999) Digestion of Streptococcus pneumoniae cell walls with its major peptidoglycan hydrolase releases branched stem peptides carrying proinflammatory activity. *J. Biol. Chem.* **274,** 12,537–12,543.
8. Bhakdi, S., Klonisch, T., Nuber, P., and Fischer, W. (1991) Stimulation of monokine production by lipoteichoic acids. *Infect. Immun.* **59,** 4614–4620.
9. Card, G.L., Jasuja, R.R., and Gustafson, G.L. (1994) Activation of arachidonic acid metabolism in mouse macrophages by bacterial amphiphiles. *J. Leukoc. Biol.* **56,** 723–728.
10. Cleveland, M.G., Gorham, J.D., Murphy, T.L., Tuomanen, E., and Murphy, K.M. (1996) Lipoteichoic acid preparations of Gram-positive bacteria induce interleukin-12 through a CD14-dependent pathway. *Infect. Immun.* **64,** 1906–1912.
11. Heumann, D., Barras, C., Severin, A., Glauser, M.P., and Tomasz, A. (1994) Gram-positive cell walls stimulate synthesis of tumor necrosis factor alpha and interleukin-6 by human monocytes. *Infect. Immun.* **62,** 2715–2721.
12. Mattsson, E., Verhage, L., Rollof, J., Fleer, A., Verhoef, J., and van Dijk, H. (1993) Peptidoglycan and teichoic acid from Staphylococcus epidermidis stimulate human monocytes to release tumour necrosis factor-alpha, interleukin-1 beta and interleukin-6. *FEMS Immunol. Med. Microbiol.* **7,** 281–287.
13. Morath, S., Geyer, A., and Hartung, T. (2001) Structure–function relationship of cytokine induction by lipoteichoic acid from Staphylococcus aureus. *J. Exp. Med.* **193,** 393–397.
14. Keller, R., Fischer, W., Keist, R., and Bassetti, S. (1992) Macrophage response to bacteria: induction of marked secretory and cellular activities by lipoteichoic acids. *Infect. Immun.* **60,** 3664–3672.
15. Riesenfeld-Orn, I., Wolpe, S., Garcia-Bustos, J.F., Hoffmann, M.K., and Tuomanen, E. (1989) Production of interleukin-1 but not tumor necrosis factor by human monocytes stimulated with pneumococcal cell surface components. *Infect. Immun.* **57,** 1890–1893.
16. Standiford, T.J., Arenberg, D.A., Danforth, J.M., Kunkel, S.L., VanOtteren, G.M., and Strieter, R.M. (1994) Lipoteichoic acid induces secretion of interleukin-8 from human blood monocytes: a cellular and molecular analysis. *Infect. Immun.* **62,** 119–125.
17. Timmerman, C.P., Mattsson, E., Martinez-Martinez, L., De Graaf, L., Van Strijp, J.A., Verbrugh, H.A., et al. (1993) Induction of release of tumor necrosis factor from human monocytes by staphylococci and staphylococcal peptidoglycans. *Infect. Immun.* **61,** 4167–4172.
18. Wang, J.E., Jorgensen, P.F., Almlof, M., Thiemermann, C., Foster, S.J., Aasen, A.O., et al. (2000) Peptidoglycan and lipoteichoic acid from Staphylococcus aureus induce tumor necrosis factor alpha, interleukin 6 (IL-6), and IL-10 production in both T cells and monocytes in a human whole blood model. *Infect. Immun.* **68,** 3965–3970.
19. Wang, Z.M., Liu, C., and Dziarski, R. (2000) Chemokines are the main proinflammatory mediators in human monocytes activated by Staphylococcus aureus, peptidoglycan, and endotoxin. *J. Biol. Chem.* **275,** 20,260–20,267.
20. Wakabayashi, G., Gelfand, J.A., Jung, W.K., Connolly, R.J., Burke, J.F. and Dinarello, C.A. (1991) Staphylococcus epidermidis induces complement activation, tumor necrosis factor and interleukin-1, a shock-like state and tissue injury in rabbits without endotoxemia. Comparison to *Escherichia coli. J. Clin. Invest.* **87,** 1925–1935.
21. Medzihtov, R. and Janeway, C.J. (2000) Innate Immunity. *N. Engl. J. Med.* **5,** 338–344.
22. Dziarski, R., Wang, Q., Miyake, K., Kirschning, C.J., and Gupta, D. (2001) MD-2 enables Toll-like receptor 2 (TLR2)-mediated responses to lipopolysaccharide and enhances TLR2-mediated responses to Gram-positive and Gram-negative bacteria and their cell wall components. *J. Immunol.* **166,** 1938–1944.
23. Akashi, S., Shimazu, R., Ogata, H., Nagai, Y., Takeda, K., Kimoto, M., et al. (2000) Cutting edge: cell surface expression and lipopolysaccharide signaling via the toll-like receptor 4-MD-2 complex on mouse peritoneal macrophages. *J. Immunol.* **164,** 3471–3475.

24. Shimazu, R., Akashi, S., Ogata, H., Nagai, Y., Fukudome, K., Miyake, K., et al. (1999) MD-2, a molecule that confers lipopolysaccharide responsiveness on Toll-like receptor 4. *J. Exp. Med.* **189**, 1777–1782.
25. Tuomanen, E., Liu, H., Hengstler, B., Zak, O., and Tomasz, A. (1985) The induction of meningeal inflammation by components of the pneumococcal cell wall. *J. Infect. Dis.* **151**, 859–868.
26. De Kimpe, S.J., Kengatharan, M., Thiemermann, C., and Vane, J.R. (1995) The cell wall components peptidoglycan and lipoteichoic acid from Staphylococcus aureus act in synergy to cause shock and multiple organ failure. *Proc. Natl. Acad. Sci. USA* **24**, 10,359–10,363.
27. De Kimpe, S.J., Hunter, M.L., Bryant, C.E., Thiemermann, C., and Vane, J.R. (1995) Delayed circulatory failure due to the induction of nitric oxide synthase by lipoteichoic acid from Staphylococcus aureus in anaesthetized rats. *Br. J. Pharmacol.* **114**, 1317–1323.
28. Kengatharan, K.M., De Kimpe, S.J., and Thiemermann, C. (1996) Role of nitric oxide in the circulatory failure and organ injury in a rodent model of Gram-positive shock. *Br. J. Pharmacol.* **119**, 1411–1421.
29. Spika, J.S., Peterson, P.K., Wilkinson, B.J., Hammerschmidt, D.E., Verbrugh, H.A., Verhoef, J., et al. (1982) Role of peptidoglycan from Staphylococcus aureus in leukopenia, thrombocytopenia, and complement activation associated with bacteremia. *J. Infect. Dis.* **146**, 227–234.
30. Marrack, P. and Kappler, J. (1990) The staphylococcal enterotoxins and their relatives. *Science* **248**, 705–711.
31. Kotb, M. (1995) Bacterial pyrogenic exotoxins as superantigens. *Clin. Microbiol. Rev.* **8**, 411–426.
32. Kotb, M. (1998) Superantigens of Gram-positive bacteria: structure-function analyses and their implications for biological activity. *Curr. Opin. Microbiol.* **1**, 56–65.
33. Calandra, T., Spiegel, L. A., Metz, C.N. and Bucala, R. (1998) Macrophage migration inhibitory factor is a critical mediator of the activation of immune cells by exotoxins of Gram-positive bacteria. *Proc. Natl. Acad. Sci. USA* **95**, 11,383–11,388.
34. Carlsson, R. and Sjogren, H.O. (1985) Kinetics of IL-2 and interferon-gamma production, expression of IL-2 receptors, and cell proliferation in human mononuclear cells exposed to staphylococcal enterotoxin A. *Cell. Immunol.* **96**, 175–183.
35. Andersson, J., Nagy, S., Björk, L., Abrams, J., Holm, S., and Andersson, U. (1992) Bacterial toxin-induced cytokine production studied at the single-cell level. *Immunol. Rev.* **127**, 69–96.
36. Ikejima, T., Dinarello, C.A., Gill, D.M., and Wolff, S.M. (1984) Induction of human interleukin-1 by a product of Staphylococcus aureus associated with toxic shock syndrome. *J. Clin. Invest.* **73**, 1312–1320.
37. Ikejima, T., Okusawa, S., van der Meer, J.W., and Dinarello, C.A. (1988) Induction by toxic-shock-syndrome toxin-1 of a circulating tumor necrosis factor-like substance in rabbits and of immunoreactive tumor necrosis factor and interleukin-1 from human mononuclear cells. *J. Infect. Dis.* **158**, 1017–1025.
38. Fast, D.J., Schlievert, P.M., and Nelson, R.D. (1989) Toxic shock syndrome-associated staphylococcal and streptococcal pyrogenic toxins are potent inducers of tumor necrosis factor production. *Infect. Immun.* **57**, 291–294.
39. Hackett, S.P. and Stevens, D.L. (1992) Streptococcal toxic shock syndrome: synthesis of tumor necrosis factor and interleukin-1 by monocytes stimulated with pyrogenic exotoxin A and streptolysin O. *J. Infect. Dis.* **165**, 879–885.
40. Jupin, C., Anderson, S., Damais, C., Alouf, J.E., and Parant, M. (1988) Toxic shock syndrome toxin 1 as an inducer of human tumor necrosis factors and gamma interferon. *J. Exp. Med.* **167**, 752–761.
41. Muller-Alouf, H., Alouf, J.E., Gerlach, D., Ozegowski, J. H., Fitting, C. and Cavaillon, J.M. (1994) Comparative study of cytokine release by human peripheral blood mononuclear cells stimulated with Streptococcus pyogenes superantigenic erythrogenic toxins, heat-killed streptococci, and lipopolysaccharide. *Infect. Immun.* **62**, 4915–4921.
42. Muller-Alouf, H., Gerlach, D., Desreumaux, P., Leportier, C., Alouf, J.E., and Capron, M. (1997) Streptococcal pyrogenic exotoxin A (SPE A) superantigen induced production of hematopoietic cytokines, IL-12 and IL-13 by human peripheral blood mononuclear cells. *Microb. Pathol.* **23**, 265–272.
43. Norrby-Teglund, A., Norgren, M., Holm, S.E., Andersson, U., and Andersson, J. (1994) Similar cytokine induction profiles of a novel streptococcal exotoxin, MF, and pyrogenic exotoxins A and B. *Infect. Immun.* **62**, 3731–3738.
44. Parsonnet, J., Hickman, R.K., Eardley, D.D., and Pier, G. B. (1985) Induction of human interleukin-1 by toxic-shock-syndrome toxin-1. *J. Infect. Dis.* **151**, 514–522.
45. Miethke, T., Wahl, C., Heeg, K., Echtenacher, B., Krammer, P.H. and Wagner, H. (1992) T cell-mediated lethal shock triggered in mice by the superantigen staphylococcal enterotoxin B: critical role of tumor necrosis factor. *J. Exp. Med.* **175**, 91–98.
46. Gjorloff, A., Fischer, H., Hedlund, G., Hansson, J., Kenney, J.S., Allison, A.C., et al. (1991) Induction of interleukin-1 in human monocytes by the superantigen staphylococcal enterotoxin A requires the participation of T cells. *Cell. Immunol.* **137**, 61–71.
47. Kotb, M., Ohnishi, H., Majumdar, G., Hackett, S., Bryant, A., Higgins, G., and Stevens, D. (1993) Temporal relationship of cytokine release by peripheral blood mononuclear cells stimulated by the streptococcal superantigen pep M5. *Infect. Immun.* **61**, 1194–1201.
48. Sriskandan, S., Evans, T.J., and Cohen, J. (1996) Bacterial superantigen-induced human lymphocyte responses are nitric oxide dependent and mediated by IL-12 and IFN-gamma. *J. Immunol.* **156**, 2430–2435.
49. Norrby-Teglund, A., Lustig, R., and Kotb, M. (1997) Differential induction of Th1 versus Th2 cytokines by group A streptococcal toxic shock syndrome isolates. *Infect. Immun.* **65**, 5209–5215.
50. Kotb, M., Norrby-Teglund, A., McGeer, A., Dorak, M.T., Khurshid, A., El-Sherbini, H., et al. (2002) Immunogenetic and molecular differences in outcomes of invasive group A streptococcal infections. *Nat. Med.* In press.
51. Tomai, M.A., Schlievert, P.M., and Kotb, M. (1992) Distinct T-cell receptor V beta gene usage by human T lymphocytes stimulated with the streptococcal pyrogenic exotoxins and pep M5 protein. *Infect. Immun.* **60**, 701–705.

52. Iwasaki, M., Igarashi, H., Hinuma, Y., and Yutsudo, T. (1993) Cloning, characterization and overexpression of a Streptococcus pyogenes gene encoding a new type of mitogenic factor. *FEBS Lett.* **331,** 187–192.
53. Norrby-Teglund, A., Newton, D., Kotb, M., Holm, S.E., and Norgren, M. (1994) Superantigenic properties of the group A streptococcal exotoxin SpeF (MF). *Infect. Immun.* **62,** 5227–5233.
54. Proft, T., Louise Moffatt, S., Berkahn, C.J., and Fraser, J.D. (1999) Identification and characterization of novel superantigens from Streptococcus pyogenes. *J. Exp. Med.* **189,** 89–102.
55. McCormick, J.K., Pragman, A.A., Stolpa, J.C., Leung, D.Y., and Schlievert, P.M. (2001) Functional characterization of streptococcal pyrogenic exotoxin J, a novel superantigen. *Infect. Immun.* **69,** 1381–1388.
56. Proft, T., Moffatt, S.L., Weller, K.D., Paterson, A., Martin, D., and Fraser, J.D. (2000) The streptococcal superantigen SMEZ exhibits wide allelic variation, mosaic structure, and significant antigenic variation. *J. Exp. Med.* **191,** 1765–1776.
57. Kamezawa, Y., Nakahara, T., Nakano, S., Abe, Y., Nozaki-Renard, J., and Isono, T. (1997) Streptococcal mitogenic exotoxin Z, a novel acidic superantigenic toxin produced by a T1 strain of Streptococcus pyogenes. *Infect. Immun.* **65,** 3828–3833.
58. Gerlach, D., Fleischer, B., Wagner, M., Schmidt, K., Vettermann, S., and Reichardt, W. (2000) Purification and biochemical characterization of a basic superantigen (SPEX/SMEZ3) from Streptococcus pyogenes. *FEMS Microbiol. Lett.* **188,** 153–163.
59. Mollick, J.A., Miller, G.G., Musser, J., Cook, R.G., Grossman, D., and Rich, R.R. (1993) A novel superantigen isolated from pathogenic strains of S. pyogenes with aminoterminal homology to staphylococcal enterotoxins B and C. *J. Clin. Invest.* **92,** 710–719.
60. Reda, K.B., Kapur, V., Goela, D., Lamphear, J.G., Musser, J.M., and Rich, R.R. (1996) Phylogenetic distribution of streptococcal superantigen SSA allelic variants provides evidence for horizontal transfer of ssa within Streptococcus pyogenes. *Infect. Immun.* **64,** 1161–1165.
61. Bohach, G.A., Fast, D.J., Nelson, R.D., and Schlievert, P.M. (1990) Staphylococcal and streptococcal pyrogenic toxins involved in toxic shock syndrome and related illnesses. *Crit. Rev. Microbiol.* **17,** 251–272.
62. Kapur, V., Reda, K.B., Li, L.L., Ho, L.J., Rich, R.R., and Musser, J.M. (1994) Characterization and distribution of insertion sequence IS1239 in Streptococcus pyogenes. *Gene* **150,** 135–140.
63. Sparwasser, T., Miethke, T., Lipford, G., Borschert, K., Hacker, H., Heeg, K., Et al. (1997) Bacterial DNA causes septic shock. *Nature* **386,** 336–337.
64. Shanley, T.P., Schrier, D., Kapur, V., Kehoe, M., Musser, J.M., and Ward, P.A. (1996) Streptococcal cysteine protease augments lung injury induced by products of group A streptococci. *Infect. Immun.* **64,** 870–877.
65. Norrby-Teglund, A. and Kotb, M. (2000) Host–microbe interactions in the pathogenesis of invasive group A streptococcal infections. *J. Med. Microbiol.* **49,** 849–852.
66. Miethke, T., Wahl, C., Regele, D., Gaus, H., Heeg, K., and Wagner, H. (1993) Superantigen mediated shock: a cytokine release syndrome. *Immunobiology* **189,** 270–284.
67. Marrack, P., Blackman, M., Kushnir, E., and Kappler, J. (1990) The toxicity of staphylococcal enterotoxin B in mice is mediated by T cells. *J. Exp. Med.* **171,** 455–464.
68. Mittrucker, H.W., Shahinian, A., Bouchard, D., Kundig, T.M., and Mak, T.W. (1996) Induction of unresponsiveness and impaired T cell expansion by staphylococcal enterotoxin B in CD28-deficient mice. *J. Exp. Med.* **183,** 2481–2488.
69. Saha, B., Harlan, D.M., Lee, K.P., June, C.H. and Abe, R. (1996) Protection against lethal toxic shock by targeted disruption of the CD28 gene. *J. Exp. Med.* **183,** 2675–2680.
70. Dinges, M.M. and Schlievert, P.M. (2001) Role of T cells and gamma interferon during induction of hypersensitivity to lipopolysaccharide by toxic shock syndrome toxin 1 in mice. *Infect. Immun.* **69,** 1256–1264.
71. Blank, C., Luz, A., Bendigs, S., Erdmann, A., Wagner, H., and Heeg, K. (1997) Superantigen and endotoxin synergize in the induction of lethal shock. *Eur. J. Immunol.* **27,** 825–833.
72. Michie, C., Scott, A., Cheesbrough, J., Beverley, P., and Pasvol, G. (1994) Streptococcal toxic shock-like syndrome: evidence of superantigen activity and its effects on T lymphocyte subsets in vivo. *Clin. Exp. Immunol.* **98,** 140–144.
73. Watanabe-Ohnishi, R., Low, D.E., McGeer, A., Stevens, D.L., Schlievert, P.M., Newton, D., et al. (1995) Selective depletion of V beta-bearing T cells in patients with severe invasive group A streptococcal infections and streptococcal toxic shock syndrome. Ontario Streptococcal Study Project. *J. Infect. Dis.* **171,** 74–84.
74. Sriskandan, S., Moyes, D., and Cohen, J. (1996) Detection of circulating bacterial superantigen and lymphotoxin-a in patients with streptococcal toxic-shock syndrome. *Lancet* **348,** 1315–1316.
75. Norrby-Teglund, A., Thulin, P., Gan, B.S., Kotb, M., McGeer, A., Andersson, J., et al. (2001) Evidence for superantigen involvement in severe group A streptococcal tissue infection. *J. Infect. Dis.* **186,** 853–860.
76. Norrby-Teglund, A., Pauksens, K., Holm, S.E., and Norgren, M. (1994) Relation between low capacity of human sera to inhibit streptococcal mitogens and serious manifestation of disease. *J. Infect. Dis.* **170,** 585–591.
77. Kaul, R., McGeer, A., Norrby-Teglund, A., Kotb, M., Schwartz, B., O'Rourke, K., et al. Streptococcal Study Group (1999) Intravenous immunoglobulin therapy for streptococcal toxic shock syndrome—a comparative observational study. *Clin. Infect. Dis.* **28,** 800–807.
78. Krieg, A.M., Yi, A.K., Matson, S., Waldschmidt, T.J., Bishop, G.A., Teasdale, R., et al. (1995) CpG DNA motifs in bacterial DNA trigger direct B-cell activation. *Nature* **374,** 546–549.
79. Klinman, D.M., Yi, A.K., Beaucage, S.L., Conover, J., and Krieg, A.M. (1996) CpG motifs present in bacterial DNA rapidly induce lymphocytes to secrete interleukin 6, interleukin 12, and interferon gamma. *Proc. Natl. Acad. Sci. USA* **93,** 2879–2883.
80. Heeg, K., Sparwasser, T., Lipford, G.B., Hacker, H., Zimmermann, S., and Wagner, H. (1998) Bacterial DNA as an evolutionary conserved ligand signalling danger of infection to immune cells. *Eur. J. Clin. Microbiol. Infect. Dis.* **17,** 464–469.

81. Hemmi, H., Takeuchi, O., Kawai, T., Kaisho, T., Sato, S., Sanjo, H., et al. (2000) A Toll-like receptor recognizes bacterial DNA. *Nature* **408**, 740–745.
82. Chatellier, S. and Kotb, M. (2000) Preferential stimulation of human lymphocytes by oligodeoxynucleotides that copy DNA CpG motifs present in virulent genes of group A streptococci. *Eur. J. Immunol.* **30**, 993–1001.
83. Rasmussen, M. and Bjorck, L. (2002) Proteolysis and its regulation at the surface of Streptococcus pyogenes. *Mol. Microbiol.* **43**, 537–544.
84. Kapur, V., Majesky, M.W., Li, L.L., Black, R.A., and Musser, J.M. (1993) Cleavage of interleukin 1 beta (IL-1 beta) precursor to produce active IL-1 beta by a conserved extracellular cysteine protease from Streptococcus pyogenes. *Proc. Natl. Acad. Sci. USA* **90**, 7676–7680.
85. Burns, E.H., Marciel, A.M., and Musser, J.M. (1996) Activation of a 66-kilodalton human endothelial cell matrix metalloprotease by Streptococcus pyogenes extracellular cysteine protease. *Infect. Immun.* **64**, 4744–4750.
86. Kapur, V., Topouzis, S., Majesky, M. W., Li, L. L., Hamrick, M. R., Hamill, R. J., et al. (1993) A conserved Streptococcus pyogenes extracellular cysteine protease cleaves human fibronectin and degrades vitronectin. *Microb. Pathog.* **15**, 327–346.
87. Herwald, H., Collin, M., Muller-Esterl, W. and Björck, L. (1996) Streptococcal cysteine proteinase releases kinins: a virulence mechanism. *J. Exp. Med.* **184**, 665–673.
88. Collin, M. and Olsén, A. (2001) Effect of SpeB and EndoS from Streptococcus pyogenes on human immunoglobulins. *Infect. Immun.* **69**, 7187–7189.
89. Ben Nasr, A.B., Herwald, H., Muller-Esterl, W., and Bjorck, L. (1995) Human kininogens interact with M protein, a bacterial surface protein and virulence determinant. *Biochem. J.* **305**, 173–180.
90. DeLa Cadena, R.A., Laskin, K.J., Pixley, R.A., Sartor, R.B., Schwab, J.H., Back, N., et al. (1991) Role of kallikrein–kinin system in pathogenesis of bacterial cell wall-induced inflammation. *Am. J. Physiol.* **260**, G213–G219.
91. Sriskandan, S. and Cohen, J. (2000) Kallikrein-kinin system activation in streptococcal toxic shock syndrome. *Clin. Infect. Dis.* **30**, 961–962.
92. Kapur, V., Maffei, J.T., Greer, R.S., Li, L.L., Adams, G.J., and Musser, J.M. (1994) Vaccination with streptococcal extracellular cysteine protease (interleukin-1 beta convertase) protects mice against challenge with heterologous group A streptococci. *Microb. Pathog.* **16**, 443–450.
93. Björck, L., Akesson, P., Bohus, M., Trojnar, J., Abrahamson, M., Olafsson, I., et al. (1989) Bacterial growth blocked by a synthetic peptide based on the structure of a human proteinase inhibitor. *Nature* **337**, 385–386.
94. Ashbaugh, C. D., Warren, H. B., Carey, V. J. and Wessels, M. R. (1998) Molecular analysis of the role of the group A streptococcal cysteine protease, hyaluronic acid capsule, and M protein in a murine model of human invasive soft-tissue infection. *J. Clin. Invest.* **102**, 550–560.
95. Kansal, R.G., McGeer, A., Low, D.E., Norrby-Teglund, A., and Kotb, M. (2000) Inverse relation between disease severity and expression of the streptococcal cysteine protease, SpeB, among clonal M1T1 isolates recovered from invasive group A streptococcal infection cases. *Infect. Immun.* **68**, 6362–6369.
96. Raeder, R., Harokopakis, E., Hollingshead, S., and Boyle, M.D. (2000) Absence of SpeB production in virulent large capsular forms of group A streptococcal strain 64. *Infect. Immun.* **68**, 744–751.
97. Raeder, R., Woischnik, M., Podbielski, A., and Boyle, M.D. (1998) A secreted streptococcal cysteine protease can cleave a surface-expressed M1 protein and alter the immunoglobulin binding properties. *Res. Microbiol.* **149**, 539–548.
98. Berge, A. and Björck, L. (1995) Streptococcal cysteine proteinase releases biologically active fragments of streptococcal surface proteins. *J. Biol. Chem.* **270**, 9862–9867.
99. Alouf, J.E. (1980) Streptococcal toxins (streptolysin O, streptolysin S, erythrogenic toxin). *Pharmacol. Ther.* **11**, 661–717.
100. Betschel, S.D., Borgia, S.M., Barg, N.L., Low, D.E., and De Azavedo, J.C. (1998) Reduced virulence of group A streptococcal Tn916 mutants that do not produce streptolysin S. *Infect. Immun.* **66**, 1671–1679.
101. Courtney, H.S., Ofek, I. and Hasty, D.L. (1997) M protein mediated adhesion of M type 24 Streptococcus pyogenes stimulates release of interleukin-6 by Hep-2 tissue culture cells. *FEMS Microbiol. Lett.* **151**, 65–70.
102. Ruiz, N., Wang, B., Pentland, A., and Caparon, M. (1998) Streptolysin O and adherence synergistically modulate proinflammatory responses of keratinocytes to group A streptococci. *Mol. Microbiol.* **27**, 337–346.
103. Wang, B., Ruiz, N., Pentland, A., and Caparon, M. (1997) Keratinocyte proinflammatory responses to adherent and nonadherent group A streptococci. *Infect. Immun.* **65**, 2119–2126.
104. Limbago, B., Penumalli, V., Weinrick, B., and Scott, J.R. (2000) Role of streptolysin O in a mouse model of invasive group A streptococcal disease. *Infect. Immun.* **68**, 6384–6390.
105. Bone, R.C. (1991) The pathogenesis of sepsis. *Ann. Intern. Med.* **115**, 457–469.
106. Cavaillon, J.M. and Adib-Conquy, M. (2000) The proinflammatory cytokine cascade, in *Update in Intensive Care and Emergency Medicine. Immune Responses in the Critically Ill* (Marschall, J.C. and Cohen, J., eds), Springer-Verlag, Berlin, New York. pp. 37–66
107. Bernhagen, J., Calandra, T., and Bucala, R. (1998) Regulation of the immune response by macrophage migration inhibitory factor: biological and structural features. *J. Mol. Med.* **76**, 151–161.
108. Wang, H., Bloom, O., Zhang, M., Vishnubhakat, J.M., Ombrellino, M., Che, J., et al. (1999) HMG-1 as a late mediator of endotoxin lethality in mice. *Science* **285**, 248–251.
109. Calandra, T., Echtenacher, B., Roy, D.L., Pugin, J., Metz, C.N., Hultner, L., et al. (2000) Protection from septic shock by neutralization of macrophage migration inhibitory factor. *Nat. Med.* **6**, 164–170.
110. Andersson, U., Wang, H., Palmblad, K., Aveberger, A.C., Bloom, O., Erlandsson-Harris, H., et al. (2000) High Mobility Group 1 Protein (HMG-1) Stimulates Proinflammatory Cytokine Synthesis in Human Monocytes. *J. Exp. Med.* **192**, 565–570.

111. Abraham, E. (1999) Why immunomodulatory therapies have not worked in sepsis. *Intensive Care Med.* **25,** 556–566.
112. Stevens, D.L., Bryant, A.E., Hackett, S.P., Chang, A., Peer, G., Kosanke, S., et al. (1996) Group A streptococcal bacteremia: the role of tumor necrosis factor in shock and organ failure. *J. Infect. Dis.* **173,** 619–626.
113. Cohen, J. (1999) Adjunctive therapy in sepsis: a critical analysis of the clinical trial programme. *Br. Med. Bull.* **55,** 212–215.
114. Fisher, C.J.J., Agosti, J.M., Opal, S.M., Lowry, S.F., Balk, R.A., Sadoff, J.C., et al. (1996) Treatment of septic shock with the tumor necrosis factor receptor:Fc fusion protein. The Soluble TNF Receptor Sepsis Study Group. *N. Engl. J. Med.* **334,** 1697–1702.
115. Raeder, R.H., Barker-Merrill, L., Lester, T., Boyle, M.D. and Metzger, D.W. (2000) A pivotal role for interferon-gamma in protection against group A streptococcal skin infection. *J. Infect. Dis.* **181,** 639–645.
116. Norrby-Teglund, A., Pauksens, K., Norgren, M., and Holm, S. (1995) Correlation between serum TNFα and IL6 levels and severity of group A streptococcal infections. *Scand. J. Infect. Dis.* **27,** 125–130.
117. Norrby-Teglund, A., Chatellier, S., Low, D.E., McGeer, A., Green, K., and Kotb, M. (2000) Host variation in cytokine responses to superantigens determine the severity of invasive group A streptococcal infection. *Eur. J. Immunol.* **30,** 3247–3255.
118. Sriskandan, S., Moyes, D., Lemm, G. and Cohen, J. (1996) Lymphotoxin-α (TNF-β) during sepsis. *Cytokine* **8,** 933–937.
119. Andersson, J. and Andersson, U. (1993) Characterization of cytokine production in infectious mononucleosis studied at a single-cell level in tonsil and peripheral blood. *Clin. Exp. Immunol.* **92,** 7–13.
120. Schrager, H.M., Alberti, S., Cywes, C., Dougherty, G.J., and Wessels, M.R. (1998) Hyaluronic acid capsule modulates M protein-mediated adherence and acts as a ligand for attachment of group A streptococcus to CD44 on human keratinocytes. *J. Clin. Invest.* **101,** 1708–1716.
121. Cywes, C., Stamenkowic, I., and Wessels, M.R. (2000) CD44 as a receptor for colonization of the pharynx by group A streptococcus. *J. Clin. Invest.* **106,** 995–1002.
122. Cywes, C. and Wessels, M.R. (2001) Group A Streptococcus tissue invasion by CD44-mediated cell signalling. *Nature* **414,** 648–652.
123. DeGrendele, H. C., Kosfiszer, M., Estess, P., and Siegelman, M. H. (1997) CD44 activation and associated primary adhesion is inducible via T cell receptor stimulation. *J. Immunol.* **159,** 2549–2553.
124. DeGrendele, H.C., Estess, P., and Siegelman, M.H. (1997) Requirement for CD44 in activated T cell extravasation into an inflammatory site. *Science* **278,** 672–675.
125. Robert, C. and Kupper, T.S. (1999) Inflammatory skin diseases, T cells, and immune surveillance. *N. Engl. J. Med.* **341,** 1817–1828.
126. Leung, D.Y., Gately, M., Trumble, A., Ferguson-Darnell, B., Schlievert, P.M., and Picker, L.J. (1995) Bacterial superantigens induce T-cell expression of the skin-selective homing receptor, the cutaneous lymphocyte-associated antigen, via stimulation of interleukine 12 production. *J. Exp. Med.* **181,** 747–753.
127. Strickland, I., Hauk, P.J., Trumble, A.E., Picker, L.J., and Leung, D.Y. (1999) Evidence for superantigen involvement in skin homing of T cells in atopic dermatitis. *J. Invest. Dermatol.* **112,** 249–253.
128. Norrby-Teglund, A., Kaul, R., Low, D.E., McGeer, A., Newton, D., Andersson, J., et al. (1996) Plasma from patients with severe invasive group A streptococcal infections treated with normal polyspecific IgG inhibits streptococcal superantigen-induced T cell proliferation and cytokine production. *J. Immunol.* **156,** 3057–3064.
129. Arad, G., Levy, R., Hillman, D., and Kaempfer, R. (2000) Superantigen antagonist protects against lethal shock and defines a new domain for T-cell activation. *Nat. Med.* **6,** 414–421.
130. Visvanathan, K., Charles, A., Bannan, J., Pugach, P., Kashfi, K., and Zabriskie, J.B. (2001) Inhibition of bacterial superantigens by peptides and antibodies. *Infect. Immun.* **69,** 875–884.
131. Norrby-Teglund, A. and Stevens, D.L. (1998) Novel therapies in streptococcal toxic shock syndrome: attenuation of virulence factor expression and modulation of the host response. *Curr. Opin. Infect. Dis.* **11,** 285–291.
132. Wang, B., Schlievert, P.M., Gaber, A.O., and Kotb, M. (1993) Localization of an immunologically functional region of the streptococcal superantigen pepsin-extracted fragment of type 5 M protein. *J. Immunol.* **151,** 1419–1429.

7

Superantigens and Bacterial DNA as Cytokine Inducers in Gram-Positive Sepsis

Klaus Heeg

1. INTRODUCTION

Gram-positive bacteria like *Staphylococcus aureus* cause severe and life-threatening infections, including systemic bacteremia (sepsis) and local infections that eventually may lead to toxic shock syndrome (TSS). In addition, staphylococci not only play an important role as a single causative agent of a systemic infection, but they also can be isolated frequently from blood cultures, together with other infectious agents, especially Gram-negative bacteria. Although major steps in the pathogenesis of Gram-negative infections have been elucidated in the last decades, it was unknown for a long time which constitutive components or induced products of staphylococci would contribute to pathogenesis of staphylococcal infections.

A major breakthrough in the general understanding of an infection was the finding that innate immune cells sense infectious danger by the recognition of conserved bacterial products or constituents via phylogenetically conserved receptors *(1,2)*. According to their counterparts in nonmammalians, they are termed Toll-like receptors (TLRs). So far, 10 distinct TLRs have been identified, of which TLR4 is mandatory for recognition of lipopolysaccharide (LPS) *(3)*. However, opposed to Gram-negative, bacteria staphylococci do not synthesize LPS (endotoxin), a key mediator in pathogenesis of infections with Gram-negative bacteria *(4)*. Therefore, other components or products of staphylococci mediate initial activation of the innate immune system, which eventually lead to inflammation and systemic cytokine syndrome (shock). Several constituents of staphylococci have been identified to exert activation of innate immune cells in a TLR-dependent manner: peptidoglycan (PepG), lipoteichoic acid (LTA) *(5)* and bacterial DNA (CpG-DNA) *(6)*. In addition, secreted products of staphylococci also play an important role in activating and regulating the innate immune system: pore-forming toxins *(7)* and superantigens *(8–10)*. This chapter focuses on two of these components: CpG-DNA and superantigens (SAgs).

2. SUPERANTIGENS

2.1. Superantigens: Mode of Action

A group of proteins has been termed Sag; they share a unique mechanism to interact with innate as well as adaptive immune cells. These features distinguish SAgs from conventional proteins and characterize an alternative pathway of antigen presentation and subsequent activation of T-cells *(11)*. According to the classical method of antigen presentation, foreign proteins are taken up by professional antigen-presenting cells, subsequently degraded in specialized intracellular compartments, and,

From: *Cytokines and Chemokines in Infectious Diseases Handbook*
Edited by: M. Kotb and T. Calandra © Humana Press Inc., Totowa, NJ

finally, presented as small peptide fragments within the groove of major histocompatibility complex (MHC) class II molecules to peptide reactive T-lymphocytes *(12)*. The fraction of reacting T-lymphocytes corresponds to the specificity of their clonally distributed T-cell receptor, representing only a minor fraction of the total antigen-reactive T-cell pool. In contrast to conventional antigen, SAgs bypass these rate-limiting steps of antigen processing and bind directly as an intact protein to MHC class II molecules on the surface of antigen-presenting cells (*see* Fig. 1) *(13–15)*. Furthermore, a SAg bound to MHC class II interacts then with regions of the β-chain of the T-cell receptor (TCR) that are encoded by the Vβ gene segments of the TCR gene locus *(16–18)*. Because the number of distinct Vβ gene segments is limited, SAgs target many more T-cells than conventional antigens. Depending of the individual SAg and the host species, individual SAgs are thus capable of reacting with up to 25% of all peripheral T-lymphocytes.

Most prominent SAgs are the staphylococcal enterotoxins (SEs) *(11)* and the streptococcal pryogenic exotoxins (SPEs) *(19)*, although many different bacteria as well as viruses have been shown to produce superantigeneic proteins. Staphylococcal enterotoxins were first detected as causative agents in staphylococcal-dependent gastroenteritis. They do not comprise a single entity. Genetically distinct staphylococcal enterotoxins have been described (SEA–SET) *(20)* that share the SAg properties yet differ in their binding affinity to MHC class II as well as in their preference for certain Vβ chains. Moreover, SAg production is not a quality of a subpopulation staphylococci, rather it is a general feature of pathogenic *Staphylococcus aureus* strains [e.g., more than 50% of *S. aureus* isolates are able to produce at least one of the SAgs *(21)*].

Although SEs have been recognized long ago, their superantigeneic properties were discovered not until the late 1980s *(22,23)*. First, it was recognized that enterotoxins are mitogenic for peripheral blood lymphocytes and, subsequently, also for certain, but not all, T-cell clones *(13)*. It was the epochal work of White et al. that correlated the selective mitogenicity of enterotoxins for T-cells to the T-cell's usage of certain Vβ encoded TCR β-chains *(24)*.

2.2. The In Vivo Response to SAg: Progression from Activation to Unresponsiveness

Introduction of SAg into mice leads to a complex pattern of concomitant and sequential reactivities that ultimately results in clonal anergy and unresponsiveness of the reactive T-cells *(25–27)*. SAg injected locally enters the draining lymph system within minutes and floats into the local lymph nodes *(28)*. There, SAg binds to MHC class II positive cells (macrophages, dendritic cells [DC] and B-cells) and subsequently activates the respective Vβ-bearing T-cells. T-Cell activation takes place within minutes because loss of L-selectin expression of the reacting T-cells can be measured after 10–15 min *(29)*. T-Cells are activated and start to initiate transcription and translation of a wide variety of cytokine mRNAs, including those for interleukin (IL)-2, tumor necrosis factor (TNF), and interferon-γ (IFN-γ) *(30)*. After 1–2 h, cytokines can be detected systemically in the sera of mice. IL-2 and TNF secretion is shut down after reaching peak values at 2–4 h *(31)*. In contrast, IL-10 production reaches its maximum after 24 h. Initial cytokine secretion is strictly dependent on T-cells, because the T-cell-specific immunosuppressive agent CsA is inhibitory and because T-cell-deficient mutant mice do not respond to SAgs *(31,32)*.

During this initial phase, cytokine release triggers wasting of mice accompanied with a transient loss of weight, symptoms that are probably brought about by the systemic action of TNF *(32)*. When very high doses of SAgs are used or when mice are presensitized to the action of TNF by D-galactosamine (D-GalN) treatment, mice succumb to lethal cytokine syndrome *(31)*. Lethal outcome is caused by the systemic action of TNF because anti-TNF monoclonal antibodies prevent death *(31)*. Moreover, TNF receptor p55 knockout (KO) mice or TNF KO mice survive SAg bolus injection. Thus, in the initial phase, Sag-induced lethality resembles that of LPS-induced lethal cytokine syndrome in that both are dependent on overshooting TNF production. In contrast to LPS-induced shock that depends on the activation of CD14- and TLR4-positive innate immune cells, Sag-induced shock critically relies on the activation of T-lymphocytes.

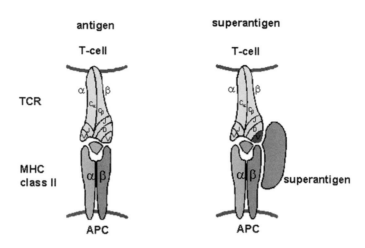

Fig. 1. Recognition of antigen and superantigen.

After initial hyperactivation, Sag-induced T-cells transit to a refractory state, where TCR triggering fails to induce further cellular responses like IL-2 secretion *(33,34)*. The refractory state is Vβ selective and followed by a stepwise and transient downregulation of TCR- and coreceptors like CD4/CD8 or CD2 *(34)*. Depending on the strength of activation, a significant proportion of T-cells undergo apoptosis. However, the remaining cells express IL-2 R and start extensive proliferation and Vβ selective expansion *(35)*. After 2 d Sag-reactive T-cells comprise more than 50% of all T-cells in secondary lymphoid organs. Thereafter, expansion ceases and most Sag-reactive T-cells die via apoptosis *(36)*. The proportion of the remaining SAg-specific Vβ expressing T-cell population is less than normal and characterized by an anergic state *(37,38)*. These T-cells fail to respond to further stimulation to SAgs as well as to conventional antigens *(39)*. Hence, after initial activation, SAgs induce long-lasting Vβ selective T-cell anergy.

2.3. SAg Effects on Innate Immune Cells (Antigen-Presenting Cells)

Superantigens activate MHC class II-expressing antigen-presenting cells (APCs) by two routes *(40)*. It has been shown that several SAg are capable of crosslinking MHC class II molecules on APC and thus induce activation and induction of APC function *(41)*. On the other hand, cytokines derived from SAg-activated T-lymphocytes critically control APC function. The latter mechanisms seems to be dominant, because blockade of T-cell-derived cytokines by the T-cell-specific immunosuppressive agent cyclosporine A (CsA) suppresses most of the effects of SAgs on APCs. Two waves of reactivities characterize the cytokine-mediated effects on APC *(42)*. Initially, effector cytokines like IFN-γ and TNF activate APCs and enhance immunostimulation as well as bactericidal effector functions of macrophages. One important first-step effector mechanism is induction of the inducible NO synthase (iNOS) *(43)*, which, in turn, enhances the bactericidal macrophage functions. Indeed, after SEB pretreatment mice display an enhanced resistance to otherwise lethal injection with Listeria monocytogenes (unpublished observations). After initial activation, regulatory cytokines like IL-10 *(44)*, which peak 24 h after SAg injection, take over control: the antigen-presentation function of APCs is inhibited *(45,46)*. In fact, APC derived from mice 24 h after treatment with SAg fail to stimulate peptide- or Sag-specific naïve T-lymphocytes.

2.4. SAg and Induction of Lethal Cytokine Syndrome

After oligoclonal activation of Sag-reactive Vβ expressing T-cells, a burst of proinflammatory cytokines is released. TNF serum levels peak after 2 h and then fall back to background values *(31)*. In contrast, IL-2 and IFN-γ levels peak later (4 h) and can still be detected after 16 h. Compared to the endotoxin response, the peak values for TNF are rather low. In normal mice, these low systemic amounts of TNF fail to induce lethal systemic responses (e.g., a lethal cytokine syndrome). If, however, the hepatic acute-phase response is blocked by prior administration of D-GalN SAg-induced TNF levels are sufficient for liver cell apoptosis and subsequent lethality *(31,47)*. Hence, SAgs, at least in an experimental model of shock, are rather inefficient to induce directly and solitarily a lethal cytokine syndrome. Nevertheless, in humans, SAgs are the key mediators of the toxic shock syndrome, which is characterized by a systemic action of locally produced superantigens *(48)*.

2.5. SAg and Its Functional Interactions with Lipopolysaccharides

Although SAg *per se* are rather poor inducers of a systemic cytokine response, their interactions with other inducers of septic shock are of immense importance. Two forms of relations can be operationally distinguished: acute synergism and sensitization to LPS.

When SAgs and LPS are given to mice concomitantly, both inducers synergize in inducing macrophage activation and production of cytokines *(49,50)*. Resulting TNF serum levels increased several-fold and mice died of lethal shock without being presensitized with D-GalN *(47)*. Thus, combined injection of SAgs and LPS leads to an acute cytokine syndrome that resembles septic shock, yet does not require artificial manipulation of mice. Interestingly, mice die after injection of SAgs and LPS at later time-points with only minor signs of disintegration of the liver *(47)*. Instead, they show apoptotic areas in the gut (large intestine) and in the hippocampus. In mice with no T-cells or mice with a suppressed T-cell system (e.g., CsA), SAgs and LPS fail to manifest this synergistic response. Synergism is also characterized by up to a 100-fold reduction of the doses of SAgs or LPS required to induce complete lethality *(47)*.

Although SAgs and LPS target different responder cells and thus induce macrophage as well as T-cell-derived TNF, this mechanism only partially explains the synergistic effects observed. Experiments using anti-IFN-γ monoclonal antibodies (mAbs) and IFN-γ receptor KO mice point to another explanation *(47)*. Because blockade of IFN-γ by mAb completely prevented synergism, this T-cell-derived cytokine seems to be a key mediator. Accordingly, SAgs induce high IFN-γ production from reacting T-cells. The mechanism of the resulting IFN-γ mediated synergism might be twofold. First, IFN-γ might synergize together with TNF and IL-6 in inducing lethal cytokine responses. Indeed, such cytokine-mediated effects have been demonstrated *(51)*. However, this mechanism does not explain elevated TNF serum levels in mice treated with SAgs and LPS. Therefore, a second mechanism could be operative. T-Cell-derived IFN-γ would activate macrophages that, in turn, now become hyperresponsive to LPS and thus produce higher amounts of TNF *(52,53)*. Hence, SAgs and LPS target different responder cells and the in vivo immune response to these stimuli is interconnected at the level of cytokines. The interconnectivity of distinct stimuli might result in stronger and synergistically enhanced responses of the innate immune system. Because both LPS and SAgs are effective not only at the local site of infection but also systemically, these interactions might occur frequently and might critically determine the fate of an infection.

2.6. SAg Induce Sensitization of Innate Immune
Cells to LPS (Shwartzman-like Reaction)

Whereas pretreatment of mice with high doses of LPS induces a transient state of hyporeactivity (LPS tolerance), injection of low doses of LPS leads to a systemic hyperreactivity toward a subsequent challenge with LPS (Shwartzman reaction) *(54)*. IL-12 and IFN-γ have been identified as key cytokines conveying sensitization *(52,54)*.

Perhaps the most prominent action of SAgs in vivo during lethal cytokine syndrome is the induction of a Shwartzman-like reaction *(55)*. When SAgs are injected into mice, they induce a transient state of hyperreactivity to LPS. The hyperreactive period starts 8 h after SAg administration and lasts for at least another 24 h. During that period, administration of LPS leads to an overshooting production of cytokines by macrophages. TNF serum levels have been observed that are up to 100-fold higher than in nonsensitized mice *(55)*. Moreover, macrophages from sensitized mice produce IFN-γ even when triggered with LPS. This tremendous storm of cytokines is, again, lethal for mice without prior pretreatment with D-GalN. The key mediator of presensitization is IFN-γ, because anti-IFN-γ mAbs completely block this Shwartzman-like reaction *(55)*. Presensitized macrophages display higher expression of CD14 molecules on their surface. This upregulation overlaps in time with the sensitized phenotype. In addition, these cells also express the chains of the IL-2 receptor complex: IL-2R-α, -β, and -γ. Upregulation of these molecules is dependent on T-cell-derived IFN-γ because anti-IFN-γ mAbs as well as CsA block these changes (unpublished observations). Surprisingly, the upregulated IL-2R complexes are functional at least in vitro, because peritoneal macrophages isolated from mice that were preinjected with SAg respond with TNF secretion upon stimulation with recombinant IL-2. Thus, presensitized macrophages not only show an enhanced responsiveness to endotoxin, but also respond to stimuli that otherwise have no direct effect on these cells.

Taken together, SAgs gain importance during infection because of their oligoclonal T-cell stimulation. It is not only the direct effect of SAgs that may eventually induce a toxic shock syndrome, but, of equal importance, it is their indirect action on innate immune cells like macrophages. The key mediator of these effects is T-cell-derived IFN-γ that critically influences macrophage function and regulates the response of these cells to other stimuli like LPS. Prominent effects of SAgs are acute synergism with LPS and induction of a Shwartzman-like reaction that sensitizes the immune system to endotoxin (*see* Fig. 2).

3. BACTERIAL DNA AS MICROBIAL PATTERN

3.1. Bacterial DNA and CpG Motifs: Historical Aspects

For a long time, DNA was considered immunologically inert; however, this notion was challenged and completely changed in the last decade. Three initially independent lines of scientific experimentation led to the formulation of the concept of immunostimulative CpG DNA. The first track started in the 1970s with the observation that *Mycobacteria* could be used to treat cancer *(56)*. In attempting to identify the underlying principle, Tokunaga and colleagues identified the active component in their mycobacterial preparations as a DNA-rich fraction; they termed it MY-1 *(57)*. My-1 not only caused tumor regression but also activated natural killed (NK) cells and induced IFN production *(58)*. They further noted that only bacterial DNA but not mammalian DNA was effective *(59)*. A breakthrough was the observation that single-stranded oligonucleotides selected from mycobacterial genomic sequences were able to mimic the effects of bacterial DNA *(60)*. This, in turn, allowed the identification of a minimal DNA motif, which induced NK activation and cytokine secretion. The motif was characterized as a six-base palindrominc sequence. The motif was most effective when the central bases were comprised of a cytosine and guanosine (CpG) *(61)*.

In analyzing the immune response of systemic lupus erythematosus (SLE), Pisetzky and colleagues reported that bacterial DNA but not mammalian DNA could be found in immune complexes in plasma of SLE patients *(62)*. They were able to show further that bacterial DNA was mitogenic for B-lymphocytes and induced polyclonal IgM responses *(63)*. Interestingly, methylation of synthetic oligonucleotides resulted in complete loss of the DNA's immunogenicity. Finally, Krieg and colleagues defined immunostimulative motifs in analyzing unexpected side effects of antisense oligonucleotides, targeted to inhibited certain endogenous and exogenous genes *(64)*. These side effects included proliferation and clonal expansion of B-cells as well as upregulation of MHC class II molecules *(65)*. In elegant work, this group defined the base sequence requirements for optimal mitogenicity on B-cells. They found that a hexameric motif in single-stranded oligonucleotides is mandatory for the immunostimulatory effects: two purins at the 5' end, centered by a CpG dinucleotide, and two pyrimidines at the 3' end (5'-Pur-Pur-CpG-Pyr-Pyr-3'). Whenever an oligonucleotide contained such an sequence motif, it was immunostimulatory on B-lymphocytes *(65,66)*.

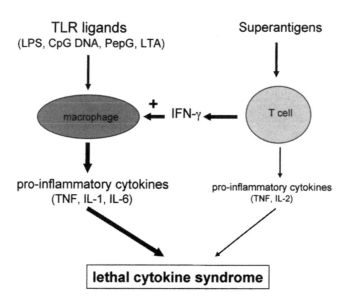

Fig. 2. Role of superantigens during sensitization to endotoxin.

3.2. CpG-Sequence Motifs Confer Immunostimulatory Activity to DNA

Although both bacterial and mammalian DNA contain CpG dinucleotides and, thus, immunostimulatory motifs, the frequency of immunoactive CpG dinucleotides is different. First, the overall frequency of CpG dinucleotides is reduced in mammalian DNA, a phenomenon that has been recognized long ago as "CpG-suppression" *(67)*. Second, most cytosine bases in mammalian DNA are methylated, whereas methylation only rarely occurs in bacterial DNA *(68)*. Therefore, it is generally accepted that "free" CpG dinucleotides of bacterial DNA represent a structural pattern that can be recognized by innate immune cells *(69)*.

Cytosine and guanosine dinucleotides are recognized by innate immune cells in the context of 5' and 3' flanking regions. For mice, a hexameric motif has been described (*see* Section 3.1) *(65)*. However, other mammalian species recognize CpG dinucleotides in the context of different flanking regions *(70–72)*. An effective motif for human cells seems to contain multiple CpG dinucleotides and flanking regions with less stringent sequence requirements. In addition to the classical CpG DNA, other DNA sequence motifs have been described that display different biological effects *(73)*. Oligonucleotides containing multiple guanosine residues activate NK cells and not macrophages and thus represent a second class of immunostimulatory DNA *(73; unpublished data)*. Moreover, DNA sequences derived from adenoviral sequences have antagonistic properties and block the action of CpG DNA *(74)*. Synthetic DNA sequences with similar characteristics have been described also *(73,75)*. Thus, the DNA molecule itself is able to interact with and signal innate immune cells at multiple levels and with different outcomes, depending on its base sequence.

3.3. CpG DNA: Uptake and Mode of Action

The mode of action of CpG DNA was primarily elucidated with synthetic oligonucleotides as a probe for immunostimulatory DNA. For some effects of CpG DNA, it is still controversial whether CpG DNA has to be taken up or whether CpG DNA exerts its effects by binding of an cell surface receptor. The latter mechanism may apply for some effects of CpG DNA on human B-lymphocytes. In contrast, it is generally accepted that the action of CpG on innate immune cells like dendritic cells (DCs) or macrophages requires cellular uptake. An involvement of specific receptors (e.g., the scavenger receptor) is still under debate *(76,77)*. Lysosomotropic substances like chloroquine or

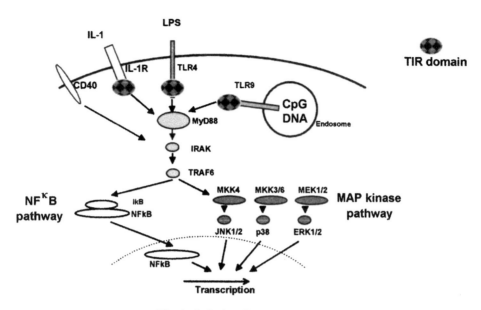

Fig. 3. CpG signaling pathways.

bafilomycin block effect of synthetic CpG DNA as well as of bacterial DNA preparations *(78–80)*. Thus, initiation of CpG-dependent signals seem to occur in the early endosomal compartment. After triggering cells with CpG DNA, signal cascades are activated within minutes *(79,80)*. Those include the MAP kinase pathway and translocation of nuclear factor (NF)-κB that induce transcription of the relevant genes.

In comparing different signal pathways, it became evident that CpG DNA triggers signal pathways, that are indistinguishable from other signal pathways like the LPS triggered pathways or IL-1R-related signaling cascades *(81)*. Moreover, it was shown that essential intracellular signal adaptor proteins like MyD88 or TRAF6 are shared by these signal pathways *(82)* (*see* Fig. 3). A major breakthrough was the description of a new receptor class that shares homology with a receptor system in *Drosophila* termed the "Toll receptor." Toll receptors are important in embryonic development and for initiation of appropriate immunological response to infection. In humans, 10 receptor homologs have been found so far (Toll-like receptor, TLR) *(3,83,84)*. All TLRs contain an intracellular domain termed "TIR," which links the TLR to the intracellular signal adaptor molecules (*see* Fig. 3). Because LPS signal transduction was attributed to TLR4 *(85,86)*, it was no major surprise when TLR9 could be identified recently as the signal transducing receptor in CpG DNA signaling *(87)*. Individual TLR receptors show distinct pattern of expression. TLR 9 is primarily expressed on B-lymphocytes, macrophages, and DCs. In humans, plasmacytoid DCs express high levels of TLR9, whereas monocytic DCs show no expression *(88)*. Interestingly, the distinct CpG motif requirements in human and mouse correlate with the respective TLR9 molecule. Thus, cells transfected with murine TLR9 are responsive to the murine CpG motif, whereas the same cells transfected with the human TLR9 molecule respond to the human CpG motif. Interestingly, preliminary evidence suggests that in contrast to TLR4 expression, TLR9 seems to be confined to the endosomal compartment. That would explain why CpG DNA has to be taken up to exert its immunostimulatory function.

3.4. CpG DNA: Effects

The most relevant effect of CpG DNA, irrespective of whether synthetic DNA or bacterial DNA is used, is its effect on APCs such as DCs or macrophages *(70,89)*. Within minutes, these cells become activated and respond with a variety of distinct effects. Rapid induction of proinflammatory cytokines

(TNF, IL-12) as well as upregulation of the antigen-presenting machinery (expression of MHC molecules and costimulatory molecules) is observed *(89,90)*. In mice, immature DCs differentiate into mature DCs and enhance their potency to present antigen to T-cells *(89)*. The initial production of proinflammatory cytokines is followed by secretion of regulatory cytokines such as IL-10. B-Cells are polyclonally activated by CpG DNA and produce IgM. NK lymphocytes respond with secretion of IFN-γ *(71)*; this response is indirect and the result of macrophage-derived IL-12 *(91)*. Finally, it was reported that CpG DNA stimulates extramedullary hemopoiesis *(92)*.

Compared to other TLR-dependent microbial patterns, stimulation with CpG DNA is most effective in inducing IL-12 *(93,94)*. This, in turn, indicates that individual signal pathways might exist that critically determine the biological valence of a TLR stimulus. One can speculate that this selective signaling could be caused by distinct TIR domain-selective intracellular signal adaptor proteins in addition to MyD88 *(95)*. Furthermore, the marked propensity of CpG DNA to induce high amounts of IL-12 classifies CPG DNA opposed to LPS or LTA as a powerful agent to assist the induction of T-cell responses *(96)*. Indeed, CpG DNA has been used as an immune adjuvant in vaccination studies with promising results (for a review, see ref. *97*). Moreover, CpG DNA not only favors T-cell activation but also directs ongoing T-cell responses to an Th1-type response characterized by IFN-γ secretion and suppression of IL-4 *(98)*. In infection models for Th2-mediated diseases (murine leishmaniasis) CpG DNA was capable of preventing induction of lethal Th2-mediated pathology and even was able to cure established Th2 illness *(99)*. It is thought that these Th1-promoting effects of CpG DNA during infection disfavor induction of undesired Th2 profiles, as in allergies. Accordingly, infection directs an immune system toward the Th1 type of reactivity via the action of CpG DNA *(100)* (*see* Fig. 4). The hygiene hypothesis of induction allergy follows this line of argument *(101)*.

3.5. CpG DNA: Pathophysiology

Because of its immunostimulatory properties, CpG DNA can cause a lethal cytokine syndrome, at least in experimental animals *(6)*. Synthetic oligonucleotides as well as bacteria-derived DNA activated innate immune cells, followed by an intensive release of proinflammatory cytokines, including TNF, IL-6, and IFN-γ *(6,102)*. This cocktail of mediators induces lethal shock. LPS nonresponder mice as well as T-cell-deficient mice are as susceptible to the CpG DNA-mediated cytokine syndrome as normal wild-type mice, indicating that, primarily, the DCs and macrophages respond to CpG DNA in a TLR4-independent fashion *(103)*. Pathophysiological effectiveness has been attributed to DNA derived from bacteria. DNA isolated from vertebrate sources (e.g., calf thymus DNA) is ineffective. However, not only prokaryotic DNA but also eukaryotic DNA might be immunostimulative. It has been reported that DNA derived from *Drosophila* is capable of inducing the production of type I interferons *(104)*. Thus, recognition of nonvertebrate foreign DNA seems to be a distinctive property of the vertebrate's innate immune system.

There are indications that DNA from different bacterial species might have not the same immunostimulatory potency on a molecular base. This might be the result of a characteristic mixture of immunostimulatory and inhibitory DNA sequence motifs within the genomic DNA of individual species. Because the immunostimulatory DNA motifs recognized by different vertebrate species differ (*see* Section 3.4) *(88)*, it is attempting to speculate that during coevolution, bacteria have been selected according to the immunoreactivity of their DNA. Accordingly, the immunostimulatory potency of DNA from individual bacteria could be different when tested with innate immune cells of a natural host compared to other species. In addition, synthetic DNA fragments from individual isolates of pathogenic bacteria show different immunostimulative properties that were linked to their pathophysiological effectiveness *(105)*.

3.6. CpG DNA and Its Relation to Other Bacterial Stimuli

Because CpG DNA triggers similar intracellular signal pathways as other TLR-related microbial stimuli like PepG or LTA, it is no surprise that a combined treatment of APCs with TLR-dependent

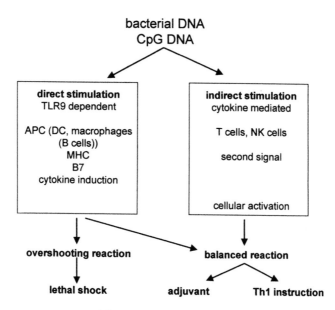

Fig. 4. Effects of CpG DNA.

stimuli would be additive. Additive effects of CpG DNA can be observed with LPS or LTA not only in vitro but also in vivo and relate to cytokine induction as well as on cellular activation and upregulation of antigen presentation *(106;* unpublished observations). Treatment of macrophages with high doses of LPS primarily induces activation, followed by a transient state of paralysis termed "LPS tolerance" *(107).* The mechanism of this effect is not yet completely understood; yet, recent data suggest that TLR4 expression might be downregulated upon stimulation with LPS *(108).* However, there are also indications that intracellular TLR-related signal cascades are affected causing a cistype of signal inhibition. Accordingly, in vitro triggering with CpG DNA induces a state of refractory toward CpG DNA, which resembles LPS tolerance. This refractory state not only affects stimulation with TLR9-dependent ligands (CpG DNA) but also the stimulatory activity of LPS or LTA (unpublished observations). Thus, in vitro, individual TLR-dependent ligands induce a state of refractoriness (tolerance), which includes also the reactivity to other TLR ligands. One could term these effects "cross-tolerance" *(109).* Because different TLRs are involved in cross-tolerance, it can be assumed that tolerance operates at the level of shared intracellular signal processing pathways.

Although cross-tolerance can be observed easily on macrophage cell lines in vitro, the mutual effects of TLR ligands might be different in vivo. It has been shown that preinjection of mice with CpG DNA does not inhibit the response to a subsequent challenge with LPS; rather, it enhances the response *(110).* These apparently contradicting findings can be explained by the different cellular tropisms of TLRs and distinct cellular responses. Although CpG DNA induces tolerance in vitro on isolated macrophages, in vivo, CpG DNA also is a strong inducer of NK-cell-derived IFN-γ. Because the enhancing effect of CpG DNA on LPS reactivity can be blocked by inhibiting IFN-γ and because IFN-γ sensitizes macrophages, one can conclude that, in vivo, the CpG DNA-mediated tolerization effects are overridden by CpG-induced IFN-γ *(110).* Thus, depending on the profile of induced cellular responses, CpG DNA might enhance or suppress cellular reactivities to other TLR ligands. These observations point to a rather complex interplay between different TLR ligands during infection.

3.7. CpG DNA and Its Regulatory Effects on Cytokine Signaling

CpG DNA activates signal cascades within innate immune cells that ultimately lead to transcription and translation of a set of response genes *(81,111,112).* This set not only is comprised of cytokine

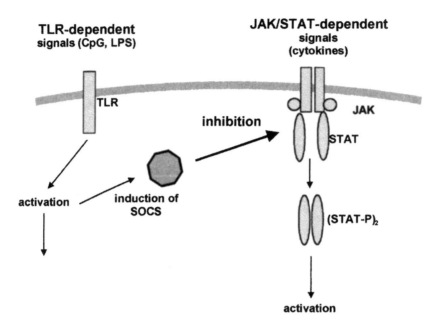

Fig. 5. CpG-mediated regulation of cytokine signaling in macrophages.

genes or genes involved in antigen presentation, but also includes genes of the family of "suppressors of cytokine signaling", (SOCS). SOCS proteins first have been described as negative regulators of the JAK–STAT signal pathway, being induced by the respective receptor ligands *(113,114)*; for example, IFN-γ signals via JAK–STAT-dependent pathways and induces the expression of SOCS1as a negative control mechanism, which, in turn, inhibits STAT-dependent signaling. In analyzing the response of macrophages, it was found that the TLR4 ligand LPS also effectively induced SOCS expression. LPS-induced SOCS proteins were effective because they inhibited the cellular responses to IFN-γ *(115)*. The same was found to be true for CpG and an LTA-mediated cellular stimulation *(116)*. Accordingly, it was shown that TLR-dependent stimulation not only induced the classical proinflammatory response genes but also negative regulators that shut off the cellular response to regulatory cytokines (*see* Fig. 5). Depending on their receptor structure and induced signaling cascades, cytokines using JAK–STAT signal pathways are critically influenced by this mechanism. Those include IFN-γ, granulocyte colony-stimulating factor, and IL-6 *(116,117)*. Because expression of SOCS proteins seems not to interfere with intracellular TLR-related signals, one has to assume that TLR stimulation induces a type of trans-regulatory response. The key target might be IFN-γ, whose activating effects on macrophages can be completely blocked by SOCS proteins.

Cis and trans negative regulation induced by TLR stimulation might have important consequences during infection. Although TLR dependent ligands interact and collaborate during initial activation of innate immune cells, the induced response also includes negative regulatory events that influence TLR signaling (cis) and cytokine signaling (trans). It is obvious that these regulatory mechanism, when triggered in a timely coordinated fashion (as in severe infections), might induce a subsequent immunosuppression or immunoparalysis. This paralysis, in turn, might critically determine the outcome of an infection.

4. CONCLUDING REMARKS

The recent years have witnessed a tremendous gain in understanding the molecular mechanisms of the interaction of bacteria with the innate immune cells. These developments not only will help to unravel the complex activating and regulatory pathophysiological event during infection but also may shade light into new pathways of a rational therapy. In this context, both superantigens and bacterial DNA are new and important players. SAgs are important during infection as a direct activator and, perhaps more important, as an indirect regulator of macrophage function. Blocking SAgs by monoclonal antibodies or by inhibiting the overshooting T-cell response might be new strategies to combat certain infections. CpG DNA, on the other hand, has extended the family of microbial pattern recognized by innate immune cells. In contrast to other TLR-dependent stimuli, the immunostimulatory capacity of CpG DNA can be exploited by using synthetic oligonucleotides as adjuvant or Th1/Th2 immunomodulators. Nevertheless, the exact role of CpG DNA during infection has still to be defined. However, synthetic inhibitory DNA sequences may allow one, in the future, to selectively inhibit bacterial CpG DNA. Finally, in elucidating the consequences of TLR-activated intracellular signal cascades and the subsequent expression of regulatory gene products, different phases of immunoreactivity during infection could be defined at a mechanistic level. Whether these new regulatory mechanisms will result in new strategies to directly manipulate an immune response during severe infection will be a rewarding task to answer in the future.

REFERENCES

1. Medzhitov, R. and Janeway, C.A. (1997) Innate immunity: impact on the adaptive immune response. *Curr. Opin. Immunol.* **9,** 4–9.
2. Medzhitov, R. and Janeway, C., Jr. (2000) The Toll receptor family and microbial recognition. *Trends Microbiol.* **8,** 452–456.
3. Akira, S., Takeda, K., and Kaisho, T. (2001) Toll-like receptors: critical proteins linking innate and acquired immunity. *Nat. Immunol.* **2,** 675–680.
4. Rietschel, E.T., Brade, H., Holst, O., Brade, L., Müller-Loennies, S., Mamat, U., et al. (1996) Bacterial endotoxin: chemical constitution, biological recognition, host response, and immunological detoxification. *Curr. Topics Microbiol. Immunol.* **216,** 39–81.
5. de Kimpe, S.J., Kengatharan, M., Thiemermann, C., and Vane, J.R. (1995) The cell wall components peptidoglycan and lipotheichoic acid from *Staphylococcus aureus* act in synergy to cause shock and multiple organ failure. *Proc. Natl. Acad. Sci. USA* **92,** 10,359–10,363.
6. Sparwasser, T., Miethke, T., Lipford, G.B., Borschert, K., Häcker, H., Heeg, K., et al. (1997) Bacterial DNA cause septic shock. *Nature* **386,** 336–337.
7. Bhakdi, S., Walev, I., Jonas, D., Palmer, M., Weller, U., Suttorp, N., et al. (1996) Pathogenesis of sepsis syndrome: possible relevance of pore- forming bacterial toxins. *Curr. Topics Microbiol. Immunol.* **216,** 101–118.
8. Marrack, P. and Kappler, J.W. (1990) The staphylococcal enterotoxins and their relatives. *Science* **248,** 705–711.
9. Rott, O. and Fleischer, B. A. (1994) superantigen as virulence factor in an acute bacterial infection. *J. Infect. Dis.* **169,** 1142–1146.
10. Dinges, M.M., Orwin, P.M., and Schlievert, P.M. (2000) Exotoxins of *Staphylococcus aureus*. *Clin. Microbiol. Rev.* **13,** 16–34.
11. Kappler, J.W., Kotzin, B.L., Herron, L., Gelfand, E.W., Bigler, R.D., Boylston, A., et al. (1989) V beta-specific stimulation of human T cells by staphylococcal toxins. *Science* **244,** 811–813.
12. Germain, R.N. and Margulies, D.H. (1993) The biochemistry and cell biology of antigen processing and presentation. *Annu. Rev. Immunol.* **11,** 403–450.
13. Fleischer, B. and Schrezenmeier, H. (1988) T cell stimulation by staphylococcal enterotoxins. Clonally variable response and requirement for major histocompatibility complex class II molecules on accessory or target cells. *J. Exp. Med.* **167,** 1697–1707.
14. Dellabona, P., Peccoud, J., Kappler, J.W., Marrack, P., Benoist, C., and Mathis, D. (1990) Superantigens interact with MHC class II molecules outside of the antigen groove. *Cell* **62,** 1115–1121.
15. Herman, A., Labrecque, N., Thibodeau, J., Marrack, P., Kappler, J.W., and Sekaly, R.P. (1991) Identification of the staphylococcal enterotoxin A superantigen binding site in the beta 1 domain of the human histocompatibility antigen HLA-DR. *Proc. Natl. Acad. Sci. USA* **88,** 9954–9958.
16. Pullen, A.M., Wade, T., Marrack, P., and Kappler, J.W. (1990) Identification of the region of T cell receptor beta chain that interacts with the self-superantigen MIs-1a. *Cell* **61,** 1365–1374.
17. Herrmann, T. and MacDonald, H.R. (1991) T cell recognition of superantigens. *Curr. Topics Microbiol. Immunol.* **174,** 21–38.
18. Irwin, M.J., Hudson, K.R., Ames, K.T., Fraser, J.D., and Gascoigne, N.R.J. (1993) T-cell receptor -chain binding to enterotoxin superantigens. *Immunol. Rev.* **131,** 61–78.
19. Norrby-Teglund, A., Newton, D., Kotb, M., Holm, S.E., and Norgren, M. (1994) Superantigenic properties of the group A streptococcal exotoxin SpeF (MF). *Infect. Immun.* **62,** 5227–5233.
20. Williams, R.J., Ward, J.M., Henderson, B., Poole, S., O'Hara, B.P., Wilson, M., et al. (2000) Identification of a novel gene cluster encoding staphylococcal exotoxin-like proteins: characterization of the prototypic gene and its protein product, SET1. *Infect. Immun.* **68,** 4407–4415.

21. Lehn, N., Schaller, E., Wagner, H., and Krönke, M. (1995) Frequency of toxic shock syndrome toxin- and enterotoxin-producing clinical isolates of *staphylococcus aureus*. *Eur. J. Clin. Microbiol. Infect. Dis.* **14,** 43–46.
22. Carlsson, R. and Sjögren, H.O. (1985) Kinetics of IL-2 and interferon-gamma production, expression of IL-2 receptors, and cell proliferation in human mononuclear cells exposed to staphylococcal enterotoxin A. *Cell Immunol.* **96,** 175–183.
23. Parsonnet, J., Hickman, R.K., Eardley, D.D., and Pier, G.B. (1985) Induction of human interleukin-1 by toxic-shock-syndrome toxin-1. *J. Infect. Dis.* **151,** 514–522.
24. White, J., Herman, A., Pullen, A.M., Kubo, R.T., Kappler, J.W., and Marrack, P. (1989) The V beta-specific superantigen staphylococcal enterotoxin B: stimulation of mature T cells and clonal deletion in neonatal mice. *Cell* **56,** 27–35.
25. Herrmann, T., Baschieri, S., Lees, R.K., and MacDonald, H.R. (1992) In vivo responses of CD4+ and CD8+ cells to bacterial superantigens. *Eur. J. Immunol.* **22,** 1935–1938.
26. Heeg,K., Miethke,T., and Wagner,H. (1996) Superantigen-mediated lethal shock: the functional state of ligand-reactive T cells. *Curr. Topics Microbiol. Immunol.* **216,** 83–100.
27. MacDonald, H.R., Lees, R.K., Baschieri, S., Herrmann, T., and Lussow, A.R. (1993) Peripheral T cell reactivity to bacterial superantigens in vivo: the response/anergy paradox. *Immunol. Rev.* **133,** 105–117.
28. Vabulas, R., Bittlingmaier, R., Heeg, K., Wagner, H., and Miethke, T. (1996) Rapid clearance of the bacterial superantigen staphylococcal enterotoxin B in vivo. *Infect. Immun.* **64,** 4567–4573.
29. Miethke, T., Wahl, C., Holzmann, B., Heeg, K., and Wagner, H. (1993) Bacterial superantigens induce rapid and TCR Vβ-selective downregulation of L-selectin (gp90-Mel14) in vivo. *J. Immunol.* **151,** 6777–6782.
30. Gaus, H., Miethke, T., Wagner, H., and Heeg, K. (1994) Superantigen-induced anergy of Vβ8+ CD4+ T cells induces functional but nonproliferative T cells in vivo. *Immunology* **83,** 333–340.
31. Miethke, T., Wahl, C., Heeg, K., Echtenacher, B., Krammer, P.H., and Wagner, H. (1992) T cell-mediated lethal shock triggered in mice by the superantigen staphylococcal enterotoxin B: critical role of tumor necrosis factor. *J. Exp. Med.* **175,** 91–98.
32. Marrack, P., Blackman, M.A., Kushnir, E., and Kappler, J.W. (1990) The toxicity of staphylococcal enterotoxin B in mice is mediated by T cells. *J. Exp. Med.* **171,** 455–464.
33. Wahl, C., Miethke, T., Heeg, K., and Wagner, H. (1993) Clonal deletion as direct consequence of an in vivo T cell response to bacterial superantigen. *Eur. J. Immunol.* **23,** 1197–1200.
34. Miethke, T., Wahl, C., Gaus, H., Heeg, K., and Wagner, H. (1994) Exogenous superantigens acutely trigger distinct levels of peripheral T cell tolerance/immunosuppression: dose-response relationship. *Eur. J. Immunol.* **24,** 1893–1902.
35. MacDonald, H.R., Baschieri, S., and Lees, R.K. (1991) Clonal expansion precedes anergy and death of V beta 8+ peripheral T cells responding to staphylococcal enterotoxin B in vivo. *Eur. J. Immunol.* **21,** 1963–1966.
36. Renno, T., Hahne, M., and MacDonald, H.R. (1995) Proliferation is a prerequisite for bacterial superantigen- induced T cell apoptosis in vivo. *J. Exp. Med.* **181,** 2283–2287.
37. Kawabe, Y. and Ochi, A. (1990) Selective anergy of V beta 8+,CD4+ T cells in Staphylococcus enterotoxin B-primed mice. *J. Exp. Med.* **172,** 1065–1070.
38. Rellahan, B.L., Jones, L.A., Kruisbeek, A.M., Fry, A.M., and Matis, L.A. (1990) In vivo induction of anergy in peripheral V beta 8+ T cells by staphylococcal enterotoxin B. *J. Exp. Med.* **172,** 1091–1100.
39. Miethke, T., Wahl, C., Heeg, K., and Wagner, H. (1993) Acquired resistance to superantigen-induced T cell shock. *J. Immunol.* **150,** 3776–3784.
40. Grossman, D., Cook, R.G., Sparrow, J.T., Mollick, J.A., and Rich, R.R. (1990) Dissociation of the stimulatory activities of staphylococcal enterotoxins for T cells and monocytes. *J. Exp. Med.* **172,** 1831–1841.
41. Chatila, T. and Geha, R.S. (1993) Signal transduction by microbial superantigens via MHC class II molecules. *Immunol. Rev.* **131,** 43–59.
42. Assenmacher, M., Löhning, M., Scheffold, A., Manz, R.A., Schmitz, J., and Radbruch, A. (1998) Sequential production of IL-2, IFN-gamma and IL-10 by individual staphylococcal enterotoxin B activated T helper lymphocytes. *Eur. J. Immunol.* **28,** 1534–1543.
43. Won, S.J., Huang, W.T., Lai, Y.S., and Lin, M.T. (2000) Staphylococcal enterotoxin A acts through nitric oxide synthase mechanisms in human peripheral blood mononuclear cells to stimulate synthesis of pyrogenic cytokines. *Infect. Immun.* **68,** 2003–2008.
44. Kusunoki, T. and Wright, S.D. (1996) Chemical characteristics of *Staphylolcoccus aureus* molecules that have CD14-dependent cell-stimulationg activity. *J. Immunol.* **157,** 5112–5117.
45. Bean, A.G., Freiberg, R.A., Andrade, S., Menon, S., and Zlotnik, A. (1993) Interleukin 10 protects mice against staphylococcal enterotoxin B-induced lethal shock. *Infect. Immun.* **61,** 4937–4939.
46. Florquin, S., Amraoui, Z., Abramowicz, D., and Goldman, M. (1994) Systemic release and protective role of IL-10 in staphylococcal enterotoxin B-induced shock in mice. *J. Immunol.* **153,** 2618–2623.
47. Blank, C., Luz, C., Bendigs, S., Wagner, H., and Heeg, K. (1997) Superantigen and endotoxin synergize in the induction of lethal shock. *Eur. J. Immunol.* **27,** 825–833.
48. Lee, V.T., Chang, A.H., and Chow, A.W. (1992) Detection of staphylococcal enterotoxin B among toxic shock syndrome (TSS-) and non-TSS-associated *Staphylococcus aureus* isolates. *J. Infect. Dis.* **166,** 911–915.
49. Stiles, B.G., Bavari, S., Krakauer, T., and Ulrich,R.G. (1993) Toxicity of staphylococcal enterotoxins potentiated by lipopolysaccharide: major histocompatibility complex class II molecule dependency and cytokine release. *Infect. Immun.* **61,** 5333–5338.
50. LeClaire, R.D., Hunt, R.E., Bavari, S., Estep, J.E., Nelson, G.O., and Wilhelmsen, C.L. (1996) Potentiation of inhaled staphylococcal enterotoxin B-induced toxicicty by lipopolysaccharide in mice. *Toxicol. Pathol.* **24,** 619–626.

51. Dinarello, C.A. (1996) Cytokines as mediators in the pathogenesis of septic shock. Curr. Topics Microbiol. Immunol. **216,** 133–167.
52. Heremans, H., van Damme, J., Dillen, C., Dijkmans, R., and Billiau, A. (1990) Interferon gamma, a mediator of lethal lipopolysaccharide-induced Shwartzman-like shock reactions in mice. *J. Exp. Med.* **171,** 1853–1869.
53. Billiau, A. (1996) Interferon-gamma: biology and role in pathogenesis. *Adv. Immunol.* **62,** 61–130.
54. Ozmen, L., Pericin, M., Hakimi, J., Chizzonite, R.A., Wysocka, M., Trinchieri, G et al. (1994) Interleukin 12, interferon gamma and tumor necrosis factor alpha are the key mediators of the generalized Shwartzman reaction. *J. Exp. Med.* **180,** 907–915.
55. Hochholzer, P., Blank, C., Bendigs, S., Wagner, H., and Heeg, K. *Superantigen-Induced Shwartzman-like Reaction: Critical Role of Interferon-gamma,* (Faist, E., ed.) Monduzzi Editore, Bologna, pp. 479–482.
56. Tokunaga, T., Yamamoto, T., and Yamamoto, S. (1999) How BCG led to the discovery of immunostimulatory DNA. *Jpn. J. Infect. Dis.* **52,** 1–11.
57. Shimada, S., Yano, O., Inoue, H., Kuramoto,E., Fukuda, T., Yamamoto, H., et al. (1985) Antitumor activity of the DNA fraction from *Mycobacterium bovis* BCG. II. Effects on various syngeneic mouse tumors. *J. Natl. Cancer Inst.* **74,** 681–688.
58. Yamamoto, S., Kuramoto, E., Shimada, S., and Tokunaga, T. (1988) In vitro augmentation of natural killer cell activity and production of interferon-alpha/beta and -gamma with deoxyribonucleic acid fraction from *Mycobacterium bovis* BCG. *Jpn. J. Cancer Res.* **79,** 866–873.
59. Yamamoto, S., Yamamoto, T., Shimada, S., Kuramoto, E., Yano, O., Kataoka, T., and Tokunaga, T. (1992) DNA from bacteria, but not from vertebrates, induces interferons, activates natural killer cells and inhibits tumor growth. *Microbiol. Immunol.* **36,** 983–997.
60. Tokunaga, T., Yano, O., Kuramoto, E., Kimura, Y., Yamamoto, T., Kataoka, T., et al. (1992) Synthetic oligonucle-otides with particular base sequences from the cDNA encoding proteins of *Mycobacterium bovis* BCG induce interferons and activate natural killer cells. *Microbiol. Immunol.* **36,** 55–66.
61. Yamamoto, T., Yamamoto, S., Kataoka, T., Komuro, K., Kohase, M., and Tokunaga, T. (1994) Synthetic oligonucle-otides with certain palindromes stimulate interferon production of human peripheral blood lymphocytes in vitro. *Jpn. J. Cancer Res.* **85,** 775–779.
62. Pisetsky, D.S., Reich, C., Crowley, S.D., and Halpern, M.D. (1995) Immunological properties of bacterial DNA. *Ann. NY Acad. Sci.* **772,** 152–163.
63. Liang, H., Nishioka, Y., Reich, C.F., Pisetsky, D.S., and Lipsky, P.E. (1996) Activation of human B cells by phosphorothioate oligonucleotides. *J. Clin. Invest.* **98,** 1119–1129.
64. Mojcik, C.F., Gourley, M.F., Klinman, D.M., Krieg, A.M., Gmelig Meyling, F., and Steinberg, A.D. (1993) Adminis-tration of a phosphorothioate oligonucleotide antisense to murine endogenous retroviral MCF env causes immune effects in vivo in a sequence-specific manner. *Clin. Immunol. Immunopathol.* **67,** 130–136.
65. Krieg, A.M., Yi, A.K., Matson, S., Waldschmidt, T.J., Bishop, G.A., Teasdale, R., et al. (1995) CpG motifs in bacterial DNA trigger direct B-cell activation. *Nature* **374,** 546–549.
66. Krieg, A.M. (1996) Lymphocyte activation by CpG dinucleotide motifs in prokaryotic DNA. *Trends Microbiol.* **4,** 73–76.
67. Bird, A.P. (1980) DNA methylation and the frequency of CpG in animal DNA. Nucleic. Acids Res. **8,** 1499–1504.
68. Shimizu, T.S., Takahashi, K., and Tomita, M. (1997) CpG distribution patterns in methylated and non-methylated species. *Gene* **205,** 103–107.
69. Krieg, A.M. and Wagner, H. (2000) Causing a commotion in the blood: immunotherapy progresses from bacteria to bacterial DNA. *Immunol. Today* **21,** 521–526.
70. Hartmann, G., Weiner, G.J., and Krieg, A.M. (1999) CpG DNA: A potent signal for growth, activation, and maturation of human dendritic cells. *Proc. Natl. Acad. Sci. USA* **96,** 9305–9310.
71. Ballas, Z.K., Rasmussen, W.L., and Krieg, A.M. (1996) Induction of NK activity in murine and human cells by CpG motifs in oligodeoxynucleotides and bacterial DNA. *J. Immunol.* **157,** 1840–1845.
72. Bauer, M., Heeg, K., Wagner, H., and Lipford, G.B. (1997) DNA activates human immune cells through a CpG se-quence dependent manner. *Immunology* **97,** 699–705.
73. Verthelyi, D., Ishii, K.J., Gursel, M., Takeshita, F., and Klinman, D.M. (2001) Human peripheral blood cells differen-tially recognize and respond to two distinct CpG motifs. *J. Immunol.* **166,** 2372–2377.
74. Krieg,A.M., Wu,T., Weeratna,R., Efler,S.M., Love-Homan,L., Yang,L., et al. (1998) Sequence motifs in adenoviral DNA block immune activation by stimulatory CpG motifs. *Proc. Natl. Acad. Sci. USA* **95,** 12,631–12,636.
75. Halpern, M.D. and Pisetsky, D.S. (1995) In vitro inhibition of murine IFN gamma production by phosphorothioate deoxyguanosine oligomers. *Immunopharmacology* **29,** 47–52.
76. Zhu, F.G., Reich, C.F., III, and Pisetsky, D.S. (2001) The role of the macrophage scavenger receptor in immune stimu-lation by bacterial DNA and synthetic oligonucleotides. *Immunology* **103,** 226–234.
77. Pearson, A.M., Rich, A., and Krieger, M. (1993) Polynucleotide binding to macrophage scavenger receptors depends on the formation of base-quartet-stabilized four-stranded helices. *J. Biol. Chem.* **268,** 3546–3554.
78. Macfarlane, D.E. and Manzel, L. (1998) Antagonism of immunostimulatory CpG—oligodeoxynucleotides by quina-crine, chloroquine, and structurally related compounds. *J. Immunol.* **160,** 1122–1131.
79. Yi, A.K. and Krieg, A.M. (1998) Rapid induction of mitogen-activated protein kinases by immune stimulatory CpG DNA. *J. Immunol.* **161,** 4493–4497.
80. Häcker, H., Mischak, H., Miethke, T., Liptay, S., Schmid, R., Sparwasser, T., et al. (1998) CpG-DNA specific activa-tion of antigen presenting cells requires stress kinase activity and is proceeded by non-specific endocytosis and endosomal maturation. *EMBO J.* **17,** 6230–6240.

81. Häcker, H. (2000) Signal transduction pathways activated by CpG-DNA. *Curr. Topics Microbiol. Immunol.* **247,** 77–92.
82. Medzhitov, R., Preston-Hurlburt, P., Kopp, E., Stadlen, A., Chen, C., Ghosh, S., et al. (1998) MyD88 is an adaptor protein in the hToll/IL-1 receptor family signaling pathways. *Mol. Cell* **2,** 253–258.
83. Chaudhary, P.M., Ferguson, C., Nguyen, V., Nguyen, O., Massa, H.F., Eby, M., et al. (1998) Cloning and characterization of two Toll/interleukin-1 receptor-like genes TIL3 and TIL4: evidence for a multi-gene receptor family in humans. *Blood* **91,** 4020–4027.
84. Rock, F.L., Hardiman,G., Timans,J.C., Kastelein,R.A., and Bazan, J.F. (1998) A family of human receptors structurally related to *Drosophila* Toll. *Proc. Natl. Acad. Sci. USA* **95,** 588–593.
85. Chow, J.C., Young, D.W., Golenbock, D.T., Christ, W.J., and Gusovsky, F. (1999) Toll-like receptor-4 mediates lipopolysaccharide-induced signal transduction. *J. Biol. Chem.* **274,** 10,689–10,692.
86. Hoshino, K., Takeuchi, O., Kawai, T., Sanjo, H., Ogawa, T., Takeda, Y., et al. (1999) Cutting edge: Toll-like receptor 4 (TLR4)-deficient mice are hyporesponsive to lipopolysaccharide: evidence for TLR4 as the Lps gene product. *J. Immunol.* **162,** 3749–3752.
87. Hemmi, H., Takeuchi, O., Kawai, T., Kaisho, T., Sato, S., Sanjo, H., et al. (2000) A Toll-like receptor recognizes bacterial DNA. *Nature* **408,** 740–745.
88. Bauer, S., Kirschning, C.J., Hacker, H., Redecke, V., Hausmann, S., Akira, S., et al. (2001) Human TLR9 confers responsiveness to bacterial DNA via species-specific CpG motif recognition. *Proc. Natl. Acad. Sci. USA* **98,** 9237–9242.
89. Sparwasser, T., Koch, E.S., Vabulas, R.M., Heeg, K., Lipford, G.B., Ellwart, J., et al. (1998) Bacterial DNA and immunostimulating CpG oligonucleotides trigger maturation and activation of murine dendritic cells. *Eur. J. Immunol.* **28,** 2045–2054.
90. Jakob, T., Walker, P.S., Krieg, A.M., Udey, M.C., and Vogel, J.C. (1998) Activation of cutaneous dendritic cells by CpG-containing oligodeoxynucleotides: a role for dendritic cells in the augmentation of Th1 responses by immunostimulatory DNA. *J. Immunol.* **161,** 3042–3049.
91. Halpern, M.D., Kurlander, R.J., and Pisetsky, D.S. (1996) Bacterial DNA induces murine interferon-gamma production by stimulation of interleukin 12 and tumor necrosis factor-alpha. *Cell Immunol.* **167,** 72–78.
92. Sparwasser, T., Hültner, L., Koch, E.S., Luz, A., Lipford, G.B., and Wagner, H. (1999) Immunostimulatory CpG-oligodeoxynucleotides cause extramedullary murine hemopoiesis. *J. Immunol.* **162,** 2368–2374.
93. Kranzer, K., Bauer, M., Lipford, G.B., Heeg, K., Wagner, H., and Lang, R. (2000) CpG oligodeoxynucleotides enhance T cell receptor-triggered IFN-gamma production and up-regulation of CD69 via induction of antigen-presenting cell-derived interferon type I and IL-12. *Immunology* **99,** 170–178.
94. Cowdery, J.S., Boerth, N.J., Norian, L.A., Myung, P.S., and Koretzky, G.A. (1999) Differential regulation of the IL-12 p40 promoter and of p40 secretion by CpG DNA and lipopolysaccharide. *J. Immunol.* **162,** 6770–6775.
95. Horng, T., Barton, G.M., and Medzhitov, R. (2001) TIRAP: an adapter molecule in the Toll signaling pathway. *Nat. Immunol.* **2,** 835–841.
96. Lipford, G.B., Bauer, M., Blank, C., Reiter, R., Wagner, H., and Heeg, K. (1997) CpG-containing synthetic oligonucleotides promote B and cytotoxic T cell responses to protein antigen: a new class of vaccine adjuvants. *Eur. J. Immunol.* **27,** 2340–2344.
97. Weeratna, R.D., McCluskie, M.J., Xu, Y., and Davis, H.L. (2000) CpG DNA induces stronger immune responses with less toxicity than other adjuvants. *Vaccine* **18,** 1755–1762.
98. Heeg, K. and Zimmermann, S. (2000) CpG DNA as a Th1 trigger. *Int. Arch. Allergy Immunol.* **121,** 87–97.
99. Zimmermann, S., Egeter, O., Hausmann, S., Lipford, G.B., Röcken, M., Wagner, H., et al. (1998) CpG oligodeoxynucleotides trigger protective and curative Th1 responses in lethal murine leishmaniasis. *J. Immunol.***160,** 3627–3630.
100. Askenase, P.W. (2000) Gee whiz: CpG DNA allergy therapy! J. Allergy Clin. Immunol. **106,** 37–40.
101. Parronchi, P., Brugnolo, F., Sampognaro, S., and Maggi,E. (2000) Genetic and environmental factors contributing to the onset of allergic disorders. *Int. Arch. Allergy Immunol.* **121,** 2–9.
102. Sparwasser, T., Miethke, T., Lipford, G.B., Erdmann, A., Häcker, H., Heeg, K., et al. (1997) Macrophages sense pathogens via DNA motifs: Induction of TNF-alpha mediated shock. *Eur. J. Immunol.* **27,** 1671–1679.
103. Wagner, H., Lipford, G.B., and Hacker, H. (2000) The role of immunostimulatory CpG-DNA in septic shock. Semin. Immunopathol. **22,** 167–171.
104. Sun, S., Kishimoto, H., and Sprent, J. (1998) DNA as an adjuvant: capacity of insect DNA and synthetic oligodeoxynucleotides to augment T cell responses to specific antigen. *J. Exp. Med.* **187,** 1145–1150.
105. Chatellier, S. and Kotb, M. (2000) Preferential stimulation of human lymphocytes by oligodeoxynucleotides that copy DNA CpG motifs present in virulent genes of group A streptococci. *Eur. J. Immunol.* **30,** 993–1001.
106. Sato, S., Nomura, F., Kawai, T., Takeuchi, O., Muhlradt, P.F., Takeda, K., et al. (2000) Synergy and cross-tolerance between toll-like receptor (TLR) 2- and TLR4-mediated signaling pathways. *J. Immunol.* **165,** 7096–7101.
107. Milner, K.C. (1973) Patterns of tolerance to endotoxin. *J. Infect. Dis.* **128,** (**Suppl.**) 237–245.
108. Nomura, F., Akashi, S., Sakao, Y., Sato, S., Kawai, T., Matsumoto, M., et al. (2000) Cutting edge: endotoxin tolerance in mouse peritoneal macrophages correlates with down-regulation of surface toll-like receptor 4 expression. *J. Immunol.* **164,** 3476–3479.
109. Lehner, M.D., Morath, S., Michelsen, K.S., Schumann, R.R., and Hartung, T. (2001) Induction of cross-tolerance by lipopolysaccharide and highly purified lipoteichoic acid via different toll-like receptors independent of paracrine mediators. *J. Immunol.* **166,** 5161–5167.
110. Cowdery, J.S., Chace, J.H., Yi, A.K., and Krieg, A.M. (1996) Bacterial DNA induces NK cells to produce IFN-gamma in vivo and increases the toxicity of lipopolysaccharides. *J. Immunol.* **156,** 4570–4575.

111. Hacker, H., Vabulas, R.M., Takeuchi, O., Hoshino, K., Akira, S., and Wagner, H. (2000) Immune cell activation by bacterial CpG-DNA through myeloid differentiation marker 88 and tumor necrosis factor Rreceptor-associated factor (TRAF)6. *J. Exp. Med.* **192,** 595–600.
112. Krieg, A.M. (2000) Signal transduction induced by immunostimulatory CpG DNA. Semin. Immunopathol. **22,** 97–105.
113. Starr, R., Willson, T.A., Viney, E.M., Murray, L.J.L., Rayner, J.R., Jenkins, B.J., et al. (1997) A family of cytokine-inducible inhibitors of signalling. *Nature* **387,** 917–921.
114. Naka, T., Narazaki, M., Hirata, M., Tomoshige, M., Minamoto, S., Aono, A., et al. (1997) Structure and function of a new STAT-induced STAT inhibitor. *Nature* **387,** 924–929.
115. Stoiber, D., Kovarik, P., Cohney, S., Johnston, J.A., Steinlein, P., and Decker, T. (1999) Lipopolysaccharide induces in macrophages the synthesis of the suppressor of cytokine signaling 3 and suppresses signal transduction in response to the activating factor IFN-gamma. *J. Immunol.* **163,** 2640–2647.
116. Dalpke, A., Opper, S., Zimmermann, S., and Heeg, K. (2000) Suppressor of cytokine signalling (SOCS)-3 is induced by CpG DNA and modulates cytokine responses in APC. *J. Immunol.* **166,** 7082–7089.
117. Teague, T.K., Schaefer, B.C., Hildeman, D., Bender, J., Mitchell, T., Kappler, J.W., et al. (2000) Activation-induced inhibition of interleukin 6-mediated T cell survival and signal transducer and activator of transcription 1 signaling. *J. Exp. Med.* **191,** 915–926.

8

Cytokines and Chemokines in Listeriosis

Michael S. Rolph and Stefan H. E. Kaufmann

1. INTRODUCTION

The mouse model of experimental *Listeria monocytogenes* infection has contributed greatly to studies on cellular immunity since its development in the 1960s by Mackaness *(1)*. It represents a highly reliable, safe, and rapid model for infection with intracellular bacteria. Indeed, many fundamental discoveries in cell-mediated immunity have been achieved using the *Listeria* model of infection. In this chapter, we concentrate specifically on the role of cytokines and chemokines in the immune response of mice to *L. monocytogenes* infection.

2. BASIC MICROBIOLOGY OF *L. MONOCYTOGENES*

Listeria monocytogenes is a Gram-positive, non-spore-forming facultatively anaerobic rod. It is a facultative intracellular bacterium, with the principal host cell being the macrophage, and hepatocytes and epithelial cells are also commonly infected. Numerous virulence factors involved in cell invasion, intracellular replication, and cell-to-cell spread have been identified. Following phagocytic uptake, the pore-forming cytolysin listeriolysin O (LLO) is produced and becomes active in the low pH of the phagosome. LLO promotes rupture of the phagosomal membrane and allows the bacterium to escape into the more benign and nutrient-rich cytoplasmic environment *(2)*. LLO is a major virulence factor, and in its absence, *L. monocytogenes* remains in the phagosome and is destroyed by cellular antimicrobial mechanisms *(3)*. Escape to the phagosome is assisted by phospholipase C molecules and a lecithinase *(4–6)*.

Within the cytoplasm, the bacteria proliferate readily with a doubling time of approximately 1 h. After 2–3 h, the bacteria begin to migrate to the periphery of the cell, utilizing host cell actin for locomotion, mediated by the actA virulence factor. At the periphery, the bacteria induce the formation of elongated filopods, which allow bacterial movement to an adjacent cell without leaving the intracellular environment *(7)*.

Although *Listeria* is widely prevalent in the environment, listeriosis is rarely a disease in humans and is most often found in sheep and cattle *(3)*. Outbreaks of listeriosis are most commonly food-borne *(8)*. The rate of infection is substantially higher in immunocompromised and pregnant individuals.

3. OVERVIEW OF IMMUNE RESPONSE TO *L. MONOCYTOGENES* INFECTION

The immune response to infection is a highly dynamic and complex process that begins within the first hours of infection and can continue several days after clearance of the pathogen. It represents a continuous process involving a wide range of biological processes, many of which are regulated by cytokines and chemokines. The *Listeria* model has been a cornerstone in elucidating the processes of cell-mediated immunity. Following intravenous infection, *L. monocytogenes* primarily infects mac-

From: *Cytokines and Chemokines in Infectious Diseases Handbook*
Edited by: M. Kotb and T. Calandra © Humana Press Inc., Totowa, NJ

rophages and hepatocytes. Although *L. monocytogenes* can readily survive within resting macrophages, bacterial death is rapid once macrophages become activated. Because interferon-γ (IFN-γ) is an essential mediator of macrophage activation, the ability of the host to produce this cytokine is a central determinant of the success of the immune response. *Listeria* infection can be controlled (but not cleared) by the innate immune response, in a process involving interleukin (IL)-12 and tumor necrosis factor (TNF) production by infected macrophages and subsequent activation of IFN-γ-producing cells such as natural killer (NK) cells *(9)*. However, T-cell activation is required for sterile clearance of bacteria. *Listeria*-specific CD4+ and CD8+ T-cells are generated rapidly following infection and can be detected as early as 4 d following infection, with maximal T-cell activity observed at 5–7 d. As a direct consequence of T cell regulatory and effector function, sterile clearance is typically observed on d 7–10. CD4+ and CD8+ T-cells activated during *L. monocytogenes* infection are overwhelmingly of the Th1/Tc1 variety, characterized by IFN-γ production and essentially no IL-4 (reviewed in refs. *10–12*).

An interesting feature of the immune response to *L. monocytogenes* is the strong CD8+ T-cell response *(13)*. The ability of *L. monocytogenes* to escape from the phagosome to the cytoplasm of resting macrophages means that bacteria-derived peptides are readily presented on major histocompatibility complex (MHC) class I molecules. Indeed, CD8+ T-cells are considerably more potent than CD4+ T-cells in controlling *L. monocytogenes* infection. Aside from these so-called conventional T-cells, γδ T-cells play a minor role in protection, but are also involved in granuloma formation *(14)*.

4. CYTOKINES AND CHEMOKINES IN INFECTION

The *Listeria* model has provided a wealth of information about the role of cytokines and chemokines in the immune response. In vitro and in vivo studies have revealed important information about the production and role of soluble mediators at all stages of the immune response. In the last 10 yr, the pace of discovery has been greatly accelerated by the application of knockout (KO) mouse technology. The cytokine response to *L. monocytogenes* is predominantly of the proinflammatory, type 1 variety with only a weak type 2 response in evidence *(15)*. In the following text, we will detail the production and role of the major cytokines and chemokines in the immune response to *L. monocytogenes*.

4.1. Cytokines in Listeriosis

4.1.1. Interleukin-1

Interleukin (IL)-1 is a proinflammatory cytokine with a broad spectrum of biological activities. There are two genes for IL-1 (IL-1α and IL-1β) with very similar biological activities despite sharing only 26% homology at the protein level. Uptake of *L. monocytogenes* induces substantial IL-1 production by macrophages *(16)*. During listeriosis, there is a significant increase in IL-1 levels in the spleen and liver *(17)*. The production of IL-1 parallels the kinetics of infection; IL-1 was detectable 24 h following infection, peaked at d 4, and fell away quite rapidly *(17)*.

Interleukin-1 contributes to protection against *L. monocytogenes* infection. Neutralization of IL-1 in *L. monocytogenes*-infected mice results in increased susceptibility *(17,18)*, whereas administration of recombinant IL-1 increases resistance *(19)*. The importance of IL-1 in resistance to *L. monocytogenes* infection was recently confirmed using mice deficient in the IL-1 receptor (IL-1R) antagonist *(20)*. IL-1R antagonist is a cytokine whose function is to inhibit the binding of IL-1 to its receptor. IL-1R antagonist KO mice were less susceptible to *L. monocytogenes* infection, whereas IL-1R-antagonist-overproducing mice were more susceptible *(20)*.

The precise mechanism of action of IL-1 in *L. monocytogenes* infection is not known. Neutralization of IL-1 reduces neutrophil accumulation at the site of infection *(21)*, and this may be a major contributor to the anti-*Listeria* activity of IL-1 because neutrophils are important effector cells during the early phase of infection *(22)*. IL-1 enhances the ability of antigen-presenting cells (APCs) to stimulate T-cells and is required for the enhanced MHC class II expression on macrophages in *L. monocytogenes* infection *(21)*. Expression of interferon (IFN)-γ is not affected by anti-IL-1 treatment and the reduced MHC class II expression appears to be the result of macrophage unresponsiveness to IFN-γ *(9)*.

4.1.2. IL-4

Interleukin-4 is the prototypic Th2 cytokine and is critically involved in regulation of the Th1/Th2 balance. The normal immune response to *L. monocytogenes* infection is dominated by a proinflammatory, Th1 response, and IL-4 is produced only transiently and in small quantities *(15)*. However, there are some circumstances under which increased IL-4 is produced during *L. monocytogenes* infection, and in such cases, the IL-4 may downregulate protective immunity.

Interleukin-4 is produced rapidly following infection of mice with *L. monocytogenes*. Using a sensitive ELISPOT assay, elevated IL-4 production could be detected as early as 10 min following infection, but 3 h later the production of IL-4 had returned to baseline levels *(23)*. NK T-cells are the most likely cellular source of this IL-4. This rapid burst of IL-4 production appears to regulate chemokine production; the peak of IL-4 production is followed by monocyte chemoattractant protein (MCP)-1 production that can be inhibited by neutralization of IL-4 *(23)*. IL-4 production by NK T cells is rapidly switched off in response to IL-12 production by *L. monocytogenes*-infected macrophages *(15)*.

Although only very little IL-4 is produced during *L. monocytogenes* infection, it may be sufficient to moderately dampen protective immunity. Neutralization of IL-4 can enhance clearance of *L. monocytogenes* in mice *(24,25)*, although this has not been consistently observed *(26,27)*.

However, there are some conditions of *L. monocytogenes* infection under which higher levels of IL-4 are produced. For example, in the absence of IFN-γ signaling, substantially increased levels of IL-4 are observed *(28,29)*. Under these circumstances of increased IL-4 production, the immune-downregulatory function of IL-4 in *L. monocytogenes* infection is more apparent. Thus, lethally infected IFN-γ-receptor-deficient mice can be rescued by treatment with anti-IL-4 antibody and can completely clear the infection *(28)*. The immune-downregulatory mechanism of IL-4 in these experiments was not fully elucidated, but was associated with decreased tumor necrosis factor (TNF) production *(28)*.

4.1.3. IL-6

Interleukin-6 is a multifunctional cytokine involved in many aspects of the immune response. High levels of IL-6 can be detected in the spleen and bloodstream of mice infected with *L. monocytogenes (30–32)*. Maximum IL-6 production occurs at d 1–3 following infection. Although numerous cell types are capable of producing IL-6, the principal cellular source of IL-6 during *L. monocytogenes* infection appears to be the macrophage *(30,31)*.

Recombinant IL-6 given as a bolus dose enhances resistance of mice to infection with *L. monocytogenes*, whereas mice treated with anti-IL-6 are more susceptible to *L. monocytogenes (33)*. The requirement for IL-6 in effective resistance to *L. monocytogenes* was confirmed following the generation of IL-6 KO mice, as these mice are substantially more susceptible to *L. monocytogenes* infection *(34,35)*.

The mechanism by which IL-6 protects is not clear. The protective effect of bolus doses of recombinant IL-6 can be abrogated by neutralization of IFN-γ or TNF *(33,36)*, suggesting that the effects of IL-6 treatment are ultimately mediated by these cytokines. Another possible mechanism of protection is neutrophil stimulation. Wild-type mice had a prominent neutrophilia within 24 h of infection, but this was not the case in IL-6 KO mice *(35)*. Furthermore, the protective effect of recombinant IL-6 was not observed in neutrophil-depleted mice *(35)*.

4.1.4. IL-10

Interleukin-10 is produced by a range of cell types including T-cells, B-cells, and APCs *(37)*. The immunobiology of IL-10 is complex and it has both stimulatory and suppressive actions on the immune response. However, for immunity to *L. monocytogenes*, it is generally immunosuppressive.

In particular, it has a potent capacity to downregulate effector and regulatory functions of monocyte/macrophages *(37)*, including listericidal activity *(38)*.

Interleukin-10 mRNA is rapidly upregulated following infection with *L. monocytogenes (39,40)*, and is not significantly regulated by T-cells, because high levels of IL-10 are produced in T-cell-deficient RAG KO mice *(40)*. Although many cells have the potential to produce IL-10 during *L. monocytogenes* infection, the macrophage is the principal source *(40)*.

Treatment of mice with recombinant IL-10 results in a marked reduction in the ability to resist *L. monocytogenes* infection *(41)*. Although immunodeficient SCID mice were able to survive *L. monocytogenes* infection until d 14, SCID mice treated with recombinant IL-10 died by d 4, with a profoundly increased bacterial burden.

More meaningful data about the role of IL-10 in *L. monocytogenes* infection have been obtained from studies utilizing neutralizing anti-IL-10 antibodies or IL-10 KO mice. IL-10 KO mice were substantially more resistant to *L. monocytogenes* infection than wild-type mice *(42)*. As early as d 2, a 10-fold reduction in bacterial load was found in the IL-10 KO mice, and these mice cleared the infection several days earlier than did the wild-type mice. Several factors could explain the increased resistance of IL-10 KO mice. First, peritoneal cells from *L. monocytogenes*-infected IL-10 KO mice produce much higher levels of inflammatory cytokines, including IL-12, IFN-γ, TNF, IL-1α, and IL-6 in response to stimulation with heat-killed *L. monocytogenes*. Second, a stronger Th1 polarization has been observed in the IL-10 KO mice, as determined by increased IFN-γ production from anti-CD3-stimulated CD4+ and CD8+ T-cells *(42)*. CD4+ T-cells from KO mice also produced less IL-4 in response to anti-CD3. However, the T-cell response of wild-type mice is almost entirely of a Th1 nature *(15)* and the importance of this latter finding for *L. monocytogenes* infection is doubtful.

Treatment of *L. monocytogenes*-infected mice with neutralizing anti-IL-10 antibody at the time of infection resulted in enhanced bacterial clearance early during infection *(43,44)*, thus confirming the results with the KO mice. However, during the later stages of infection, the clearance of bacteria in the anti-IL-10 treated mice was actually delayed compared with that of control mice *(43)*. In this experiment, anti-IL-10 was only given once, at the time of infection, and this may explain the results at later time-points.

Finally, IL-10 is involved in the increased susceptibility of neonatal mice to *L. monocytogenes* infection. Following infection of adult and neonatal mice with LD_{90} *L. monocytogenes*, neonatal mice produced much higher levels of IL-10 *(44)*. Neutralization of IL-10 markedly improved resistance of neonatal mice, compared with the moderate effect of anti-IL-10 in adult mice. Thus, the increased susceptibility of neonates to *L. monocytogenes* infection may be at least partly explained by overproduction of IL-10.

4.1.5. IL-12

Interleukin-12 is a critical cytokine in the development of protective IFN-γ responses during infection with intracellular bacteria. IL-12 production typically occurs early during *L. monocytogenes* infection and does not require T-cells *(45)*. Production of IL-12 is predominantly by macrophages and is induced following infection with live bacteria, as well as in response to bacterial products such as lipoteichoic acid *(46)* and bacterial DNA *(47)*. IL-12, together with TNF, is an essential factor in inducing NK cell production of IFN-γ *(48)*. Although IL-12 is clearly produced in large amounts by infected macrophages, the earliest source of IL-12 may be dendritic cells (DCs), which express IL-12 p40 mRNA as early as 3 h following infection of mice with *L. monocytogenes (49)*.

The importance of IL-12 in IFN-γ-mediated protection against *L. monocytogenes* has also been demonstrated in vivo. Neutralization of IL-12 in both immunocompetent and SCID mice exacerbated infection and converted a sublethal infection to a lethal one. This was associated with decreased I-A^d expression and increased bacterial burden. These effects could be reversed by concomitant treatment with IFN-γ, suggesting that IL-12 regulates IFN-γ production in vivo via a pathway similar to that already described in vitro *(48)*. Similar results were obtained with IL-12 p35 KO mice. IFN-γ production in the response of these mice to *L. monocytogenes* infection was impaired and they were consequently unable to control infection as efficiently as wild-type mice *(50)*.

4.1.6. IL-13

Interleukin-13 is a Th2 cytokine sharing a number of functions with IL-4 *(51)*. Flesch et al. *(52)* investigated the effect of recombinant IL-13 on the course of *L. monocytogenes* infection. Although IL-13 is typically considered to downregulate cell-mediated immunity in much the same way as IL-4, treatment of mice with IL-13 protected the mice from *L. monocytogenes* challenge. This was associated with an increased number of IL-12-producing cells early in infection and increased NK cell activity. Evidence from other model systems indeed suggests that IL-13 can activate phagocytes in the absence of inflammation. This could represent the underlying mechanisms of antilisterial effects of IL-13 treatment.

4.1.7. IL-15

Interleukin-15 is a cytokine sharing considerable biological activity with IL-2, although it has a considerably broader pattern of cellular expression. Following oral *L. monocytogenes* infection, IL-15 is produced rapidly (within 24 h) by intestinal epithelial cells and may stimulate IFN-γ production by intraepithelial lymphocytes *(53)*. This cytokine has been found to promote memory responses in other systems, and its role in long-term protection against *L. monocytogenes* remains to be clarified.

4.1.8. TNF

Tumor necrosis factor is a pleiotropic molecule that is required for protective immunity against intracellular pathogens, but it is also a major mediator of immunopathology *(11,54)*. Macrophages rapidly produce TNF following infection with *L. monocytogenes* *(55)*. Similarly, TNF is produced rapidly in vivo following *L. monocytogenes* infection. Maximal levels of TNF mRNA and protein were found 1 d after infection and remained high throughout the course of the infection *(56,57)*. The macrophage was the principal source of TNF.

Early studies using neutralizing antibodies demonstrated the absolute requirement for TNF for effective control of *L. monocytogenes* infection *(56,58–60)*. These results were subsequently confirmed using gene-targeted mice deficient in TNF-R1 *(61,62)* or TNF and lymphotoxin-α *(63,64)*. In the *Listeria* model, impaired TNF signaling presents one of the most extreme phenotypes—the mice are exquisitely susceptible *(61,62)*, with a 500-fold increase in LD_{50} *(65)*. Signaling through TNF-R1 accounts entirely for the listericidal effect of TNF, because mice deficient in TNF-R2 are as resistant to *L. monocytogenes* infection as wild-type (WT) mice *(66)*.

The proposed effects of TNF in *L. monocytogenes* infection are wide ranging *(67–69)*, but despite intensive study, the molecular mechanism underlying the critical role for TNF has not been elucidated. Endres et al. *(70)* conducted an extensive analysis of the immune response in *L. monocytogenes*-infected TNF-R1 KO mice, but were unable to explain the extreme susceptibility of these mice. No difference between WT and TNF-R1 KO mice was found in the following immune parameters: granulocyte and monocyte influx; oxidative burst formation; expression of inflammatory cytokines including IL-10, IL-12, TNF, and IFN-γ; activation status of macrophages *(70)*.

Bone-marrow-derived cells are the targets for TNF-mediated listericidal activity. Bone marrow chimeras prepared by reconstituting irradiated WT mice with TNF-R1 KO bone marrow cells were as susceptible as TNF-R1 KO mice, whereas irradiated TNF-R1 KO mice reconstituted with WT bone marrow cells were as resistant as WT mice. Thus, TNF-R1 signaling on bone-marrow-derived cells is essential for TNF-mediated listericidal activity, whereas TNF-R1 signaling on parenchymal cells is of minimal importance *(70)*.

4.1.9. IFN-γ

Interferon-γ is essential for controlling infection with intracellular pathogens, including *L. monocytogenes (11,54)*. Although much attention has been given to the importance of T-cell-derived

IFN-γ, maximal IFN-γ mRNA expression in the spleens of *L. monocytogenes*-infected C57BL/6 mice is seen at d 1–2 and decreases markedly at later time-points *(71)*. The upregulation of IFN-γ following infection is extremely rapid; within 1 h, a significant upregulation is observed *(72)*. The source of IFN-γ during the early phase was assumed to be NK cells, but other cells such as macrophages, DCs, and NK T-cells may also be involved.

Studies in the SCID mouse model have suggested that NK cells are the major source of early IFN-γ production. Detailed in vitro studies from the Unanue Group demonstrated the following pathway: macrophages infected with *L. monocytogenes* produce a range of cytokines, including IL-12 and TNF, these acting to stimulate IFN-γ production by NK cells *(9)*.

In recent years, it has become apparent that macrophages and dendritic cells, following appropriate stimulation, are capable of producing significant levels of IFN-γ *(73,74)*. When T-cell-deficient (Rag-2 KO) mice are infected with *L. monocytogenes*, early IFN-γ production is not substantially reduced compared to that seen in normal mice. Traditional thinking was that NK cells were responsible for this early IFN-γ production. However, when NK cells were depleted from *L. monocytogenes*-infected RAG KO mice, there was no reduction in IFN-γ production *(75)*. Subsequent in vitro analysis suggested that both DCs and monocytes were the source of IFN-γ and that production was critically dependent on IL-12 *(75)*.

Treatment of mice with recombinant IFN-γ protects mice from *L. monocytogenes (76)*, and endogenous IFN-γ is essential for effective control of primary infection *(77,78)*. The principal listericidal function of IFN-γ is considered to be its potent ability to activate macrophages. A critical function of IFN-γ appears to be its ability to prevent pathogen escape from the phagosome to the cytosol *(79)*. Escape to the cytosol is considered to be an important pathogen defense mechanism, allowing the bacterium to avoid the harsh environment of the phagolysosome.

Interferon-γ stimulates numerous potent listericidal mechanisms. In particular, nitric oxide and reactive oxygen species are important in the control of *L. monocytogenes* infection *(80–82)*. Both of these listericidal pathways are crucially regulated by IFN-γ *(83)*.

4.1.10. Osteopontin

Osteopontin is a secreted glycoprotein regulator of inflammation and biomineralization. Mice deficient in osteopontin are markedly more susceptible to *L. monocytogenes* infection *(84)*. The increased susceptibility of osteopontin KO mice is associated with decreased production of IL-12 and IFN-γ and increased IL-10 production.

4.1.11. Other Cytokines

Recently, a novel cytokine receptor, designated T-cell cytokine receptor (TCCR), was identified by homology screening *(85)*. Signaling through this receptor is critical for the generation of Th1 immunity, and TCCR-deficient mice are markedly more susceptible to *L. monocytogenes* infection than WT mice *(85)*. The TCCR ligand has not yet been identified, but it is clearly important for resistance to *L. monocytogenes*.

Interleukin-18 is structurally related to IL-1, but functionally more closely related to IL-12. It is produced mainly by antigen-presenting cells and acts in synergy with IL-12 for Th1 cell differentiation *(86)*. During infection with the intracellular pathogens *Mycobacterium tuberculosis*, *Salmonella typhimurium*, and *Yersinia enterocolitica*, IL-18 regulates production of IFN-γ, TNF, and nitric oxide and contributes to protection *(87–89)*. These results suggest that IL-18 will turn out to be an important cytokine during *L. monocytogenes* infection.

4.2. Chemokines in Listeriosis

Chemokines are small, secreted molecules that exert chemotactic function on certain cell types *(90)*. Although the production and role of chemokines in *L. monocytogenes* infection has not been extensively studied, they are clearly important in regulating the immune response to *L. monocytogenes*.

Infection of macrophages with *L. monocytogenes* induces chemokine expression, including macrophage inflammatory protein (MIP)-1α, MIP-1β, MIP-2, KC, interferon-inducible protein (IP)-10, and RANTES *(91)*. MCP-1 induction was also observed, but only when infected macrophages were also treated with IFN-γ. Hepatocytes also responded to *L. monocytogenes* infection with chemokine production, but produced a more limited range; MCP-1 and KC, but not MIP-2 and MIP-1α *(68)*. Rapid chemokine induction was also observed following in vivo infection. Within 1–3 h of infection, mRNA for MCP-1, MIP-1α, MIP-2, KC, and IP-10 was detected in the liver of infected mice *(68)*.

A limited number of studies have focused on specific chemokines in *L. monocytogenes* infection. In a number of cases, the biological role of chemokines has been investigated by focusing on their receptor rather than the ligand.

4.2.1. MIP-1α

Macrophage inflammatory protein-1α is produced in the liver *(68)* and spleen *(90)* of *L. monocytogenes*-infected mice. Maximal MIP-1α expression in the spleen was detected at d 7, a time that coincides with maximal T-cell activation. A protective role for CD8+ T-cell-derived MIP-1α was postulated on the basis of adoptive transfer experiments *(92)*. Following transfer, *L. monocytogenes*-immune CD8+ T-cells from MIP-1α KO mice mediate much less protection than CD8+ T-cells from WT mice. It was postulated that MIP-1α was involved in the homing of CD8+ T-cells to the site of infection *(92)*.

4.2.2. MCP-1 and CCR2

Macrophage inflammatory protein-1 is a chemokine with potent chemotactic activity for monocytes. It is produced very early following *L. monocytogenes* infection, and its production is regulated by NK T-cell-derived IL-4 *(23)*. MCP-1 signals through the CCR2 chemokine receptor. CCR2 KO mice are extremely susceptible to *L. monocytogenes* infection, and this may be a result of a failure to induce macrophage migration into the site of infection *(93)*. This indicates a potentially important role for MCP-1 in resistance to *L. monocytogenes* infection, although it should be noted that there are numerous other ligands for CCR2 besides MCP-1, including MCP-2, 3, 4, and 5 *(90)*.

Paradoxically, transgenic mice expressing MCP-1 under the control of the mouse mammory tumor virus long terminal repeat (MMTV-LTR) were also more susceptible to *L. monocytogenes* infection, despite having very high levels of MCP-1 production *(94)*. It was hypothesized that this may have been the result of desensitization of circulating monocytes to MCP-1 *(95)*.

4.2.3. CCR5

The CCR5 chemokine receptor binds MIP-1α, MIP-1β, and RANTES, all of which are produced by *L. monocytogenes*-infected macrophages *(91)*. CCR5 KO mice are mildly impaired in their ability to resist *L. monocytogenes (96)*. It should be noted that these results do not preclude a more important role for MIP-1α and RANTES, as these chemokines can signal through receptors in addition to CCR5 *(96)*.

4.2.4. IL-8

Interleukin-8 is a chemokine involved in neutrophil recruitment and is released by *L. monocytogenes*-infected neutrophils *(97)*. Mice deficient in the IL-8 receptor homolog exhibit an unusual response to infection with *L. monocytogenes*. The mice showed enhanced resistance to *L. monocytogenes* infection during the early phase (d 1–4) of infection. However, some of the KO mice suffered from an inability to fully clear the infection *(98)*.

4.2.5. ATAC/Lymphotactin

Activation-induced, T cell-derived, and chemokine-related cytokine (ATAC) (lymphotactin) is the sole member of the C class of chemokines and exhibits chemotactic activity for CD4+ and CD8+ T-lymphocytes *(99)*. We have recently examined expression of this molecule in *L. monocytogenes* infection and found that it is strongly produced by NK cells and CD8+ T-lymphocytes *(100)*.

5. CONCLUSIONS

The mouse model of listeriosis has been a cornerstone for studies into the role of soluble mediators in cell-mediated immunity. In this chapter, we have attempted to summarize current knowledge about cytokines and chemokines in listeriosis. It is obvious from the discussion that numerous cytokines participate in the regulation and expression of the immune response against *L. monocytogenes*. Thus far, three major approaches have been employed, namely, (1) bolus administration of recombinant cytokines, (2) depletion of cytokines using either neutralizing antibodies or by gene knockout technology, (3) determination of cytokines by enzyme-linked immunosorbent assay and EliSpot assay, or by polymerase chain reation assays. These approaches have led to the identification of a large number of cytokines and chemokines during listeriosis. However, it is likely that the picture remains incomplete. In particular, depletion of, and treatment with, individual cytokines does not reveal at which stage of infection the particular cytokine is induced and becomes functional. A more global approach is required, which can now be achieved by transcriptome analysis *(101)*. Cytokine and chemokine microarrays will provide an excellent tool for such studies and provide new insights into the intricate crosstalk of the cytokine/chemokine repertoire involved in the immune response.

REFERENCES

1. Mackaness, G.B. (1971) Resistance to intracellular infection. *J. Infect. Dis.* **123**, 439–445.
2. Cossart, P. and Lecuit, M. (1998) Interactions of Listeria monocytogenes with mammalian cells during entry and actin-based movement: bacterial factors, cellular ligands and signaling. *EMBO J.* **17**, 3797–3806.
3. Southwick, F.S. and Purich, D.L. (1996) Intracellular pathogenesis of listeriosis. *New Engl. J. Med.* **334**, 770–776.
4. Camilli, A., Goldfine, H., and Portnoy, D.A. (1991) Listeria monocytogenes mutants lacking phosphatidylinositol-specific phospholipase C are avirulent. *J. Exp. Med.* **173**, 751–754.
5. Geoffroy, C., Raveneau, J., Beretti, J.L., Lecroisey, A., Vazquez-Boland, J.A., Alouf, J.E., et al. (1991) Purification and characterization of an extracellular 29-kilodalton phospholipase C from Listeria monocytogenes. *Infect. Immun.* **59**, 2382–2388.
6. Leimeister-Wachter, M., Domann, E., and Chakraborty, T. (1991) Detection of a gene encoding a phosphatidylinositol-specific phospholipase C that is co-ordinately expressed with listeriolysin in Listeria monocytogenes. *Mol. Microbiol.* **5**, 361–366.
7. Cossart, P. and Bierne, H. (2001) The use of host cell machinery in the pathogenesis of *Listeria monocytogenes*. *Curr. Opin. Immunol.* **13**, 96–103.
8. Schuchat, A., Deaver, K.A., Wenger, J.D., Plikaytis, B.D., Mascola, L., Pinner, R.W., et al. (1992) Role of foods in sporadic listeriosis. I. Case-control study of dietary risk factors. The Listeria Study Group. *JAMA* **267**, 2041–2045.
9. Unanue, E.R. (1997) Studies in listeriosis show the strong symbiosis between the innate cellular system and the T-cell response. *Immunol. Rev.* **158**, 11–25.
10. Edelson, B.T. and Unanue, E.R. (2000) Immunity to Listeria infection. *Curr. Opin. Immunol.* **12**, 425–431.
11. Schaible, U.E., Collins, H.L., and Kaufmann, S.H. (1999) Confrontation between intracellular bacteria and the immune system. *Adv. Immunol.* **71**, 267–377.
12. North, R.J. and Conlan, J.W. (1998) Immunity to Listeria monocytogenes. *Chem. Immunol.* **70**, 1–20.
13. Pamer, E.G., Sijts, A.J., Villanueva, M.S., Busch, D.H., and Vijh, S. (1997) MHC class I antigen processing of Listeria monocytogenes proteins: implications for dominant and subdominant CTL responses. *Immunol. Rev.* **158**, 129–136.
14. Mombaerts, P., Arnoldi, J., Russ, F., Tonegawa, S., and Kaufmann, S.H.E. (1993) Different roles of α/β and γ/δ T cells in immunity against an intracellular bacterial pathogen. *Nature* **365**, 53–56.
15. Kaufmann, S.H., Emoto, M., Szalay, G., Barsig, J., and Flesch, I.E. (1997) Interleukin-4 and listeriosis. *Immunol Rev.* **158**, 95–105.
16. Kurt-Jones, E.A., Virgin, H.W.T., and Unanue, E.R. (1986) In vivo and in vitro expression of macrophage membrane interleukin 1 in response to soluble and particulate stimuli. *J. Immunol.* **137**, 10–14.
17. Havell, E.A., Moldawer, L.L., Helfgott, D., Kilian, P.L., and Sehgal, P.B. (1992) Type I IL-1 receptor blockade exacerbates murine listeriosis. *J. Immunol.* **148**, 1486–1492.
18. Rogers, H.W., Sheehan, K.C., Brunt, L.M., Dower, S.K., Unanue, E.R., and Schreiber, R.D. (1992) Interleukin 1 participates in the development of anti-Listeria responses in normal and SCID mice. *Proc. Natl. Acad. Sci. USA* **89**, 1011–1015.
19. Czuprynski, C.J. and Brown, J.F. (1987) Recombinant murine interleukin-1 alpha enhancement of nonspecific antibacterial resistance. *Infect. Immun.* **55**, 2061–2065.
20. Hirsch, E., Irikura, V.M., Paul, S.M., and Hirsh, D. (1996) Functions of interleukin 1 receptor antagonist in gene knockout and overproducing mice. *Proc. Natl. Acad. Sci. USA* **93**, 11,008–11,013.
21. Rogers, H.W., Tripp, C.S., Schreiber, R.D., and Unanue, E.R. (1994) Endogenous IL-1 is required for neutrophil recruitment and macrophage activation during murine listeriosis. *J. Immunol.* **153**, 2093–2101.
22. Rogers, H.W. and Unanue, E.R. (1993) Neutrophils are involved in acute, nonspecific resistance to Listeria monocytogenes in mice. *Infect. Immun.* **61**, 5090–5096.

23. Flesch, I.E., Wandersee, A., and Kaufmann, S.H. (1997) IL-4 secretion by CD4+ NK1+ T cells induces monocyte chemoattractant protein-1 in early listeriosis. *J. Immunol.* **159**, 7–10.
24. Texeira, H.C. and Kaufmann, S.H. (1994) Role of NK1.1+ cells in experimental listeriosis. NK1+ cells are early IFN-gamma producers but impair resistance to Listeria monocytogenes infection. *J. Immunol.* **152**, 1873–1882.
25. Haak-Frendscho, M., Brown, J.F., Iizawa, Y., Wagner, R.D., and Czuprynski, C.J. (1992) Administration of anti-IL-4 monoclonal antibody 11B11 increases the resistance of mice to Listeria monocytogenes infection. *J. Immunol.* **148**, 3978–3985.
26. Nishikawa, S., Miura, T., Sasaki, S., and Nakane, A. (1996) The protective role of endogenous cytokines in host resistance against an intragastric infection with Listeria monocytogenes in mice. *FEMS Immunol. Med. Microbiol.* **16**, 291–298.
27. Samsom, J.N., Annema, A., Langermans, J.A., and van Furth, R. (1998) Endogenous interleukin-4 does not suppress the resistance against a primary or a secondary Listeria monocytogenes infection in mice. *Scand. J. Immunol.* **47**, 369–374.
28. Szalay, G., Ladel, C.H., Blum, C., and Kaufmann, S.H. 1996 IL-4 neutralization or TNF-alpha treatment ameliorate disease by an intracellular pathogen in IFN-gamma receptor-deficient mice. *J. Immunol.* **157**, 4746–4750.
29. Nakane, A., Nishikawa, S., Sasaki, S., Miura, T., Asano, M., Kohanawa, M., et al. (1996) Endogenous interleukin-4, but not interleukin-10, is involved in suppression of host resistance against Listeria monocytogenes infection in interferon-depleted mice. *Infect. Immun.* **64**, 1252–1258.
30. Nakane, A., Numata, A., and Minagawa, T. (1992) Endogenous tumor necrosis factor, interleukin-6, and gamma interferon levels during Listeria monocytogenes infection in mice. *Infect. Immun.* **60**, 523–528.
31. Liu, Z. and Cheers, C. (1993) The cellular source of interleukin-6 during Listeria infection. *Infect. Immun.* **61**, 2626–2631.
32. Liu, Z., Simpson, R.J., and Cheers, C. (1992) Recombinant interleukin-6 protects mice against experimental bacterial infection. *Infect. Immun.* **60**, 4402–4406.
33. Liu, Z., Simpson, R.J., and Cheers, C. (1994) Role of IL-6 in activation of T cells for acquired cellular resistance to Listeria monocytogenes. *J. Immunol.* **152**, 5375–5380.
34. Kopf, M., Baumann, H., Freer, G., Freudenberg, M., Lamers, M., Kishimoto, T., et al. 1994 Impaired immune and acute-phase responses in interleukin-6-deficient mice. *Nature* **368**, 339–342.
35. Dalrymple, S. A., Lucian, L. A., Slattery, R., McNeil, T., Aud, D. M., Fuchino, S., et al. (1995) Interleukin-6-deficient mice are highly susceptible to Listeria monocytogenes infection: correlation with inefficient neutrophilia. *Infect. Immun.* **63**, 2262–2268.
36. Liu, Z., Simpson, R.J., and Cheers, C. (1995) Interaction of interleukin-6, tumour necrosis factor and interleukin-1 during Listeria infection. *Immunology* **85**, 562–567.
37. Moore, K.W., de Waal Malefyt, R., Coffman, R.L., and O'Garra, A. (2001) Interleukin-10 and the interleukin-10 receptor. *Annu. Rev. Immunol.* **19**, 683–765.
38. Blauer, F., Groscurth, P., Schneemann, M., Schoedon, G., and Schaffner, A. (1995) Modulation of the antilisterial activity of human blood-derived macrophages by activating and deactivating cytokines. *J. Interferon Cytokine Res.* **15**, 105–114.
39. Wagner, R.D., and Czuprynski, C.J. (1993) Cytokine mRNA expression in livers of mice infected with Listeria monocytogenes. *J. Leukocyte Biol.* **53**, 525–531.
40. Flesch, I.E., and Kaufmann, S.H. (1994) Role of macrophages and alpha beta T lymphocytes in early interleukin 10 production during Listeria monocytogenes infection. *Int. Immunol.* **6**, 463–468.
41. Kelly, J.P. and Bancroft, G.J. (1996) Administration of interleukin-10 abolishes innate resistance to Listeria monocytogenes. *Eur. J. Immunol.* **26**, 356–364.
42. Dai, W.J., Kohler, G., and Brombacher, F. (1997) Both innate and acquired immunity to *Listeria monocytogenes* infection are increased in IL-10-deficient mice. *J. Immunol.* **158**, 2259–2267.
43. Wagner, R.D., Maroushek, N.M., Brown, J.F., and Czuprynski, C.J. (1994) Treatment with anti-interleukin-10 monoclonal antibody enhances early resistance to but impairs complete clearance of *Listeria monocytogenes* infection in mice. *Infect. Immun.* **62**, 2345–2353.
44. Genovese, F., Mancuso, G., Cuzzola, M., Biondo, C., Beninati, C., Delfino, D., et al. (1999) Role of IL-10 in a neonatal mouse listeriosis model. *J. Immunol.* **163**, 2777–2782.
45. Tripp, C.S., Gately, M.K., Hakimi, J., Ling, P., and Unanue, E.R. (1994) Neutralization of IL-12 decreases resistance to Listeria in SCID and C.B-17 mice. Reversal by IFN-gamma. *J. Immunol.* **152**, 1883–1887.
46. Cleveland, M.G., Gorham, J.D., Murphy, T.L., Tuomanen, E., and Murphy, K.M. (1996) Lipoteichoic acid preparations of gram-positive bacteria induce interleukin-12 through a CD14-dependent pathway. *Infect. Immun.* **64**, 1906–1912.
47. Chace, J.H., Hooker, N.A., Mildenstein, K.L., Krieg, A.M., and Cowdery, J.S. (1997) Bacterial DNA-induced NK cell IFN-gamma production is dependent on macrophage secretion of IL-12. *Clin. Immunol. Immunopathol.* **84**, 185–193.
48. Tripp, C.S., Wolf, S.F., and Unanue, E.R. (1993) Interleukin 12 and tumor necrosis factor alpha are costimulators of interferon gamma production by natural killer cells in severe combined immunodeficiency mice with listeriosis, and interleukin 10 is a physiologic antagonist. *Proc. Natl. Acad. Sci. USA* **90**, 3725–3729.
49. Liu, T., Nishimura, H., Matsuguchi, T., and Yoshikai, Y. (2000) Differences in interleukin-12 and -15 production by dendritic cells at the early stage of *Listeria monocytogenes* infection between BALB/c and C57 BL/6 mice. *Cell Immunol.* **202**, 31–40.
50. Brombacher, F., Dorfmuller, A., Magram, J., Dai, W.J., Kohler, G., Wunderlin, A., et al. (1999) IL-12 is dispensable for innate and adaptive immunity against low doses of Listeria monocytogenes. *Int. Immunol.* **11**, 325–332.
51. McKenzie, A.N. (2000) Regulation of T helper type 2 cell immunity by interleukin-4 and interleukin-13. *Pharmacol. Ther.* **88**, 143–151.

52. Flesch, I.E., Wandersee, A., and Kaufmann, S.H. *1997* Effects of IL-13 on murine listeriosis. *Int. Immunol.* **9**, 467–474.
53. Hirose, K., Suzuki, H., Nishimura, H., Mitani, A., Washizu, J., Matsuguchi, T., et al. (1998) Interleukin-15 may be responsible for early activation of intestinal intraepithelial lymphocytes after oral infection with *Listeria monocytogenes* in rats. *Infect. Immun.* **66**, 5677–5683.
54. Kaufmann, S.H.E. (1998) Immunity to intracellular bacteria, in *Fundamental Immunology* (Paul, W.E., ed.), Lippincott-Raven, New York.
55. Kuhn, M. and Goebel, W. (1994) Induction of cytokines in phagocytic mammalian cells infected with virulent and avirulent Listeria strains. *Infect. Immun.* **62**, 348–356.
56. Havell, E.A. (1987) Production of tumor necrosis factor during murine listeriosis. *J. Immunol.* **139**, 4225–4231.
57. Poston, R.M. and Kurlander, R.J. (1992) Cytokine expression in vivo during murine listeriosis. Infection with live, virulent bacteria is required for monokine and lymphokine messenger RNA accumulation in the spleen. *J. Immunol.* **149**, 3040–3044.
58. Nakane, A., Minagawa, T., and Kato, K. (1988) Endogenous tumor necrosis factor (cachectin) is essential to host resistance against *Listeria monocytogenes* infection. *Infect. Immun.* **56**, 2563–2569.
59. Havell, E.A. (1989) Evidence that tumor necrosis factor has an important role in antibacterial resistance. *J. Immunol.* **143**, 2894–2899.
60. Beretich, G.R., Jr., Carter, P.B., and Havell, E.A. (1998) Roles for tumor necrosis factor and gamma interferon in resistance to enteric listeriosis. *Infect. Immun.* **66**, 2368–2373.
61. Pfeffer, K., Matsuyama, T., Kundig, T.M., Wakeham, A., Kishihara, K., Shahinian, A., et al. (1993) Mice deficient for the 55 kd tumor necrosis factor receptor are resistant to endotoxic shock, yet succumb to *L. monocytogenes* infection. *Cell* **73**, 457–467.
62. Rothe, J., Lesslauer, W., Lotscher, H., Lang, Y., Koebel, P., Kontgen, F., et al. 1993 Mice lacking the tumour necrosis factor receptor 1 are resistant to TNF-mediated toxicity but highly susceptible to infection by *Listeria monocytogenes*. *Nature* **364**, 798–802.
63. Eugster, H.P., Muller, M., Karrer, U., Car, B.D., Schnyder, B., Eng, V.M., et al. (1996) Multiple immune abnormalities in tumor necrosis factor and lymphotoxin- alpha double-deficient mice. *Int. Immunol.* **8**, 23–36.
64. Pasparakis, M., Alexopoulou, L., Episkopou, V., and Kollias, G. (1996) Immune and inflammatory responses in TNF alpha-deficient mice: a critical requirement for TNF alpha in the formation of primary B cell follicles, follicular dendritic cell networks and germinal centers, and in the maturation of the humoral immune response. *J. Exp. Med.* **184**, 1397–1411.
65. White, D.W., Badovinac, V.P., Fan, X., and Harty, J.T. (2000) Adaptive immunity against *Listeria monocytogenes* in the absence of type I tumor necrosis factor receptor p55. *Infect. Immun.* **68**, 4470–4476.
66. Peschon, J.J., Torrance, D.S., Stocking, K.L., Glaccum, M.B., Otten, C., Willis, C.R., et al. (1998) TNF receptor-deficient mice reveal divergent roles for p55 and p75 in several models of inflammation. *J Immunol.* **160**, 943–952.
67. Wherry, J.C., Schreiber, R.D., and Unanue, E.R. 1991 Regulation of gamma interferon production by natural killer cells in scid mice: roles of tumor necrosis factor and bacterial stimuli. *Infect. Immun.* **59**, 1709–1715.
68. Barsig, J., Flesch, I.E., and Kaufmann, S.H. (1998) Macrophages and hepatocytic cells as chemokine producers in murine listeriosis. *Immunobiology* **199**, 87–104.
69. Zhan, Y. and Cheers, C. (1998) Control of IL-12 and IFN-gamma production in response to live or dead bacteria by TNF and other factors. *J. Immunol.* **161**, 1447–1453.
70. Endres, R., Luz, A., Schulze, H., Neubauer, H., Futterer, A., Holland, S.M., et al. (1997) Listeriosis in p47(phox–/–) and TRp55–/– mice: protection despite absence of ROI and susceptibility despite presence of RNI. *Immunity* **7**, 419–432.
71. Poston, R.M. and Kurlander, R.J. (1991) Analysis of the time course of IFN-gamma mRNA and protein production during primary murine listeriosis. The immune phase of bacterial elimination is not temporally linked to IFN production in vivo. *J. Immunol.* **146**, 4333–4337.
72. Iizawa, Y., Brown, J.F., and Czuprynski, C.J. (1992) Early expression of cytokine mRNA in mice infected with *Listeria monocytogenes*. *Infect. Immun.* **60**, 4068–4073.
73. Puddu, P., Fantuzzi, L., Borghi, P., Varano, B., Rainaldi, G., Guillemard, E., et al. (1997) IL-12 induces IFN-gamma expression and secretion in mouse peritoneal macrophages. *J. Immunol.* **159**, 3490–3497.
74. Munder, M., Mallo, M., Eichmann, K., and Modolell, M. (1998) Murine macrophages secrete interferon gamma upon combined stimulation with interleukin (IL)-12 and IL-18: A novel pathway of autocrine macrophage activation. *J. Exp. Med.* **187**, 2103–2108.
75. Ohteki, T., Fukao, T., Suzue, K., Maki, C., Ito, M., Nakamura, M., et al. (1999) Interleukin 12-dependent interferon gamma production by CD8alpha+ lymphoid dendritic cells. *J. Exp. Med.* **189**, 1981–1986.
76. Kiderlen, A.F., Kaufmann, S.H.E., and Lohmann-Mathes, M.L. (1984) Protection of mice against the intracellular bacterium *Listeria monocytogenes* by recombinant immune interferon. *Eur. J. Immunol.* **14**, 964–967.
77. Huang, S., Hendriks, W., Althage, A., Hemmi, S., Bluethmann, H., Kamijo, R., et al. (1993) Immune response in mice that lack the interferon-gamma receptor. *Science* **259**, 1742–1745.
78. Buchmeier, N.A. and Schreiber, R.D. (1985) Requirement of endogenous interferon-gamma production for resolution of *Listeria monocytogenes* infection. *Proc. Natl. Acad. Sci. USA* **82**, 7404–7408.
79. Portnoy, D.A., Schreiber, R.D., Connelly, P., and Tilney, L.G. (1989) Gamma interferon limits access of *Listeria monocytogenes* to the macrophage cytoplasm. *J. Exp. Med.* **170**, 2141–2146.
80. Beckerman, K.P., Rogers, H.W., Corbett, J.A., Schreiber, R.D., McDaniel, M.L., and Unanue, E.R. (1993) Release of nitric oxide during the T cell-independent pathway of macrophage activation. Its role in resistance to *Listeria monocytogenes*. *J. Immunol.* **150**, 888–895.

81. Muller, M., Althaus, R., Frohlich, D., Frei, K., and Eugster, H.P. (1999) Reduced antilisterial activity of TNF-deficient bone marrow-derived macrophages is due to impaired superoxide production. *Eur. J. Immunol.* **29,** 3089–3097.

82. Shiloh, M.U., MacMicking, J.D., Nicholson, S., Brause, J.E., Potter, S., Marino, M., et al. (1999) Phenotype of mice and macrophages deficient in both phagocyte oxidase and inducible nitric oxide synthase. *Immunity* **10,** 29–38.

83. Ding, A.H., Nathan, C.F., and Stuehr, D.J. (1988) Release of reactive nitrogen intermediates and reactive oxygen intermediates from mouse peritoneal macrophages. Comparison of activating cytokines and evidence for independent production. *J. Immunol.* **141,** 2407–2412.

84. Ashkar, S., Weber, G.F., Panoutsakopoulou, V., Sanchirico, M.E., Jansson, M., Zawaideh, S., et al. (2000) Eta-1 (osteopontin): an early component of type-1 (cell-mediated) immunity. *Science* **287,** 860–864.

85. Chen, Q., Ghilardi, N., Wang, H., Baker, T., Xie, M.H., Gurney, A., et al. (2000) Development of Th1-type immune responses requires the type I cytokine receptor TCCR. *Nature* **407,** 916–920.

86. Lebel-Binay, S., Berger, A., Zinzindohoue, F., Cugnenc, P., Thiounn, N., Fridman, W. H., et al. (2000) Interleukin-18: biological properties and clinical implications. *Eur. Cytokine Network* **11,** 15–26.

87. Sugawara, I., Yamada, H., Kaneko, H., Mizuno, S., Takeda, K., and Akira, S. (1999) Role of interleukin-18 (IL-18) in mycobacterial infection in IL-18-gene-disrupted mice. *Infect. Immun.* **67,** 2585–2589.

88. Bohn, E., Sing, A., Zumbihl, R., Bielfeldt, C., Okamura, H., Kurimoto, M., et al. (1998) IL-18 (IFN-gamma-inducing factor) regulates early cytokine production in, and promotes resolution of, bacterial infection in mice. *J. Immunol.* **160,** 299–307.

89. Dybing, J.K., Walters, N., and Pascual, D.W. (1999) Role of endogenous interleukin-18 in resolving wild-type and attenuated *Salmonella typhimurium* infections. *Infect. Immun.* **67,** 6242–6248.

90. Rossi, D. and Zlotnik, A. (2000) The biology of chemokines and their receptors. *Annu. Rev. Immunol.* **18,** 217–242.

91. Flesch, I.E., Barsig, J., and Kaufmann, S.H. (1998) Differential chemokine response of murine macrophages stimulated with cytokines and infected with *Listeria monocytogenes*. *Int Immunol.* **10,** 757–765.

92. Cook, D.N., Smithies, O., Strieter, R.M., Frelinger, J.A., and Serody, J.S. 1999 CD8+ T cells are a biologically relevant source of macrophage inflammatory protein-1 alpha in vivo. *J. Immunol.* **162,** 5423–5428.

93. Kurihara, T., Warr, G., Loy, J., and Bravo, R. (1997) Defects in macrophage recruitment and host defense in mice lacking the CCR2 chemokine receptor. *J. Exp. Med.* **186,** 1757–1762.

94. Rutledge, B.J., Rayburn, H., Rosenberg, R., North, R.J., Gladue, R.P., Corless, C.L., et al. (1995) High level monocyte chemoattractant protein-1 expression in transgenic mice increases their susceptibility to intracellular pathogens. *J. Immunol.* **155,** 4838–4843.

95. Gu, L., Rutledge, B., Fiorillo, J., Ernst, C., Grewal, I., Flavell, R., et al. (1997) In vivo properties of monocyte chemoattractant protein-1. *J Leukocytr Biol.* **62,** 577–580.

96. Zhou, Y., Kurihara, T., Ryseck, R.P., Yang, Y., Ryan, C., Loy, J., et al. (1998) Impaired macrophage function and enhanced T cell-dependent immune response in mice lacking CCR5, the mouse homologue of the major HIV-1 coreceptor. *J. Immunol.* **160,** 4018–4025.

97. Arnold, R. and Konig, W. (1998) Interleukin-8 release from human neutrophils after phagocytosis of *Listeria monocytogenes* and *Yersinia enterocolitica*. *J. Med. Microbiol.* **47,** 55–62.

98. Czuprynski, C.J., Brown, J.F., Steinberg, H., and Carroll, D. (1998) Mice lacking the murine interleukin-8 receptor homologue demonstrate paradoxical responses to acute and chronic experimental infection with *Listeria monocytogenes*. *Microb. Pathog.* **24,** 17–23.

99. Dorner, B., Muller, S., Entschladen, F., Schroder, J. M., Franke, P., Kraft, R., et al. (1997) Purification, structural analysis, and function of natural ATAC, a cytokine secreted by CD8(+) T cells. *J. Biol. Chem.* **272,** 8817–8823.

100. Dorner, B.G., Scheffold, A., Rolph, M.S., Huser, M.B., Kaufmann, S.H.E., Radbruch, A., et al. (2002) MIP-1α, MIP-1β, RANTES, and ATAC/lymphotostin function together with IFN-γ as type 1 cytokines. *Proc. Natl. Acad. Sci. USA.* **99,** 6181–6186.

101. Cohen, P., Bouaboula, M., Bellis, M., Baron, V., Jbilo, O., Poinot-Chazel, C., et al. 2000 Monitoring cellular responses to *Listeria monocytogenes* with oligonucleotide arrays. *J. Biol. Chem.* **275,** 11,181–11,190.

IV
Cytokines in Mycobacterial Infections

9

Regulation of Cytokines and Chemokines in Human *Mycobacterium tuberculosis* Infection

Zahra Toossi and Jerrold J. Ellner

1. INTRODUCTION

Tuberculosis (TB) continues to scourge mankind with a mortality of approx 3 million and an incidence of 10 million new cases each year *(1)*. One-third of the world population is infected with *Mycobacterium tuberculosis* (MTB), which signifies both the success of this intracellular pathogen in the establishment of infection in humans and the lack of effective available means of prevention of infection. A complete understanding of the interface of MTB with the human immune response is critical to the development of immunotherapies and effective vaccines in the fight against TB.

Recent research indicates that intense cytokine and chemokine responses ensue upon MTB infection of the primary cell type targeted by the pathogen, human alveolar macrophages. Subsequent to infection, the innate immune response comprised of newly recruited white blood cells and both proinflammatory and anti-inflammatory cytokines is initiated *in situ*. As the local immune response matures, the cellular constituents and the cytokine and chemokine profile of the tuberculous lesion change over time. The full development of anti-MTB immune responsiveness, which involves T-cells, a Th1 cytokine profile, and macrophage activation, finally allows the control of MTB infection in 95% of infected individuals *(2)*. However, ultimately in a small group (5%) of those who have mounted effective anti-MTB immunity, mechanisms of immunosurveillance against MTB are lost, resulting in active TB (reactivation TB). Dysregulations of cytokines and chemokines during active TB and at sites of MTB infection have been documented, which correlate with the intensity of MTB infection and the advancement of disease *(3)*. However, these features of active TB further underscores the role of a coordinated immune response in the success of containment of MTB infection.

This chapter summarizes data accumulated over recent years on cytokine and chemokine responses induced by MTB, their cross-regulation at sites of infection, and their role in containment of MTB infection. Further, the significance of cytokine and chemokine dysregulation in pathogenesis of TB are described, and a potential role for immunotherapies to fortify or inhibit particular responses is defined.

2. INDUCTION OF CYTOKINES AND CHEMOKINES DURING PRIMARY MTB INFECTION

Mycobacterium tuberculosis induces immune cells to produce cytokines and chemokines through both phagocytic and nonphagocytic interactions and through a multitude of mycobacterial protein and nonprotein moieties. Autoinduction and amplification loops allow the predominant expression of a group of molecules at sites of MTB infection that varies at different time-points. Functionally,

From: *Cytokines and Chemokines in Infectious Diseases Handbook*
Edited by: M. Kotb and T. Calandra © Humana Press Inc., Totowa, NJ

cytokines and chemokines may either act in synergy or antagonize one another. However, at any stage of infection, the balance of macrophage-activating versus macrophage-deactivating molecules may impact on the balance between containment versus extension and dissemination of MTB infection.

The recruitment of blood mononuclear and polymorphonuclear (PMN) cells that mediate inflammation and, ultimately, are important to the development of protective immunity at sites of MTB infection is orchestrated by chemokines *(4)*. Specifically, interleukin (IL)-8 *(5)*, monocyte chemoattractant protein-1 (MCP-1) *(6)*, and growth-related gene product (GRO)-α *(7,8)* are promptly induced by MTB in alveolar macrophages and allow the recruitment of PMN cells, monocytes, natural killer (NK) cells, and γδ T-cells. The recruited PMN and mononuclear cells generate secondary waves of chemokines once exposed to MTB and its products *in situ*. For example, MTB induces PMN cells to release IL-8, GROα-, and MCP-1 *(9,10)*. However, it is of note that on a per cell basis, monocyte/macrophages produce more chemokines than PMN cells. Thus, the evolution of the chemokine profile *in situ* may be mainly determined by the profile of molecules induced by MTB in newly recruited monocytes and alveolar macrophages. It appears that in comparison to other β-chemokines, MCP-1 is preferentially induced by MTB in macrophages *(6)*. Further, amplifying loops may lead to excess production of certain chemokines. For example, the release of MCP-1 and IL-8, but not macrophage inflammatory protein (MIP)-1α, was induced by tumor necrosis factor (TNF)-α *(11,12)*. Therefore, the expression of TNF-α, which is documented to occur during all stages of MTB infection *(13)*, provides a mechanism for continuous recruitment of monocytes and PMN cells to tuberculous lesions.

A prominent feature of MTB infection, which likely is important in the pathogenesis of TB, is the profuse induction of proinflammatory cytokines in monocyte/macrophages *(11)* and PMN cells. Early studies indicated that purified protein derivative (PPD) of MTB induces the proinflammatory cytokines interleukin (IL)-1β and TNF-α *(14,15)* in monocyte/macrophages. Importantly, major secretory components of actively replicating MTB, such as the 30-kDa antigen *(16)* and the 58-kDa antigen *(17)*, and mycobacterial cell wall lipoarabinomannan (LAM) *(18)*, strongly induce TNF-α. Interestingly, the 30-kDa antigen is a fibronectin-binding protein *(19)*, and its interaction with fibronectin enhances the production of TNF-α by monocytes *(16)*. Other antigens of MTB *(17)* also induce TNF-α and IL-1β. Other proinflammatory cytokines, such as IL-6 and granulocyte–macrophage colony-stimulating factor (GM-CSF), are also induced by MTB and its components. In addition, MTB strongly induces the expression of IL-12 in mononuclear phagocytes, which is critical to the development of a Th1 response *(20)*.

However, mechanisms to turn off *in situ* MTB-induced inflammation are also operative early on, in part secondary to the effects of the inflammatory cytokines themselves and partly induced by MTB and its components. For example, IL-10 is induced in response to TNF-α, and by MTB *(22,23)*. Further, MTB *(24)* and its cell wall LAM *(25)* are potent inducers of transforming growth factor (TGF)-β. The effect of LAM on induction of TGF-β appears to be dominant over induction of the proinflammatory cytokines (TNF-α, IL-1β, and IL-6), and IL-10 *(25)*. Recently, mycobacterial 30-kDa antigen also has been shown to induce TGF-α (Hirsch, unpublished data). Further, through binding and activation of plasminogen *(26)*, MTB may also be involved in conversion of latent (L) TGF-β to the bioactive form of this cytokine *(27)*. However, in addition to being anti-inflammatory cytokines, IL-10 and TGF-β, are also macrophage deactivating and suppressive of T-cell responses *(28)*.

With the recruitment of NK cells, γδ T-cells, and, finally, αβ T-cells to sites of MTB-infection, an MTB-directed immune response appears and gradually strengthens *in situ*, in which the Th1 cytokines, IL-2 and interferon (IFN)-γ are expressed. In animal models of MTB infection, infiltration by CD4 and CD8 cells and the development of Th1 response is coincident with the disappearance of active MTB replication and establishment of MTB latency *(29)*. IL-2 is critical to the clonal expansion of MTB-reactive T-cells, and IFN-γ activates macrophages against MTB *(11)*. In humans, evidence for a definitive role for Th1 cytokines in the containment of mycobacterial diseases derives from fatal mycobacterial infections seen in subjects lacking genes for IFN-γ receptor (R) *(30)* or IL-

12R *(31)*. Once matured, the Th1 response counteracts macrophage deactivation by molecules such as TGF-β and IL-10, which are already present *in situ*, and, finally, control of MTB replication becomes possible. Lack of IL-4 at sites of primary MTB infection *(32)* undermines a role for Th2 cytokines in cross-regulation of the developing Th1 response.

3. DYSREGULATIONS OF CYTOKINES AND CHEMOKINES DURING ACTIVE TB AND AT SITES OF MTB INFECTION

Dysregulation of cytokine networks during TB involve both depressed TH1 cytokines and excessive production of monocyte cytokines. Both in vivo and in vitro evidence support the contention that patients with active pulmonary tuberculosis are suppressed in cell-mediated immune responses to antigens of MTB. Delayed-type skin test reactivity to PPD is lost in 17–25% of patients, and about 60% have low T-cell blastogenic responses to PPD. Low T-cell responses correlate with skin test anergy and the severity of pulmonary TB *(11,33)*. The Th1 cytokines (IL-2 and IFN-γ), responses are blunted in response to MTB in patients with active pulmonary TB *(11)*, but remain strong in paucibacillary TB *(34)*. The low production of IFN-γ is associated with lower responsiveness to IL-12 *(35)* and decreased expression of IL-12R *(36)*. On the other hand, the stimulated release of TNF-α *(37)*, IL-1β *(15)*, and IL-6 *(37)* in blood mononuclear cells from TB patients are upregulated during active TB. Monocytes from patients with active TB express TGF-β spontaneously and have an enhanced capacity to produce this cytokine upon in vitro stimulation by products of MTB *(33, 38)*. Abrogation of TGF-β both by neutralizing antibody and by natural inhibitors corrects low MTB-induced T-cell responses *(33,39)*. Also, expression of both IL-12 and IL-12R *(35,36)* improve upon neutralization of TGF-β. On the other hand, MTB antigen-induced IL-10 levels were either similar *(33)* or only slightly elevated *(40)* in cultures of peripheral blood mononuclear cells (PBMCs) from patients with tuberculosis as compared to healthy PPD skin test reactive subjects. However, in both studies the antibody to IL-10 corrected low T-cell responses of patients. These data suggest either a greater sensitivity of T-cells from TB patients to IL-10 or cooperativity between cytokines in modulation of Th1 responses. Interestingly, whereas high TGF-β and IL-10 production by mononuclear cells from TB patients corrects by the third month of antituberculous chemotherapy, a more sustained defect in production of IFN-γ can be observed *(40)*, suggesting a possible primary T-cell defect during TB. Recent studies indicate that during TB, both CD4 and non-CD4 cells undergo apoptosis *(41)*.

Studies of human mononuclear cells from sites of active MTB infection are less frequent but very helpful in understanding the role of cytokines and chemokines during the spectrum of MTB infection. For example, increased production of TNF-α and IFN-γ in pleural fluid and by pleural mononuclear cells from patients with TB pleuritis *(34,41)* may indicate that this form of postprimary TB, which is self-resolving and usually smear and culture negative (in the human immunodeficiency virus [HIV]-uninfected host) at the time of diagnosis, is associated with a successful, although not complete, anti-MTB immune responsiveness *in situ*. On the other hand, a greater frequency of IFN-γ producing cells in broncho-alveolar lavage (BAL) of patients with pulmonary TB as compared to healthy PPD reactive subjects in the face of a similar capacity to produce this cytokine *(42)* most likely indicates a relative suppression of the function of MTB reactive T-cells *in situ* during TB. In support of this, lower IFN-γ responses of bronchoalveolar cells (BACs) from a limited number of TB patients improved upon treatment of TB *(43)*. Furthermore, administration of IFN-γ to a limited number of subjects with drug-resistant TB proved to be beneficial *(44)*. However, production of "adequate" amounts of IFN-γ may be only one of several components contributing to successful anti-MTB responses in vivo. Another macrophage-activating cytokine, TNF-α, is increased in BAL fluid from TB patients *(43)*. On the other hand, in contrast to previous studies in which no *(42)* or variable amounts *(43)* of TGF-β were found in the BAL fluid of TB patients, an augmentation of TGF-β activity in BAL fluid of TB patients as compared to healthy subjects has been recently described *(45)*. More studies, however, are needed to clarify the role of TGF-β at sites of MTB infection. Whether the immunopathogenesis of reactivation TB in humans involves an *in situ* shift of Th1 to Th2 cytokine production is not known. However, excess expression of Th2 cytokines by blood cells is not a feature of pulmonary *(33)* or lymph node TB *(46)*.

Recent studies have also characterized dysregulations in patterns of chemokines at sites of MTB infection. For example, MIP-1α is limited, but MCP-1 is excessive in pleural fluid of patients with pleural TB, regardless of HIV infection *(47)*. The same pattern can be seen in the BAL fluid of patients with pulmonary TB *(6)*. Excessive IL-8 activity has been also found in the BAL fluid from TB patients *(48)*. However, the significance of these chemokine imbalances in the pathogenesis of TB is not yet clear.

Histopathological studies of tuberculous lesions from patients with TB have established associations between the architecture of tuberculous granuloma and *in situ* cytokine and chemokine expression. For example, expression of GM-CSF, TNF-α, and IL-8 by granulomas correlate with the presence of florid granulomatous lesions, the absence of central necrosis, and the presence of neutrophil infiltration *(49)*, respectively. On the other hand, TGF-β, but not TNF-α or IFN-γ, has been identified in lung lesions of patients with active TB *(50)*, in association with Langhans' giant cells and epithelioid cells *(38)* . However, excess TGF-β *in situ* may reflect the stage of the granulomatous response, as observed in MTB-infected mice *(51)*.

Recent studies have indicated that the cytokine profile may vary according to the clinical form of TB. For example, whereas IL-10 was found to be the predominant macrophage-deactivating cytokine in the BAL fluid of children with miliary TB, TGFβ was found to predominate in children with pulmonary TB *(32)*. Also, the frequency of circulating CD4 and CD8 mononuclear cells expressing IL-4 was higher in cavitary as opposed to noncavitary TB *(52)*, indicating a possible role for Th2 responses in tissue destruction. Other studies indicate that genetic polymorphisms of cytokine responses may also influence the form of TB *(53)*. However, the influence of disease severity on capacity of expression of TH1 cytokines by blood mononuclear cells in vitro has been well documented *(33,54)*.

4. CROSS-MODULATION OF CYTOKINE EXPRESSION AND ACTION IN MTB INFECTION

Interactive stimulatory and/or inhibitory pathways established between cytokines or chemokines may result in potentiation or attenuation of the effects of each molecule on immune responses. As noted earlier, cytokines and chemokines may regulate their own production or the production of one another by the creation of amplification loops. Cytokines such as TNF-α *(55)* and TGF-β *(27)* upregulate their own production, thereby allowing a mechanism for predominance over other cytokines. Also, they may synergize or counteract the effects of one another, thus assuring the expression of a particular immunologic event at a time *in situ*. However, the interaction of cytokines and their net balance with regard to macrophage activation (or deactivation) and immune stimulation (or suppression) ultimately determines the success of the host immune response at sites of active infection.

The interaction of TGF-β and IL-12 in the regulation of MTB-induced IFN-γ production of PBMCs from patients with pulmonary TB and by MTB has been recently investigated extensively. Expression of both IL-12 p40 and p35 mRNA in response to MTB was suppressed by TGF-β *(35)*. However, TGF-β also interfered with the activity of IL-12 in the enhancement of MTB-induced IFN-γ mRNA expression and cytokine production *(35)*. In PBMCs of TB patients, the main effect of TGF-β on IL-12 appeared to be counter to the action of IL-12-induced IFN-γ production in response to MTB *(35)*. This may be the result of TGF-β-mediated modulation of IL-12R *(36)*.

A regulatory role for interleukin IL-12 in the production of TGF-β has been suggested, but remains controversial. In the human cell lines K562 and A549 and in primary human monocytes and macrophages, exogenous IL-12 downregulates TGF-β mRNA expression *(56)*. Other monocyte/macrophage cytokines, including IL-10, TNF-α, IL-1β, or IL-6, do not affect TGF-β expression (Toossi, unpublished data). Further, the effect of IL-12 on TGF-β expression appears to be mediated through

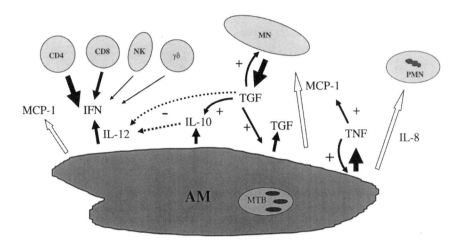

Fig. 1. Model of cytokine and chemokine production by mononuclear cells at sites of *M. tuberculosis* (MTB) infection. MTB-infected alveolar macrophages (AM) produce chemokines (e.g., IL-8, MCP-1). Recruitment by chemokines (empty arrow) of polymorphonuclear cells (PMN), monocytes (MN), natural killer cells (NK), and, eventually, CD4 and CD8 cells to MTB infected sites of infection is associated with cytokine production (black arrow). Amplification (+) and inhibition (–) loops between cytokines and chemokines occur. IFN-γ produced by all classes of lymphocytes ultimately limits MTB growth.

modulation of TGF-β promoter *(56)*. Thus, the critical role of IL-12 in the early activation of the immune response to MTB may include down-modulation of TGF-β gene activity.

An amplifying interaction of TGF-β and IL-10 on MTB-stimulated production of IFN-γ has been described that may impede Th1 responses during MTB infection. Both exogenous IL-10 and TGF-β independently suppress the production of MTB antigen-induced IFN-γ in human mononuclear cells *(23)*. However, synergistic suppression of IFN-γ in cultures containing both rTGF-β and rIL-10 was only seen when the responder cell population was enriched for monocytes and when cells were pre-treated with rTGF-β but not with rIL-10. Also, neutralization of both endogenous TGF-β and IL-10 enhanced PPD-induced IFN-γ in PBMC in a synergistic manner. Further, TGF-β induced monocyte IL-10 production but not IL-10R expression. At sites of active MTB infection, these interactions may be conducive to suppression of TH1 responses. (*See* Fig. 1.)

5. CYTOKINE IMMUNOMODULATION IN TB

Several pilot studies have investigated the potential use of immunotherapies in TB; however, no large clinical studies have been performed to address the usefulness of cytokine immunotherapies in TB. To date no immunotherapy directed at modulation of chemokine responses has been reported likely because the biological profile of these molecules are still largely unknown.

The rationale for inhibition of TGF-β during TB is based on the excessive activity of this immuno-suppressive/macrophage-deactivating cytokine systemically and at sites of MTB infection. It appears that a vicious cycle is created *in situ*, in which MTB replication and TGF-β production in tissues augment one another. In addition, autoinduction assures excess activity of TGF-β. To a certain extent, the lack of a rapid expression of protective responses (IFN-γ and IL-2) at sites of active MTB infection in patients who are receiving antituberculous chemotherapy may be explained by excess TGF-β. In other diseases, sustained and excessive production of TGF-β is clearly associated with extensive fibrosis and tissue damage *(57)*. Fibrosis and cavity formation are features of active TB *(2)*. Thus, immunotherapies based on inhibition of production and/or action of TGF-β may be particularly help-ful as adjuncts to antituberculous chemotherapy in tuberculosis. The natural inhibitors of TGF-β (decorin and LAP) act by binding to the bioactive, mature, form of TGF-β and thus reduce the bioavailability of TGF-β. These natural inhibitors of TGF-β were effective in the restoration of MTB antigen-induced T-cell functions in patients with pulmonary TB and in enhancing MTB growth con-tainment by monocytes of healthy subjects *(39)*. More recently, we also examined the activity of systemic leukocyte alkaline phosphatase (LAP) administration on local immune responses of mice infected by BCG by aerosolization and found that LAP treatment improved IFN-γ expression and decreased MTB growth in the pulmonary tissues of these animals *(58)*. However, the TGF-β–inhibi-tors have not been assessed as immunotherapy in human TB.

The basis for the use of anti-inflammatory agents, such as corticosteroids, as adjuncts in the man-agement of patients with TB is the notion that excess TNF-α may be involved not only in the tissue destruction *(59)*, and therefore organ dysfunction, but also in enhancement of MTB replication *(60)*. The mechanism of action of corticosteroids is through activation of nuclear glucocorticoid receptors, which then can form close physical association with nuclear factor-κB (NF-κB), which upregulates the transcription of TNF-α *(61)*. Another mechanism may be through upregulation of production of the cytoplasmic inhibitor of NF-κB, I-κBα *(62)*. Other agents that can transcriptionally inhibit TNF-α are thalidomide *(63)* and pentoxyfylline *(64)*. A recent controlled study indicated that thalidomide when added to antituberculous regimen for 2–3 wk not only improved the systemic symptoms and weight gain of patients with pulmonary TB but also increased their T-cell responses to MTB *(65)*.

Use of exogenous Th1 cytokines in the immunotherapy of TB has also been assessed recently. Administration of recombinant IFN-γ to a group of HIV-uninfected patients with disseminated *Myco-bacterium avium* disease that was refractory to chemotherapy was found to be beneficial *(66)*. In another mycobacterial disease, leprosy, IFN-γ decreased the bacillary burden but was associated with a high incidence of untoward side effects *(67)*. IFN-γ has been successfully used in the treatment of an immunocompromised patient with MDR tuberculosis *(68)*. A small trial of aerosolized IFN-γ in patients with drug-resistant TB showed that treatment was well tolerated and associated with clinical and microbiologic improvements *(44)*. However, the usefulness of IFN-γ in the immunotherapy of TB awaits the completion of larger studies. Precedence for enhancement of antimycobacterial immune response employing IL-2 comes from studies using recombinant IL-2 in leprosy *(69)*. In a recent study, low-dose recombinant IL-2 was administered to patients with drug-sensitive and drug-resis-tant TB *(70)*. Minimal side effects were observed and improvement in both clinical and microbio-logic parameters were noted. Further, an increase in the size of the tuberculin skin test and enhancement of T-cell responses in the group who responded clinically to IL-2 were observed. Again, the use of IL-2 in clinical TB awaits data from already completed studies (Johnson, unpublished).

REFERENCES

1. Nunn, P. (2001) The global control of tuberculosis: what are the prospects? *Scand. J. Infect. Dis.* **33**, 329–332.
2. Toossi, Z. and Ellner, J. (1992) Tuberculosis, in *Infectious Diseases* (Gorbach, S.L., Bartlett, J.G., and Blacklow, N.R. eds.), Lippincott, Philadelphia, pp. 1238 –1245.
3. Ellner, J.J. (1997) Review: the immune response in human tuberculosis—implications for tuberculosis control. *J. In-fect. Dis.* **176**, 1351–1359.
4. Rollins, B.J., Yoshimura, T., Leonard, E.J., and Pober, J.S. (1990) Cytokine-activated human endothelial cells synthe-size and secrete a monocyte chemoattractant, MCP-1/JE. *Am. J. Pathol.* **136**, 1229–1233.
5. Zhang, Y., Broser, M., Cohen, H., Bodkin, M., Law, K., Reibman, J., et al. (1995) Enhanced interleukin-8 release and gene expression in macrophages after exposure to *Mycobacterium tuberculosis* and its components. *J. Clin. Invest.* **95**, 586–592.
6. Sadek, M.I., Sada, E., Toossi, Z., Schwander, S.K., and Rich, E.A. (1998) Chemokines induced by infection of mono-nuclear phagocytes with mycobacteria and present in lung alveoli during active pulmonary tuberculosis. *Am. J. Respir. Cell. Mol. Biol.* **19**, 513–521.
7. Riedel, D.D. and Kaufmann, S.H. (1997) Chemokine secretion by human polymorphonuclear granulocytes after stimu-lation with *Mycobacterium tuberculosis* and lipoarabinomannan. *Infect. Immun.* **65**, 4620–4623.
8. Zhang, Y., Nakata, K., Weiden, M., and Rom, W.N. (1995) *Mycobacterium tuberculosis* enhances human immunode-ficiency virus-1 replication by transcriptional activation at the long terminal repeat. *J. Clin. Invest.* **95**, 2324–2331.

9. Zhang, Y. and Rollins, B.J. (1995) A dominant negative inhibitor indicates that monocyte chemoattractant protein 1 functions as a dimer. *Mol. Cell. Biol.* **15,** 4851–4855.

10. Kasahara, K., Sato, I., Ogura, K., Takeuchi, H., Kobayashi, K., and Adachi, M. (1998) Expression of chemokines and induction of rapid cell death in human blood neutrophils by *Mycobacterium tuberculosis.* *J.Infect. Dis.* **178,** 127–137.

11. Toossi, Z. (1996) Cytokine circuits in tuberculosis. *Infect. Agents Dis.* **5,** 98–107.

12. Goebeler, M., Kilian, K., Gillitzer, R., Kunz, M., Yoshimura, T., Brocker, E.B., et al. (1999) The MKK6/p38 stress kinase cascade is critical for tumor necrosis factor-alpha-induced expression of monocyte-chemoattractant protein-1 in endothelial cells. *Blood* **93,** 857–865.

13. Toossi, Z., Mayanja-Kizza, H., Hirsch, C.S., Edmonds, K.L., Spahlinger, T., Hom, D.L., et al. (2000) Impact of tuber-culosis (TB) on HIV-1 activity in dually infected patients. *Clin. Exp. Immunol.* **122,** 1–7.

14. Valone, S.E., Rich, E.A., Wallis, R.S., and Ellner, J.J. (1988) Expression of tumor necrosis factor in vitro by human mononuclear phagocytes stimulated with whole *Mycobacterium bovis* BCG and mycobacterial antigens. *Infect. Immun.* **56,** 3313–3315.

15. Wallis, R.S., Fujiwara, H., and Ellner, J.J. (1986) Direct stimulation of monocyte release of interleukin 1 by mycobac-terial protein antigens. *J. Immunol.* **136,**193–196.

16. Aung, H., Toossi, Z., Wisnieski, J.J., Wallis, R.S., Culp, L.A., Phillips, N.B., et al. (1996) Induction of monocyte expression of tumor necrosis factor alpha by the 30-kD alpha antigen of Mycobacterium tuberculosis and synergism with fibronectin. *J. Clin. Invest.* **98,**1261–1268.

17. Wallis, R.S., Paranjape, R., and Phillips, M. (1993) Identification by two-dimensional gel electrophoresis of a 58-kilodalton tumor necrosis factor-inducing protein of Mycobacterium tuberculosis. *Infect. Immun.* **61,** 627–632.

18. Balcewicz-Sablinska, M.K., Keane, J., Kornfeld, H., and Remold, H.G. (1998) Pathogenic Mycobacterium tuberculo-sis evades apoptosis of host macrophages by release of TNF-R2, resulting in inactivation of TNF- alpha. *J. Immunol.* **161,** 2636–2641.

19. Abou-Zeid, C., Ratliff, T.L., Wiker, H.G., Harboe, M., Bennedsen, J., and Rook, G.A. (1988) Characterization of fibronectin-binding antigens released by *Mycobacterium tuberculosis* and *Mycobacterium bovis* BCG. *Infect. Immun.* **56,** 3046–3051.

20. Fulton, S.A., Johnsen, J.M., Wolf, S.F., Sieburth, D.S., and Boom, W.H. (1996) Interleukin-12 production by human monocytes infected with *Mycobacterium tuberculosis:* role of phagocytosis. *Infect. Immun.* **64,** 2523–2531.

21. Wanidworanun, C. and Strober, W. (1993) Predominant role of tumor necrosis factor-alpha in human monocyte IL-10 synthesis. *J. Immunol.* **151,** 6853–6861.

22. Barnes, P.F., Chatterjee, D., Abrams, J.S., Lu, S., Wang, E., Yamamura, M., et al. (1992) Cytokine production induced by Mycobacterium tuberculosis lipoarabinomannan. Relationship to chemical structure. *J. Immunol.* **149,** 541–547.

23. Othieno, C., Hirsch, C.S., Hamilton, B.D., Wilkinson, K., Ellner, J.J., and Toossi, Z. (1999) Interaction of Mycobacte-rium tuberculosis-induced transforming growth factor beta1 and interleukin-10. *Infect. Immun.* **67,** 5730–5735.

24. Hirsch, C.S., Yoneda, T., Averill, L., Ellner, J.J., and Toossi, Z. (1994) Enhancement of intracellular growth of *Myco-bacterium tuberculosis* in human monocytes by transforming growth factor-beta 1. *J. Infect. Dis.* **170,** 1229–1237.

25. Dahl, K.E., Shiratsuchi, H., Hamilton, B.D., Ellner, J.J., and Toossi, Z. (1996) Selective induction of transforming growth factor beta in human monocytes by lipoarabinomannan of *Mycobacterium tuberculosis.* *Infect. Immun.* **64,** 399–405.

26. Monroy, V., Amador, A., Ruiz, B., Espinoza-Cueto, P., Xolalpa, W., Mancilla, R., et al. (2000) Binding and activation of human plasminogen by *Mycobacterium tuberculosis.* *Infect. Immun.* **68,** 4327–4330.

27. Toossi, Z. and Ellner, J.J. (1998) The role of TGF beta in the pathogenesis of human tuberculosis. *Clin. Immunol. Immunopathol.* **87,** 107–114.

28. Toossi, Z., Hirsch, C.S., Hamilton, B.D., Knuth, C.K., Friedlander, M.A., and Rich, E.A. (1996) Decreased production of TGF-beta 1 by human alveolar macrophages compared with blood monocytes. *J. Immunol.* **156,** 3461–3468.

29. Howard, A.D., and Zwilling, B.S. (1998) Cytokine production by CD4 and CD8 T cells during the growth of *Mycobac-terium tuberculosis* in mice. *Clin. Exp. Immunol.* **113,** 443–449.

30. Newport, M.J., Huxley, C.M., Huston, S., Hawrylowicz, C.M., Oostra, B.A., Williamson, R., et al. (1996) A mutation in the interferon-gamma-receptor gene and susceptibility to mycobacterial infection. *N. Engl. J. Med.* **335,** 1941–1949.

31. Ottenhoff, T.H., Kumararatne, D., and Casanova, J.L. (1998) Novel human immunodeficiencies reveal the essential role of type-I cytokines in immunity to intracellular bacteria. *Immunol. Today* **19,** 491–494.

32. Aubert-Pivert, E.M., Chedevergne, F.M., Lopez-Ramirez, G.M., Colle, J.H., Scheinmann, P.L., Gicquel, B.M., et al. (2000) Cytokine transcripts in pediatric tuberculosis: a study with bronchoalveolar cells. *Tuberc. Lung Dis.* **80,** 249–258.

33. Hirsch, C.S., Hussain, R., Toossi, Z., Dawood, G., Shahid, F., and Ellner, J.J. (1996) Cross-modulation by transforming growth factor beta in human tuberculosis: suppression of antigen-driven blastogenesis and interferon gamma produc-tion. *Proc. Natl. Acad. Sci. USA* **93,** 3193–3198.

34. Barnes, P.F., Lu, S., Abrams, J.S., Wang, E., Yamamura, M., and Modlin, R.L. (1993) Cytokine production at the site of disease in human tuberculosis. *Infect. Immun.* **61,** 3482–3489.

35. Toossi, Z., Mincek, M., Seeholtzer, E., Fulton, S.A., Hamilton, B.D., and Hirsch, C.S. (1997) Modulation of IL-12 by transforming growth factor-beta (TGF-beta) in *Mycobacterium tuberculosis*-infected mononuclear phagocytes and in patients with active tuberculosis. *J. Clin. Lab. Immunol.* **49,** 59–75.

36. Barnes, P.F. and Wizel, B. (2000) Type 1 cytokines and the pathogenesis of tuberculosis. *Am. J. Respir. Crit. Care Med.* **161,** 1773–1774.

37. Ogawa, T., Uchida, H., Kusumoto, Y., Mori, Y., Yamamura, Y., and Hamada, S. (1991) Increase in tumor necrosis factor alpha- and interleukin-6-secreting cells in peripheral blood mononuclear cells from subjects infected with *Myco-bacterium tuberculosis. Infect. Immun.* **59,** 3021–3025.

38. Toossi, Z., Gogate, P., Shiratsuchi, H., Young, T., and Ellner, J.J. (1995) Enhanced production of TGF-beta by blood monocytes from patients with active tuberculosis and presence of TGF-beta in tuberculous granulomatous lung lesions. *J. Immunol.* **154,** 465–473.

39. Hirsch, C.S., Ellner, J.J., Blinkhorn, R., and Toossi, Z. (1997) In vitro restoration of T cell responses in tuberculosis and augmentation of monocyte effector function against *Mycobacterium tuberculosis* by natural inhibitors of transforming growth factor beta. *Proc. Natl. Acad. Sci. USA* **94,** 3926–3931.

40. Hirsch, C.S., Toossi, Z., Othieno, C., Johnson, J.L., Schwander, S.K., Robertson, S., et al. (1999) Depressed T-cell interferon-gamma responses in pulmonary tuberculosis: analysis of underlying mechanisms and modulation with therapy. *J. Infect. Dis.* **180,** 2069–2073.

41. Hirsch, C.S., Toossi, Z., Johnson, J.L., Luzze, H., Ntambi, L., Peters, P., et al. (2001) Augmentation of Apoptosis and Interferon-gamma Production at Sites of Active *Mycobacterium tuberculosis* infection in human tuberculosis. *J. Infect. Dis.* **183,** 779–788.

42. Schwander, S.K., Torres, M., Sada, E., Carranza, C., Ramos, E., Tary-Lehmann, M., et al. (1998) Enhanced responses to Mycobacterium tuberculosis antigens by human alveolar lymphocytes during active pulmonary tuberculosis. *J. Infect. Dis.* **178,** 1434–1445.

43. Condos, R., Rom, W.N., Liu, Y.M., and Schluger, N.W. (1998) Local immune responses correlate with presentation and outcome in tuberculosis. *Am. J. Respir. Crit. Care Med.* **157,** 729–735.

44. Condos, R., Rom, W.N., and Schluger, N.W. (1997) Treatment of multidrug-resistant pulmonary tuberculosis with interferon- gamma via aerosol. *Lancet* **349,** 1513–1515.

45. Somoskovi, A., Zissel, G., Zipfel, P.F., Ziegenhagen, M.W., Klaucke, J., Haas, H., et al. (1999) Different cytokine patterns correlate with the extension of disease in pulmonary tuberculosis. *Eur Cytokine Network* **10,** 135–142.

46. Lin, Y., Zhang, M., Hofman, F.M., Gong, J., and Barnes, P.F. (1996) Absence of a prominent Th2 cytokine response in human tuberculosis. *Infect. Immun.* **64,** 1351–1356.

47. Toossi, Z., Johnson, J.L., Kanost, R.A., Wu, M., Luzze, H., Peters, P., et al. (2001) Increased replication of HIV-1 at sites of *Mycobacterium tuberculosis* infection: potential mechanisms of viral activation. *J. Acquir. Immune Defic. Syndr.* **28,**1–8.

48. Kurashima, K., Mukaida, N., Fujimura, M., Yasui, M., Nakazumi, Y., Matsuda, T., et al. (1997) Elevated chemokine levels in bronchoalveolar lavage fluid of tuberculosis patients. *Am. J. Respir. Crit. Care Med.* **155,**1474–1477.

49. Bergeron, A., Bonay, M., Kambouchner, M., Lecossier, D., Riquet, M., Soler, P., et al. (1997) Cytokine patterns in tuberculous and sarcoid granulomas: correlations with histopathologic features of the granulomatous response. *J. Immunol.* **159,** 3034–3043.

50. Aung, H., Toossi, Z., McKenna, S.M., Gogate, P., Sierra, J., Sada, E., et al. (2000) Expression of transforming growth factor-beta but not tumor necrosis factor-alpha, interferon-gamma, and interleukin-4 in granulomatous lung lesions in tuberculosis. *Tuberc. Lung Dis.* **80,** 61–67.

51. Hernandez-Pando, R., Orozco, H., Arriaga, K., Sampieri, A., Larriva-Sahd, J., and Madrid-Marina, V. (1997) Analysis of the local kinetics and localization of interleukin-1 alpha, tumour necrosis factor-alpha and transforming growth factor-beta, during the course of experimental pulmonary tuberculosis. *Immunology* **90,** 607–617.

52. van Crevel, R., Karyadi, E., Preyers, F., Leenders, M., Kullberg, B.J., Nelwan, R.H., et al. (2000) Increased production of interleukin 4 by CD4+ and CD8+ T cells from patients with tuberculosis is related to the presence of pulmonary cavities. *J. Infect. Dis.* **181,** 1194–1197.

53. Wilkinson, R.J., Patel, P., Llewelyn, M., Hirsch, C.S., Pasvol, G., Snounou, G., et al. (1999) Influence of polymorphism in the genes for the interleukin (IL)-1 receptor antagonist and IL-1beta on tuberculosis. *J. Exp. Med.* **189,** 1863–1874.

54. Dlugovitzky, D., Bay, M.L., Rateni, L., Urizar, L., Rondelli, C.F., Largacha, C., et al. (1999) In vitro synthesis of interferon-gamma, interleukin-4, transforming growth factor-beta and interleukin-1 beta by peripheral blood mononuclear cells from tuberculosis patients: relationship with the severity of pulmonary involvement. *Scand. J. Immunol.* **49,** 210–217.

55. Zhu, W., Downey, J.S., Gu, J., Di Padova, F., Gram, H., and Han, J. (2000) Regulation of TNF expression by multiple mitogen-activated protein kinase pathways. *J. Immunol.* **164,** 6349–6358.

56. Wilkinson, K.A., Aung, H., Wu, M., and Toossi, Z. (2000) Modulation of transforming growth factor beta-1 gene expression by interleukin-12. *Scand. J. Immunol.* **52,** 271–277.

57. Border, W.A., Noble, N.A., Yamamoto, T., Harper, J.R., Yamaguchi, Y., Pierschbacher, M.D., et al. (1992) Natural inhibitor of transforming growth factor-beta protects against scarring in experimental kidney disease. *Nature* **360,** 361–364.

58. Wilkinson, K.A., Martin, T.D., Reba, S.M., Aung, H., Redline, R.W., Boom, W.H., et al. (2000) Latency-associated peptide of transforming growth factor beta enhances mycobacteriocidal immunity in the lung during mycobacterium bovis BCG infection in C57BL/6 mice. *Infect. Immun.* **68,** 6505–6508.

59. Rook, G.A., and Hernandez-Pando, R. (1996) The pathogenesis of tuberculosis. *Annu. Rev. Microbiol.* **50,** 259–284.

60. Byrd, T.F. (1997) Tumor necrosis factor alpha (TNFalpha) promotes growth of virulent Mycobacterium tuberculosis in human monocytes iron-mediated growth suppression is correlated with decreased release of TNFalpha from iron- treated infected monocytes. *J. Clin. Invest.* **99,** 2518–2529.

61. Baeuerle, P.A. and Baichwal, V.R. (1997) NF-kappa B as a frequent target for immunosuppressive and anti-inflammatory molecules. *Adv. Immunol.* **65,** 111–137.

62. Scheinman, R.I., Cogswell, P.C., Lofquist, A.K., and Baldwin, A.S., Jr. (1995) Role of transcriptional activation of I kappa B alpha in mediation of immunosuppression by glucocorticoids. *Science* **270,** 283–286.

63. Tavares, J.L., Wangoo, A., Dilworth, P., Marshall, B., Kotecha, S., and Shaw, R.J. (1997) Thalidomide reduces tumour necrosis factor-alpha production by human alveolar macrophages. *Respir. Med.* **91,** 31–39.

64. Zabel, P., Schade, F.U., and Schlaak, M. (1993) Inhibition of endogenous TNF formation by pentoxifylline. *Immunobiology* **187,** 447–463.

65. Tramontana, J.M., Utaipat, U., Molloy, A., Akarasewi, P., Burroughs, M., Makonkawkeyoon, S., et al. (1995) Thalidomide treatment reduces tumor necrosis factor alpha production and enhances weight gain in patients with pulmonary tuberculosis. *Mol. Med.* **1,** 384–397.

66. Holland, S.M., Eisenstein, E.M., Kuhns, D.B., Turner, M.L., Fleisher, T.A., Strober, W., et al. (1994) Treatment of refractory disseminated nontuberculous mycobacterial infection with interferon gamma. A preliminary report. *N. Engl. J. Med.* **330,** 1348–1355.

67. Nathan, C.F., Kaplan, G., Levis, W.R., Nusrat, A., Witmer, M.D., Sherwin, S.A., et al. (1986) Local and systemic effects of intradermal recombinant interferon-gamma in patients with lepromatous leprosy. *N. Engl. J. Med.* **315,** 6–15.

68. Raad, I., Hachem, R., Leeds, N., Sawaya, R., Salem, Z., and Atweh, S. (1996) Use of adjunctive treatment with interferon-gamma in an immunocompromised patient who had refractory multidrug-resistant tuberculosis of the brain. *Clin. Infect. Dis.* **22,** 572–574.

69. Kaplan, G., Sampaio, E.P., Walsh, G.P., Burkhardt, R.A., Fajardo, T.T., Guido, L.S., et al. (1989) Influence of Mycobacterium leprae and its soluble products on the cutaneous responsiveness of leprosy patients to antigen and recombinant interleukin 2. *Proc. Natl. Acad. Sci. USA* **86,** 6269–6273.

70. Johnson, B.J., Ress, S.R., Willcox, P., Pati, B.P., Lorgat, F., Stead, P., et al. (1995) Clinical and immune responses of tuberculosis patients treated with low-dose IL-2 and multidrug therapy. *Cytokines Mol. Ther.* **1,** 185–196.

10

Cytokines and Chemokines in Protective and Inflammatory Responses to Infection with Nontuberculous Mycobacteria

Stefan Ehlers

1. INTRODUCTION

Mycobacteria other than *M. tuberculosis* and *M. leprae* are potentially pathogenic environmental micro-organisms *(1)*. Nontuberculous mycobacteria (NTM) comprise an increasing number of species *(2)*. Because of improved methods of isolation and cultivation, and to more refined diagnostic methods such as 16SrRNA sequencing *(3,4)*, more than 50 hitherto uncharacterized new species have been discovered in the past two decades. In most diagnostic laboratories, the most prevalent, clinically relevant nontuberculous species isolated is *M. avium*, but *M. kansasii*, *M. genavense*, *M. xenopi*, and *M. abscessus* also occur with relative frequency *(5,6)*. Many species (*M. avium*, *M. scrofulaceum*, *M. malmoense*) primarily cause lymphadenitis, particularly in children *(7)*; some species (*M. kansasii*, *M. avium*, *M. intracellulare*, *M. malmoense*, *M. xenopi*) are mostly found in pulmonary disease *(1,7)*. Disseminated infections have most frequently been described with *M. avium*, *M. kansasii*, *M. genavense*, *M. malmoense*, and *M. celatum (8)*.

In view of the fact that encounter with these ubiquitous species is unavoidable, they relatively rarely cause disease. Some apparently immunocompetent hosts develop localized infections, for the most part at the port of entry or the draining lymph node, but further spread is arrested although the mycobacteria are not eliminated. Typical patients affected by this entity are children with lymphadenitis and older women with bronchopneumonia *(7,9–12)*. More frequently, these opportunistic mycobacterial species cause endobronchial disease on the basis of pre-existing pulmonary disorders, such as chronic obstructive pulmonary disease, bronchiectasis, or chronic bronchitis because of smoking *(11,13,14)*. Thus, a local disturbance in innate mucosal defense systems seems to be a necessary prerequisite not only for colonization but also for locally invasive disease with a chronic inflammatory component.

Disseminated disease with NTM occurs whenever T-cell-mediated macrophage activation is severely compromised, e.g., during high-dose immunosuppression, idiopathic CD4$^+$ lymphocytopenia, or, most prominently, during advanced-stage acquired immunodeficiency syndrome (AIDS), where a drop of CD4+ T-cells below 50/mm^3 is in up to 50% of cases accompanied by disseminated *M. avium* or *M. genavense* infection *(15–18)*. The realization that a defect along the T-cell–macrophage activation axis (*see* Fig. 1) invariably leads to disseminated NTM infection made researchers postulate that at least some of the cases of disseminated NTM disease without evidence of human immunodeficiency virus (HIV) infection might be accounted for by a genetically determined immunodeficiency affecting this axis. The search for these genetic predispositions has been highly

From: *Cytokines and Chemokines in Infectious Diseases Handbook*
Edited by: M. Kotb and T. Calandra © Humana Press Inc., Totowa, NJ

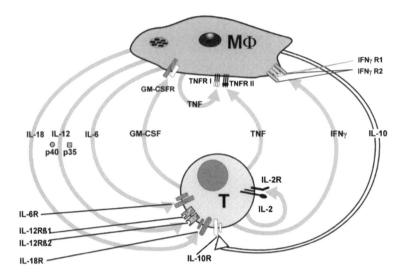

Fig. 1. Cytokine regulation of antimycobacterial immune responses. Macrophages (Φ) are the major host cells for mycobacteria. Cytokines induced during infection with mycobacteria initiate intracellular signals following interaction with specific receptors. Infected macrophages secrete IL-6, IL-12 (a heterodimer of p35 and p40 chains), and IL-18 that act as costimulators for T-cells that bear cytokine-specific heterodimeric receptors. Activated T-cells secrete IL-2, which is an autocrine growth factor. Effector T-cells produce IFN-γ, the central macrophage-activating cytokine, that binds to IFN-γR1 and generates intracellular signals via IFN-γR2. Effector T-cells also secrete granulocyte–macrophage which activates macrophages. Tumor necrosis factor is produced both by T-cells and macrophages and stimulates macrophages mostly through TNFRI. IL-10 derived from macrophages suppresses T-cell effector functions.

successful in human patients, and microsatellite mapping and subsequent sequencing of candidate genes has revealed a number of loss-of-function mutations in the interleukin-12/interferon-γ (IL-12/IFN-γ) pathway of macrophage activation *(19)*. A parallel and converging approach has been to use the mouse model of infection, because it shares many properties of disease progression and immunopathology *(20–22)*. In particular, experimental infection with NTM in gene-deficient (knockout [KO]) mice has been a useful tool to characterize the pathogenesis of disseminated disease and to generate new candidate genes that may be defective in patients with no currently known immunodeficiency.

2. LESSONS FROM MACROPHAGES IN VITRO: FIRST CLUES IN A COMPLEX RESPONSE

2.1. Cytokines

In a reductionist approach to identifying cytokines and chemokines that may be involved in the control of NTM infections, numerous investigations have focused on the consequences of infection in macrophages in vitro, using *M. avium* as the most commonly occurring, clinically relevant NTM species. For instance, IL-2, IL-7, and macrophage colony-stimulating factor (M-CSF) were shown to reduce mycobacterial replication under specific conditions *(23–25)*, and IL-12 was demonstrated to stimulate natural killer (NK) cells, which, in turn, activate macrophages to inhibit intracellular growth of *M. avium (26)*. Most of the in vitro studies, however, have yielded highly controversial results. For example, the addition of tumor necrosis factor (TNF), interferon -γ (IFN-γ) or granulocyte–macrophage colony-stimulating factor (GM-CSF) was found to have mycobacteriostatic or mycobacteriocidal effects in some studies, whereas it had no effect in others *(23,27–30)*. Similarly, IL-6 and neutralization of IL-10 were reported to have either growth-enhancing properties or no effect on *M. avium* replication *(27,31–34)*.

These highly discrepant results may be explained by the inherent difficulties in standardizing this type of experiment. In particular, the timing of exposure of macrophages to stimulating and inhibiting cytokines often determines the ultimate effect on macrophage function; this is particularly true for TNF, IFN-γ, and IL-10 *(35–38)*. *M. avium* downregulates the expression of IFN-γ receptors and thereby presumably modulates the macrophage response to IFN-γ *(39)*. Furthermore, the choice of host cell and the differentiation state of the host cell (cell line, primary monocyte or macrophage, in the case of human cells: the choice of donor) and the choice of NTM organism (virulent or avirulent strain, hemolytic or nonhemolytic, smooth opaque, transparent, or rough morphotype) all critically influence the cytokine profile induced or the susceptibility to cytokine stimulation *(40–46)*. The intramacrophage signaling cascades regulating distinct cytokine profiles induced by different species and morphotypes of NTM are only beginning to be uncovered *(47,47a)*. It is important to emphasize that in in vitro culture, macrophage activation often leads to secretion and accumulation of TGF-β1, nitric oxide (NO), and prostaglandin E_2 (PGE_2) *(48–50)*. These mediators may modulate the secretion of other cytokines and thereby determine the extent of intracellular parasitism *(50,51)*. Similarly, IL-6 antagonizes TNF-induced mycobacteriostatic activities in macrophages *(52)* and suppresses T-cell responses *(53)*. In conclusion, direct comparison between published results from different investigators is extremely difficult, and only few general truths may be distilled from these studies.

One common theme that has emerged from a few studies is that some strains or morphotypes may replicate less in vivo (in mouse models) or in vitro (in macrophage cultures), because they induce higher amounts of TNF, IL-12p40, IL-18, IFN-γ, or GM-CSF, which serve to activate the macrophage to effectively reduce mycobacterial growth *(54–59)*. This correlation holds true for a number of *M. avium* strains, but is by no means valid for all of them and may differ already when mouse or human macrophages are used as host cells. An example is illustrated in Fig. 2: *M. avium* strain TMC724 is highly virulent in mice, but replicates only poorly in human macrophages, yet induces only small amounts of TNF in these host cells. On the other hand, strain SE01 is intermediately virulent in mice, but replicates very well in human macrophages despite its capacity to induce large amounts of TNF. Therefore, there is no simple and direct correlation between cytokine induction/ responsiveness and virulence of different *M. avium* morphotypes. It appears to be generally true, however, that TNF does not play a critical role in controlling the growth of avirulent strains, so that for these strains, other intrinsic, antimycobacterially active mechanisms of the macrophage are more important *(46,47a)*. However, because of the substantial variability of in vitro studies, the clinical relevance of whether cytokines are induced in host cells or whether mycobacteriostasis is achieved in a given culture system remains questionable and more detailed analyses in vivo are required.

A number of studies have sought to shed light on the mycobacteriostatic and mycobacteriocidal pathways operative in activated macrophages. Apoptosis of host cells, induced by cytokines or other metabolic products, may restrict intracellular mycobacterial growth *(60–62)* and prevent the spread of infection *(63)*. Moreover, IFN-γ-mediated activation of murine macrophages results in acidification and maturation of *M. avium*-containing phagolysosomes *(64)*. In an elegant model system addressing the question of whether acidified phagolysomes are sufficient to inhibit *M. avium* growth, murine bone-marrow-derived macrophages were infected with *M. avium* and then coinfected with *Coxiella burnetii*. The majority of phagocytosed mycobacteria colocalized to the *C. burnetii*-containing vacuole, which maintained its acidic properties. In coinfected macrophages, the growth of *M. avium* was not impaired following fusion with the acidified vacuole, revealing that acidification of the phagosome is not sufficient to kill *M. avium (65)*. Practically all strains of *M. avium* are resistant to nitric oxide *(66)*, but it is unknown in how far this applies to other NTM species. Enhanced production of reactive oxygen intermediates may be relevant in controlling growth of some strains or morphotypes, but not others *(30,67)*. Nutrient, particularly iron, deprivation within the phagolysosome is another attractive mechanism by which activated macrophages may inhibit the growth of certain NTM species *(68)*. Elucidation of the effector pathways by which cytokines regulate antimycobacterial activities of the macrophage will remain an important goal in future studies.

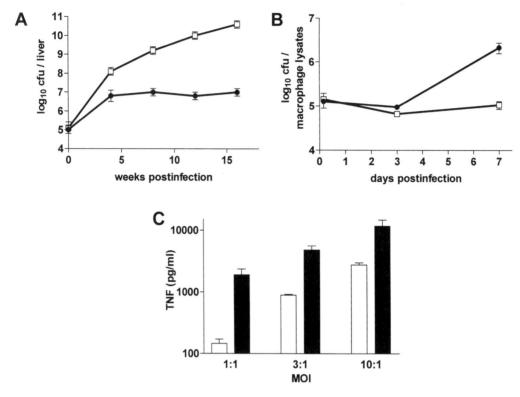

Fig. 2. Complexity of in vivo and in vitro behavior of different *M. avium* strains. (**A**) Development of colony-forming units (cfu) in the liver of immunocompetent C57BL/6 mice intravenously infected with *M. avium*. The highly mouse-virulent strain TMC724 (open squares) grows progressively, whereas the intermediate mouse-virulent strain SE01 (filled circles) reaches a plateau. (**B**) Development of cfu counts in human macrophages infected with *M. avium*. Strain TMC724 (open squares) persists but does not multiply, whereas strain SE01 (filled circles) grows progressively. (**C**) TNF secretion of human macrophages infected 20 h previously with *M. avium* at indicated multiplicities of infection (MOIs). The low-replicating strain TMC724 (white bars) induces low-level TNF secretion, whereas the highly replicating strain SE01 (black bars) induces high-level TNF production.

Finally, some diagnostic and therapeutic applications that have emerged from in vitro macrophage stimulation are worth mentioning. In several studies involving patients with localized *M. avium* infections, mycobacterium-stimulated peripheral blood mononuclear cells (PBMCs) produced higher amounts of IL-10, but lower concentrations of IFN-γ, IL-12, and TNF compared to PBMCs from healthy controls *(69–71)*. Interestingly, stimulation with IFN-γ, TNF, or GM-CSF resulted in the increase of intracellular concentration of azithromycin and was associated with significant augmentation of antimycobacterial activity compared with the effects of azithromycin or ofloxacin alone *(72,73)*. This finding may explain some of the beneficial effects seen in combined immunochemotherapy in patients.

2.2. Chemokines

Very few studies have addressed the production of chemokines in response to NTM infection in vitro. A human alveolar epithelial cell line was found to secrete macrophage chemoattractant protein (MCP)-1 upon interaction with viable, but not heat-killed *M. avium*, and this was postulated to provide a mechanism for recruitment of macrophages to early sites of implantation *(74)*. *M. avium* infection of intestinal epithelial cell lines was associated with a delay in IL-8 and RANTES production, and this finding was interpreted as reflecting an evasion mechanism of *M. avium* *(75)*. The mycobacterial cell wall component lipoarabinomannan (LAM) was shown to induce expression of MCP-3 in human monocytes, and this effect was inhibited by IL-10 or IL-13 *(76)*.

Because *M. avium* is a common opportunistic pathogen in AIDS patients, coinfection studies with HIV were performed to address the possible cross-regulation of bacterial and viral replication. Following infection with *M. avium*, CCR5 (a coreceptor for HIV entry) expression was increased at both the mRNA level and on the surface of macrophages. Upregulation of CCR5 by *M. avium* was not paralleled by an increase in the T-cell tropic coreceptor, CXCR4 *(77)*. The increased production of TNF, together with elevated expression of CCR5, provide potential mechanisms for enhanced infection and replication of HIV-1 by macrophages in *M. avium*-infected cells and tissues. Consequently, treating *M. avium* may inhibit not only the *M. avium*-induced pathology but also limit the viral burden *(78)*.

3. LESSONS FROM ANIMAL MODELS: MANIPULATING THE HOST TO CHARACTERIZE PATHOGENETIC PATHWAYS

3.1. IL-12 / IFN-γ Pathway

Most experimental studies on the pathogenesis of NTM have been performed in mice using *M. avium*. There is abundant evidence from these experiments, using either gene-targeted mice or cytokine neutralization/supplementation, that IL-12 (p70) and IFN-γ are crucial mediators in restricting mycobacterial growth *(79–81)*.

By neutralizing IL-12 activity during different stages of infection, IL-12 was determined to be involved in the induction but not in the expression of acquired cell-mediated immunity, similar to what was found for IL-6 *(82,83)*. In particular, IL-12 plays a crucial role in the development of T-cells capable of producing IFN-γ *(84)*. Thus, treatment of *M. avium*-infected mice with IL-12 induced CD4+ T-cells with a greater capacity to produce IFN-γ and to confer protection against *M. avium (85,86)*. By a similar mechanism, IL-12 was found to have adjuvant properties when used in conjunction with subunit vaccines against *M. avium*, enhancing, at least initially, the protective efficacy of subunit vaccines *(87)*. BALB/c mice were shown to have decreased IL-12 production, and IL-12 therapy resulted in long-lasting reduction of mycobacterial loads in these mice *(88)*. Following IL-12 administration, there was also evidence of NK cell activation *(84)*. This mechanism may explain the requirement for IL-12 in the T-cell-independent pathway of resistance against *M. avium* present in SCID mice *(80)*.

More recently, mice with targeted mutations in either the IL-12p35 or the IL-12p40 or in both genes were infected with *M. avium*. These mice had significantly increased bacterial loads in all organs examined *(85;* Ehlers, unpublished data). IL-12p40 KO mice and IL-12-depleted mice also had dramatically reduced granulomatous infiltration early during infection, but did develop circumscript granulomas during later stages of infection *(79,85;* Ehlers unpublished data), although these contained many foamy macrophages rather than the typical epithelioid cells *(see* Fig. 3 E,F). The capacity to form granulomas in IL-12 KO mice may be because IL-18, and possibly other mediators such as IL-23, may induce residual levels of IFN-γ *(89,90)*. It is also interesting to note that IL-12 and IL-18 levels are apparently reduced in the susceptible mouse strain, BALB/c, yet increased in a resistant mouse strain, DBA/2 *(91)*. Indeed, DNA encoding IL-18 during intranasal infection with *M. avium* in BALB/c mice resulted in a significant reduction of the bacterial burden, presumably because a persistent production of IFN-γ was induced *(92)*.

Adjunctive IL-12 was demonstrated to promote clearance of *M. avium* in mice induced by chemotherapy with clarithromycin or rifabutin *(93,94)*. This effect is dependent on endogenous IFN-γ, but adjunctive IFN-γ itself failed to significantly enhance antibiotic-induced clearance of mycobacteria *(94)*.

Neutralization of IFN-γ in mice leads to exacerbation of *M. avium* infection both in the early T-cell-independent phase and in the subsequent T-cell-dependent phase *(81)*. Similarly, during long-term infection, a spontaneously occurring abrupt cessation of IFN-γ production is associated with an increase in bacterial numbers *(95)*.

T-Cells within granulomas were directly shown to secrete IFN-γ in murine *M. avium* infection *(96)*. In sheep infected with *M. paratuberculosis*, the lepromatous manifestation is accompanied by low levels of IFN-γ, whereas in the tuberculoid form, higher levels of IFN-γ are found *(97)*. Exogenously administered IFN-γ augmented *M. intracellulare* clearance in mice, in part by suppressing production of PGE_2 *(98)*. However, virulent strains of *M. avium* may resist the antimycobacterial mechanisms induced in IFN-γ-activated granuloma macrophages. Because IFN-γ KO mice were able to restrict growth of less virulent strains of *M. avium*, albeit at a higher plateau than wild-type mice, it was speculated that there may be IFN-γ-independent, yet T-cell-dependent signals required for the effective control of mycobacterial replication inside macrophages *(99)*.

Mycobacterium avium-infected IFN-γ KO mice are severely deficient in granuloma formation and show, instead, a highly dysregulated hyperinflammatory response characterized by massive mixed cellular infiltrations with a high percentage of neutrophils *(100*; Ehlers, unpublished data) (Fig. 3G,H). This may be because all mycobacterial infections in IFN-γ KO mice cause a severe remodeling of the hematopoietic system with significant neutrophilia *(101)*. This increased inflammatory cell influx may partially be caused by the reduced levels of nitric oxide in these mice. In fact, iNOS KO mice and mice treated with a pharmacologic inhibitor of iNOS activity show an increased inflammatory response with increased recruitment of lymphocytes, monocytes, and neutrophils *(102,103)*. Generally, mice deficient for IL-12 are less severely affected, in terms of overall bacterial load or excessive inflammatory cell influx, during *M. avium* infection than IFN-γ KO mice, and succumb to infection much later than IFN-γ KO mice *(100*; Ehlers, unpublished data). IL-12 KO mice remain capable of forming granulomas, albeit in a delayed fashion, whereas mice deficient for IFN-γ completely lack the capacity to form circumscript mononuclear cell foci (Fig. 3E–H).

Recently, two studies made use of IFN-γ KO mice to investigate whether several newly described mycobacterial species would also replicate more extensively in vivo when the IFN-γ pathway of macrophage activation is impaired *(104,105)*. In these studies, *M. genavense*, *M. branderi*, *M. celatum*, *M. xenopi*, *M. conspicuum*, *M. malmoense*, *M. bohemicum*, and *M. interiectum* behaved in a similar fashion as clinical isolates of *M. avium*. The either grew progressively or persisted at plateau levels in the livers and spleens of immunocompetent mice, and their growth was increased in IFN-γ KO mice. *M. heidelbergense* and *M. intermedium* were eliminated in immunocompetent mice, but persisted in IFN-γ KO mice. *M. confluentis* and *M. lentiflavum* were eradicated even in the absence of IFN-γ, revealing that at least with some nontuberculous species, other predisposing conditions or as yet unidentified defects, presumably at the macrophage level, must be responsible for productive infection. Interestingly, nontuberculous mycobacterial species differed widely in their capacity to induce splenomegaly and lymphadenopathy in IFN-γ KO mice, suggesting that some strains will cause clinical disease more rapidly than others. This study provides a first experimental basis for the contention that IFN-γ is a crucial determinant of infection outcome with most, but not all, opportunistic mycobacterial species *(104)*.

3.2. IL-12/IFN-γ-Induced Putative Mechanisms of Bacteriostasis

Nitric oxide (NO) is induced by IFN-γ and was shown to be a critical efector mechanism against *M. tuberculosis* infection in mice *(106)*. However, NO is not involved in the bacteriostatic mechanisms of macrophages against *M. avium (66,102)*. In contrast, NO levels induced during the natural course of infection may even serve to exacerbate *M. avium* infection by causing suppression of the immune response. Indeed, iNOS KO mice had increased survival of $CD4^+$ T-cells, higher IFN-γ levels in the serum, and reduced bacterial loads at 4 mo postinfection *(102)*. NO was shown to regu-

---

Fig. 3. *(opposite page)* Granuloma formation in the liver of immunocompetent and gene-targeted mice. Mice were infected with highly mouse-virulent strain *M. avium* TMC724 by the intravenous route. A, B, C, E, G: Hematoxylin and eosin stain; D, F, H: Ziehl–Neelsen stain. Original magnification: (64×). **(A)** Well-formed granuloma 5 wk postinfection in C576BL/6 mice. **(B)** Disintegrating granuloma with multiple apoptotic cells

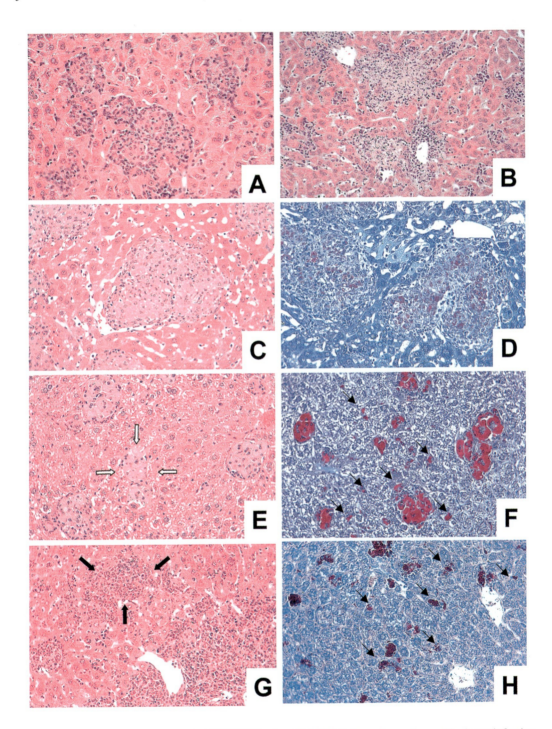

and central necrosis 5 wk postinfection in TNF-RI KO mice. **(C,D)** Well-formed granulomas 12 wk postinfection in C57BL/6 mice. All acid-fast bacteria are contained within granulomas. **(E,F)** Circumscript, well-demarcated lesions with mostly foamy macrophages (white arrows in **E**) 12 wk postinfection in IL-12p35/p40 KO mice. Note several macrophages and Kupffer cells filled with acid-fast bacteria outside of granulomatous lesions (arrows in **F**). **(G,H)** Mixed cellular infiltrations with foamy macrophages and numerous, often eosinophilic granulocytes (black arrows in **G**) 12 wk postinfection in IFN-γ KO mice. Note several macrophages and Kupffer cells filled with acid-fast bacteria outside of diffuse lesions (arrows in **H**).

late the number, size, and cellular composition of *M. avium*-induced granulomas by modulating the cytokine and chemokine profile within infected tissues, specifically by decreasing TNF, IL-12, IFN-γ, IL-10, and IP-10 *(103)*.

Oxygen radicals were also proposed to have mycobacteriostatic effects *(67)*. However, the p47(phox–/–) mouse which is defective in generating reactive oxidants, had bacterial loads similar to wild-type mice and normal granuloma formation and cytokine responses to *M. avium (107)*.

3.3. IL-10

The role of IL-10 in experimental *M. avium* infection is highly controversial. Some experiments neutralizing IL-10 in vivo by repeated administration of specific monoclonal antibodies showed that resistance to *M. avium* was augmented by this treatment, whereas others documented no effect on the course of infection *(32,34,108)*. Mice deficient in IL-10 were marginally more susceptible to *M. bovis* BCG very early during infection *(109,110)*. *M. avium*-infected IL-10 KO mice had increased numbers of IFN-γ-secreting T-cells and reduced bacterial load in the liver and lung early during infection, but this effect was short-lived *(111)*. Other investigators using IL-10 KO mice have been unable to confirm a significant role of IL-10 in interfering with antibacterial protection against *M. avium (112*; Ehlers, unpublished data). However, when neutralizing anti-IL-10 antibodies were combined with antimycobacterial chemotherapy in *M. avium*-infected mice, improved clearance was observed *(113)*.

Investigations on the role of IL-10 in the inflammatory response to NTM are still lacking. Our own preliminary data suggest that, in the absence of IL-10, there is significant exacerbation of tissue pathology, similar to that occurring in models of autoimmune diseases (Ehlers, unpublished data).

3.4. TNF

In vivo cytokine neutralization experiments have clearly demonstrated that IFN-γ and TNF act in a synergistic fashion in the induction of bacteriostasis against *M. avium*. More particularly, IFN-γ was found to be involved in the priming of TNF secretion *(81)*. Neutralization of TNF significantly increased the mycobacterial burden *(114,115)*. Lack of the major signalling component of the TNF receptor, TNF-RI, was found to have no or only a marginal effect on bacterial replication in *M. avium*-infected mice *(116,117)*. Administration of an antagonist TNF-RII antibody to *M. avium*-infected mice inhibited the bacterial growth in the spleen, so that membrane or soluble TNF-RII may also be functionally involved in controlling infection *(118)*.

The TNF-RI is critically required for timely granuloma formation, confirming previous studies with *M. avium* and M. bovis Bacillus Calmette-Guérin (BCG) infection in which TNF was neutralized and granuloma formation aborted *(116,119–121)*. TNF-RI is crucial for granuloma maintenance, because in its absence, incipient granulomas disintegrate (Fig. 3B). The ensuing significant pathology causes death of *M. avium*-infected TNF-RI KO mice *(116)*. These mice were found to have an excessive T-cell response, as evidenced by high levels of IFN-γ and increased numbers of T-cells in the granulomas, and this T-cell-mediated granuloma disintegration could be prevented by treatment with anti-IL-12 *(122)*. These studies provide further evidence of how tightly protective and inflammatory events need to be regulated in order to prevent an otherwise excessive and detrimental inflammatory response. They also reveal a previously underestimated role for TNF in downmodulating inflammation in response to NTM infection.

3.5. Colony Stimulating Factors

In the beige mouse model of infection, a significant reduction in the number of viable *M. avium* was observed in blood, liver, and spleen of mice treated with a combination of recombinant GM-CSF and azithromycin or amikacin compared with control mice or those treated with rGM-CSF or antimicrobials alone *(123*; Ehlers, unpublished data). Administration of recombinant G-CSF promoted an extensive blood neutrophilia but failed to improve the course of *M. avium* infection in C57BL/6 or beige mice. rG-CSF administration also failed to improve the efficacy of a triple chemotherapeutic regimen *(112)*.

3.6. Chemokines

As with studies using macrophages in vitro, there is a paucity of data on chemokine production in vivo in response to NTM. A preparation of LAM (although not specifically derived from nontuberculous mycobacteria), when inoculated intranasally into mice, induced increases in the lung concentrations of MIP-2 and GRO-α *(124)*. In a model system using bead-immobilized purified protein derivative from *M. tuberculosis* to induce pulmonary granulomas in preimmunized mice, the following chemokine transcripts were found to be induced: γ-interferon-inducible protein (IP-10), monokine induced by IFN-γ (MIG), macrophage inflammatory protein-2 (MIP-2), lipopolysaccharide-induced chemokine (LIX), rodent growth-related oncogene homolog (KP), macrophage inflammatory protein-1α (MIP-1α) and -1β (MIP-1β), lymphotactin, MCP-1, MCP-5, monocyte-derived chemokine (MDC), and thymus and activation-related chemokine (TARC), C10. Other transcripts were found to be constitutively expressed: lungkine, secondary lymphoid-tissue chemokine (SLC), EBI1-ligand chemokine (ELC), fractalkine, MIP-1γ, and stromal cell derived factor-1α (SDF1-α). In this system, chemokines displayed characteristic temporal patterns of expression. CXC (IP-10, MIG, MIP-2, LIX) and certain CC (MCP-1, MCP-5, MIP-1α, MIP-1β) chemokines were produced maximally within 1–2 d. Lymphotactin displayed peak expression later *(125)*.

When *M. avium*-infected beige mice were examined, they had a lower MIP-1β and MIP-2 expression in the lungs than wild-type controls. The enhanced susceptibility of beige mice, which is particularly evident in the first few weeks of infection, may therefore be the result of defective recruitment of neutrophils or other cells responsive to these chemokines *(126)*.

3.7. A Note on the Use of Mouse Models for NTM Infection

Intravenous infection in mice is an adequate model for investigating the course of disseminated infection with NTM and has yielded significant insight into the roles different cytokines play in the protective and inflammatory response to infection with different NTM species. Aerosol infection with, for example, *M. avium*, however, does not adequately reflect the typical endobronchial disease (i.e., the localized form of NTM pneumonia present in patients with pre-existing pulmonary damage). On the other hand, aerosol infection with *M. avium* does lead to pulmonary pathology similar to that present in human tuberculosis (TB) patients, with caseating necrosis of the granulomatous lesions *(121)*. Therefore, this model lends itself to the investigation of the cause for granuloma necrosis and tissue pathology, and it was recently found that CD4[+] T-cells and IFN-γ, but not iNOS, are critical mediators in this form of mycobacteria-induced immunopathology *(100)*. There was excessive inflammation in both IFN-γ and iNOS KO mice, showing that dysregulation of the inflammatory response was likely mediated by a lack of nitric oxide; however, IFN-γ mediated necrosis was speculated to be the result of IFN-γ-induced chemokines, such as IP-10 and MIG, which have profound angiostatic effects and may cause localized hypoxia *(127)*.

4. LESSONS FROM HUMAN PATIENTS: FROM THE CLINIC TO DEFECTIVE GENES AND BACK TO IMMUNOTHERAPY

Careful investigation of unusual immunologic phenotypes in patients with disseminated NTM disease has led to the discovery of a number of genetic defects in the IL-12/IFN-γ pathway of macrophage activation in these patients. These comprise defects in the regulation of IL-12 secretion, mutations in the IL-12p40 gene, and various defects in IL-12Rβ1, IFN-γR1, IFN-γR2, and a STAT1 mutation.

Complete IFN-γ receptor deficiency is caused by frame-shift mutations creating premature stop codons in the genes for IFN-γR1 or IFN-γR2 *(128–133)*. These defects are associated with a complete absence of IFN-γ responsiveness in affected patients who characteristically have severe disseminated NTM infections [in one case, even arising from *M. smegmatis*, *(130)*] involving virtually every organ. Disease onset is very early in life, typically in small children, and infections are usually fatal if untreated. Because antibiotic therapy does not completely eradicate NTMs, recurrent infections establish a very poor prognosis. Histologic examination reveals poorly differentiated multibacillary lesions *(131,134,135)*. Interestingly, delayed-type hypersensitivity (DTH) responses were reported to be normal in disseminated BCG infection in these patients, suggesting that IFN-γ may not be necessary for DTH responses to mycobacteria in humans.

Partial IFN-γR deficiencies are characterized by a partial loss of IFN-γ responsiveness and may arise from a premature stop codon in the proximal intracellular protein domain, missense mutations, small in-frame deletions or insertions, or aberrant splicing events *(136–139)*. Mutant proteins are still expressed on the surface but cannot signal [e.g., because of the absence of JAK1 and STAT1 docking sites *(19)*]. This deficiency is found in an autosomal dominant form in which heterozygosity confers residual responsiveness to IFN-γ. There is also an autosomal recessive form of partial IFN-γR1 deficiency in which, again, IFN-γ responsiveness is diminished but not abolished. The clinical phenotype of affected patients is generally milder and characterized by a later onset. Histologically, mature, well-demarcated, and paucibacillary granulomas are found *(137)*. For unknown reasons, many of the patients with partial IFN-γR deficiencies suffer from NTM osteomyelitis *(140–142)*. Because IFN-γ plays a role in the regulation of itself and IL-12, PBMCs of these patients produce lower levels of TNF, IFN-γ, and IL-12 in response to PHA *(143)*.

All autosomal recessive mutations in the genes encoding IL-12p40 or IL-12Rβ1 described so far preclude expression of the respective proteins *(144–147)*. All patients suffer from disseminated NTM or BCG infection, and most also have severe *Salmonella* infections. Histologically, the appearance of well-organized and mature tuberculoid granulomas was documented *(144,145)*, suggesting that IL-12-dependent IFN-γ secretion is not necessary for granuloma formation. In vitro studies showed that patients' T-lymphocytes were not completely deficient in IFN-γ production, likely explaining the often milder clinical phentoype compared to patients with complete IFN-γ receptor deficiencies *(144,145,147,148)*. As with IFN-γR deficiencies, DTH reactions to PPD were reported to be normal in IL-12Rβ1-deficient patients. There have also been reports of abnormal IL-12 regulation in familial disseminated *M. avium* infection, and this has led to the discovery of IL-12-independent IFN-γ secretion pathways, although not all of them have been defined at the molecular level *(148,150)*. Generally speaking, defects in IL-12 secretion and/or IL-12R expression show considerable heterogeneity in terms of clinical outcome of nontuberculous infection, even among affected members of the same family *(151,152)*.

So far, no genuine deficiency in IFN-γ production has been detected in humans. In a recent clinical report, no production of IFN-γ was found despite normal IL-12R expression, but this could be attributed to a defective activation pathway for STAT-1, -3, and -5 by IL-12 in this patient *(153)*. In a publication describing a heterozygous germline human STAT-1 mutation, nuclear accumulation of gamma-activating factor (GAF) but not of interferon-stimulated gamma factor 3 (ISGF-3) was found to be impaired following stimulation of macrophages by interferons. Because only antimycobacterial but not antiviral defenses were deficient in macrophages with the STAT-1 mutation, this finding reveals for the first time that interferon-induced antimycobacterial mechanisms are channeled through GAF *(154)*.

4.1. Therapeutic Implications

Interferon-γ has been in various clinical trials for infectious diseases since the mid-1980s. Long-term follow-up of patients with chronic granulomatous disease who have received over 10 yr of IFN-γ has shown no unexpected toxicity *(155,156)*. In all trials involving *M. avium* infection, benefits have only been significant when concurrent antimycobacterial chemotherapy was given *(157,158)*. On the other hand, there have also been reports that IFN-γ has no effect in HIV-infected *M. avium* patients *(159)*. In a cohort comprised of HIV-negative patients with abnormal IL-12 production, idiopathic CD4 lymphocytopenia, and partial IFN-γR deficiencies, the cure rate was 60% when antimycobacterial chemotherapy was combined with subcutaneous IFN-γ *(155,160)*. Subcutaneous IFN-γ was also effective in patients with refractory pulmonary disease, and best results were observed in patients with noncavitary disease *(161,162)*. In a study using aerosolized IFN-γ, treatment converted smears to negative, although cultures remained positive for *M. avium (163)*.

Interleukin-12 has successfully been used as an adjuvant to a standard antituberculotic medication in patients suffering from progressive clinical tuberculosis *(164)*, but there have been only few attempts using IL-12 as adjuvant treatment in NTM infections so far. In one patient whose pulmonary *M. abscessus* infection was refractory to IFN-γ treatment, low-dose IL-12 was successful and led to sputum conversion *(165)*. IL-12 can be quite toxic, and this has been particularly evident in the setting of IFN-γ deficiency in a mouse model *(166)*. Further studies defining safe dosage and application intervals will be necessary to include IL-12 therapy in the "standard" immunotherapeutic armamentarium against NTM infection.

Granulocyte–macrophage colony-stimulating factor has also been used in some NTM patients. Although no significant effect on mycobacteremia was documented, activation of blood monocytes was noted in treated AIDS patients, as evidenced by enhanced mycobactericidal activity in vitro *(167)*, although others failed to observe this effect *(168)*. An anecdotal report on the use of GM-CSF in *M. kansasii* infection also showed increased activation of monocytes and improved control in vitro *(169)*.

5. PERSPECTIVE

This chapter has summarized data on cytokine induction/cytokine responsiveness in human patients, mouse models, and in vitro macrophage infections with NTM (*see* Table 1). There is now solid evidence from the mouse model of infection that several cytokines, such as IFN-γ, IL-12, IL-6, and TNF play important roles in immunity to NTM infections. Thus far, patients with disseminated NTM infections have only been found to have defects in the IL-12/IFN-γ pathway. Evidence for genetic defects in localized NTM disease is entirely lacking, and a recent study in older HIV-negative women without pre-existing lung disease who had localized *M. avium* pneumonia found no association with any known form of IFN-γR1-deficiency *(170)*.

The purpose of this chapter is to emphasize the likelihood that further genetic scrutiny of NTM patients will lead to the discovery of more, as yet unknown anomalies involving the pathways of macrophage recruitment and activation. These defects may again account for only the disseminated infections, but they may also lie at the core of some localized forms of disease. NTM infections may thus provide a unique opportunity for discovering cytokine/chemokine defects that may subsequently turn out to be critically involved also in the pathogenesis of other infectious diseases *(171)*.

This chapter has also documented that very little is known about the role of chemokines in NTM infections. However, it is likely that the relevance of chemokines recruiting mononuclear cells into the granuloma will prove to be substantial, for a number of reasons: (1) IFN-γ by itself has very little antimycobacterial activity in vitro and in vivo, yet has shown promise in adjunctive therapy; (2) many chemokines are induced by IFN-γ and a coordinated granulomatous response is essential for containing NTM infections.

Most critically, however, the mechanisms by which NTM are killed or inhibited in their growth are still completely unknown. The identification of the signaling pathways involved is only now beginning. The dissection of IFN-γ-induced inflammatory and protective events should ultimately lead to more specific forms of immunotherapy targeting the mycobactericidal mechanisms directly.

ACKNOWLEDGMENTS

Work in my laboratory is funded by grants SFB 367-C9, SFB 470-A6, and SFB 415-C7 from the Deutsche Forschungsgemeinschaft, a grant from the Medical University of Lubeck (Focus on Innate Defense Mechanisms against Infection), and the National Genome Research Network. I would like to thank C. Keller and A. Blumenthal for critically reading the manuscript and I. Bouchain for designing Fig. 1.

Table 1
Role of Cytokines and Chemokines in NTM Infection in Humans and Mice

Cytokine/ receptor	Effect on resistance/immunity	Effect on inflammation	Clinical disease when deficient	Ref.
IL-6	T: induction of T-cell immunity increased N: induction of T-cell immunity decreased	ND	Not known	82, 83
IL-10	N: reduced bacterial load N plus chemotherapy: improved clearance KO: marginally or no reduced bacterial load	KO: increased	Not known	32, 34, 108,113, Ehlers (unpublished)
IL-12	T: induction of T-cell immunity increased N: induction of T-cell immunity decreased KO: severely reduced resistance HD: severely reduced resistance HT: improved bacterial clearance	KO: delayed, circumscript granuloma formation HD: mature granulomas	Disseminated NTM infection	79–82, 84, 85, 87, 94, 149, 150, 164
IL-12Rβ2	HD: severely reduced resistance	HD: circumscript granulomas	Disseminated NTM infection	144–147
I-18	T: enhanced resistance	ND	Not known	92
TNF	N: impaired resistance	N: delayed or absent granuloma formation	Not known	114, 115, 120
TNFRI	KO: marginally or no increased bacterial load	KO: delayed granuloma formation; fatal granuloma disintegration	Not known	116, 117, 121, 122
TNFRII	N: growth inhibition in spleen	ND	Not known	118, 95, 98–100,
IFN-γ	T: increased macrophage activation N: impaired resistance KO: dramatic exacerbation of bacterial loads HT: improved bacterial clearance when combined with chemotherapy	KO: delayed response; then dysregulated mixed cellular infiltrate	Not known	115,155, 157, 158, 160–163, Ehlers (unpublished)
IFN-γRI/ IFN-γRII	HD: high bacterial load	HD: no circumscript granulomas, multi-bacillary lesions	HD: disseminated, often fatal infection	128–131, 133–139
G-CSF	T: improved clearance HT: clinical benefit	ND	Not known	123, 167, 169

Summary of results from studies using treatment with (T) or neutralization of (N) or gene detect: (KO) of a gene cytokine in mice or from treatment in human patients (HT) or from human immunodeficiencies (HD). ND: not determined.

REFERENCES

1. Woods, G.L. and Washington, J.A. (1987) Mycobacteria other than *Mycobacterium tuberculosis:* review of microbiologic and clinical aspects. *Rev. Infect. Dis.* **9,** 275–294.
2. Harmsen, D., Rothganger, J., Singer, C., Albert, J., and Frosch, M. (1999) Intuitive hypertext-based molecular identification of micro-organisms. *Lancet* **353,** 291.
3. Rogall, T., Wolters, J., Flohr, T., and Bottger, E.C. (1990) Towards a phylogeny and definition of species at the molecular level within the genus *Mycobacterium. Int. J. Syst. Bacteriol.* **40,** 323–330.
4. Boddinghaus, B., Rogall, T., Flohr, T., Blocker, H., and Bottger, E.C. (1990) Detection and identification of mycobacteria by amplification of rRNA. *J. Clin. Microbiol.* **28,** 1751–1759.

5. Falkinham, J.O., III (1996) Epidemiology of infection by nontuberculous mycobacteria. *Clin. Microbiol. Rev.* **9**, 177–215.
6. Horsburgh, C.R., Jr. (1996) Epidemiology of disease caused by nontuberculous mycobacteria. *Semin. Respir. Infect.* **11**, 244–251.
7. Wolinsky, E. (1992) Mycobacterial diseases other than tuberculosis. *Clin. Infect. Dis.* **15**, 1–10.
8. Horsburgh, C.R., Jr. (1999) The pathophysiology of disseminated *Mycobacterium avium* complex disease in AIDS. *J. Infect. Dis.* **179**, S461–S465.
9. Rosenzweig, D.Y. (1996) Nontuberculous mycobacterial disease in the immunocompetent adult. *Semin. Respir. Infect.* **11**, 252–261.
10. Hazra, R., Robson, C.D., Perez-Atayde, A.R., and Husson, R.N. (1999) Lymphadenitis due to nontuberculous mycobacteria in children: presentation and response to therapy. *Clin. Infect. Dis.* **28**, 123–129.
11. Shinners, D. and Yeager, H. (1999) Nontuberculous mycobacterial infection: clinical syndromes and diagnosis, in *Tuberculosis and Nontuberculous Mycobacterial Infections* (Schlossberg, D., ed.), W.B. Saunders, Philadelphia, pp. 341–350.
12. Iseman, M.D. (1989) *Mycobacterium avium* complex and the normal host: the other side of the coin. *N. Engl. J. Med.* **321**, 896–898.
13. Olivier, K.N. (1998) Nontuberculous mycobacterial pulmonary disease. *Curr. Opin. Pulm. Med.* **4**, 148–153.
14. Griffith, D.E. (1997) Nontuberculous mycobacteria. *Curr. Opin. Pulm. Med.* **3**, 139–145.
15. Inderlied, C.B., Kemper, C.A., and Bermudez, L.E. (1993) The *Mycobacterium avium* complex. *Clin. Microbiol. Rev.* **6**, 266–310.
16. Hartmann, P. and Plum, G. (1999) Immunological defense mechanisms in tuberculosis and MAC-infection. *Diagn. Microbiol. Infect. Dis.* **34**, 147–152.
17. Benator, D.A. and Gordin, F.M. (1996) Nontuberculous mycobacteria in patients with human immunodeficiency virus infection. *Semin. Respir. Infect.* **11**, 285–300.
18. Tortoli, E., Brunello, F., Cagni, A.E., Colombrita, D., Dionisio, D., Grisendi, L., et al. (1998) *Mycobacterium genavense* in AIDS patients, report of 24 cases in Italy and review of the literature. *Eur. J. Epidemiol.* **14**, 219–224.
19. Dorman, S.E. and Holland, S.M. (2000) Interferon-gamma and interleukin-12 pathway defects and human disease. *Cytokine Growth Factor Rev.* **11**, 321–333.
20. Cooper, A.M., Appelberg, R., and Orme, I.M. (1998) Immunopathogenesis of *Mycobacterium avium* infection. *Front Biosci.* **3**, 141–148.
21. Saunders, B.M. and Cooper, A.M. (2000) Restraining mycobacteria: role of granulomas in mycobacterial infections. *Immunol. Cell Biol.* **78**, 334–341.
22. Hansch, H.C., Smith, D.A., Mielke, M.E., Hahn, H., Bancroft, G.J., and Ehlers, S. (1996) Mechanisms of granuloma formation in murine Mycobacterium avium infection: the contribution of CD4+ T cells. *Int. Immunol.* **8**, 1299–1310.
23. Bermudez, L.E. and Young, L.S. (1988) Tumor necrosis factor, alone or in combination with IL-2, but not IFN-gamma, is associated with macrophage killing of *Mycobacterium avium* complex. *J. Immunol.* **140**, 3006–3013.
24. Rose, R.M., Fuglestad, J.M., and Remington, L. (1991) Growth inhibition of *Mycobacterium avium* complex in human alveolar macrophages by the combination of recombinant macrophage colony-stimulating factor and interferon-gamma. *Am. J. Respir. Cell Mol. Biol.* **4**, 248–254.
25. Tantawichien, T., Young, L.S., and Bermudez, L.E. (1996) Interleukin-7 induces anti-*Mycobacterium avium* activity in human monocyte-derived macrophages. *J. Infect. Dis.* **174**, 574–582.
26. Bermudez, L.E., Wu, M., and Young, L.S. (1995) Interleukin-12-stimulated natural killer cells can activate human macrophages to inhibit growth of *Mycobacterium avium*. *Infect. Immun.* **63**, 4099–4104.
27. Appelberg, R. and Orme, I.M. (1993) Effector mechanisms involved in cytokine-mediated bacteriostasis of *Mycobacterium avium* infections in murine macrophages. *Immunology* **80**, 352–359.
28. Toba, H., Crawford, J.T., and Ellner, J.J. (1989) Pathogenicity of *Mycobacterium avium* for human monocytes: absence of macrophage-activating factor activity of gamma interferon. *Infect. Immun.* **57**, 239–244.
29. Bermudez, L.E. and Young, L.S. (1990) Recombinant granulocyte-macrophage colony-stimulating factor activates human macrophages to inhibit growth or kill *Mycobacterium avium* complex. *J. Leukoc. Biol.* **48**, 67–73.
30. Suzuki, K., Lee, W.J., Hashimoto,T., Tanaka,E., Murayama, T., Amitani, R., et al. (1994) Recombinant granulocyte-macrophage colony-stimulating factor (GM-CSF) or tumour necrosis factor-alpha (TNF-alpha) activate human alveolar macrophages to inhibit growth of *Mycobacterium avium* complex. *Clin. Exp. Immunol.* **98**, 169–173.
31. Denis, M. and Gregg, E.O. (1991) Recombinant interleukin-6 increases the intracellular and extracellular growth of *Mycobacterium avium*. *Can. J. Microbiol.* **37**, 479–483.
32. Denis, M., Ghadirian, E. (1993) IL-10 neutralization augments mouse resistance to systemic *Mycobacterium avium* infections. *J. Immunol.* **151**, 5425–5430.
33. Shiratsuchi, H., Hamilton, B., Toossi, Z., and Ellner, J.J. (1996) Evidence against a role for interleukin-10 in the regulation of growth of *Mycobacterium avium* in human monocytes. *J. Infect. Dis.* **173**, 410–417.
34. Sano, C., Sato, K., Shimizu, T., Kajitani, H., Kawauchi, H., and Tomioka, H. (1999) The modulating effects of proinflammatory cytokines interferon-gamma (IFN-gamma) and tumour necrosis factor-alpha (TNF-alpha), and immunoregulating cytokines IL-10 and transforming growth factor-beta (TGF-beta), on anti-microbial activity of murine peritoneal macrophages against *Mycobacterium avium*-intracellulare complex. *Clin. Exp. Immunol.* **115**, 435–442.
35. Appelberg, R. (1995) Opposing effects of interleukin-10 on mouse macrophage functions. *Scand. J. Immunol.* **41**, 539–544.
36. Eriks, I.S. and Emerson, C.L. (1997) Temporal effect of tumor necrosis factor alpha on murine macrophages infected with *Mycobacterium avium*. *Infect. Immun.* **65**, 2100–2106.

37. Shiratsuchi, H., Johnson, J.L., and Ellner, J.J. (1991) Bidirectional effects of cytokines on the growth of *Mycobacterium avium* within human monocytes *J. Immunol.* **146,** 3165–3170.

38. Gomez-Flores, R., Tamez-Guerra, R., Tucker, S.D., and Mehta, R.T. (1997) Bidirectional effects of IFN-gamma on growth of *Mycobacterium avium* complex in murine peritoneal macrophages. *J. Interferon Cytokine Res.* **17,** 331–336.

39. Hussain, S., Zwilling, B.S., and Lafuse, W.P. (1999) *Mycobacterium avium* infection of mouse macrophages inhibits IFN-gamma Janus kinase-STAT signaling and gene induction by down-regulation of the IFN-gamma receptor. *J. Immunol.* **163,** 2041–2048.

40. Carvalho de Sousa, J.P. and Rastogi, N. (1992) Comparative ability of human monocytes and macrophages to control the intracellular growth of *Mycobacterium avium* and *Mycobacterium tuberculosis:* effect of interferon-gamma and indomethacin. *FEMS Microbiol. Immunol.* **4,** 329–334.

41. Shiratsuchi, H., Johnson, J.L., Toba, H., and Ellner, J.J. (1990) Strain- and donor-related differences in the interaction of *Mycobacterium avium* with human monocytes and its modulation by interferon-gamma *J. Infect. Dis.* **162,** 932–938.

42. Bradbury, M.G. and Moreno,C. (1993) Effect of lipoarabinomannan and mycobacteria on tumour necrosis factor production by different populations of murine macrophages. *Clin. Exp. Immunol.* **94,** 57–63.

43. Blanchard, D.K., Michelini-Norris, M.B., and Djeu, J.Y. (1991) Interferon decreases the growth inhibition of *Mycobacterium avium*-intracellulare complex by fresh human monocytes but not by culture-derived macrophages. *J.Infect.Dis.* **164,** 152–157.

44. Rudnicka, W., Brzychcy, M., Klink, M., Lopez, A.G., Fonteyne, P.A., Rusch-Gerdes, S., et al. (1999) The production of nitric oxide and tumor necrosis factor by murine macrophages infected with mycobacterial strains differing by hemolytic activity. *Microbiol.Immunol.* **43,** 637–644.

45. Fattorini, L., Xiao, Y., Li, B., Santoro, C., Ippoliti, F., and Orefici, G. (1994) Induction of IL-1 beta, IL-6, TNF-alpha, GM-CSF and G-CSF in human macrophages by smooth transparent and smooth opaque colonial variants of *Mycobacterium avium*. *J. Med. Microbiol.* **40,** 129–133.

46. Appelberg, R., Sarmento, A., and Castro, A.G. (1995) Tumour necrosis factor-alpha (TNF-alpha) in the host resistance to mycobacteria of distinct virulence. *Clin. Exp. Immunol.* **101,** 308–313.

47. Reiling, N., Blumenthal, A., Flad, H.D., Ernst, M., and Ehlers, S. (2001) Mycobacteria-induced TNF-alpha and IL-10 formation by human macrophages is differentially regulated at the level of mitogen-activated protein kinase activity. *J.Immunol.* **167,** 3339–3345.

47a. Blumenthal, A., Ehlers, S., Ernst, M., Flad, H.-D., and Reiling, N. (2002) Control of mycobacterial replication in human macrophages: roles of extracellular signal-regulated kinases 1 and 2 and p38 mitogen-activated protein kinase pathways. *Infect. Immun.* **70,** 4961–4967.

48. Tomioka, H., Sato, K., Maw, W.W., and Saito, H. (1995) The role of tumor necrosis factor, interferon-gamma, transforming growth factor-beta, and nitric oxide in the expression of immunosuppressive functions of splenic macrophages induced by *Mycobacterium avium* complex infection. *J. Leukocyte Biol.* **58,** 704–712.

49. Tomioka, H., Maw, W.W., Sato, K., and Saito, H. (1996) The role of tumour necrosis factor-alpha in combination with interferon-gamma or interleukin-1 in the induction of immunosuppressive macrophages because of *Mycobacterium avium* complex infection. *Immunology* **88,** 61–67.

50. Bermudez, L.E. (1993) Production of transforming growth factor-beta by *Mycobacterium avium*-infected human macrophages is associated with unresponsiveness to IFN-gamma. *J. Immunol.* **150,** 1838–1845.

51. Venkataprasad, N., Shiratsuchi, H., Johnson, J.L., and Ellner, J.J. (1996) Induction of prostaglandin E2 by human monocytes infected with *Mycobacterium avium* complex—modulation of cytokine expression. *J. Infect. Dis.* **174,** 806–811.

52. Bermudez, L.E., Wu, M., Petrofsky, M., and Young, L.S. (1992) Interleukin-6 antagonizes tumor necrosis factor-mediated mycobacteriostatic and mycobactericidal activities in macrophages. *Infect. Immun.* **60,** 4245–4252.

53. VanHeyningen, T.K., Collins, H.L., and Russell, D.G. (1997) IL-6 produced by macrophages infected with *Mycobacterium* species suppresses T cell responses. *J. Immunol.* **158,** 330–337.

54. Sarmento, A.M. and Appelberg, R. (1995) Relationship between virulence of *Mycobacterium avium* strains and induction of tumor necrosis factor alpha production in infected mice and in in vitro-cultured mouse macrophages. *Infect. Immun.* **63,** 3759–3764.

55. Furney, S.K., Skinner, P.S., Roberts, A.D., Appelberg, R., and Orme, I.M. (1992) Capacity of *Mycobacterium avium* isolates to grow well or poorly in murine macrophages resides in their ability to induce secretion of tumor necrosis factor. *Infect. Immun.* **60,** 4410–4413.

56. Shiratsuchi, H. and Ellner, J.J. (2001) Expression of IL-18 by *Mycobacterium avium*-infected human monocytes; association with *M. avium* virulence. *Clin. Exp. Immunol.* **123,** 203–209.

57. Shiratsuchi, H., Toossi, Z., Mettler, M.A., and Ellner, J.J. (1993) Colonial morphotype as a determinant of cytokine expression by human monocytes infected with *Mycobacterium avium*. *J. Immunol.* **150,** 2945–2954.

58. Beltan, E., Horgen, L., and Rastogi, N. (2000) Secretion of cytokines by human macrophages upon infection by pathogenic and non-pathogenic mycobacteria. *Microb. Pathol.* **28,** 313–318.

59. von Grunberg, P.W. and Plum, G. (1998) Enhanced induction of interleukin-12(p40) secretion by human macrophages infected with *Mycobacterium avium* complex isolates from disseminated infection in AIDS patients. *J. Infect. Dis.* **178,** 1209–1212.

60. Pais, T.F. and Appelberg, R. (2000) Macrophage control of mycobacterial growth induced by picolinic acid is dependent on host cell apoptosis. *J. Immunol.* **164,** 389–397.

61. Flad, H.D., Grage-Griebenow, E., Scheuerer, B., Durrbaum-Landmann, I., Petersen, F., Brandt, E., et al. (1998) The role of cytokines in monocyte apoptosis. *Res. Immunol.* **149,** 733–736.

62. Balcewicz-Sablinska, M.K., Gan, H., and Remold, H.G. (1999) Interleukin 10 produced by macrophages inoculated

with *Mycobacterium avium* attenuates mycobacteria-induced apoptosis by reduction of TNF-alpha activity. *J. Infect. Dis.* **180,** 1230–1237.

63. Fratazzi, C., Arbeit, R.D., Carini, C., Balcewicz-Sablinska, M.K., Keane, J., Kornfeld, H., et al. (1999) Macrophage apoptosis in mycobacterial infections. *J. Leukocyte Biol.* **66,** 763–764.

64. Schaible, U.E., Sturgill-Koszycki, S., Schlesinger, P.H., and Russell, D.G. (1998) Cytokine activation leads to acidification and increases maturation of *Mycobacterium avium*-containing phagosomes in murine macrophages. *J. Immunol.* **160,** 1290–1296.

65. Gomes, M.S., Paul, S., Moreira, A.L., Appelberg, R., Rabinovitch, M., and Kaplan, G. (1999) Survival of *Mycobacterium avium* and *Mycobacterium tuberculosis* in acidified vacuoles of murine macrophages. *Infect. Immun.* **67,** 3199–3206.

66. Doi, T., Ando, M., Akaike, T., Suga, M., Sato, K., and Maeda, H. (1993) Resistance to nitric oxide in *Mycobacterium avium* complex and its implication in pathogenesis. *Infect. Immun.* **61,** 1980–1989.

67. Sarmento, A. and Appelberg, R. (1996) Involvement of reactive oxygen intermediates in tumor necrosis factor alpha-dependent bacteriostasis of *Mycobacterium avium*. *Infect. Immun.* **64,** 3224–3230.

68. Gomes, M.S., Boelaert, J.R., and Appelberg, R. (2001) Role of iron in experimental *Mycobacterium avium* infection. *J. Clin. Virol.* **20,** 117–122.

69. Nylen, O., Berg-Kelly, K., and Andersson, B. (2000) Cervical lymph node infections with non-tuberculous mycobacteria in preschool children: interferon gamma deficiency as a possible cause of clinical infection. *Acta Paediatr.* **89,** 1322–1325.

70. Vankayalapati, R., Wizel, B., Samten, B., Griffith, D.E., Shams, H., Galland, M.R., et al. (2001) Cytokine profiles in immunocompetent persons infected with *Mycobacterium avium* complex. *J. Infect. Dis.* **183,** 478–484.

71. Greinert, U., Schlaak, M., Rusch-Gerdes, S., Flad, H.D., and Ernst, M. (2000) Low in vitro production of interferon-gamma and tumor necrosis factor-alpha in HIV-seronegative patients with pulmonary disease caused by nontuberculous mycobacteria. *J. Clin. Immunol.* **20,** 445–452.

72. Bermudez, L.E., Inderlied, C., and Young, L.S. (1991) Stimulation with cytokines enhances penetration of azithromycin into human macrophages. *Antimicrob. Agents Chemother.* **35,** 2625–2629.

73. Onyeji, C.O., Nightingale, C.H., Tessier, P.R., Nicolau, D.P., and Bow, L.M. (1995) Activities of clarithromycin, azithromycin, and ofloxacin in combination with liposomal or unencapsulated granulocyte-macrophage colony-stimulating factor against intramacrophage *Mycobacterium avium*-Mycobacterium intracellulare. *J. Infect. Dis.* **172,** 810–816.

74. Rao, S.P., Hayashi, T., and Catanzaro, A. (2000) Release of monocyte chemoattractant protein (MCP)-1 by a human alveolar epithelial cell line in response to *Mycobacterium avium*. *FEMS Immunol. Med. Microbiol.* **29,** 1–7.

75. Sangari, F.J., Petrofsky, M., and Bermudez, L.E. (1999) *Mycobacterium avium* infection of epithelial cells results in inhibition or delay in the release of interleukin-8 and RANTES. *Infect. Immun.* **67,** 5069–5075.

76. Vouret-Craviari, V., Cenzuales, S., Poli, G., and Mantovani, A. (1997) Expression of monocyte chemotactic protein-3 in human monocytes exposed to the mycobacterial cell wall component lipoarabinomannan. *Cytokine* **9,** 992–998.

77. Wahl, S.M., Greenwell-Wild, T., Peng, G., Hale-Donze, H., Doherty, T.M., Mizel, D., et al. (1998) *Mycobacterium avium* complex augments macrophage HIV-1 production and increases CCR5 expression. *Proc. Natl. Acad. Sci. USA* **95,** 12,574–12,579.

78. Wahl, S.M., Greenwell-Wild, T., Peng, G., Hale-Donze, H., and Orenstein, J.M. (1999) Co-infection with opportunistic pathogens promotes human immunodeficiency virus type 1 infection in macrophages. *J. Infect. Dis.* **179,** S457–S460.

79. Saunders, B.M., Zhan, Y., and Cheers, C. (1995) Endogenous interleukin-12 is involved in resistance of mice to *Mycobacterium avium* complex infection. *Infect. Immun.* **63,** 4011–4015.

80. Castro, A.G., Silva, R.A., and Appelberg, R. (1995) Endogenously produced IL-12 is required for the induction of protective T cells during *Mycobacterium avium* infections in mice. *J. Immunol.* **155,** 2013–2019.

81. Appelberg, R., Castro, A.G., Pedrosa, J., Silva, R.A., Orme, I.M., and Minoprio, P. (1994) Role of gamma interferon and tumor necrosis factor alpha during T-cell-independent and -dependent phases of *Mycobacterium avium* infection. *Infect. Immun.* **62,** 3962–3971.

82. Leal, I.S., Smedegard, B., Andersen, P., and Appelberg, R. (1999) Interleukin-6 and interleukin-12 participate in induction of a type 1 protective T-cell response during vaccination with a tuberculosis subunit vaccine. *Infect. Immun.* **67,** 5747–5754.

83. Appelberg, R., Castro, A.G., Pedrosa, J., and Minoprio, P. (1994) Role of interleukin-6 in the induction of protective T cells during mycobacterial infections in mice. *Immunology* **82,** 361–364.

84. Silva, R.A., Pais, T.F., and Appelberg, R. (1998) Evaluation of IL-12 in immunotherapy and vaccine design in experimental *Mycobacterium avium* infections. *J. Immunol.* **161,** 5578–5585.

85. Silva, R.A., Florido, M., and Appelberg, R. (2001) Interleukin-12 primes CD4+ T cells for interferon-gamma production and protective immunity during *Mycobacterium avium* infection. *Immunology* **103,** 368–374.

86. Kang, B.Y., Chung, S.W., Lim, Y.S., Kim, E.J., Kim, S.H., Hwang, S.Y., and Kim, T.S. (1999) Interleukin-12-secreting fibroblasts are more efficient than free recombinant interleukin-12 in inducing the persistent resistance to *Mycobacterium avium* complex infection. *Immunology* **97,** 474–480.

87. Silva, R.A., Pais, T.F., and Appelberg, R. (2000) Effects of interleukin-12 in the long-term protection conferred by a *Mycobacterium avium* subunit vaccine. *Scand. J. Immunol.* **52,** 531–533.

88. Kobayashi, K., Yamazaki, J., Kasama, T., Katsura, T., Kasahara, K., Wolf, S.F., and Shimamura, T. (1996) Interleukin (IL)-12 deficiency in susceptible mice infected with *Mycobacterium avium* and amelioration of established infection by IL-12 replacement therapy. *J. Infect. Dis.* **174,** 564–573.

89. Muller, U., Kohler, G., Mossmann, H., Schaub, G.A., Alber, G., Di Santo, J.P., et al. (2001) IL-12-independent IFN-gamma production by T cells in experimental Chagas' disease is mediated by IL-18. *J. Immunol.* **167,** 3346–3353.

90. Oppmann, B., Lesley, R., Blom, B., Timans, J.C., Xu, Y., Hunte, B., et al. (2000) Novel p19 protein engages IL-12p40 to form a cytokine, IL-23, with biological activities similar as well as distinct from IL-12. *Immunity* **13,** 715–725.
91. Kobayashi, K., Nakata, N., Kai, M., Kasama, T., Hanyuda, Y., and Hatano, Y. (1997) Decreased expression of cytokines that induce type 1 helper T cell/interferon-gamma responses in genetically susceptible mice infected with *Mycobacterium avium. Clin. Immunol. Immunopathol.* **85,** 112–116.
92. Kim, S.H., Cho, D., and Kim, T.S. (2001) Induction of in vivo resistance to *Mycobacterium avium* infection by intramuscular injection with DNA encoding interleukin-18. *Immunology* **102,** 234–241.
93. Bermudez, L.E., Petrofsky, M., Wu, M., and Young, L.S. (1998) Clarithromycin significantly improves interleukin-12-mediated anti-*Mycobacterium avium* activity and abolishes toxicity in mice. *J. Infect. Dis.* **178,** 896–899.
94. Doherty, T.M. and Sher, A. (1998) IL-12 promotes drug-induced clearance of *Mycobacterium avium* infection in mice. *J. Immunol.* **160,** 5428–5435.
95. Gilbertson, B., Zhong, J., and Cheers, C. (1999) Anergy, IFN-gamma production, and apoptosis in terminal infection of mice with *Mycobacterium avium. J. Immunol.* **163,** 2073–2080.
96. Sacco, R.E., Jensen, R.J., Thoen, C.O., Sandor, M., Weinstock, J., Lynch, R.G., et al. (1996) Cytokine secretion and adhesion molecule expression by granuloma T lymphocytes in *Mycobacterium avium* infection. *Am. J. Pathol.* **148,** 1935–1948.
97. Burrells, C., Clarke, C.J., Colston, A., Kay, J.M., Porter, J., Little, D., et al. (1999) Interferon-gamma and interleukin-2 release by lymphocytes derived from the blood, mesenteric lymph nodes and intestines of normal sheep and those affected with paratuberculosis (Johne's disease). *Vet. Immunol. Immunopathol.* **68,** 139–148.
98. Edwards, C.K., III, Hedegaard, H.B., Zlotnik, A., Gangadharam, P.R., Johnston, R.B., Jr., and Pabst, M.J. (1986) Chronic infection due to *Mycobacterium intracellulare* in mice: association with macrophage release of prostaglandin E2 and reversal by injection of indomethacin, muramyl dipeptide, or interferon-gamma. *J. Immunol.* **136,** 1820–1827.
99. Florido, M., Goncalves, A.S., Silva, R.A., Ehlers, S., Cooper, A.M., and Appelberg, R. (1999) Resistance of virulent *Mycobacterium avium* to gamma interferon-mediated antimicrobial activity suggests additional signals for induction of mycobacteriostasis. *Infect. Immun.* **67,** 3610–3618.
100. Ehlers, S., Benini, J., Held, H.D., Roeck, C., Alber, G., and Uhlig, S. (2001) αβTCR+ cells and IFNγ, but not iNOS, are critical for granuloma necrosis in a mouse model of mycobacteria-induced pulmonary immunopathology. *J. Exp. Med.* **194,** 1847–1859
101. Murray, P.J., Young, R.A., and Daley, G.Q. (1998) Hematopoietic remodeling in interferon-gamma-deficient mice infected with mycobacteria. *Blood* **91,** 2914–2924.
102. Gomes, M.S., Florido, M., Pais, T.F., and Appelberg, R. (1999) Improved clearance of *Mycobacterium avium* upon disruption of the inducible nitric oxide synthase gene. *J. Immunol.* **162,** 6734–6739.
103. Ehlers, S., Kutsch, S., Benini, J., Cooper, A., Hahn, C., Gerdes, J., et al. (1999) NOS2-derived nitric oxide regulates the size, quantity and quality of granuloma formation in *Mycobacterium avium*-infected mice without affecting bacterial loads. *Immunology* **98,** 313–323.
104. Ehlers, S. and Richter, E. (2001) Differential requirement for interferon-gamma to restrict the growth of or eliminate some recently identified species of nontuberculous mycobacteria in vivo. *Clin. Exp. Immunol.* **124,** 229–238.
105. Ehlers, S. and Richter, E. (2000) Gamma interferon is essential for clearing *Mycobacterium genavense* infection. *Infect. Immun.* **68,** 3720–3723.
106. MacMicking, J.D., North, R.J., LaCourse, R., Mudgett, J.S., Shah, S.K., and Nathan, C.F. (1997) Identification of nitric oxide synthase as a protective locus against tuberculosis. *Proc. Natl. Acad. Sci. USA* **94,** 5243–5248.
107. Segal, B.H., Doherty, T.M., Wynn, T.A., Cheever, A.W., Sher, A., and Holland, S.M. (1999) The p47(phox–/–) mouse model of chronic granulomatous disease has normal granuloma formation and cytokine responses to *Mycobacterium avium* and *Schistosoma mansoni* eggs. *Infect. Immun.* **67,** 1659–1665.
108. Bermudez, L.E. and Champsi, J. (1993) Infection with *Mycobacterium avium* induces production of interleukin-10 (IL-10), and administration of anti-IL-10 antibody is associated with enhanced resistance to infection in mice. *Infect. Immun.* **61,** 3093–3097.
109. Jacobs, M., Brown, N., Allie, N., Gulert, R., and Ryffel, B. (2000) Increased resistance to mycobacterial infection in the absence of interleukin-10. *Immunology* **100,** 494–501.
110. Murray, P.J. and Young, R.A. (1999) Increased antimycobacterial immunity in interleukin-10-deficient mice. *Infect. Immun.* **67,** 3087–3095.
111. Roach, D.R., Martin, E., Bean, A.G., Rennick, D.M., Briscoe, H., and Britton, W.J. (2001) Endogenous inhibition of antimycobacterial immunity by IL-10 varies between mycobacterial species. *Scand. J. Immunol.* **54,** 163–170.
112. Goncalves, A.S. and Appelberg, R. (2001) Effects of recombinant granulocyte-colony stimulating factor administration during *Mycobacterium avium* infection in mice. *Clin. Exp. Immunol.* **124** 239–247.
113. Silva, R.A., Pais, T.F., and Appelberg, R. (2001) Blocking the receptor for IL-10 improves antimycobacterial chemotherapy and vaccination. *J. Immunol.* **167,** 1535–1541.
114. Bala, S., Hastings, K.L., Kazempour, K., Inglis, S., and Dempsey, W.L. (1998) Inhibition of tumor necrosis factor alpha alters resistance to *Mycobacterium avium* complex infection in mice. *Antimicrob. Agents Chemother.* **42,** 2336–2341.
115. Appelberg, R., Castro, A.G., Pedrosa, J., Silva, R.A., Orme, I.M., and Minoprio, P. (1994) Role of gamma interferon and tumor necrosis factor alpha during T-cell-independent and -dependent phases of *Mycobacterium avium* infection. *Infect. Immun.* **62,** 3962–3971.
116. Ehlers, S., Benini, J., Kutsch, S., Endres, R., Rietschel, E.T., and Pfeffer, K. (1999) Fatal granuloma necrosis without exacerbated mycobacterial growth in tumor necrosis factor receptor p55 gene-deficient mice intravenously infected with *Mycobacterium avium Infect. Immun.* **67,** 3571–3579.

117. Silva, R.A., Gomes, M.S., and Appelberg, R. (2000) Minor role played by type I tumour necrosis factor receptor in the control of *Mycobacterium avium* proliferation in infected mice. *Immunology* **99,** 203–207.
118. Corti, A., Fattorini, L., Thoresen, O.F., Ricci, M.L., Gallizia, A., Pelagi, M., et al. (1999) Upregulation of p75 tumor necrosis factor alpha receptor in *Mycobacterium avium*-infected mice: evidence for a functional role. *Infect. Immun.* **67,** 5762–5767.
119. Kindler, V., Sappino, A.P., Grau, G.E., Piguet, P.F., and Vassalli, P. (1989) The inducing role of tumor necrosis factor in the development of bactericidal granulomas during BCG infection. *Cell* **56,** 731–740.
120. Smith, D., Hansch, H., Bancroft, G., and Ehlers, S. (1997) T-cell-independent granuloma formation in response to *Mycobacterium avium:* role of tumour necrosis factor-alpha and interferon-gamma. *Immunology* **92,** 413–421.
121. Benini, J., Ehlers, E.M., and Ehlers, S. (1999) Different types of pulmonary granuloma necrosis in immunocompetent vs. TNFRp55-gene-deficient mice aerogenically infected with highly virulent *Mycobacterium avium J. Pathol.* **189,** 127–137.
122. Ehlers, S., Kutsch, S., Ehlers, E.M., Benini, J., and Pfeffer, K. (2000) Lethal granuloma disintegration in mycobacteria-infected TNFRp55–/– mice is dependent on T cells and IL-12. *J. Immunol.* **165,** 483–492.
123. Bermudez, L.E., Martinelli, J., Petrofsky, M., Kolonoski, P., and Young, L.S. (1994) Recombinant granulocyte–macrophage colony-stimulating factor enhances the effects of antibiotics against *Mycobacterium avium* complex infection in the beige mouse model. *J. Infect. Dis.* **169,** 575–580.
124. Juffermans, N.P., Verbon, A., Belisle, J.T., Hill, P.J., Speelman, P., van Deventer, S.J., et al. (2000) Mycobacterial lipoarabinomannan induces an inflammatory response in the mouse lung. A role for interleukin-1. *Am. J. Respir. Crit. Care Med.* **162,** 486–489.
125. Qiu, B., Frait, K.A., Reich, F., Komuniecki, E., and Chensue, S.W. (2001) Chemokine expression dynamics in mycobacterial (type-1) and schistosomal (type-2) antigen-elicited pulmonary granuloma formation. *Am. J. Pathol.* **158,** 1503–1515.
126. Florido, M., Appelberg, R., Orme, I.M., and Cooper, A.M. (1997) Evidence for a reduced chemokine response in the lungs of beige mice infected with *Mycobacterium avium. Immunology* **90,** 600–606.
127. Oppenheim, J.J., Zack Howard, O.M., and Goetzl, E. (2001) Chemotactic factors, neuropeptides, and other ligands for seven transmembrane receptors, in *Cytokine Reference* (Oppenheim, J.J. and Feldmann, M. eds.), Academic, San Diego, CA, pp. 985–1021.
128. Altare, F., Jouanguy, E., Lamhamedi, S., Doffinger, R., Fischer,A., and Casanova, J.L. (1998) Mendelian susceptibility to mycobacterial infection in man. *Curr. Opin. Immunol.* **10,** 413–417.
129. Vesterhus, P., Holland, S.M., Abrahamsen, T.G., and Bjerknes, R. (1998) Familial disseminated infection due to atypical mycobacteria with childhood onset. *Clin. Infect. Dis.* **27,** 822–825.
130. Pierre-Audigier, C., Jouanguy, E., Lamhamedi, S., Altare, F., Rauzier, J., Vincent, V., et al. (1997) Fatal disseminated *Mycobacterium smegmatis* infection in a child with inherited interferon gamma receptor deficiency. *Clin. Infect. Dis.* **24,** 982–984.
131. Dorman, S.E. and Holland, S.M. (1998) Mutation in the signal-transducing chain of the interferon-gamma receptor and susceptibility to mycobacterial infection. *J. Clin. Invest.* **101,** 2364–2369.
132. Remus, N., Reichenbach, J., Picard, C., Rietschel, C., Wood, P., Lammas, D., et al. (2001) Impaired interferon gamma-mediated immunity and susceptibility to mycobacterial infection in childhood. *Pediatr. Res.* **50,** 8–13.
133. Roesler, J., Kofink, B., Wendisch, J., Heyden, S., Paul, D., Friedrich, W., et al. (1999) Listeria monocytogenes and recurrent mycobacterial infections in a child with complete interferon-gamma-receptor (IFNgammaR1) deficiency: mutational analysis and evaluation of therapeutic options. *Exp. Hematol.* **27,** 1368–1374.
134. Emile, J.F., Patey, N., Altare, F., Lamhamedi, S., Jouanguy, E., Boman, F., et al. (1997) Correlation of granuloma structure with clinical outcome defines two types of idiopathic disseminated BCG infection. *J. Pathol.* **181,** 25–30.
135. Jouanguy, E., Altare, F., Lamhamedi, S., Revy, P., Emile, J.F., Newport, M., et al. (1996) Interferon-gamma-receptor deficiency in an infant with fatal bacille Calmette–Guerin infection. *N. Engl. J. Med.* **335,** 1956–1961.
136. Doffinger, R., Altare, F., and Casanova, J.L. (2000) Genetic heterogeneity of Mendelian susceptibility to mycobacterial infection. *Microbes Infect.* **2,** 1553–1557.
137. Jouanguy, E., Lamhamedi-Cherradi, S., Lammas, D., Dorman, S.E., Fondaneche, M.C., Dupuis, S., et al. (1999) A human IFNGR1 small deletion hotspot associated with dominant susceptibility to mycobacterial infection. *Nat. Genet.* **21,** 370–378.
138. Jouanguy, E., Lamhamedi-Cherradi, S., Altare, F., Fondaneche, M.C., Tuerlinckx, D., Blanche, S., et al. (1997) Partial interferon-gamma receptor 1 deficiency in a child with tuberculoid bacillus Calmette–Guerin infection and a sibling with clinical tuberculosis. *J. Clin. Invest.* **100,** 2658–2664.
139. Doffinger, R., Jouanguy, E., Dupuis, S., Fondaneche, M.C., Stephan, J.L., Emile, J.F., et al. (2000) Partial interferon-gamma receptor signaling chain deficiency in a patient with bacille Calmette-Guerin and *Mycobacterium abscessus* infection. *J. Infect. Dis.* **181,** 379–384.
140. Arend, S.M., Janssen, R., Gosen, J.J., Waanders, H., de Boer, T., Ottenhoff, T.H., et al. (2001) Multifocal osteomyelitis caused by nontuberculous mycobacteria in patients with a genetic defect of the interferon-gamma receptor. *Neth. J. Med.* **59,** 140–151.
141. Villella, A., Picard, C., Jouanguy, E., Dupuis, S., Popko, S., Abughali, N., et al. (2001) Recurrent Mycobacterium avium osteomyelitis associated with a novel dominant interferon gamma receptor mutation. *Pediatrics* **107,** E47.
142. Allende, L.M., Lopez-Goyanes, A., Paz-Artal, E., Corell, A., Garcia-Perez, M.A., Varela, P., et al. (2001) A point mutation in a domain of gamma interferon receptor 1 provokes severe immunodeficiency. *Clin. Diagn. Lab Immunol.* **8,** 133–137.
143. Holland, S.M., Dorman, S.E., Kwon, A., Pitha-Rowe, I.F., Frucht, D.M., Gerstberger, S.M., et al. (1998) Abnormal regulation of interferon-gamma, interleukin-12, and tumor necrosis factor-alpha in human interferon-gamma receptor 1 deficiency. *J. Infect. Dis.* **178,** 1095–1104.

144. Altare, F., Durandy, A., Lammas, D., Emile, J.F., Lamhamedi, S., Le Deist, F., et al. (1998) Impairment of mycobacterial immunity in human interleukin-12 receptor deficiency. *Science* **280**, 1432–1435.

145. de Jong, R., Altare, F., Haagen, I.A., Elferink, D.G., Boer, T., Breda Vriesman, P.J., et al. (1998) Severe mycobacterial and Salmonella infections in interleukin-12 receptor-deficient patients. *Science* **280**, 1435–1438.

146. Sakai, T., Matsuoka, M., Aoki, M., Nosaka, K., and Mitsuya, H. (2001) Missense mutation of the interleukin-12 receptor beta1 chain-encoding gene is associated with impaired immunity against *Mycobacterium avium* complex infection. *Blood* **97**, 2688–2694.

147. Altare, F., Lammas, D., Revy, P., Jouanguy, E., Doffinger, R., Lamhamedi, S., et al. (1998) Inherited interleukin 12 deficiency in a child with bacille Calmette–Guerin and Salmonella enteritidis disseminated infection. *J. Clin. Invest.* **102**, 2035–2040.

148. Verhagen, C.E., de Boer, T., Smits, H.H., Verreck, F.A., Wierenga, E.A., Kurimoto, M., et al. (2000) Residual type 1 immunity in patients genetically deficient for interleukin 12 receptor beta1 (IL-12Rbeta1): evidence for an IL-12Rbeta1-independent pathway of IL-12 responsiveness in human T cells. *J. Exp. Med.* **192**, 517–528.

149. Frucht, D.M. and Holland, S.M. (1996) Defective monocyte costimulation for IFN-gamma production in familial disseminated *Mycobacterium avium* complex infection: abnormal IL-12 regulation. *J. Immunol.* **157**, 411–416.

150. Frucht, D.M., Sandberg, D.I., Brown, M.R., Gerstberger, S.M., and Holland, S.M. (1999) IL-12-independent costimulation pathways for interferon-gamma production in familial disseminated *Mycobacterium avium* complex infection. *Clin. Immunol.* **91**, 234–241.

151. Elloumi-Zghal, H., Barbouche, M.R., Chemli, J., Bejaoui, M., Harbi, A., Snoussi, N., et al. (2002) Clinical and genetic heterogeneity of inherited autosomal recessive susceptibility to disseminated *Mycobacterium bovis* bacille Calmette–Guerin infection. *J. Infect. Dis.* **185**, 1468–1475.

152. Picard, C., Fieschi, C., Altare, F., Al Jumaah, S., Al Hajjar, S., Feinberg, J., et al. (2002) Inherited interleukin-12 deficiency: IL12B genotype and clinical phenotype of 13 patients from six kindreds. *Am. J. Hum. Genet.* **70**, 336–348.

153. Gollob, J.A., Veenstra, K.G., Jyonouchi, H., Kelly, A.M., Ferrieri, P., Panka, D.J., et al. (2000) Impairment of STAT activation by IL-12 in a patient with atypical mycobacterial and staphylococcal infections. *J. Immunol.* **165**, 4120–4126.

154. Dupuis, S., Dargemont, C., Fieschi, C., Thomassin, N., Rosenzweig, S., Harris, J., et al. (2001) Impairment of mycobacterial but not viral immunity by a germline human STAT1 mutation. *Science* **293**, 300–303.

155. Holland, S.M., Eisenstein, E.M., Kuhns, D.B., Turner, M.L., Fleisher, T.A., Strober, W., et al. (1994) Treatment of refractory disseminated nontuberculous mycobacterial infection with interferon gamma. A preliminary report. *N. Engl. J. Med.* **330**, 1348–1355.

156. Gallin, J.I., Farber, J.M., Holland, S.M., and Nutman T.B. (1995) Interferon-gamma in the management of infectious diseases. *Ann. Intern. Med.* **123**, 216–224.

157. Squires, K.E., Brown, S.T., Armstrong, D., Murphy, W.F., and Murray, H.W. (1992) Interferon-gamma treatment for *Mycobacterium avium*-intracellular complex bacillemia in patients with AIDS. *J. Infect. Dis.* **166**, 686–687.

158. Squires, K.E., Murphy, W.F., Madoff, L.C., and Murray, H.W. (1989) Interferon-gamma and *Mycobacterium avium*-intracellulare infection. *J. Infect. Dis.* **159**, 599–600.

159. Lauw, F.N., Der Meer, J.T., de Metz, J., Danner, S.A., and van Der, P.T. (2001) No beneficial effect of interferon-gamma treatment in 2 human immunodeficiency virus-infected patients with *Mycobacterium avium* complex infection. *Clin. Infect. Dis.* **32**, e81–e82.

160. Holland, S.M. (1996) Therapy of mycobacterial infections. *Res. Immunol.* **147**, 572–581.

161. Holland, S.M. (2000) Cytokine therapy of mycobacterial infections. *Adv. Intern. Med.* **45**, 431–452.

162. Holland, S.M. (2000) Treatment of infections in the patient with Mendelian susceptibility to mycobacterial infection. *Microbes. Infect.* **2**, 1579–1590.

163. Chatte, G., Panteix, G., Perrin-Fayolle, M., and Pacheco, Y. (1995) Aerosolized interferon gamma for *Mycobacterium avium*-complex lung disease. *Am. J. Respir. Crit. Care Med.* **152**, 1094–1096.

164. Greinert, U., Ernst, M., Schlaak, M., and Entzian, P. (2001) Interleukin-12 as successful adjuvant in tuberculosis treatment. *Eur. Respir. J.* **17**, 1049–1051.

165. Holland, S.M. and Dorman, S.E. (1998) Successful IL-12 therapy in interferon gamma refractory pulmonary *M. abscessus*. AFMR (abstract).

166. Car, B.D., Eng, V.M., Schnyder, B., LeHir, M., Shakhov, A.N., Woerly, G., et al. (1995) Role of interferon-gamma in interleukin 12-induced pathology in mice. *Am. J. Pathol.* **147**, 1693–1707.

167. Kemper, C.A., Bermudez, L.E., and Deresinski, S.C. (1998) Immunomodulatory treatment of *Mycobacterium avium* complex bacteremia in patients with AIDS by use of recombinant granulocyte-macrophage colony-stimulating factor. *J. Infect. Dis.* **177**, 914–920.

168. Cinti, S., Coffey, M., Sullivan, A., and Kazanjian, P. (1999) Killing of Mycobacterium avium by neutrophils and monocytes from AIDS patients treated with recombinant granulocyte–macrophage colony-stimulating factor. *J. Infect. Dis.* **180**, 229–233.

169. Bermudez, L.E., Kemper, C.A., and Deresinski, S.C. (1994) Dysfunctional monocytes from a patient with disseminated *Mycobacterium kansasii* infection are activated in vitro and in vivo by GM-CSF. *Biotherapy* **8**, 135–142.

170. Huang, J.H., Oefner, P.J., Adi, V., Ratnam, K., Ruoss, S.J., Trako, E., et al. (1998) Analyses of the NRAMP1 and IFN-gammaR1 genes in women with *Mycobacterium avium*-intracellulare pulmonary disease. *Am. J. Respir. Crit. Care Med.* **157**, 377–381.

171. Holland, S.M. (2001) Immune deficiency presenting as mycobacterial infection. *Clin. Rev. Allergy Immunol* **20**, 121–137.

11

Human Interleukin-12–Interferon-γ Axis in Protective Immunity to Mycobacteria

Claire Fieschi, Stéphanie Dupuis,
Capucine Picard, and Jean-Laurent Casanova

1. INTRODUCTION

The genus *Mycobacterium* comprises more than 85 species of Gram-positive acid-fast aerobic bacilli. *M. tuberculosis* is the agent of tuberculosis, which preferentially affects lungs and lymph nodes; *M. leprae* is responsible for leprosy, a disease of peripheral nerves and skin; and *M. ulcerans* is the agent of cutaneous Buruli ulcer. These three species are the most pathogenic of the known mycobacteria, but not all infected individuals develop clinical disease. The remaining mycobacterial species are environmental and poorly pathogenic in humans. However, environmental mycobacteria (EM) and Bacille Calmette–Guérin (BCG) vaccine substrains may be responsible for severe infections in patients with impaired immunity. Thus, even following infection with a virulent species, the appearance of clinical mycobacterial disease implies that host defenses have failed.

Studies of mouse models of mycobacterial infection have established that interleukin (IL)-12 and interferon (IFN)-γ are crucial for protective immunity. The depletion of these molecules in mice induced by IL-12-specific or IFN-γ-specific antibodies renders animals highly vulnerable to BCG, *M. avium*, and *M. tuberculosis (1)*. Studies in IL-12 (and IL-12-receptor) *(2,3)* and IFN-γ (and IFN-γ-receptor) *(4,5)* knockout (KO) mice support these findings. Although a number of other cytokines appear to be important for mouse defenses against mycobacteria, IL-12 and IFN-γ are the key cytokines, as IL-12 KO and IFN-γ KO mice die within 7 *(2)* and 3 *(4)* wk after intravenous *M. tuberculosis* inoculation, respectively.

There is a body of evidence that IL-12 and IFN-γ play an important role in mycobacterial immunity in humans. Here, we begin by considering the immunological basis of IL-12 and IFN-γ production and regulation in healthy individuals. We then review studies that have assessed the secretion of and cellular responses to IL-12 and IFN-γ in vivo or ex vivo during mycobacterial infections, mostly tuberculosis. Finally, we review inherited disorders of the IL-12–IFN-γ axis, which lead to severe EM, BCG, and, occasionally *M. tuberculosis* diseases. Overall, these data demonstrate the central role of the human IL-12–IFN-γ axis in protective immunity against mycobacterial species of high and low virulence.

2. THE IL-12 IFN-γ AXIS IN HUMANS

2.1 The Interleukin-12 Pathway

Interleukin-12 is a disulfide-linked glycosylated heterodimer, IL-12p70. It consists of two sub-units, IL-12 p35 and IL-12 p40, encoded by the *IL12A* and *IL12B* genes, located on 3p12 and 5q31, respectively *(6)*. Interleukin-12 is secreted by activated antigen-presenting cells (dendritic cells and

From: *Cytokines and Chemokines in Infectious Diseases Handbook*
Edited by: M. Kotb and T. Calandra © Humana Press Inc., Totowa, NJ

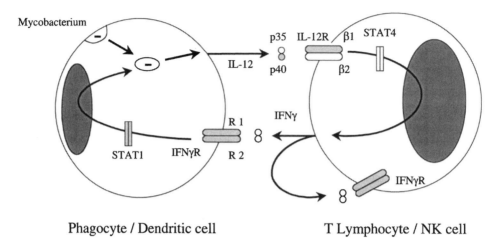

Fig. 1. Cells involved in IFN-γ-mediated immunity. IL-12 is principally secreted by phagocytes and dendritic cells and binds to a heterodimeric receptor consisting of β1- and β2-chains, which is specifically expressed on NK and T-lymphocytes. IFN-γ is secreted by NK and T-lymphocytes and binds to a ubiquitous receptor made of two chains: a ligand-binding (IFN-γR1) and a signaling-associated chain (IFN-γR2). STAT-1 is phosphorylated in response to IFN-γ and is translocated to the nucleus as a homodimer (*see* Fig. 3). Genetic etiologies of Mendelian susceptibility to mycobacterial infection: five molecules (in gray) have been found to be mutated in certain patients with severe mycobacterial infection.

monocytes macrophages) and polymorphonuclear cells (*see* Fig. 1). The secretion of IL-12 p70 is highly regulated, particularly at the transcriptional level; p35 is ubiquitously produced, whereas p40 is inducible. IL-12 p70 production is induced by various microbial stimuli, including mycobacteria. Other stimuli include CD154 (CD40 ligand) and IL-12 itself.

The cell surface, high-affinity IL-12 receptor consists of two noncovalently linked type I transmembrane proteins subunits, IL-12Rβ1 and IL-12Rβ2. The *IL12RB1* gene is located on 19p13, whereas the *IL12RB2* gene is located on 1p31. IL-12Rβ1 is detected on the surface of T-cells and NK cells and activated B-cells and dendritic cells. IL-12Rβ2 production and expression is limited to activated T-cells and NK cells, which respond to IL-12 by secreting IFN-γ. IL-4, IL-10 and transforming growth factor (TGF)-β downregulate β2 expression, whereas IL-18 and IFN-γ help to maintain levels of the high-affinity receptor on the surface of activated cells.

The binding of IL-12 to its receptor leads to activation of the two receptor-associated tyrosine kinases, JAK2 and TYK2. TYK2 is associated with IL-12Rβ1, and JAK2 is associated with IL-12Rβ2. These two members of the Janus kinase (JAK) family phosphorylate tyrosine residues in the cytoplasmic domain of IL-12Rβ2. Various members of the STAT family may be activated by the IL-12 receptor, but STAT-4 dimers probably account for the vast majority of IFN-γ production, based on the phenotype of mice in which the *STAT4* gene has been disrupted. Activated STAT-4 dimers are translocated to the nucleus, where they bind to specific DNA sequences, thereby regulating the transcription of IL-12-inducible genes such as those encoding IFN-γ, the IL-18 receptor, IL-12Rβ2, and IL-12 itself (*see* Fig. 2).

2.2. The Interferon-γ Pathway

The gene encoding IFN-γ (*IFNG*) is located on 12q15. Biologically active IFN-γ is a noncovalently linked, homodimeric, glycosylated protein *(7)*. IFN-γ is produced principally by NK cells and T-cells. Mononuclear phagocytes and dendritic cells also seem to produce IFN-γ, but in smaller amounts. IFN-γ production is induced not only by IL-12 *(7)* but also by other cytokines such as IL-1β *(8)*, IL-18 *(9)*, IL-23 *(10)*, and tumor necrosis factor (TNF)-α *(7)*.

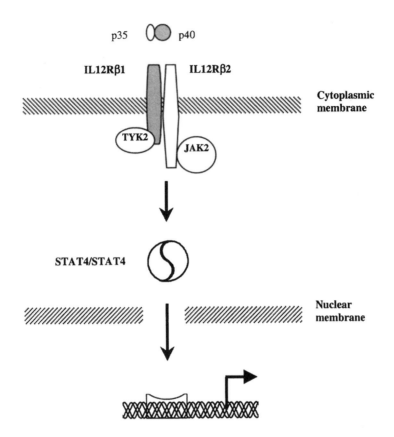

Fig. 2. IL-12 signaling pathway. Binding of IL-12 to the IL-12 receptor induces phosphorylation of TYK2 and JAK-2, thus activating the signal transducing protein STAT-4. This protein dislocates from the receptor and translocates as homodimer to the nucleus, where it acts as a transcriptional activator, binding to specific DNA response elements in the promoter region of IL-12-inducible genes. Two molecules (in gray) in the signaling pathway have been found to be mutated in patients with severe mycobacterial infection.

The high-affinity IFN-γ receptor is tetrameric and consists of two R1 (ligand-binding) and two R2 (signal transduction) chains. The *IFNGR1* gene is located on 6q23, and the *IFNGR2* gene is located on 21q22. Both subunits are type I glycoproteins containing a cellular domain with tyrosines. Homodimeric IFN-γ dimerizes two IFN-γR1 molecules, and recruits two molecules of IFN-γR2. IFN-γR1 expression is constitutive and ubiquitous. The regulation and trafficking of IFN-γR2 are less well understood, and although IFN-γR2 expression is also ubiquitous, it may be downregulated or upregulated in various cell types. The intracellular domains of IFN-γR1 and IFN-γR2 have no intrinsic kinase activity, but IFN-γR1 and IFN-γR2 are constitutively associated with JAK-1 and JAK-2. IFN-γ binding induces the formation of a tetramer (two R1 chains and two R2 chains), JAK-1 and JAK-2 transactivate themselves and one another and phosphorylate tyrosine residues in IFN-γR1. This creates a docking site for STAT-1, and JAKs phosphorylate the tyrosine residues of docked STAT-1. The phosphorylated STAT-1 molecules then dissociate from the receptor and form homodimeric complexes. These complexes are then rapidly translocated to the nucleus, where they bind to specific DNA sequences, known as gamma-activating sequence (GAS) elements, in the promoters of IFN-γ-inducible genes (*see* Fig. 3). The genes activated fall into two classes: IFN-γ-induced immediate-early genes, such as interferon regulatory factor 1 (IRF-1), and IFN-γ-regulated intermediate genes, such as human leukocyte antigens (HLAs).

2.3. The IL-12-IFN-γ Axis

Although the molecular mechanisms that govern the production of and response to IL-12 and IFN-γ have been unraveled in recent years, little is known about the basis of the IL-12–IFN-γ axis in cells and tissues in vivo. It is clear that the two major cytokines of the axis amplify each other, as IL-12 induces IFN-γ secretion by T-cells and NK cells, and IFN-γ induces IL-12 production by antigen-presenting cells (*see* Fig. 1). However, the respective roles of the various cell subsets involved in the production of and response to IL-12 and IFN-γ are unclear. In tissues, it is probably within granulomas that activated macrophages secrete IL-12 and other proinflammatory cytokines and differentiate into epithelioid and giant cells. The surrounding lymphocytes are recruited by the secreted cytokines and chemokines and activated, resulting in their differentiation into IFN-γ-producing T-cells.

3. IL-12 AND IFN-γ IN PATIENTS WITH MYCOBACTERIAL INFECTIONS

As a first approach to exploring the role of the human IL-12–IFN-γ axis in immunity to mycobacteria, several investigators have assessed levels of cytokines and their receptors in vivo. They have also measured in vitro the production of, and response to, cytokines by stimulating mononuclear blood cells from infected patients.

3.1. In Situ *Detection of Cytokines and Receptors in Mycobacterial Diseases*

Fenhalls et al. *(11)* used *in situ* hybridization with a specific mRNA probe to investigate the presence of IFN-γ in tuberculous granulomas from the lungs of patients undergoing lobectomy for severe tuberculous hemoptysis. Histopathological studies showed granulomatous lesions in all patients and the persistence of acid-fast bacilli despite 2 mo of antimycobacterial treatment. Two of the five patients studied tested positive for IFN-γ and negative for IL-4 by *in situ* hybridization. The three remaining patients produced both IFN-γ and IL-4. The cytokine profiles of these patients are therefore heterogeneous: IFN-γ is detected in all granulomas, but some contain IL-4, whereas others do not. Zhang et al. *(12)* used reverse transcription–polymerase chain reaction (RT-PCR) to compare levels of IFN-γ and IL-12Rβ2 mRNA in lymph nodes from tuberculous patients with those from patients with benign follicular hyperplasia. IFN-γ and IL-12Rβ2 mRNA levels were markedly higher in tuberculous lymph nodes than in lymph nodes from patients with benign follicular hyperplasia. Patients with lepromatous leprosy have weak cell-mediated immunity, with immature granulomas and a progressive form of disseminated disease, whereas patients with tuberculoid leprosy have strong cell-mediated immunity with mature granulomas and are able to restrict and to eliminate *M. leprae*. Kim et al. *(13)* studied IL-12-receptor production in these two polar forms of leprosy. IL-12R production in cutaneous leprosy lesions correlates with the type of cell-mediated immunity: IL-12Rβ2 mRNA is absent from lepromatous lesions, but present in tuberculoid lesions. IL-12Rβ1 mRNA levels are similar in lepromatous and tuberculoid lesions. Finally, these studies *in situ* suggest that the cytokines and receptors comprising the IL-12–IFN-γ axis are detectable at the site of mycobacterial disease.

3.2. IL-12-IFN-γ *Axis Exploration in Broncho-alveolar lavage*

Cytokine levels should be evaluated in broncho-alveolar lavage (BAL) because the cytokine-producing cells are directly in contact with tuberculous lesions. Taha et al. *(14)* measured IL-12R levels in the BAL of patients with active tuberculosis and compared them with those in healthy controls: they found that there were significantly more cells containing IL-12Rβ1 mRNA and IL-12Rβ2 mRNA in tuberculous patients than in healthy controls. *In situ* hybridization and immunohistochemistry studies carried out in parallel showed that the majority of IL-12Rβ1- and IL-12β2-positive cells were also CD8 positive. Taha et al. *(15)* also compared the levels of IL-12 and IFN-γ mRNA in BAL from patients with active tuberculosis with those in BAL from patients with inactive tuberculosis. They showed, by *in situ* hybridization, that a significantly higher proportion of BAL cells contained IL-12

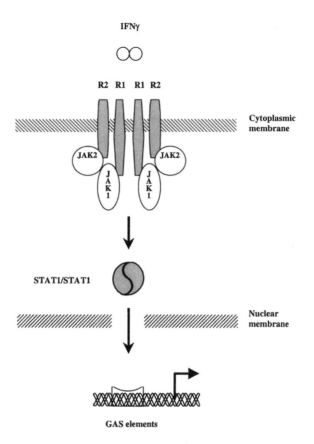

Fig. 3. Genetic defects in the IFN-γ-signaling pathway. IFN-γ is a homodimer that binds to and dimerizes IFN-γR1 molecules. Upon dimerization, IFN-γR2 molecules are recruited to form a tetramer that brings together IFN-γR1- and IFN-γR2-associated JAK-1 and JAK-2 kinases, respectively. Phosphorylation of IFN-γR1 allows the docking of STAT-1, a latent cytosolic monomer. The two STAT-1 molecules recruited and subsequently phosphorylated are released into the cytosol, where they dimerize and are translocated to the nucleus. Three molecules (in gray) in the signaling pathway have been found to be mutated in patients with severe mycobacterial infection.

and IFN-γ mRNA in patients with active tuberculosis than in patients with inactive tuberculosis patients (8% IFN-γ mRNA-positive cells versus 4%). These results were consistent with those previously published by Robinson et al. *(16)*. Somoskovi et al. *(17)* compared IFN-γ levels in the BAL of patients with various clinical forms of pulmonary tuberculosis (mild, moderate, severe) and in healthy controls; they found that IFN-γ levels were significantly higher in patients with tuberculosis. Thus, levels of the cytokines and receptors involved in the IL-12–IFN-γ axis appear to be significantly higher in the BAL of tuberculosis than in that of control subjects.

3.3. Cytokine Levels in Pleural Fluid

Tuberculous pleurisy is generally thought to result from the rupture of small foci of pneumonitis into the pleural space. The cells responsible for the immune response to mycobacterial infection are released *de facto* into the pleural space, and many authors have quantified the levels of cytokines in the pleural fluid in patients with tuberculosis. Cytokine levels in the pleural effusion are thought to reflect the production of lymphocytes and other immune cells released by pulmonary tissue. IFN-γ levels in pleural effusion were first reported to be high in patients with tuberculosis in 1988 *(18)*. These findings have since been confirmed by other studies *(19–23)*. Chen et al. *(22)* showed that

IFN-γ levels were significantly higher in the pleural effusion of patients with tuberculosis (mean 664 pg/mL) than in the pleural effusions patients with noninfectious diseases, such as malignant effusion (mean: 0.7 pg/mL). Zhang et al. *(24)* determined IL-12 levels in the pleural effusion of patients with tuberculosis and patients with malignant pleural effusion. They used an enzyme-linked immunosorbent assay (ELISA) that detected both IL-12p40 and IL-12p70. The mean concentration of IL-12 was 585 ± 89 pg/mL in patients with tuberculous pleurisy and significantly higher than in patients with malignant pleural effusion (123 ± 35 pg/mL). Mean IL-12p70 levels were 165 ± 28 pg/mL in patients with tuberculous pleurisy, whereas this molecule was undetectable in patients with malignant pleural effusions. Vankayalapati et al. determined IL-18 and IFN-γ levels in the pleural effusions of patients with tuberculous and nontuberculous effusion (malignant, trauma, or bacterial) *(25)*. Pleural IL-18 levels were significantly higher in patients with tuberculosis (278 ± 53 pg/mL) than in patients with pleural effusions of nontuberculous origin (106 ± 17 pg/mL), and IFN-γ levels in pleural effusion displayed parallel progressions (1573 ± 414 vs 59 ± 40 pg/mL). Thus, as in *in situ* studies and in BAL, levels of IL-12 and IFN-γ are high in the pleurisy of patients with tuberculous.

3.4. Cytokine Levels in Serum

As tuberculosis is a systemic infection, several investigators have measured cytokine levels in the serum. Verbon et al. *(26)* found IFN-γ levels to be high (0–450 pg/mL: mean: 22 pg/mL) in the sera of 81 patients with tuberculosis before the initiation of antibiotic treatment. IFN-γ was undetectable in the sera of control subjects and other patients in remission after infection (after the completion of treatment). IFN-γ levels were significantly higher (mean 46 pg/mL) in patients with general symptoms than in those without such symptoms (mean 29 pg/mL), and this finding was confirmed by another study *(27)*. IFN-γ levels do not correlate with the location of the disease (pulmonary or extrapulmonary), and low levels of IFN-γ do not rule out a diagnosis of tuberculosis *(22,26,27)*. Chen et al. confirmed these findings *(22)* and showed that serum IFN-γ levels in patients with tuberculosis were significantly higher than those in patients with lung cancer. High levels of IFN-γ in the sera of patients with active tuberculosis probably result from intense and sustained IFN-γ production during tuberculosis.

Investigators have also determined serum levels of IL-12 and IL-18 in tuberculous patients, as both of these cytokines are involved in IFN-γ production during mycobacterial infection. Verbon et al. *(26)*, found no detectable IL-12p70 in the sera of patients and controls, and there was no significant difference in IL-12p40 levels between patients with active tuberculosis and controls. Yamada et al. *(27)* measured serum IL-18 concentration in patients with tuberculosis. Patients with tuberculosis have higher levels of IL-18 (424 ± 516 pg/mL) than do healthy matched controls (140 ± 89 pg/mL). High levels of cytokines in the sera of patients with active tuberculous disease probably account for the systemic immune response to the infection.

3.5. Cytokine Production by Cultured Cells During Mycobacterial Infection

The first studies of IFN-γ production by peripheral blood mononuclear cells (PBMC) in human tuberculosis date back to 1985 *(28)*. Zhang et al. *(29)* determined IFN-γ concentrations in the supernatants of heat-killed *M. tuberculosis*-stimulated PBMCs. IFN-γ levels were significantly lower in tuberculous patients than in healthy tuberculin reactors, and these lower levels were not associated with lower levels of IL-12. These abnormalities in IFN-γ levels in stimulated PBMCs were abolished following the completion of antibiotic treatment in most patients. Schwander et al. *(30)* confirmed these findings: they showed that PBMCs from tuberculous patients had a lower than normal proliferative response to both mycobacterial (purified protein derivative [PPD]) and nonmycobacterial antigens (candida, tetanus toxoid) and that IFN-γ levels in the supernatants of PPD-stimulated PBMCs from tuberculous patients were one-seventh those in healthy controls (median: 927 vs 6790 pg/mL, respectively). Other investigators have studied the cellular type of IFN-γ-producing cells; CD8 T-cells seem to be largely responsible for IFN-γ production *(31,32)*. Dlugovitzky et al. *(33)* confirmed the decrease in IFN-γ production by stimulated PBMCs and showed that the proliferative response of PBMCs was weaker in patients with severe disease (mean: 5358 vs 18075 cpm). This was also confirmed in children with tuberculosis *(34)*. However, Vankayalapati et al. *(35)* demonstrated that in *M. avium* infection with normal proliferative response, *M. avium*-activated PBMCs produced significantly less IFN-γ in patients than in positive skin test controls. Dlugovitzky et al. *(36)* also showed in a later study that IL-12 levels in the supernatants of *M. tuberculosis*-activated PBMCs were significantly higher for PBMCs from patients with severe disease than for PBMCs from control subjects or patients with moderate tuberculosis.

Zhang et al. *(12)* have shown that 20–30% of freshly isolated PBMCs from healthy tuberculin reactors are IL-12Rβ1+, whereas only 2–3% of PBMCs are IL-12Rβ1+ in patients with tuberculosis. IL-12Rβ1 production increased in parallel in both patients (mean $18 \pm 8\%$ of stimulated PBMCs) and healthy tuberculin reactors (mean: $46 \pm 6\%$) after *M. tuberculosis* stimulation. IL-12Rβ2 is not expressed at the surface of PBMCs from healthy tuberculin reactors or tuberculosis patients, but the production of this molecule is induced by *M. tuberculosis*. However, the percentage of cells acquiring IL-12Rβ2 expression is significantly lower in tuberculosis patients than in healthy tuberculin reactors ($10 \pm 3\%$ vs $37 \pm 3\%$). This expression of both the IL-12Rβ2 and IL-12Rβ1 chains, resulting in a functional IL-12R, is correlated with IFN-γ levels in the supernatant of cultured PBMCs from tuberculosis patients and healthy tuberculin reactors (433 ± 105 vs 3132 ± 260 pg/mL).

Kim et al. *(13)* studied the IL-12-mediated induction of IFN-γ production in T-cells from leprosy patients activated by *M. tuberculosis* or *M. leprae*. T-cells from patients with tuberculoid lesions produced similar levels of IFN-γ after activation by *M. tuberculosis* and after activation by *M. leprae*, whereas T-cells from patients with lepromatous lesions produced large amounts of IFN-γ after *M. tuberculosis* activation and very small amounts after *M. leprae* activation. The lack of response to *M. leprae* is confirmed by the absence of STAT-4 activation (DNA binding and phosphorylation) in IL-12-activated PBMCs from patients with lepromatous lesions, whereas PBMCs from patients with tuberculoid lesions respond to *M. leprae* stimulation. Similarly, the lack of response to *M. leprae* in lepromatous patients is confirmed by the absence of IL-12Rβ2 induction at the surface of activated PBMCs. Thus, T-cells from mycobacteria-infected patients seem to secrete very little IFN-γ in vitro upon mycobacterial stimulation. This is consistent with the hypothesis that IFN-γ-producing T-cells are preferentially recruited to the site of the disease. Alternatively, mycobacteria may themselves induce T-cell anergy in vivo.

4. GENETIC DEFECTS IN THE IL-12 AND IFN-γ PATHWAYS

The high levels of IL-12 and IFN-γ observed in the course of various mycobacterial diseases suggest that this axis is involved in antimycobacterial immunity. The observation of severe disease caused by Bacillus Calmette–Guerin (BCG), environmental mycobacteria, and *M. tuberculosis* in patients lacking IL-12- or IFN-γ-mediated immunity supports and extends this conclusion. Mendelian predisposition to mycobacterial disease is a heterogeneous syndrome, the limits of which are poorly defined. Otherwise healthy patients develop severe disease as a result of BCG and environmental mycobacteria in the absence of immunodeficiency. To date, various mutations have been found in five genes in patients with the syndrome (*see* Fig. 1) and these mutations define nine different diseases.

4.1 Interferon-γ Receptor Deficiency

4.1.1. Complete IFN-γR1 and IFN-γR2 Deficiency

Complete IFN-γR1 deficiency was the first genetic etiology to be identified *(37,38)*. Other patients have been described since these early reports *(39–42)*. Mutations in the *IFNGR1* gene are recessive and cause a loss of function. They preclude cell surface expression of the IFN-γR1-binding chain or the binding of IFN-γ to the surface-expressed mutated receptors *(43)*. Complete IFN-γ receptor signaling chain (IFN-γR2) deficiency has also been reported *(44)*. Clinical and histopathological phenotypes of complete IFN-γR2 deficiency are marked by disseminated environmental mycobacterial or BCG diseases and poorly limited multibacillary granulomas.

A lack of cellular responses to IFN-γ has been demonstrated in vitro in patients with complete IFN-γR deficiency, and the mutant alleles have been shown to cause an impaired cellular response to IFN-γ in experiments involving the complementation of defective cells with the wild-type *IFNGR1* or *IFNGR2* gene. IFN-γ levels are high in the sera of patients with such defects, because of a lack of binding of the cytokine to its receptor, in contrast to other deficiencies and unexplained mycobacterial diseases *(45)*.

4.1.2. Partial IFN-γR1 and IFN-γR2 Deficiency

Two siblings with partial, as opposed to complete, recessive IFN-γR1 deficiency have also been reported *(46)*. A homozygous recessive missense mutation causing an amino acid substitution in the extracellular domain of the ligand-binding chain was identified. This mutation probably only reduces the affinity of the encoded receptor for its ligand. A 20-yr-old patient was found to have partial, as opposed to complete, IFN-γR2 deficiency. A missense mutation was found in the extracellular domain of the encoded receptor *(47)*.

Twenty patients from unrelated kindreds were found to have a dominant form of partial IFN-γR1 deficiency *(48,49)*. These patients have a small heterozygous frame-shift deletion in *IFNGR1* exon 6, downstream from the segment encoding the transmembrane domain, resulting in the production of a truncated chain. The encoded receptors can reach the cell surface because the leader, extracellular, and transmembrane domains are conserved and IFN-γ binding is normal. Despite the normal dimerization of IFN-γR1 subunits and tetramerization with two IFN-γR2 subunits, IFN-γ signaling is impossible because of the lack of a cellular domain. The receptors also accumulate at the cell surface because of the lack of an intracellular recycling site. Position 818 of this *IFNGR1* mutation is the first small deletion hot spot to be identified in the human genome.

These defects predispose the individual to infection, not only with nontuberculous mycobacteria (environmental and BCG vaccines), but also with *M. tuberculosis*, as one of the siblings with partial IFN-γR1 deficiency, who was not vaccinated with BCG, developed symptomatic primary tuberculosis. The granulomas are well circumscribed and differentiated, paucibacillary, and tuberculoid. The clinical and histopathological phenotypes are milder than those of complete IFN-γR deficiency.

4.2. Partial STAT-1 Deficiency

Two patients in two unrelated kindreds have been found to have a heterozygous missense mutation in the *STAT1* gene *(50)*. The mutation is located in the tail segment of STAT-1. The resulting mutant STAT-1 molecule is nonfunctional because the tyrosine in position 701 cannot be phosphorylated. This prevents the cytosolic release of IFN-γR1-associated STAT-1 molecules, impairing STAT-1 dimerization and nuclear translocation. The severity of the clinical phenotype is similar to that of partial dominant IFN-γR1 deficiency, with curable mycobacterial disease and mature granulomas. The cell lines of patients with partial IFN-γR or STAT-1 deficiency display a weak cellular response to IFN-γ, as detected by STAT-1 phosphorylation. In each case, the mutant alleles have been shown to be responsible for this impaired cellular response to IFN-γ. Individuals with deficiencies in the IFN-γ pathway *(see* Fig. 3) may be classified into groups based on genotype and clinical and cellular phenotype, and the correlation between the various features suggests that IFN-γ-mediated cell activation is a genetically controlled quantitative trait that determines the outcome of mycobacterial infection in humans *(51)*.

4.3. Complete IL-12 p40 and IL-12Rβ1 Deficiency

A child with a recessive mutation in the gene-encoding IL-12 p40 (*IL12B*) has been reported *(52)*. The mutation consists of a homozygous frame-shift deletion of 4.4 kb encompassing two coding exons. Following stimulation of blood cells in vitro, much less IFN-γ was produced than was produced in the blood cells of a control subject. This impaired IFN-γ secretion was complemented in a dose-dependent manner with exogenous recombinant IL-12, implying that IFN-γ deficiency is not a primary event but a consequence of inherited IL-12 deficiency.

Mutations in the gene encoding the β1-subunit of the IL-12 receptor have been identified in other children *(53–57)*. All patients were homozygous for recessive mutations (nonsense, missense, and splice mutations). The families were from different countries and the mutations differed from each other. All of these mutations preclude the expression of IL-12Rβ1 at the surface of activated T-cells, and specific antibodies do not detect the affected subunit in flow cytometry. The clinical phenotype appears to be less severe than that of children with complete IFN-γR deficiency. Two siblings with the same mutation were recently reported to display different phenotypes: One child suffered BCGitis after BCG vaccination, whereas the other was resistant to BCG despite several inoculations, but developed peritoneal tuberculosis *(57)*. In patients with complete IL-12Rβ1 deficiency, IFN-γ secretion in vitro by otherwise functional NK cells and T-cells has been demonstrated to be impaired. In patients with IL-12Rβ1 or IL-12 p40 deficiency *(see* Fig. 2), impaired IFN-γ production is probably responsible for mycobacterial disease, and residual, IL-12-independent, IFN-γ-mediated immunity probably accounts for the milder clinical and histological phenotype.

5. CONCLUSION

Consistent with studies in the mouse model, several studies in humans have suggested that the IL-12–IFN-γ axis is essential for protective immunity against mycobacteria. Evidence consistent with this notion was provided by the observation of high levels of IL-12 and IFN-γ and their receptors in patients with mycobacterial disease, both at the site of the disease (granulomas, BAL, pleurisy) and in the bloodstream (serum levels). Conclusive evidence was provided by the observation of severe cases of BCG, environmental mycobacterial, and *M. tuberculosis* infection in patients with inherited deficiency of the IL-12–IFN-γ axis. The apparent rarity of other infections in patients with inherited impairment of IL-12–IFN-γ axis suggests that this axis plays a "specific" role in the immune response to mycobacteria.

It is unclear whether mycobacterial disease develops in apparently healthy individuals despite an intact IL-12–IFN-γ axis or because of undetectable variations in the IL-12–IFN-γ axis. If the IL-12–IFN-γ axis is intact, immunity mediated by other important cytokines or chemokines may be impaired. Alternatively, IL-12–IFN-γ-mediated immunity in the patients may be weaker than that in healthy resistant individuals. The development of mycobacterial disease probably results in part from several inherited host disorders, affecting various immunological pathways, including the IL-12–IFN-γ axis. Further genetic dissection of immunity to mycobacteria in patients with mycobacterial diseases should provide further insight into these issues *(58)*.

REFERENCES

1. Flynn, J.L. and Chan, J. (2001) Immunology of tuberculosis. *Annu. Rev. Immunol.* **19,** 93–122.
2. Cooper, A.M., Magram, J., Ferrante, J., and Orme, I.M. (1997) Interleukin-12 (IL-12) is crucial to the development of protective immunity in mice intravenously infected with Mycobacterium tuberculosis. *J. Exp. Med.* **186,** 39–45.
3. Wu, C., Ferrante, J., Gately, M.K., and Magram, J. (1997) Characterization of IL-12 receptor beta1 chain (IL-12Rbeta1)-deficient mice: IL-12Rbeta1 is an essential component of the functional mouse IL-12 receptor.*J. Immunol.* **159,**1658–1665.
4. Dalton, D.K., Pitts-Meek, S., Keshav, S., Figari, I.S., Bradley, A., and Stewart, T.A. (1993) Multiple defects of immune cell function in mice with disrupted interferon-gamma gene. *Science* **259,** 1739–1742.
5. Huang, S., Hendriks, W., Althage, A., Hemmi, S., Bluethmann, H., Kamijo, R., et al. (1993) Immune response in mice that lack the interferon-gamma receptor. *Science* **259,** 1742–1745.
6. Gately, M.K., Renzetti, L.M., Magram, J., Stern, A.S., Adorini, L., Gubler, U., et al. (1998) The interleukin-12/interleukin-12 receptor system: role in normal and pathologic immune response. *Annu. Rev. Immunol.* **16,** 495–521.
7. Boehm, U., Klamp, T., Groot, M., and Howard, J.C. (1997) Cellular response to interferon-γ. *Annu. Rev. Immunol.* **15,** 749–795.
8. Cooper, M.A., Fehniger, T.A., Ponnappan, A., Mehta, V., Wewers, M.D., and Caliguri, M.A. (2001) Interleukin-1β costimulates interferon-γ production by human natural killer cells. *Eur. J. Immunol.* **31,** 792–801.
9. Okamura, H., Tsutsi, H., Komatsu, T., Yutsudo, M., Hakura, A., Tanimoto, T., et al. (1995) Cloning of a new cytokine that induces IFN-γ production by T cells. *Nature* **378,** 88–91.

10. Oppmann, B., Lesley, R., Blom, B., Timans, J.C., Xu, Y., Hunte, B., et al. (2000) Novel p19 protein engages IL-12p40 to form a cytokine, IL-23, with biological activities similar as well as distinct from IL-12. *Immunity* **13**, 715–725.
11. Fenhalls, G., Wong, A., Bezuidenhout, J., Van Helden, P., Bardin, P., and Lukey, P.T. (2000) In situ production of gamma interferon, interleukin-4, and tumor necrosis factor alpha mRNA in human lung tuberculous granulomas. *Infect. Immun.* **68**, 2827–2836.
12. Zhang, M., Gong, J., Presky, D.H., Xue, W., and Barnes, P.F. (1999) Expression of the IL-12 receptor β1 and β2 subunits in human tuberculosis. *J. Immunol.* **162**, 2441–2447.
13. Kim, J., Uyemura, K., Van Dyke, M.K., Legaspi, A.J., Rea, T.H., Shuai, K., et al. (2001) A role for IL-12 receptor expression and signal transduction in host defense in leprosy. *J. Immunol.* **167**, 779–786.
14. Taha, R.A., Minshall, E.M., Olivenstein, R., Ikahu, D., Wallaert, B., Tsicopoulos, A., et al. (1999) Increased expression of IL-12 receptor mRNA in active pulmonary tuberculosis and sarcoidosis. *Am. J. Respir. Crit. Care Med.* **160**, 1119–1123.
15. Taha, R.A., Kotsimbos, T.C., Song, Y.L., Menzies, D., and Hamid, Q. (1997) IFN-γ and IL-12 are increased in active compared with inactive tuberculosis. *Am. J. Respir. Crit. Care Med.* **155**, 1135–1139.
16. Robinson, D.S., Ying, S., Taylor, I.K., Wangoo, A., Mitchell, D.M., Kay, A.B., et al. (1994) Evidence for a Th1-like bronchoalveolar T-cell subset and predominance of interferon-gamma gene activation in pulmonary tuberculosis. *Am. J. Respir. Crit. Care Med.* **149**, 989–993.
17. Somoskovi, A., Zissel, G., Zipfel, P.F., Ziegenhagen, M.W., Klaucke, J., Haas, H., et al. (1999) Different cytokine patterns correlate with the extension of disease in pulmonary tuberculosis. *Eur. Cytokine Network* **10**, 135–142.
18. Ribera, E., Ocana, I., Martinez-Vazquez, J.M., Rossell, M., Espanol, T., and Ruibal, A. (1988) High level of interferon gamma in tuberculous pleural effusion. *Chest* **93**, 308–311.
19. Wongtim, S., Silachamroon, U., Ruxrungtham, K., Udompanich, V., Limthongkul, S., Charoenlap, P., et al. (1999) Interferon gamma for diagnosing tuberculous pleural effusions. *Thorax* **54**, 921–924.
20. Yamada, Y., Nakamura, A., Hosoda, M., Kato, T., Asano, T., Tonegawa, K., et al. (2001) Cytokines in pleural liquid for diagnosis of tuberculous pleurisy. *Respir. Med.* **95**, 577–581.
21. Villegas, M.V., Labrada, L.A., and Saravia, N.G. (2000) Evaluation of polymerase chain reaction, adenosine deaminase, and interferon-gamma in pleural fluid for the differential diagnosis of pleural tuberculosis. *Chest* **118**, 1355–1364.
22. Chen, Y.-M., Yang, W.-K., Whang-Peng, J., Tsai, C.-M., and Perng, R-P. (2001) An analysis of cytokine status in the serum and effusions of patients with tuberculous and lung cancer. *Lung Cancer* **31**, 25–30.
23. Hirsch, C.S., Toossi, Z., Johnson, J.L., Luzze, H., Ntambi, L., Peters, P., et al. (2001) Augmentation of apoptosis and interferon-gamma production at sites of active *Mycobacterium tuberculosis* infection in human tuberculosis. *J. Infect. Dis.* **183**, 779–788.
24. Zhang, M., Gately, M.K., Wang, E., Gong, J., Wolf, S.F., Lu, S., et al. (1994) Interleukin-12 at the site of disease in tuberculosis. *J. Clin. Invest.* **93**, 1733–1739.
25. Vankayalapati, R., Wisel, B., Weis, S.E., Samten, B., Girard, W.M., and Barnes, P.F. (2000) Production of interleukin-18 in human tuberculosis. *J. Infect. Dis.* **182**, 234–239.
26. Verbon, A., Juffermans. N., Van Deventer, S.J.H., Speelman, P., Van Deutekom, H., and Van der Poll, T. (1999) Serum concentrations of cytokines in patients with active tuberculosis and after treatment. *Clin. Exp. Immunol.* **115**, 110–113.
27. Yamada, G., Shijubo, N., Shigehara, K., Okamura, H., Kurimoto, M., and Abe, S. (2000) Increased levels of circulating interleukin-18 in patients with advanced tuberculosis. *Am. J. Respir. Crit. Care Med.* **161**, 1786–1789.
28. Onwubalili, J.K., Scott, G.M., and Robinson, J.A. (1985) Deficient immune interferon production in tuberculosis. *Clin. Exp. Immunol.* **59**, 405–413.
29. Zhang, M., Lin, Y., Iyer, D.V., Gong, J., Abrams, J.S., and Barnes, P.F. (1995) T-cell cytokine responses in human infection with *Mycobacterium tuberculosis*. *Infect. Immun.* **63**, 3231–3234.
30. Schwander, S.K., Torres, M., Sada, E., Carranza, C., Ramos, E., Tary-Lehmann, M., et al. (1998) Enhanced responses to *Mycobacterium tuberculosis* antigens by human alveolar lymphocytes during active pulmonary tuberculosis. *J. Infect. Dis.* **178**, 1434–1445.
31. Shams, H., Wizel, B., Weis, S.E., Samten, B., and Barnes, P.F. (2001) Contribution of CD8(+) T cells to gamma interferon production in human tuberculosis. *Infect. Immun.* **69**, 3497–3501.
32. Cho, S., Mehra, V., Thoma-Uszynski, S., Stenger, S., Serbina, N., Mazzaccaro, R.J., et al. (2000) Antimicrobial activity of MHC class I-restricted CD8+ T cells in human tuberculosis. *Proc. Natl. Acad. Sci. USA* **97**, 12210–12215.
33. Dlugovitzky, D., Bay, M.L., Rateni, L., Urizar, L., Rondelli, C.F., Largacha, C., et al. (1999) In vitro synthesis of interferon-gamma, interleukin-4, transforming growth factor-beta and interleukin-1 beta by peripheral blood mononuclear cells from tuberculosis patients: relationship with the severity of pulmonary involvement. *Scand. J. Immunol.* **49**, 210–217.
34. Swaminathan, S., Gong, J., Zhang, M., Samten, B., Hanna, L.E., Narayanan, P.R., et al. (1999) Cytokine production in children with tuberculous infection and disease. *Clin. Infect. Dis.* **28**, 1290–1293.
35. Vankayalapati, R., Wisel, B., Samten, B., Griffith, D.E., Shams, H., Galland, M.R., et al. (2001) Cytokine profiles in immunocompetent persons infected with *Mycobacterium avium* complex. *J. Infect. Dis.* **183**, 478–484.
36. Dlugovitzky, D., Bay, M.L., Rateni, L., Fiorenza, G., Vietti, L., et al. (2000) Influence of disease severity on nitrite and cytokine production by peripheral blood mononuclear cells (PBMC) from patients with pulmonary tuberculosis (TB). *Clin. Exp. Immunol.* **122**, 343–349.
37. Newport, M.J., Huxley, C.M., Huston, S., Hawrylowicz, C.M., Oostra, B.A., Williamson, R., et al. (1996) A mutation in the interferon-gamma-receptor gene and susceptibility to mycobacterial infection. *N. Engl. J. Med.* **335**, 1941–1949.
38. Jouanguy, E., Altare, F., Lamhamedi, S., Revy, P., Emile, J.F., Newport, M., et al. (1996) Interferon-gamma-receptor deficiency in an infant with fatal bacille Calmette–Guérin infection. *N. Engl. J. Med.* **335**, 1956–1961.

39. Pierre-Audigier, C., Jouanguy, E., Lamhamedi, S., Altare, F., Rauzier, J., Vincent, V., et al. (1997) Fatal disseminated Mycobacterium smegmatis infection in a child with inherited interferon gamma receptor deficiency. *Clin. Infect. Dis.* **24**, 982–984.

40. Roesler, J., Kofink, B., Wendisch, J., Heyden, S., Paul, D., Friedrich, W., et al.(1999) Listeria monocytogenes and recurrent mycobacterial infections in a child with complete interferon-gamma-receptor (IFNgammaR1) deficiency: mutational analysis and evaluation of therapeutic options. *Exp. Hematol.* **27**, 1368–1374.

41. Cunningham, J.A., Kellner, J.D., Bridge, P.J., Trevenen, C.L., Mcleod, D.R., and Davies, H.D. (2000) Disseminated bacille Calmette-Guerin infection in an infant with a novel deletion in the interferon-gamma receptor gene. *Int. J. Tuberc. Lung Dis.* **4**, 791–794.

42. Allende, L.M., Lopez-Goyanes, A., Paz-Artal, E., Corell, A., Garcia-Perez, M.A., Varela, P., et al. (2001) A point mutation in a domain of gamma interferon receptor 1 provokes severe immunodeficiency. *Clin. Diagn. Lab Immunol.* **8**, 133–137.

43. Jouanguy, E., Dupuis, S., Pallier, A., Döffinger, R., Fondanèche, M-C., Fieschi, C., et al. (2000) In a novel form of complete IFNγR1 deficiency, cell-surface receptors fail to bind IFNγ. *J. Clin. Invest.* **105**, 1429–1436.

44. Dorman, S.E. and Holland, S.M. (1998) Mutation in the signal-transducing chain of the interferon-gamma receptor and susceptibility to mycobacterial infection. *J. Clin. Invest.* **101**, 2364–2369.

45. Fieschi, C., Dupuis, S., Picard, C., Smith, C.I., Holland, S.M., and Casanova, J.L. (2001) High levels of interferon gamma in the plasma of children with complete interferon gamma receptor deficiency. *Pediatrics* **107**, E48.

46. Jouanguy, E., Lamhamedi-Cherradi, S., Altare, F., Fondanèche, M-C., Tuerlinckx, D., Blanche, S., et al. (1997) Partial interferon-gamma receptor 1 deficiency in a child with tuberculoid bacillus Calmette–Guérin infection and a sibling with clinical tuberculosis. *J. Clin. Invest.* **100**, 2658–2664.

47. Döffinger, R., Jouanguy, E., Dupuis, S., Fondanèche, M.C., Stephan, J.L., et al. (2000) Partial interferon-(receptor signaling chain deficiency in a patient with Bacille Calmette–Guérin and *Mycobacterium abscessus* infection. *J. Infect. Dis.* **181**, 379–384.

48. Jouanguy, E., Lamhamedi-Cherradi, S., Lammas, D., Dorman, S.E., Fondanèche, M-C., Dupuis, S., et al. (1999) A human IFNGR1 small deletion hotspot associated with dominant susceptibility to mycobacterial infection. *Nat. Genet.* **21**, 370–378.

49. Villella, A., Picard, C., Jouanguy, E., Dupuis, S., Popko, S., Abughali, N., et al. (2001) Recurrent *Mycobacterium avium* osteomyelitis associated with a novel dominant interferon gamma receptor mutation. *Pediatrics* **107**, E47.

50. Dupuis, S., Dargemont, C., Fieschi, C., Thomassin, N., Rosenzweig, S., Harris, J., et al. (2001). Impairment of mycobacterial but not viral immunity by a germline human STAT1 mutation. *Science* **293**, 300–303.

51. Dupuis, S., Döffinger, R., Picard, C., Fieschi, C., Altare, F., Jouanguy, E., et al. (2000). Human interferon-γ-mediated immunity is a genetically controlled continuous trait that determines the outcome of mycobacterial invasion. *Immunol. Rev.* **178**, 129–137.

52. Altare, F., Lammas, D., Revy, P., Jouanguy, E., Döffinger, R., Lamhamedi, S., et al. (1998). Inherited interleukin 12 deficiency in a child with bacille Calmette-Guérin and Salmonella enteritidis disseminated infection. *J. Clin. Invest.* **102**, 2035–2040.

53. Altare, F., Durandy, A., Lammas, D., Emile, J-F., Lamhamedi, S., Le Deist, F., et al. (1998). Impairment of mycobacterial immunity in human interleukin-12 receptor deficiency. *Science* **280**, 1432–1435.

54. De Jong, R., Altare, F., Haagen, I.A., Elferink, D.G., De Boer, T., Van Breda Vriesman, P.J.C., et al. (1998) Severe mycobacterial and salmonella infections in interleukin-12-receptor-deficient patients. *Science* **280**, 1435–1438.

55. Aksu, G., Tirpan, C., Cavusoglu, C., Soydan, S., Altare, F., Casanova, J.L., et al. (2001) *Mycobacterium fortuitum-chelonae* complex infection in a child with complete interleukin-12 receptor beta 1 deficiency. *Pediatr. Infect. Dis. J.* **20**, 551–553.

56. Sakai, T., Matsuoka, M., Aoki, M., Nosaka, K., and Mitsuya, H. (2001) Missense mutation of the interleukin-12 receptor beta1 chain-encoding gene is associated with impaired immunity against *Mycobacterium avium* complex infection. *Blood* **97**, 2688–2694.

57. Altare, F., Ensser, A., Breiman, A., Reichenbach, J., Baghdadi, J.E., Fischer, A., et al. (2001) Interleukin-12 receptor beta1 deficiency in a patient with abdominal tuberculosis. *J. Infect. Dis.* **184**, 231–236.

58. Casanova, J.L. and Abel, L. (2002). Genetic dissection of immunity to mycobacteria: the human model. *Annu. Rev Immunol.* **20**, 581–620.

12

Role of Th1 Cytokines in Host Defenses Against *Mycobacterium leprae*

Elizabeth Pereira Sampaio, Milton Ozorio Moraes, M. Cristina Vidal Pessolani, and Euzenir Nunes Sarno

1. LEPROSY: CLINICAL FEATURES

Leprosy, a chronic inflammatory disease caused by *Mycobacterium leprae*, an obligate intracellular pathogen, has existed throughout recorded history. Isolation of patients was the norm until the time of discovery of the first effective chemotherapeutic drug, dapsone (4,4'-diaminodiphenylsulfone) in treating the patients.

Leprosy provides an ideal model to address the role of T-cell subsets in human disease in that it presents a spectrum of clinical forms that primarily depend on the host's immune response (*see* Fig. 1). At one end of the spectrum lie tuberculoid patients (TT forms) with single skin lesions, a low number of bacteria, the presence of both in vivo (lepromin skin test) and in vitro cell-mediated immune (CMI) responses, and low specific antibody levels. Lepromatous patients (LL), on the other hand, demonstrate a high bacterial load, numerous lesions, high levels of antibodies, together with negative lepromin skin test and absence of specific immune response. Within these two extremes, a continuous clinical and histopathological spectrum termed "borderline leprosy" (BT, borderline tuberculoid; BB, borderline borderline; BL, borderline lepromatous) is most often seen (*see* Fig. 1). In recent years, the disease has been defined more simply as either paucibacillary (PB) or multibacillary (MB) to qualify the patient for a particular drug-treatment regimen according to the detection of bacteria in the slit smears or to the number of skin lesions. It is multibacillary leprosy that is believed to be the most highly infectious form because of the large number of bacilli found in its secretions *(1)*.

Histopathological aspects of leprosy lesions have been found to be characteristic of patients representing each group. Tuberculoid lesions reveal the presence of inflammatory infiltrates with a predominance of CD4+ T-cells, well-formed granulomas at the site of the lesion, differentiated macrophages, and a thickened epidermis as opposed to the lepromatous form, distinguished by the presence of the Unna layer, the preponderance of CD8+ T-cells, the absence of granuloma formation, and a flattened epidermis *(1)*. There is increasing evidence that, along with the dermis, the epidermis is a seat of intense immunological reactivity *in situ*. In addition to an increase in epidermal thickness at the tuberculoid pole (BT, TT), there can be seen an expression of human leukocyte antigen-DR (HLA-DR) via keratinocytes, an increase in the number of Langerhans' cells, and the presence of T-cells in the epidermal cell layer *(2–4)* in addition to an enhanced expression of the adhesion molecules (ICAM-1 and LFA-1) and the interferon (IFN)-γ-inducible protein (IP-10) in the epidermis *(5)*. None of these parameters are detected in the lepromatous forms (BL, LL).

In addition to its characteristic skin lesions, leprosy can also be looked upon as a neurological disease. Leprosy polyneuropathy is the most commonly treatable neuropathy in the world. It is esti-

From: *Cytokines and Chemokines in Infectious Diseases Handbook*
Edited by: M. Kotb and T. Calandra © Humana Press Inc., Totowa, NJ

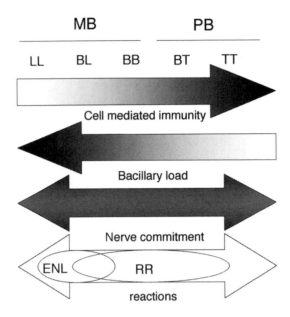

Fig. 1. Schematic representation of the clinical forms of leprosy according to the Ridley and Jopling classi-fication. The presence of CMI response to *M. leprae* dictates the clinical outcome of the disease. Multibacillary (MB) patients show low/absent in vitro and in vivo immune response to the bacteria, high bacillary load, and numerous skin lesions, whereas paucibacillary (PB) patients show absence of bacteria, few lesions, and the presence of CMI. Nerve commitment is observed in all clinical forms. During the natural course of leprosy, patients may develop reactions that are inflammatory episodes that interrupt disease chronic stability. Reac-tions are divided in type I, or reversal reaction (RR), and type II, or erythema nodosum leprosum (ENL). RR occurs in BT, BB, and BL patients, whereas ENL is observed in BL and LL forms.

mated that one-third of all diagnosed patients present nerve disabilities that are progressive and irre-versible, even after completion of multidrug therapy (MDT). Blindness, deformities, and disfigure-ment can occur across the entire spectrum of the disease, not even sparing those with localized skin lesions (*see* Fig. 1). This is the main reason why leprosy continues to represent a major social stigma. Although MDT is an unquestionably potent instrument for leprosy control, it has, by no means, exercised any significant impact on the development of disabilities. It has been suggested that sub-clinical neural damage may actually take place in virtually all patients and that some 30% of the nerve fibers may have already been destroyed before any sensory impairment becomes detectable (*6*). New insights into the mechanism(s) involved in nerve invasion by *M. leprae* and the subsequent inflammatory-mediated nerve injury will be of the utmost importance in designing new effective measures to prevent future nerve damage from occurring in leprosy at all.

2. EPIDEMIOLOGY

In 1982, WHO's study group on chemotherapy for leprosy recommended that the MDT treatment regimen be administered to individuals infected with leprosy. MDT involves the use of rifampicin (600 mg once per month), clofazimine (300 mg once per month, and 50 mg per day), and dapsone (100 mg per day) to be carried out for 12–24 mo in individuals with MB leprosy and for 6 mo (rifampi-cin and dapsone) in those with PB leprosy. The absolute goal of the WHO-supported MDT program was to reduce the leprosy prevalence rate to less than 1/10,000 worldwide. To this end, in 1997, WHO recommended an additional chemotherapeutic drug regimen which included the administra-tion of a single dose of antibiotics (600 mg rifampicin, 400 mg ofloxacin, and 100 mg minocycline [ROM]) to PB patients with a single lesion.

Since the adoption of MDT in 1982, there has been a very significant 85% reduction in the global prevalence of leprosy. However, WHO's original goal to eliminate leprosy as a global public health care problem by the year 2000 (prevalence below 1 per 10,000) has had to be postponed to the year 2005. In 1999, the number of registered cases was 795,000, with a global prevalence of 1.4 per 10,000 individuals. There still remains about 20 countries in which the prevalence rate far exceeds this figure, namely India, which accounts for nearly 80% of all registered cases worldwide, in addition to Brazil, Indonesia, and Bangladesh, which are also burdened with disproportionately high numbers of leprosy patients. Thus, it is of critical importance to maximize the effectiveness of identifying new cases in these high-prevalence countries and enrolling these individuals in MDT programs in a timely manner.

3. INFECTION AND TRANSMISSION

With regard to leprosy infection *per se*, it is generally acknowledged that a much greater number of individuals is infected with *M. leprae* at any given time than will ever develop the disease. Thus, it could be assumed that the majority probably undergo self-cure prior to any of the disease's symptoms being detected. Likewise, some individuals who develop symptoms usually associated with the PB form (TT leprosy) may also undergo self-cure even in the absence of MDT.

It has been demonstrated that, as compared to the population as a whole, household contacts of leprosy patients are at higher risk of developing the disease *(7)*. The lapse between infection and the onset of disease has been demonstrated to be within a 5–10 yr time frame. Although leprosy is rarely seen in infants less than 3 yr of age, at the other extreme, the onset of symptoms after infection has occurred can take as long as 30 yr. Despite the fact that the respiratory route of infection is being looked upon with increasing favor, it would rather appear that exposure of any mucosal surface to *M. leprae* organisms is deserving of consideration.

In terms of reservoirs, most consider that leprosy is uniquely a human disease. Even though the nine-banded armadillo (*Dasypus nomencinctus*) in the United States and Mexico is frequently infected or at least serum positive for *M. leprae*, there appears to be a very low incidence of documented transmission of *M. leprae* from armadillos kept as pets to pet owners.

Many attempts to protect against *M. leprae* infection have been made by employing *M. bovis* Bacille Calmette–Guérin (BCG). Several studies have shown that BCG vaccination in humans induced a protective immune response against *M. leprae* infection *(8)* that was even greater than the one afforded against tuberculosis itself *(9)*. Multiple BCG intakes increased protection, whereas the addition of killed *M. leprae* to BCG did not seem to improve BCG efficacy *(9,10)*. Moreover, BCG vaccination and immunotherapy with heat-killed *M. leprae* plus BCG, used as an adjunctive to MDT, have led to the clinical and bacteriological improvement of lepromatous leprosy symptoms and the induction of granuloma formation *(11,12)*. BCG has been shown to have adjuvant properties *(13)* that ultimately result in the upgrading of the immune response (CMI), leading to the clearance of bacteria and protection.

4. GENOMICS AND MOLECULAR BIOLOGY

Leprosy infection is a pathology with no available experimental models capable of reproducing many of the most relevant phenomena observed in the human disease. *M. leprae*, a Gram-positive bacillus, was the first etiologic agent to be implicated as the causative agent of an infectious disease, as described by Hansen in 1873 *(14)*. Having the longest doubling time of all known bacteria (approx 14 d), it remains one of the few pathogenic bacterium that has yet to be grown in vitro. Its most characteristic feature is the presence of mycolic acids that reduce the permeability of the bacterial cell wall as well as being responsible for the acid-fast staining of the bacilli.

A pioneering discovery by Shepard *(15)* was the ability to infect the mouse hind footpad with *M. leprae*, which, because of the low temperature of the footpad, grows 100-fold over a period of 7–9 mo. This system provided an opportunity to screen *M. leprae* for drug susceptibility. The discovery of the susceptibility of the nine-banded armadillo to infection by *M. leprae (16)* supported a means of obtaining large quantities of the bacteria from the spleen and liver after an 18- to 24-mo infection period. Most recently, nude (*nu/nu*) mice have been used to obtain significant quantities of physiologically active *M. leprae* for detailed genetic and physiological studies. In these mice, hind footpad infection yields 10^{10} *M. leprae* in 9–12 mo.

Sequencing of the *M. leprae* genome was initiated in 1991 and a fully sequenced and annotated genome is already available *(17)*. The bacterial isolate sequenced came from an armadillo passaged strain. The genome is circular, it contains 3.3 Mb compared with the 4.4-Mb chromosome of *M. tuberculosis,* and possesses ~1,600 open reading frames, whereas *M. tuberculosis* has approx 4000 *(18)*. Thus, functional gene density is considerably lower in the *M. leprae* than it is in the *M. tuberculosis* genome. The *M. leprae* genome contains a great number of noncoding or pseudogene sequences and it is surprising that this "junk DNA" has been retained. The distribution of the 1116 pseudogenes is random, and if these are excluded, 1604 potentially active genes remain, of which 1439 are common to both pathogens. Comparative proteome analysis detected only 391 soluble protein species in *M. leprae (19)* compared with approx 1800 proteins in *M. tuberculosis,* indicating that the pseudogenes are translationally inert. There appear to be very few differences in *M. leprae* genomes from different strains, and this genome sequence conservation has hampered studies on transmission of specific strains within communities or countries.

The availability of the genome sequences of both bacteria allowed the identification of 165 genes in *M. leprae* not present in *M. tuberculosis,* 29 for which functions can be attributed. These genes may code for antigens that can be used as specific diagnostic tools in the near future and/or for virulence factors that might contribute to the unique biology and infective properties of the leprosy bacillus. Several of these *M. leprae*-specific genes will need to be further evaluated for their absence in a diversity of other mycobacterial species. Genes within the RD1 region of *M. tuberculosis,* such as ESAT-6 (early secretory antigen-6) and CFP (culture filtrate protein)-10, encode antigens recognized by T-cells from patients with tuberculosis but not BCG-vaccinated individuals *(20,21)*. Likewise, identification of similar proteins in *M. leprae* may pave the way for their future use as diagnostic reagents *(22)*.

In that sense, immunological assays using ESAT-6 of *M. leprae* for stimulation of the patients' T-cells in vitro are being conducted. In addition, new sets of proteins antigens, associated with the cell wall and from the cytoplasm, are being fractionated from armadillo-derived *M. leprae* and purified to remove all nonspecific immunosuppressive lipoglycans and lipids. They are being used to develop improved skin test antigens to be applied in leprosy endemic areas *(23)*. Ideally, these new diagnostic methods will reveal infection long before clinical symptoms are recognizable. If so, then MDT can be initiated sooner, with an increasing likelihood that both the prevalence and incidence of leprosy can be further reduced.

5. PATHOGENESIS

Phagocytosis of mycobacteria by macrophages occurs via the mannose receptor, the complement receptors (CR) 1, 3, and 4 and the scavenger receptors *(24–26)*. Other candidates are Fc receptors and the fibronectin-binding protein *(27,28)*. Whether *M. leprae* within the phagosome secretes antigens that traffic to the macrophage cytoplasm for class I presentation and/or stimulates class II presentation from within the endosome is, as yet, unknown. Recent studies of macrophage antigen processing makes it likely that uptake of *M. leprae* by these cells will lead to antigen presentation by both class I and class II pathways *(29)*.

The mycobacterial cell envelope contains a extraordinarily high proportion of complex glycolipids, and their biochemical resolution, with the consequent availability of the purified components, has allowed a more systematic study of the immunomodulatory properties of these molecules. In general, several of the mycobacterial components (proteins, lipids, adjuvant-active components detected in the cell wall) have been shown to either induce or suppress cellular functions in vitro and contribute to disease pathogenesis.

Lipoarabinomannann (LAM), a molecule with similarity to Gram-negative bacterial lipopolysaccharide (LPS), is secreted in copious amounts during infection with both *M. leprae* and *M. tuberculosis*. Although it has, on the one hand, been shown to be an effective stimulator for releasing inflammatory cytokines (tumor necrosis factor-α [TNF-α], interleukin-1β [IL-1β]) from human cells *(30,31)*, which appears to be related to the extent of mannose capping in the nonreducing termini of LAM *(32)*, it has been described also as inhibiting macrophage function and interferon (IFN)-γ-induced monocyte activation *(33,34)*.

Aside from LAM, PGL-1 (phenolic glycolipid 1), an abundant glycolipid present on the surface of *M. leprae* as well as free in the infected tissue, is unique to *M. leprae* and has been shown to suppress T-cell responses and IFN-γ production *(35,36)*, in addition to modulate TNF-α production by monocytes in vitro *(37)*.

An additional feature that has been demonstrated for *M. tuberculosis* is the inhibition of phagosome–lysosome fusion in human macrophages and to reside in a compartment with endosomal characteristics *(38)*. Mycobacterial-containing phagosomes fail to acidify by exclusion of the vesicular proton-ATPase *(39)*. Whether the same mechanisms are operative following *M. leprae* entry into macrophages is not known.

To date, several *M. leprae* proteins have been characterized, and a number of the antigens responsible for inducing T-cell responses in tuberculoid patients and household contacts have also been identified, including 70 kDa, 65 kDa, 45 kDa, 35 kDa, 18 kDa, and 10 kDa (the *M. leprae* GroES homolog), among others. Another protein—a 22kDa, designated major membrane protein (MMP)-II—constitutes a bacterioferritin, an iron-rich protein that likely plays a role in the intracellular existence of *M. leprae (40,41)*.

In addition to residing inside macrophages, *M. leprae* attaches to and invades Schwann cells (SCs), cells that form the myelin sheath of peripheral nerves. *M. leprae* has been found within the nerve structures in all forms of leprosy. Nevertheless, the bacillary load does not seem to be the direct cause for the nerve lesion. The overwhelming majority of the bacilli are found in the SC cytoplasm, but *M. leprae* can also be found in endothelial cells and fibroblasts localized within the endoneurium. The segmental demyelination so frequently observed could be the result of SC destruction, although this is not a constant finding and preserved SC have also been seen covering demyelinated fibers *(42)*.

The neurotropism of *M. leprae* may be attributed to its affinity for the G-domain of the α-chain of laminin-2, an extracellular matrix protein that is present in the basal lamina of SCs *(43)*. In turn (*see* Fig. 2), the *M. leprae*–laminin-α2 complex binds to α/β-dystroglycan complexes expressed on the surface of the SC *(44)*. Other candidate (co)receptors may include integrins, which are also able to bind to laminin-2, and an as yet uncharacterized 25-kDa phosphoprotein expressed by SC, to which *M. leprae* has been reported to bind *(45)*. At the other end, mycobacterial receptors may function as critical surface adhesins for the G-domain of laminin-α2 (*see* Fig. 2). A 21-kDa laminin-binding receptor, a histone like protein (Hlp), has been identified on *M. leprae (46,47)*. Moreover, PGL-I has recently been shown to bind laminin-2 and mediate the binding of *M. leprae* to SC *(48)*.

Myobacterium leprae proliferate extensively in SC surrounding peripheral nerves, but whether bacterial gene products or metabolites or the ensuing immune responses contribute to nerve damage within lesions is unknown. *M. leprae*–SC interaction may result in loss of SC properties, which may affect the ability of SCs to adhere to each other, to associate and interact with axons, and, finally, to the lack of myelin production, among others. In any event, *M. leprae* also elicits the production of TNF-α and IFN-γ by T-cells and macrophages (and perhaps by Schwann cells), both of which are associated with a strong inflammatory response.

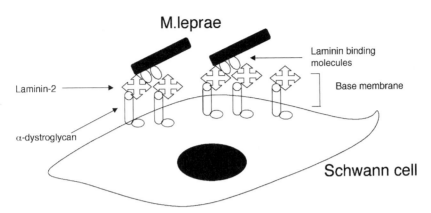

Fig. 2. Attachment of *M. leprae* to Schwann cells. The *M. leprae*-laminin-α2 complex binds to α/β-dystroglycan complexes expressed on the surface of the SCs that seems to mediate bacterial binding and entry into the cell.

6. IMMUNOLOGICAL STATUS

Without doubt, bacterial infections serve as a highly appropriate model in an effort to better understand the mechanisms involved in tissue damage because human diseases caused by mycobacteria occur whether or not specific, detectable CMI is present.

It has been well established that host immunity to *M. leprae* dictates the clinical outcome of the disease *(49,50)*. Lepromatous patients are thus unable to release IFN-γ in response to *M. leprae*, leading to the inability of these individuals to activate monocytes and destroy the bacteria *(51)*.

The crucial role of CD4[+] T-helper cells in orchestrating cell-mediated immunity has led to the belief that macrophage activation via cytokines secreted from major histocompatibility complex (MHC) class II-restricted, antigen-specific CD4 T-cells is the principal mechanism of protection against intracellular microbes. Intracellular mycobacterial elimination and granuloma formation require the differentiation of macrophages into epithelioid cells, the contribution of CD4 and CD8 T-lymphocytes, and the production of cytokines, such as IFN-γ and TNF-α *(52)*. IFN-γ activates antimicrobial mechanisms in macrophages; in mouse models, it induces nitric oxide synthase, leading to the production of nitric oxide, a powerful microbicidal molecule *(53)*.

The concept that IFN-γ production and consequent development of effective CMI results in bacilli elimination was confirmed in humans following the identification of disseminated mycobacterial infection in individuals with inherited IFN-γ receptor (IFN-γR1) deficiency *(54)*, as well as in mice *(55)*.

In leprosy, the emergence of *M. leprae*-specific IFN-γ-producing cells has been associated with protection in healthy household contacts *(56)*. The induction of IFN-γ secretion has been also described as a major effect of BCG infection, both in experimental models *(57)* and, more recently, in humans *(58)* and has been associated with its protective effects. Upon BCG vaccination, it has been demonstrated that household contacts of leprosy patients presented positive proliferative T-cell response as well as high IL-2 and IFN-γ production toward several mycobacterial antigens in vitro *(59)*. Moreover, it was demonstrated that systemic BCG administration at the peak of *M. leprae* infection modifies the evolution of the immune inflammatory response initially induced by *M. leprae* in the mouse footpad *(60)*. Coinfected mice presented a more effective clearance of *M. leprae* and enhanced expression of TNF-α and IFN-γ mRNA in the infected tissue.

Believed to be another important mediator of protection against infections, TNF-α is an inducible cytokine covering a wide range of proinflammatory and immunostimulatory activities *(61)*. The protective role of TNF-α has been suggested in earlier studies in which immunization against this cytokine in mice blocked granuloma formation in response to *M. bovis* (BCG) infection *(62)* and that

TNF-α increased the resistance against *M. avium* infection *(63)*. TNF-α knockout mice experiments also showed TNF-α to be essential for the control of *M. tuberculosis* and *Trypanosoma brucei* infection *(64,65)*.

In a previous study, it was recently demonstrated that enhanced production of TNF-α and IFN-γ as well as decreased production of IL-10 occurred in TT leprosy patients in response to *M. leprae* in vitro *(59)*, supporting a role of the aforementioned cytokines in protection and of IL-10 in the induction and/or maintenance of the anergy in lepromatous leprosy *(66)*. Moreover, detection of serum TNF-α has also been described in BT/TT forms *(67,68)*, patients with PB leprosy were found to express TNF-α mRNA in blood mononuclear cells *(69)*; and in vitro TNF-α production was enhanced in tuberculoid when compared to lepromatous (LL/BL) patients *(70)*.

Recent studies have focused on the cytokine profile of reactive T-cells. Following what was first described in the mouse model *(71)*, it has been proposed recently that the two stable polar forms of leprosy reflect the dominance of the two major T-cell subpopulations. The hypothesis that the spectrum of leprosy reflects the balance between T-helper (Th1 and Th2) cell populations activated by the mycobacterium *(72)* is indeed exciting. Yamamura et al. *(73)* have shown a predominant expression of type 2 cytokines mRNA (IL-4 and IL-10) in lepromatous lesions, hence favoring the humoral response, whereas the type 1 cytokines (IL-2 and IFN-γ) predominate in tuberculoid lesions. The secreted cytokines of Th1 and Th2 cell types can mutually regulate and inhibit each other's functions *(74)*. Therefore, the fine balance between the cytokines is important in the resulting nature of the host's resistance against the pathogen.

In fact, leprosy is not a stable disease in any of its clinical forms, so much that the above-described polar forms are rarely diagnosed in the Clinic Units. The in vivo importance of the described Th subsets has been shown in murine models of bacterial and parasitic infections, where they have been associated with protection or immunopathology. Such distinct T-cell subsets have been more difficult to identify in the human system, on which most studies have shown a mixed cytokine pattern. In a recent report *(75)*, the functional properties of CD4+CD8– T-cell clones isolated from skin lesions and blood of leprosy patients across the spectrum demonstrated substantial heterogeneity. A variety of patterns of cytokine secretion distinct from those of Th1, Th2, or Th0 (CD4+ T-cells with an intermediate cytokine profile) was evident, although no striking correlation with clinical status was apparent. Clones isolated from the blood were, in general, distinct from those isolated from the skin and showed a more restricted cytokine secretion profile. Noteworthy was the large number of clones from skin which secreted neither IL-2 nor IL-4, but large amounts of TNF-α and IFN-γ. In another study *(76)*, following the analysis of cytokine mRNA expression by reverse transcription–polymerase chain reaction (RT-PCR) and cytokine secretion in in vitro stimulated mononuclear cells of leprosy patients, it was found that around 50% of all individuals showed a Th0-like mixed-cytokine pattern, irrespective of the clinical status of leprosy or the antigen used.

7. CYTOTOXIC ACTIVITY AS AN EFFECTOR MECHANISM IN MYCOBACTERIAL INFECTION

In recent years, however, the important contribution of CD8+ T-cells and NK cells in acquired resistance to, at least, particular mycobacterial species and the role of TCR γδ cells in antimycobacterial immunity *(77)* have been indicated. In human leprosy patients, a CD8 type 1 and type 2 cell has also been described. So, as showed by Salgame et al. *(78)*, CD8+ clones from lepromatous lesions characteristically produced IL-4 (type 2 cells).

Moreover, studies in mice and humans have demonstrated the mycobacterial induction of antigen-specific, MHC-restricted CD4+ and CD8+ cytolytic T-cells *(79,80)*. In addition to functioning as a source of cytokines *(80,81)*, induction of killing of *M. tuberculosis*-infected target cells by the cytotoxic T-cell seems to be mediated through apoptosis *(82)*, a phenomena that, although still controversial, may well correlate with the elimination of the bacteria in phagocytes *(82,83)* and with the resolution of infection *(84)*.

An additional mechanism by which T-cells contribute to host defense against microbial pathogens is through the release of the antimicrobial granulysin. It has been recently demonstrated that granulysin and perforin (present in the cytotoxic granules of CD8$^+$ T-cells) act synergistically to kill intracellular *M. tuberculosis (85)*. Ochoa et al. *(86)* demonstrated a higher frequency of granulysin-expressing CD4$^+$ T-cells in tuberculoid leprosy lesions as compared to lepromatous. Given that the release of granulysin can also induce apoptosis of human cells *(87)*, it can possibly provide a mechanism for clearing infected cells from the site of infection.

More recently, a novel class of T-cell receptor ligands and antigen-presentation molecules have entered the scene. T-Cells can also recognize nonpeptide ligands such as mycobacterial mycolic acids, lipoarabinomannan, and isopentenyl-phosphate groups *(88,89)*. Lipid and glycolipid ligands can be presented by non-MHC-encoded but MHC-like molecules CD1. The presence of CD1$^+$ dendritic cells at sites of *M. leprae* infection has been associated with an improved clinical outcome *(90)*. It is completely unclear, however, to what extent these novel T-cell receptor ligands precisely contribute to protective immunity or immunopathology in naturally occurring chronic infection in humans.

The availability of knockout (KO) mice strains provided, on the other hand, intriguing additional information. Neither perforin, granzyme, nor CD1d KO mice *(91,92)* showed increased susceptibility to infection with *M. tuberculosis*, suggesting that, at least, CD8 cells may exert their effects through the secretion of IFN-γ *(93)* rather than/in addition to a cytotoxic mechanism (like the demonstration of CD1-restricted CD8 T-cells) *(93,94)*. The use of tetramers for identification of MHC class I-restricted epitopes within mycobacterial antigens will allow the detection of antigen-specific CD8$^+$ T-cells (or for CD1 cells) in the blood of patients and vaccinated donors *(80,95,96)*.

8. IS THERE ONLY ONE MECHANISM TO EXPLAIN NONRESPONSIVENESS IN LEPROSY?

Although there have been several attempts to understand immunosuppression in leprosy, the exact mechanism(s) of nonresponse remains unclear. Cellular anergy observed in lepromatous patients appears to be *M. leprae*-specific because the immune response against other antigens is largely normal *(97)*. Following the initial speculation on the role of suppressor T-cells *(98,99)*, other mechanisms have also been considered.

As related to Th1/Th2 response, whereas there is accumulated information available on the role of Th2 cells to inhibit Th1 cell function, it is not clear what mechanisms actually lead to the preferential differentiation of Th2 cells in response to bacterial antigens instead of the Th1 population. It has been postulated that the nature of the antigen, the type of antigen-presenting cell (APC), or the type of cytokine (either IL-12 or IL-4) present initially in the microenvironment of the infected tissue may all play a role *(100)*.

It has been proposed that human leukocyte antigen (HLA) genes are important genetic factors in leprosy. It has now become evident that these HLA genes do not determine susceptibility to leprosy *per se* but rather control the type of leprosy that develops upon infection of susceptible individuals. Interestingly, among the susceptible individuals, those with HLA-DR3 develop tuberculoid leprosy more often, whereas those with HLA-DQ1, develop the lepromatous form more often *(101)*. Although HLA alleles may play a role in controlling the development of the type of leprosy, genetic predisposition is only one factor in the complex process leading to disease, the end result of which is probably dependent on the interplay of several host genes.

Most intriguing is the recovery of specific *M. leprae* responsiveness that has been identified in some lepromatous patients in several experiments in which (1) the addition of IL-2 in patients' culture was able to restore the *M. leprae* unresponsiveness in some patients *(102)*, (2) preincubation of patients' culture without any stimulus reversed the specific T-cell unresponsiveness *(103)*, (3) there was the presence of *M. leprae* reactive T-cells in lepromatous patients during reactions *(104,105)*; (4) upgrading aspects in the lepromatous lesions with increasing numbers of CD4$^+$ cells were observed following PPD, rIFN-γ, and rIL-2 intradermal injection *(106)*, (5) there was the emergence of specific CMI in some long-term treated lepromatous patients *(107)*, and (6) unresponsiveness to *M. leprae* could also be overcome in vitro by stimulation of PBMCs with *M. leprae* components *(108)*. In these patients, at least some T cell clones potentially reactive to *M. leprae* have not been deleted. So, other mechanisms that might be able to explain immune tolerance must have been at work.

The concept that tolerance might exist at different levels in vivo was first proposed by Arnold et al. *(109)*. In this scheme, anergy was considered as a single stage from which cells could be rescued. Other stages included receptor downmodulation and deletion. It has been argued that anergy is a slightly slower form of T-cell death by apoptosis. Peripheral deletion of T-cells may involve engagement of Fas and Fas ligand or the TNF receptor by TNF *(110,111)*, a phenomenon that was recently proposed to apply to leprosy, tuberculosis, or *Trypanosoma cruzi* infection *(112–114)*. Alternatively, it is conceivable that deeper states of anergy, representing repeated antigen stimulation, might lead to a more rapid elimination of the cells by way of homeostatic mechanisms other than Fas- or TNF-mediated killing. Indeed, cells anergized either in the presence of IL-10 or by repeated injection of superantigens have been demonstrated *(66,115)*.

Lepromatous patients carry a high load of bacilli that may play a role in the in vivo induction of immune tolerance. As mentioned earlier, mycobacterial components, such as PGL-1 and other LPS-like molecules, seem to have a role in inhibiting T-cell and macrophage function *(33,35)*. On the other hand, secreted factors from adherent cells of lepromatous patients inhibit the proliferation of lymphocytes isolated from healthy individuals *(116,117)*. These factors were identified as IL-10 and prostaglandin E_2 (PGE_2) *(117)*.

In a recent work, major alterations in the expression of signal transduction molecules in lepromatous leprosy (LL) patients were observed. Zea et al. *(118)* have reported a decreased T-cell-receptor ζ-chain expression, decreased $p56^{lck}$ tyrosine kinase, and a loss of nuclear transcription factor NF-κB p65.

In another study, the low responsiveness observed in LL patients could be attributed to low levels of expression of B7-1 and CD28 in the PBMCs and also in the lesions *(119,120)*. Moreover, the lymphocyte proliferative response induced by *M. leprae* in tuberculoid patients was inhibited with anti-B7-1 antibody. Such accessory molecules, like CTLA-4 *(121)*, have also been implicated in the induction of tolerance in experimental models.

Interleukin-10 has been described as a potent antagonist of cutaneous T-cell-mediated immune responses, as it suppress the proliferation of $CD4^+$ T-cells (Th1-type cells) as well as the macrophage's ability to express MHC class II molecules *(122)*, the inflammatory responses, and the production of TNF-α both in vivo and in vitro *(123)*. IL-10 was found to be enhanced in lepromatous patients, suggesting that it could mediate immunosuppression in leprosy *(59,66,124)*. In this connection, it was demonstrated by Sieling et al. *(66)* that the major source of IL-10 is not lymphocytes but monocyte/macrophages triggered by *M. leprae*. IL-10 together with IL-4 can suppress multiple components of CMI, including macrophages themselves.

In a similar way, transforming growth factor (TGF)-β, a cytokine with downregulatory properties on T-cell and monocyte functions, has been detected more abundantly in lepromatous than in tuberculoid lesions (Foss, unpublished observations). In addition to monocytes, another subset of $CD4^+$ T-cells (Th3 cells) has been described to produce TGF-β and to be related to induction of tolerance and/or suppression of Th1 activities *(125,126)*. TGF-β inhibits IFN-γ production but seems to favor IL-10 secretion *(127)*.

The importance of macrophages in directing the immune response to *M. leprae* appears to include the secretion of IL-12, a heterodimeric cytokine that promotes CMI *(128)*. In another set of experiments, recombinant IL-12 (rIL-12) induced a proliferative response to *M. leprae* in the PBMCs of about 50% of the unresponsive lepromatous patients. It was particularly effective when used in combination with anti-IL-10 *(129,130)*. *M. leprae* infection can induce the production of IL-12 and IL-18 *(129,131)* by macrophages, which, together, can potentially promote the development of a Th1 response *(132,133)*.

9. INTERINDIVIDUAL DIFFERENCES IN CYTOKINE PRODUCTION

Cytokine release in the microenvironment neighboring the site of the lesion is a critical component in controlling the nature (cell-mediated versus humoral response), severity, and duration of the response against the infectious agent. The production of cytokines and expression of receptors is under tight but complex biological control, including negative and positive feedback by the cytokines themselves.

It has been proposed that in humans, a great diversity in the profile of cytokines secreted by T-cells is a common finding in that it presents as a dynamic system that would very likely lead to a continuous spectrum of response, in which Th1 and Th2 cells would merely represent the opposite extremes *(134)*. In addition, the interindividual differences in cytokine production will add another variable to the complex of non linear interactions present in the cytokine network *(135)* that will have the potential to influence the various immune and inflammatory responses in several diseases.

It is then possible that the outcome of *M. leprae* infection would, in any case, lead to the resolution of infection following the induction of IL-12, IL-18, TNF-α and IFN-γ cytokines. However, in some individuals, their genetic background would provide the scenario for a lower initial response, (innate and/or specific immune response), allowing for subsequent bacterial multiplication and then the establishment of different levels of nonresponsiveness that are present across the spectrum of leprosy. With regard to genetic background *per se*, a variety of other immunogenetic polymorphisms seems to be implicated in human infectious diseases, cytokine genes being the more relevant ones. Polymorphisms in a number of cytokine genes, such as IFN-γ, IL-10, IL-4, and TNF-α may well explain the differing patterns of response observed in lepromatous versus tuberculoid patients.

The location of TNF-α within the MHC has prompted much speculation about the role of TNF-α genes in the etiology of HLA-linked diseases. Molvig et al. *(136)* showed stable individual variations in TNF-α secretion by human monocytes stimulated with LPS. Low- and high-TNF-α producers were detected and it was speculated that individual susceptibility to Gram-negative infection might be dependent on these variations. It was also demonstrated that culture supernatants from LPS-stimulated monocytes or mitogen-stimulated blood mononuclear cells from HLA-DR3 individuals have higher TNF-α activity than those from DR-2 individuals.

10. TNF-α GENE POLYMORPHISM

The variability of the host response to infection has been demonstrated to be genetically controlled in animal models and, more recently, in humans as well. Genes such as human natural resistance associated macrophage protein 1 (*NRAMP1*) and TNF-α, capable of bridging both innate and adaptive immune responses, may be involved in the resistance to mycobacteria. In recent studies, an association of susceptibility to leprosy and the *NRAMP1* haplotypes was found among Vietnamese leprosy families *(137,138)*, which for the first time, provided evidence in support of a potential role for a non-HLA gene and the development of disease.

Polymorphisms have been described in several cytokine genes, including those encoding for TNF-α. Of the 17 described polimorphic variations, to date, only three biallelic variations in the TNF-α gene promoter, respectively at positions –308, –238 (G→A substitution), and –863 (C→A), were related *(139–141)*, but not unequivocally demonstrated *(142,143)*, to differential expression of the gene and secretion of the protein. The presence of the –308 mutant allele (TNF2) seems to influence the clinical course of cerebral malaria, mucocutaneous leishmaniasis, and meningococcal disease, all syndromes related to enhanced TNF-α levels *(141,144,145)*. Experiments with gene reporter assays and evaluation of TNF-α production in vitro have demonstrated enhanced induction of TNF-α in TNF-α2 carriers *(139,141)*.

Inflammatory reaction is an essential step of the defense mechanisms of the body. It activates the immediate nonspecific antimicrobial effectors and it is clearly required in the initiation of antigen-specific immune responses. So far, it is clear that the inflammation induced *in situ* by these cytokines is required for a successful antimicrobial response. As mentioned earlier, IFN-γ and TNF-α exert a crucial role in granuloma formation and clearance of the bacteria. To determine whether this response was related to a genetic predisposition in leprosy, the typing of TNF-α polymorphism has been performed in different groups of patients. An association of the TNF2 mutant allele with the development of lepromatous leprosy was demonstrated previously in an Indian population *(146)*. Within a Brazilian population, the frequency of the TNF2 allele has more recently been found to be increased in healthy controls (heterozygous individuals) as compared to leprosy patients *(147)*, implying that the presence of TNF2 could be a predisposing genetic factor against development of the disease. Although not significant, the proportion of TNF2 was enhanced in paucibacillary (PB) versus multibacillary (MB) patients *(147)*. Moreover, analysis of lepromin skin test reaction among TNF2 carriers and noncarriers, in PB leprosy, showed enhanced induration size of the in the former group of patients *(148)*. Once the TNF2 allele alters the level of TNF-α gene transcription and the generation of the protein, the presence of TNF2 may then increase the resistance of the host to local infection by increasing the production of TNF-α at the infection site in parallel to an enhanced risk of disease if local immune defenses fails. The persistence of the mutation in healthy control individuals may indicate a selective advantage on the part of TNF2 carriers *(149)*. Because TNF-α promotes antimicrobial mechanisms, it is possible that the TNF2 allele is maintained because heterozygotes possess an optimal level of TNF-α response against a broad range of infections. Accordingly, in vitro studies showed that healthy TNF2 heterozygotes released enhanced amounts of TNF-α in response to LPS when compared to the noncarriers *(150)*.

11. REACTIONAL STATES IN LEPROSY

In the course of leprosy, a reasonable proportion of patients (mostly borderline patients) will develop reactional episodes of acute inflammation, accompanied or not by systemic symptoms, affecting the skin and nerves. These reactional states are classified as Type I (RR, which occurs in BT, BB, and BL patients) or Type II (ENL, which occurs in BL and LL patients) reaction depending on the clinical characteristics of the acute episode and its immune background *(151–153)*. Both the precipitating factors and the physiopathological mechanisms involved in reactions remain ill-defined. In light of the current knowledge, these acute episodes of immunological and inflammatory responses are most likely associated with changes in immune reactivity that seem to be occurring in both types of reaction.

Clinically, patients with RR present with new inflamed lesions might present systemic symptoms and other signs of acute inflammation that could lead to nerve function impairment. Both the previous and the new lesions show histological features characteristic of a tuberculoid lesion. ENL is characterized by the appearance of crops of painful, erythematous, subcutaneous nodules, not related to the former leprosy lesions, associated or not with systemic manifestations of pyrexia, malaise, lymphadenopathy, neuritis, arthralgia, and loss of weight. Fragmented bacteria is a common finding in the reactional tissue.

Histologically, reactional lesions contain dense cellular infiltrate, composed predominantly of CD4+ T-cells, monocytes, and neutrophils (only seen on Type II reaction). It is also accompanied by increases in epidermal thickness, keratinocyte MHC class II antigen expression, the number of epidermal Langerhans' cells, and the presence of intraepithelial T-cells in the reactional lesion *(154–156)*. The presence of Langerhans' cells in the dermis (only seen in RR), disappearance of the Unna layer, enhanced expression of intracellular adhesion molecule (ICAM-1) on the keratinocytes, and expression of leukocyte function antigen 1 (LFA-1) have also been described. In RR, also characterized by granuloma formation and the presence of differentiated macrophages, likewise found in the previous anergic lesion, the inflammatory infiltrate reaches the upper dermis and sometimes even touches the basal layer, whereas during ENL, lesions contain dense cellular infiltrates extending from the lower dermis to the subcutaneous fat.

Another important observation refers to the fact that histological changes seen in the epidermis are quite similar in both RR and ENL, despite the differences in the extent of immune reactivation that seem to happen in both types of reaction. Although the outcome of this reactivation seems to be the elimination of bacilli or its constituents, peripheral irreversible nerve damage may occur in a significant number of patients.

The occurrence of reactions is considered a clinical emergency, and anti-inflammatory treatment must be promptly initiated. RR patients are treated with steroids (prednisone), 1 mg/kg weight, and ENL patients are treated preferentially with thalidomide (300 mg/d) or pentoxifylline (a methylxantine derivative), associated or not with steroids *(157–159)*. Thalidomide must not be administered to females of child-bearing age *(160)*.

12. IMMUNOLOGICAL REACTIVITY AND CYTOKINE PRODUCTION DURING LEPROSY REACTIONS

One may speculate that reactions occur in the course of leprosy when a patient develops increased cell-mediated immune response against *M. leprae*, when the patient's clinical state could move toward the tuberculoid end of the spectrum. These acute inflammatory episodes are often seen to evolve in MB patients, who are unable to respond properly to *M. leprae*. They comprise spontaneously-occurring events that do not take place in any other known disease and offer unique opportunity for studying the changes that occur in an individual's immunological response during the course of a chronic infection.

Notwithstanding the application of the Th1×Th2 paradigm to the polar spectrum of leprosy *(73)*, the occurrence of reactions provides new insights into the mechanisms of immunological regulation during host–pathogen interaction, demonstrating that reactional episodes might, in fact, represent an immune-inflammatory breakthrough even in a previous un(low)responder patient. The potential for patients developing Type I or Type II reaction depends on multifactorial variables that necessarily include genetic features, HLA haplotype, immunological background, and bacillary load, among others. This is particularly true in light of the observation that ENL is most often experienced by lepromatous patients (BL/LL forms), whereas BB patients more often develop RR. Interestingly, in BL patients, both types of reaction occur at a similar frequency rate *(161)*.

The RR patients are able to respond in vitro to *M. leprae* and in vivo to the lepromin skin test *(105)*. Re-emergence of CMI associated to upregulation of IFN-γ production has been largely accepted in a reversal reaction *(162,163)*. An initial low-responsive state (Th2 cytokine profile) typically migrates to a high-responsive profile (Th1 cytokines), an indication that these patients are then capable of performing mRNA syntheses and cytokine secretion *(163,164)*. This present status thereafter leads to granulogenesis and to enhanced macrophage microbicidal activity. Furthermore, CMI response detected during RR has been associated with enhanced bacterial clearance (systemic bacterial load) when compared to unreactional MB patients *(165)*. Thus, RR episodes occurring in unresponsive MB patients may represent a unique moment in the course of leprosy infection during which breakage of the anergic state takes place.

Nevertheless, regulation of the immune response that is underway during ENL is not yet fully understood. Although the Type II reaction is thought to be the result of immune complex-mediated injury *(166,167)*, some authors have showed a transient increase in *M. leprae*-specific CMI response during ENL *(104,168)*. More recently, several groups have indeed demonstrated that the re-emergence of the immune response in lepromatous patients seems to occur in both types of reaction *(69,169–171)*.

The ultimate concern in leprosy research must be the identification of inflammatory cytokines involved in the induction of tissue damage. Once the occurrence of systemic manifestations and of neuritis are more often seen during reactions, it has been hypothesized that upregulation of Th1 response in these patients leads also to the immunopathology associated to reactions.

Evidence implicating TNF-α as a pivotal molecule in this process exists. TNF-α seems to be a natural anti-infectious agent involved in bacterial resistance, which, depending on the quantity and the time period over which its production is sustained, may exert either a beneficial or deleterious effect *(61)*. TNF-α and IL-1β levels have been reported to be elevated in the sera of ENL patients *(172,173)* and in the lesions of ENL *(69,174)* and RR patients *(175)*. Further support for the role of TNF in the local and systemic manifestations of reaction was provided from studies that showed thalidomide (the drug of choice for treatment of ENL) to inhibit LPS- and mycobacteria-induced TNF-α production by monocytes in vitro *(176)*. Moreover, higher TNF-α secretion was detected in untreated reactional patients (ENL) as compared to thalidomide-treated patients, normal individuals, or lepromatous patients without ENL *(70,177,178)*; treatment with thalidomide reduced serum TNF-α levels and the histological manifestations observed *in situ* in ENL patients *(179)*. Additionally, pentoxifylline, a previously known TNF-α inhibitor *(180)*, has been shown to be useful for treating ENL *(181,182)*. Clinical improvement following anti-inflammatory treatment paralleled the decrease in TNF-α levels detected both in serum samples and from stimulated cells in vitro, and TNF-α mRNA expression at the lesion site *(174,183)*. Because reactivation of the cellular immune response has been suggested, the participation of other immuno-inflammatory cytokines that may be related to augmentation/inhibition of TNF-α production should also be considered. It has been reported that (1) intradermal injection of rIFN-γ into lepromatous patients could trigger ENL through the amplification of *M. leprae*-induced TNF-α production both in vivo and in vitro *(177)*, as well as decreased bacterial load and viability in these same patients *(177,184,185)*, (2) IFN-γ protein was detected in the serum of some ENL patients *(179)*, and (3) in addition to TNF-α, an enhanced expression of IFN-γ mRNA at the lesion site (and in the blood) was observed during the reaction (ENL) as compared to before the reaction *(69)*.

In addition to IFN-γ, a role for cell–cell contact (monocyte-activated T-cell) in the amplification of *M. leprae*-induced TNF-α secretion has been suggested *(186)*. On the other hand, the participation of NK cells or γδ T-cells as a source for IFN-γ (or TNF-α) *in situ* cannot be formally excluded. In synergy with that, it has been shown that IL-12 plays a major role in innate as well as in adaptive immunity and inflammation and induces (together with TNF-α) the early production of IFN-γ by NK cells and even uncommitted bystander T-cells *(128,187)*. IFN-γ and IL-12 may be considered important mediators to control immune responses against intracellular bacteria. Moreover, these cytokines might be a contributing factor in the deleterious effects classically attributed to TNF-α. The notion that their overwhelming or unbalanced production can contribute to undesirable inflammatory side effects must be validated. Several data point to IL-12 as playing a critical role in the pathogenesis of Th1-mediated autoimmune diseases *(188)*. In line with these findings, in vitro and in vivo detection of IL-12 production in the resistant forms of leprosy *(129,132)* has been recently demonstrated. Further results confirmed that the majority of patients expressed IFN-γ and IL-12 mRNA in the skin while undergoing reaction *(69)*. Kinetic studies performed in vitro showed early and enhanced *M. leprae*-induced TNF-α production (mRNA and protein) from ENL patients' cell cultures followed by a delayed IL-10 response (Sampaio, unpublished data). Hence, the data favor the idea that, in an unresponsive patient, induction of IFN-γ can overcome the patient's unresponsiveness by inhibiting IL-10 and augmenting IL-12 production. Again, it can be hypothesized that IL-10 is working as a potent immunosuppressor of Th1 responses, whereas a breakthrough of this steady state can transiently revert the low immunological profile to a highly responsive inflammatory condition.

Alternatively, the possibility cannot be excluded that transient IFN-γ production by Th2 cells is operative in ENL patients' lesions as opposed to a more established production of IFN-γ (and TNF-α) by Th1 clones in RR *(189)*. It was recently reported that IL-12 induced the differential expression of the β2 subunit of the IL-12 receptor (IL-12Rβ2) on established Th1 and Th2 cells *(190)*. It has been suggested that the IL-12-induced transient upregulation of the IL-12Rβ2 transcripts in Th2 clones may account for the transient production of IFN-γ in cells with an established Th2 phenotype *(191)*. Quantification of IL-12R transcripts and of subtle differences in mRNA expression (IFN-γ, TNF-α, IL-12) between ENL and RR *in situ* need to be further investigated.

The occurrence of sequential ENL and RR in one individual patient indicates further that both reactions share similar immunological backgrounds. Similar cytokine mRNA profiles were observed in the lesions of the same patient during RR and ENL, although the presence of γδ T-cells was detected in RR but not in ENL lesions *(192)*. Thus, the definition of the type of response observed clinically and histologically may result from the temporary stimulation of different T-cell subpopulations, under the selection of different antigens by the antigen-presenting cells (APCs), taking place in a microenvironment in which the amount of live and dead bacteria fluctuates in the course of the chronic infection. Follow-up evaluation of cytokine mRNA expression in reactional skin indicated further that improvement of patients' clinical symptoms following in vivo administration of antiinflammatory treatment (either prednisone, thalidomide, or pentoxifylline) was associated with the decreased expression of TNF-α *(174,183)*, IFNγ, and IL-12 *(183)* mRNAs, whereas worsening of their clinical conditions correlated to the maintenance of cytokine mRNAs levels *(see* Fig. 3). Therefore, monitoring of cytokine mRNA expression *in situ* may allow early indication of occurrence and evolution of reactional inflammation in leprosy.

13. NERVE DAMAGE DURING REACTIONS

From the point of view of clearing the bacteria, upgrading responses might be considered beneficial. However, the inflammation in nerve tissue may turn into permanent damage and disability if not treated adequately. A finding of considerable clinical importance is that many patients, even after MDT and lacking viable *M. leprae*, nevertheless present with significant nerve damage and persistent neuritis. Whether this is caused by dead bacteria or the attempt to clear the bacteria or their components is not clear. Steroid therapy administered prior to the onset of significant nerve damage is often able to prevent these permanent disabling symptoms. However, in some cases, prompt and adequate oral prednisone seems to have very little effect on the recovery of persistent nerve lesions *(193,194)*. It is known that successful axonal regeneration occurs exclusively within the endoneurial tubes lined by SC basal laminae *(195)* and that degradation and remodeling of extracellular matrices are important aspects of the regenerative process *(196)*. Therefore, it will be important to pursue new therapeutic interventions capable of promoting axonal regeneration in these patients, such as the use of neurotrophic factors, antimetalloproteinases, and vitamin B_{12}, once they are available for clinical trials.

Several pathogenic mechanisms may be responsible for nerve damage in leprosy, including biochemical interference of *M. leprae* with host cell metabolism, mechanical damage resulting from the large influx of cells and fluid, or immunological damage. Antigen-specific T-cell-mediated hypersensitivity to *M. leprae* antigens is associated with the pathogenesis of nerve lesion in the tuberculoid forms of leprosy and it is observed more frequently during acute reversal reactions *(6)*. However, the mechanism of nerve damage in the lepromatous forms of the disease is still unknown. Because reactions are accompanied by an increased CMI response and because acute nerve damage particularly occurs during these episodes, a role for the immunoinflammatory response deserves particular consideration *(197)*. The expression of TNF-α mRNA and protein in the skin and nerves of RR patients *(175)* points to a central role of TNF-α in the pathophysiology of nerve damage in leprosy.

There is evidence that TNF-α contributes to the pathogenesis of neurological autoimmune diseases such as multiple sclerosis and experimental allergic encephalomyelitis, among others *(198)*. It has been pointed out that this cytokine exerts damaging effects on oligodendrocytes, the myelinproducing cell of the central nervous system, and myelin itself *(199,200)*, and has a central role in augmenting inflammatory demyelination. In rat SCs, combination of TNF-α and TGF-β has been reported to cause significant SC detachment and lysis *(201)*.

In addition to the proposed direct effect of TNF-α in neural injury across the entire spectrum of leprosy, re-emergence of antigen-specific CD4+ T-cells has been considered to have a role both in protection as well as leading to immunopathology *(see* Fig. 4). CD4+ T-cells are more abundant in skin lesions of patients with reaction, and the anatomical location of CD4+ T-cells containing cytotoxic granules has been reported *(162)*. In addition, murine SCs have already been shown to function

Th1 Cytokines in Host Defenses

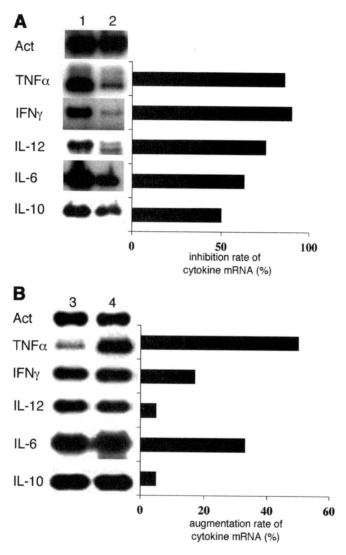

Fig. 3. Inhibition/augmentation rates of cytokine mRNA expression in leprosy reactional tissue. Follow-up analysis by semiquantitative reverse transcription–polymerase chain reaction (RT-PCR) of TNF-α, IL-6, IFN-γ, IL-10, and IL-12 mRNA expression in biopsies obtained at the onset of the reaction episode and during anti-inflammatory treatment. Following hybridization to specific internal oligonucleotides, X-ray films were analyzed by densitometry and the relative amounts of cytokine mRNA in the tissue were compared between samples from each patient. Variation rates (%) in mRNA expression were established after comparison of the intensity of PCR bands between treated and reactional biopsies in the same individual. (A) Downregulation of cytokine mRNA expression following thalidomide treatment correlated with improvement of patient´s clinical conditions. (B) Persistent cytokine message expression after 7 d of pentoxifylline treatment correlated with maintenance of inflammation in vivo in one patient.

as APCs for CD8[+] cytotoxic T-cells in a MHC class I-restricted, mycobacterial antigen-dependent manner *(202)*. It was also demonstrated that expression of HLA class II on human SCs and that IFN-γ and TNF-α action as well as *M. leprae* invasion resulted in upregulation of MHC class II by rodent SCs *(203,204)*. Thus, SCs may be actively involved in the immunopathology of leprosy neuritis by presenting *M. leprae* antigens to cytotoxic T-cells *(42)*.

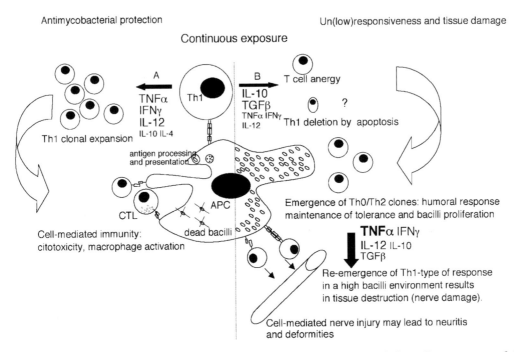

Fig. 4. The dual role of Th1 responses in leprosy: protection and immunopathology. Re-emergence of the immune responses during the natural course of disease leads to cellular activation and expression of activation molecules at the lesion site in parallel to an exacerbated inflammatory response and tissue damage.

As an alternative mechanism, expression of the neural cell adhesion molecule (N-CAM), also called CD56, on both target and effector cells has been hypothesized to be of importance. In addition to NK cells, N-CAM expression has also been observed on some CD4[+] T-cells in relation to multiple sclerosis *(205)*. These cells were able to kill N-CAM-positive oligodendrocytes in an antigen-independent manner *(206)*. It was also revealed that coadhesion via other molecules (CD54 and CD11a) was essential for establishing target lysis. As proposed by Spierings *(207)*, this mechanism may also be involved in leprosy neuritis, because cells derived from inflamed neural tissue show increased N-CAM expression when compared to peripheral T-cells. These hypotheses are currently under investigation.

14. FINAL CONSIDERATIONS

In considering the *M. leprae* genome, one could say that this mycobacterium is a dying pathogen. On the other hand, the overall characteristics discussed herein may well suggest that *M. leprae* evolution's within the human host is so long and intimate that mycobacterium evolution has been reduced to the amount of information sufficient enough to achieve infection and ensure perpetuation of the species. Thus, because of its extraordinary long generation time, *M. leprae* developed silent mechanisms of entry and survival within unusual cells (Schwann cells) that although it does not guarantee 100% of the individuals to be infected, for the few in whom infection actually succeeds, it warrants bacilli maintenance and dissemination. That is another of its feature that makes leprosy so unique and that requires special efforts to control, eliminate, and eradicate it.

It is obvious that the study of lepromatous versus tuberculoid forms is a common generalization of the infection and disease progression because clinical manifestations are the outcome of a very slow and complicated interaction between the bacterium and the host. In this regard, it is still a difficult task to define whether the lepromatous polar form (LL) is (1) the end process of a gradual evolution toward downregulation of the specific immune response (that has gone through several intermediate phases) or (2) the outcome of host–pathogen interaction that, since the beginning, is predetermined to experience an immunological shutdown.

Considering that inflammatory reactions interrupt the clinical course of leprosy, it might be suggested that the disease exhibits an unique immunological pattern that is based on complex interactions between cells and secreted factors that may well represent a dynamic but chaotic behavior *(135)*. In this model, nonlinearities in cytokine interactions implicate that the output is not necessarily proportionally related to the input. It is, therefore, postulated that continuous exposition of patients to *M. leprae* leads to infection that in some individuals evolve to the tuberculoid pole because of an early and strong immunity (Th1 response) that controls bacilli replication (TT and BT forms), whereas in others, because of delayed and/or absent immune response, it slowly evolves to a level of higher bacillary load and inactivation of macrophage functions, leading to more profound levels of non response and, ultimately, to the establishment of a Th2 profile (lepromatous pole). Up to this moment in the course of disease, it does not mean that Th1 responses were completely shutdown. The rate of immune reactivity in this phase might define the clinical outcome (borderline forms). In fact, at this stage (when rescue of specific CMI is more easily achieved), immune reactivity can emerge naturally, as the so-called reactions. Depending on the number of bacteria, MHC restriction, and spatial/temporal cell-type activation, this immune reactivation is clinically observed as RR or ENL. It is noteworthy to consider that as a result of the chaotic regulation of cytokine secretion *(135,208)*, even a subtle activation process may trigger an exacerbated inflammatory response. Thus, the definition of key cytokines/mediators that serve as immunological markers of these different states can definitely contribute to a better understanding of this paradigmatic but still mysterious disease.

REFERENCES

1. Ridley, D.S. and Jopling, W.H. (1966) Classification of leprosy according to immunity: a five group system. *Int. J. Lepr.* **34**, 255–273.
2. Van Voorhis, W.C., Kaplan, G., Sarno, E.N., Horwitz, M.A., Steinman, R.M., Levis, W.R., et al. (1982) The cutaneous infiltrates of leprosy. Cellular characteristics and the predominant T-cell phenotype. *N. Engl. J. Med.* **307**, 1593–1597.
3. Narayanan, R.B., Bhutani, L.K., Sharma, A.K., and Nath, I. (1983) T Cell subsets in leprosy lesions: in situ characterization using monoclonal antibodies. *Clin. Exp. Immunol.* **51**, 421–429.
4. Modlin, R.L., Hofman, F.M., Taylor, C.R., and Rea, T.H. (1983) T-Lymphocyte subsets in the skin lesions of patients with leprosy. *J. Am. Acad. Dermatol.* **8**, 182–189.
5. Kaplan, G., Nusrat, A., Sarno, E.N., Job, C.K., McElrath, J., Porto, J.A., et al. (1987) Cellular responses to the intradermal injection of recombinant human γ-interferon in lepromatous leprosy patients. *Am. J. Pathol.* **128**, 345–353.
6. Pearson, J.M. and Ross, W.F. (1975) Nerve involvement in leprosy—pathology, differential diagnosis and principals of management. *Lepr. Rev.* **46**, 199–212.
7. Godal, T., Lofgren, M., and Negassi, K. (1972) Immune response to *M. leprae* of healthy leprosy contacts. *Int. J. Lepr.* **40**, 243–250.
8. Convit, J.P., Smith, G., Zuniga, M., Sampson, C., Ulrich, M., Plata, J.A., et al. (1993) BCG vaccination protects against leprosy in Venezuela: a case-control study. *Int. J. Lepr.* **61**, 185–191.
9. Karonga Prevention Trial Group (1996) Ramdomised controlled trial of single BCG, repeated BCG, or combined BCG and killed Mycobacterium leprae vaccine for prevention of leprosy and tuberculosis in Malawi. *Lancet* **348**, 17–24.
10. Convit, J., Sampson, C., and Zuniga, M. (1992) Immunoprophylatic trial with combined *Mycobacterium leprae*/BCG vaccine against leprosy: preliminary results. *Lancet* **339**, 446–450.
11. Rada, E., Ulrich, M., Aranzazu, N., Rodriguez, V., Centeno, M., Gonzalez, I., et al. (1997) A follow-up study of multibacillary Hansen's disease on patients treated with multidrug therapy (MDT) + immunotherapy (IMT). *Int. J. Lepr.* **65**, 320–327.
12. Rada, E., Ulrich, M., Aranzazu, N., Santaella, C., Gallinoto, M., Rodriguez, V., et al. (1994) A longitudinal study of immunologic reactivity in leprosy patients treated with immunotherapy. *Int. J. Lepr.* **62**, 552–558.
13. Stewart-Tull, D.E.S. (1983) Immunologically important constituents of mycobacteria: adjuvants, in *The Biology of the Mycobacteria* (Ratledge, C. and Stanford, J., eds.), Academic London, pp. 3–84.
14. Hansen, G.H.A. (1874) Undersogelser aandende spedalskhedens aasager. *Norsk Magazin Laegervidenskaben 4* (Suppl.) 1–88.
15. Shepard, C.C. (1960) The experimental disease that follows the injection of human leprosy bacilli into foot pads of mice. *J. Exp. Med.* **112**, 445–454.
16. Kirchheimer, W.F. and Storrs, E.E. (1971) Attempts to establish the armadillo (*Dasypus novemcinctus*) as a model for the study of leprosy. I. Report of lepromatoid leprosy in an experimentally infected armadillo. *Int. J. Lepr.* **39**, 693–702.
17. Cole, S.T., Eigimeir, K., Parkhill, J., James, K.D., Thomson, N.R., Wheeler, P.R., et al. (2001) Massive gene decay in the leprosy bacillus. *Nature* **409**, 1007–1011.

18. Cole, S.T., Brosch R., Parkhill, J., Hornsby, T., Jagels, K., Lacroix, C., et al. (1998) Deciphering the biology of Mycobacterium tuberculosis from the complete genome sequence. *Nature* **393**, 537–544.
19. Marques, M.A.M., Chitalli, S., Brennan, P.J., and Pessolani, M.C.V. (1998) Mapping and identification of the major cell wall-associated components of *Mycobacterium leprae*. *Infect. Immun.* **66**, 2625–2631.
20. Ravn, P., Demissie, A., Eguale, T., Wondwosson, H., Lein, D., Amoudy, H.A., et al. (1999) Human T cell responses to the ESAT-6 antigen from *Mycobacterium tuberculosis*. *J. Infect. Dis.* **179**, 637–645.
21. Arend, S.M., Geluk, A., van Meijgaarden, K.E., van Dissel, J.P., Theisen, M., Andersen, P., et al. (2000) Antigenic equivalence of human T-cell responses to *Mycobacterium tuberculosis*-specific RD1-encoded protein antigens ESAT-6 and culture filtrate protein 10 and to mixtures of synthetic peptides. *Infect. Immun.* **68**, 3314–3321.
22. Dockrell, H.M., Brahmbhatt, S., Robertson, B.D., Britton, S., Fruth, U., Gebre, N., et al. (2000) A postgenomic approach to identification of *Mycobacterium leprae*-specific peptides as T-cell reagents. *Infect. Immun.* **68**, 5846–5855.
23. Manandhar, R., LeMaster, J.W., Butlin, C.R., Brennan, P.J., and Roche, P.W. (2000) Interferon-gamma responses to candidate leprosy skin-test reagents detect exposure to leprosy in an endemic population. *Int. J. Lepr.* **68**, 40–48.
24. Schlesinger, L.S. and Horwitz, M.A. (1991) Phagocytosis of *Mycobacterium leprae* by human monocyte-derived macrophages is mediated by complement receptors CR1 (CD35), CR3 (CD11b/CD18), and CR4 (CD11c/CD18) and IFN-γ activation inhibits complement receptor function and phagocytosis of this bacterium. *J. Immunol.* **147**, 1983–1994.
25. Zimmerli, S., Edwards, S., and Ernst, J.D. (1996) Selective receptor blockade during phagocytosis does not alter the survival and growth of *Mycobacterium tuberculosis* in human macrophages. *Am. J. Respir. Cell. Mol. Biol.* **15**, 760–770.
26. Schorey, J.S., Carroll, M.C., and Brown, E.J. (1997) A macrophage invasion mechanism of pathogenic mycobacteria. *Science* **277**, 1091–1093.
27. Thole, J.E.R., Shoningh, R., and Janson, A.A.M. (1992) Molecular and immunological analysis of a fibronectin-binding protein antigen secreted by *Mycobacterium leprae*. *Mol. Microbiol.* **6**, 153–163.
28. Polat, G.L., Laufer, J., Fabian, I., and Passwell, J.H. (1993) Cross-linking of monocyte plasma membrane Fcα, Fcγ or mannose receptors induces TNF production. *Immunology* **80**, 287–292.
29. Rodriguez, A., Regnault A., Kleijmeer, M., Ricciardi-Castagnoli, P., and Amigorena, S. (1999) Selective transport of internalized antigens to the cytosol for MHC class I presentation in dendritic cells. *Nat. Cell Biol.* **1**, 362–369.
30. Barnes, P.F., Chatterjee, D, Abrams, J.S., Lu, S., Wang, E., Yamamura, M., et al. (1992) Cytokine production induced by *Mycobacterium tuberculosis* lipoarabinomannan. Relationship to chemical structure. *J. Immunol.* **149**, 541–547.
31. Sampaio, E.P., Moreira, A.L., Sarno, E.N., Malta, A.M., and Kaplan, G. (1992) Prolonged treatment with recombinant interferon induces erythema nodosum leprosum in lepromatous leprosy patients. *J. Exp. Med.* **175**, 1729–1737.
32. Chatterjee, D., Roberts, A.D., Lowell, K., Brennan, P.J., and Orme, L.M. (1992) Structural basis of capacity of lipoarabinomannan to induce secretion of tumor necrosis factor. *Infect. Immun.* **60**, 1249–1251.
33. Moreno, C., Mehlert, A., and Lamb, J. (1988) The inhibitory effects of mycobacterial lipoarabinomannan and polysaccharides upon polyclonal and monoclonal human T cell proliferation. *Clin. Exp. Immunol.* **74**, 206–210.
34. Adams, L.B., Fukutomi, Y., and Krahenbuhl, J.L. (1993) Regulation of murine macrophage effector functions by lipoarabinomannan from mycobacterial strains with different degrees of virulence. *Infect. Immun.* **61**, 173–181.
35. Mehra, V., Brennan, P.J., Rada, E., Convit, J., and Bloom, B.R. (1984) Lymphocyte suppression in leprosy induced by unique *M. leprae* glycolipid. *Nature* **308**, 194–196.
36. Prasad, H.K., Mishra, R.S., and Nath, I. (1987) Phenolic glycolipid-I of *Mycobacterium leprae* induces general suppression of in vitro concanavalin A responses unrelated to leprosy type. *J. Exp. Med.* **165**, 239–244.
37. Charlab R., Sarno E.N., Chaterjee, D., and Pessolani, M.C.V. (2001) Effect of unique *Mycobacterium leprae* phenolic glycolipid (PGL-1) on tumor necrosis factor production by human mononuclear cells. *Lepr. Rev.* **96**, 63–69.
38. Malik, Z.A., Denning, G.M., and Kusner, D.J. (2000) Inhibition of Ca^{2+} signaling by *Mycobacterium tuberculosis* is associated with reduced phagosome-lysosome fusion and increased survival within human macrophages. *J. Exp. Med.* **191**, 287–302.
39. Sturgill-Koszycki, S., Schlesinger, P.H., Chakraborty, P., Haddix, P.L., Collins, H.L., Fok, A.K., et al. (1994) Lack of acidification in *Mycobacterium* phagosomes produced by exclusion of the vesicular proton-ATPase. *Science* **263**, 678–681.
40. Pessolani, M.C.V., Smith, D.R., Rivoire, B., McCormick, J., Hefta, S.A., Cole, S.T., and Brennan, P.J. (1994) Purification, characterization, gene sequence and significance of a bacterioferritin from *Mycobacterium leprae*. *J. Exp. Med.* **180**, 319–327.
41. Sampaio, E.P., Pereira, G.M.B., Pessolani, M.C.V., and Sarno, E.N. (1994) Interaction of the leprosy bacillus and the human host: relevant components and mechanism of disease. *Ciência Cultura* **46**, 462–471.
42. Spierings, E., Boer, T., Zulianello, L., and Ottenhoff, T.H.M. (2000) Novel mechanisms in the immunopathogenesis of leprosy nerve damage: the role of Schwann cells, T cells and Mycobacterium leprae. *Immunol. Cell Biol.* **78**, 349–355.
43. Rambukkana, A., Salzer, J.L., Yurchenco, P.D., and Tuomanen, E.I. (1997) Neural targeting of Mycobacterium leprae mediated by the G domain of the laminin-alpha2 chain. *Cell* **88**, 811–821.
44. Rambukkana, A., Yamada, H., and Zanazzi, G. (1998) Role of alpha dystroglycan as a Schwann cell receptor for *Mycobacterium leprae*. *Science* **282**, 2076–2079.
45. Suneetha, L.M., Satish, P.R., Korula, R.J., Suneetha, S.K., Job, C.K., and Balasubramanian, A.S. (1998) *Mycobacterium leprae* binds to a 25-kDa phosphorylated glycoprotein of human peripheral nerve. *Neurochem. Res.* **23**, 907–911.
46. Shimoji, Y., Ng, V., Matsumura, K., Fischetti, V.A., and Rambukkana, A. (1999) A 21-kDa surface protein of *Mycobacteium leprae* binds peripheral nerve laminin-2 and mediates Schwann cell invasion. *Proc. Natl. Acad. Sci. USA* **96**, 9857–9862.
47. Marques, M.A.M., Mahapatra, S., Sarno, E.N., Nandan, D., Dick, T., Brennan, P.J., et al. (2000) Bacterial and host-derived cationic proteins bind alpha2-laminins and enhance *Mycobacterium leprae* attachment to human Schwann cells. *Microbes Infect.* **2**, 1407–1417.

48. Ng, V., Zanazzi, G., Timpl, R., Talts, J.F., Salzer, J.L., Brennan, P.J., et al. (2000) Role of the cell wall phenolic glycolipid-1 in the peripheral nerve predilection of *Mycobacterium leprae*. *Cell* **103**, 511–524.
49. Bjune, G., Barnetson, R.S.C., Ridley, D.S., and Kronvall, G. (1976) Lymphocyte transformation test in leprosy: correlation of the response with inflammation of lesions. *Clin. Exp. Immunol.* **25**, 85–94.
50. Godal, T. (1984) Immunology of leprosy: some aspects of the role of the immune system in the pathogenesis of the disease. *Lepr. Rev.* **55**, 407–414.
51. Nogueira, N., Kaplan, G., Levy., E.N., Sarno, E.N., Kushner, P., Granelli-Piperno, A., et al. (1983) Defective gamma interferon production in leprosy. Reversal with antigen and interleukin-2. *J. Exp. Med.* **158**, 165–171.
52. Chensue, S.W., Warmington, K., Ruth, J., Lincoln, P., Kuo, M.-C., and Kunkel, S.L. (1994) Cytokine responses during mycobacterial and schistosomal antigen-induced pulmonary granuloma formation: production of Th1 and Th2 cytokines and relative contribution of tumor necrosis factor. *Am. J. Pathol.* **145**, 1105–1113.
53. MacMicking, J.D., North, R.J., LaCourse, R., Mudgett, J.S., Shah, S.K., and Nathan, C.F. (1997) Identification of nitric oxide synthase as a protective locus against tuberculosis. *Proc. Natl. Acad. Sci. USA* **94**, 5243–5248.
54. Hill, A.V. (1998) The immunogenetics of human infectious diseases. *Annu. Rev. Immunol.* **16**, 593–617.
55. Cooper, A.M., Dalton, D.K., Stewart, T.A., Griffin, J.P., Russell, D.G., and Orme, I.M. (1993) Disseminated tuberculosis in interferon-γ gene-disrupted mice. *J. Exp. Med.* **178**, 2243–2247.
56. Sampaio, E.P., Moreira, A.L., Kaplan, G., Alvim, M.F.S., Duppre, N.C., Miranda, C.F., et al. (1991) *Mycobacterium leprae*-induced interferon- production by household contacts of leprosy patients: association with the development of disease. *J. Infect. Dis.* **164**, 990–993.
57. Kawamura, I., Tsukada, H., Yoshikawa, H., Fujita, M., Nomoto, K., and Mitsuyama, M. (1992) IFN-gamma-producing ability as a possible marker for the protective T cells against *Mycobacterium bovis* BCG in mice. *J. Immunol.* **148**, 2887–2893.
58. Ravn, P., Boesen, H., Pedersen, B.K., and Andersen, P. (1997) Human T cell responses induced by vaccination with *Mycobacterium bovis* bacillus Calmette–Guerin. *J. Immunol.* **158**, 1949–1955.
59. Lima, M.C.B.S., Pereira, G.M.B., Rumjanek, F.D., Gomes, H.M., Duppre, N.C., Sampaio, E.P., et al. (2000) Immunological cytokine correlates of protective immunity and pathogenesis in leprosy. *Scand. J. Immunol.* **51**, 419–428.
60. Aarestrup, F.M., Sampaio, E.P., Moraes, M.O., Albuquerque, E.C.A., Castro, A.P.V., and Sarno, E.N. (2000) Experimental Mycobacterium leprae infection in BALB/c mice: effect of BCG administration on TNF-α production and granuloma development. *Int. J. Lepr.* **68**, 156–166.
61. Beutler, B.A. (1999) The role of tumor necrosis factor in health and disease. *J. Rheumatol.* **26**(Suppl. 57), 16–21.
62. Kindler, V., Sappino, A.-P., Grau, G.E., Piguet, P.F., and Vassali, P. (1989) The inducing role of tumor necrosis factor in the development of bactericidal granulomas during BCG infection. *Cell* **56**, 731–740.
63. Smith, D.A., Hansch, H. G. R., Bancroft, G. J., and Ehlers, S. (1997) T Cell independent granuloma formation in response to *Mycobacterium avium*—role of tumor necrosis factor-α and interferon-γ. *Immunology* **92**, 413–421.
64. Flynn, J. L., Goldstein, M. M., Chan, J., Triebold, K. J., Pfeffer, K., Lowenstein, C. J., et al. (1995) Tumor necrosis factor-α is required in the protective immune response against *Mycobacterium tuberculosis* in mice. *Immunity* **2**, 561–572.
65. Magez, S., Radwanska, M., Beschin, A., Sekikawa, K., and De Baetselier, P. (1999) Tumor necrosis factor alpha is a key mediator in the regulation of experimental Trypanosoma brucei infections. *Infect. Immun.* **67**, 3128–3132.
66. Sieling, P.A., Abrams, J.S., Yamamura, M., Barnes, P.F., and Modlin, R.L. (1993) Immunosuppressive roles for IL-10 and IL-4 in human infection. In vitro modulation of T-cell responses in leprosy. *J. Immunol.* **150**, 5501–5510.
67. Pisa, P., Mengistu, G., Soder, O., Ottenhoff, T.H.M., Hanson, M., and Kiessling, R. (1990) Serum tumour necrosis factor levels and disease dissemination in leprosy and leishmaniasis. *J. Infect. Dis.* **161**, 988–991.
68. Silva, C.L. and Foss, N.T. (1989) Tumor necrosis factor in leprosy patients. *J. Infect. Dis.* **159**, 787–790.
69. Moraes, M.O., Sarno, E.N., Almeida, A.S., Saraiva, B.C.C., Nery, J.A.C., and Sampaio, E.P. (1999) Cytokine gene expression in leprosy: a possible role for IFN-γ and IL-12 in reactions (RR and ENL). *Scand J. Immunol.* **50**, 541–549.
70. Barnes, P.F., Chatterjee, D., Brennan, P.J., Rea, T.H., and Modlin, R.L. (1992) Tumor necrosis factor production in patients with leprosy. *Infect. Immun.* **60**, 1441–1446.
71. Mosmann, T.R., Cherwinski, H., Bond, M.W., Gildlin, M.A., and Coffman, R.L. (1986) Two types of murine helper T cell clone. Definition according to profiles of lymphokines activities and secreted proteins. *J. Immunol.* **136**, 2348–2357.
72. Ramos, T., Zalcberg-Quintana, I., Appelberg, R., Sarno, E.N., and Silva, M.T. (1989) T-Helper cell subpopulations and the immune spectrum of leprosy. *Int. J. Lepr.* **57**, 73–81.
73. Yamamura, M., Uyemura, U., Deans, R., Weinberg, K., Rea, T.H., Bloom, B., et al. (1991) Defining protective responses to pathogens: cytokine profiles in leprosy lesions. *Science* **254**, 277–279.
74. Maggi, E., Parronchi, P., Manetti, R., Simonelli, C., Piccinni, M.P., Santoni, R., et al. (1992) Reciprocal regulatory role of IFN-γ and IL-4 on the in vitro development of human TH1 and TH2 clones. *J. Immunol.* **148**, 2142–2147.
75. Howe, R.C., Wondimu, A., Demisse, A., and Frommel, D. (1995) Functional heterogeneity among CD4+ T cell clones from blood and skin lesions of leprosy patients. Identification of T-cell clones distinct from Th0, Th1 and Th2. *Immunology* **84**, 585–594.
76. Misra, N., Murtaza, A., Walker, B., Narayanan, N.P.S., Misra, R.S., Ramesh, V., et al. (1995) Cytokine profile of circulating T cells of leprosy patients reflects both indiscriminate and polarized T-helper subsets: T-helper phenotype is stable and uninfluenced by related antigens of *Mycobacterium leprae*. *Immunology* **86**, 97–103.
77. Follows, G.A., Munk, M.E., Gatrill, A.J., Conradt, P., and Kaufmann, S.H.E. (1992) Gamma interferon and interleukin 2, but not interleukin 4, are detectable in γδ T-cell cultures after activation with bacteria. *Infect. Immun.* **60**, 1229–1231.
78. Salgame, P., Abrams, J.S., Clayberger, C., Goldstein, H., Convit, J., Modlin, R.L., et al. (1991) Differing lymphokine profiles of functional subsets of human CD4 and CD8 T cell clones. *Science* **254**, 279–282.

79. Mutis, T., Cornelisse, Y.E., and Ottenhoff, T.H.M. (1993) Mycobacteria induce CD4⁺ T cells that are cytotoxic and display Th1-like cytokine secretion profile: heterogeneity in cytotoxic activity and cytokine secretion levels. *Eur. J. Immunol.* **23**, 2189–2195.
80. Smith, S.M. and Dockrell, H.M. (2000) Role of CD8⁺ T cells in mycobacterial infections. *Immunol. Cell Biol.* **78**, 325–333.
81. Serbina, N.V. and Flynn, J.F. (1999) Early emergence of CD8⁺ T cells primed for production of type 1 cytokines in the lungs of *Mycobacterium tuberculosis*-infected mice. *Infect. Immun.* **67**, 3980–3988.
82. Oddo, M., Renno T., Attinger, A., Bakker, T., MacDonald, H.R., and Meylan, P.R.A. (1998) Fas ligand-induced apoptosis of infected human macrophages reduces the viability of intracellular *Mycobacterium tuberculosis*. *J. Immunol.* **22**, 5448-5454.
83. Molloy, A., Laochumroonvoporang, P., and Kaplan, G. (1994) Apoptosis, but not necrosis, of infected monocytes is coupled with killing of intracellular bacillus Calmette–Guerin. *J. Exp. Med.* **180**, 1499–1509.
84. Serbina, N.V. Liu, C-C., Sanga, C.A., and Flynn, J.F. (2000) CD8⁺ CTL from lungs of *Mycobacterium tuberculosis*-infected mice express perforin in vivo and lyse infected macrophages. *J. Immunol.* **165**, 353–363.
85. Stenger, S., Hanson, D., Teitelbaum, R., Dewan, P., Niasi, K.R., Froelich, C.J., et al. (1998) An antimicrobial activity of cytolitic T cells mediated by granulysin. *Science* **282**, 121–125.
86. Ochoa, M.-T., Stenger, S., Sieling, P.A., Uszynski, S.T., Sabet, S., Cho, S., et al. (2001) T cell release of granulysin contributes to host defense in leprosy. *Nat. Med.* **7**, 174–179.
87. Gamen, S., Hanson, D.A., Kaspar, A., Naval, J., and Krensky, A.M. (1998) Granulysin-induced apoptosis. I. Involvement of at least two distinct pathways. *J. Immunol.* **161**, 1758–1764.
88. Sieling, P.A., Chatterjee, D., Porcelli, S.A., and Modlin, R.L. (1995) CD1-restricted T cell recognition of microbial lipoglycans. *Science* **269**, 227–230.
89. Porcelli, S.A. and Modlin, R.L. (1999) The CD1 system: antigen-presenting molecules for T cell recognition of lipids and glycolipids. *Annu. Rev. Immunol.* **17**, 297–329.
90. Sieling, P.A., Jullien, D., Dahlem, M., Tedder, T.F., Rea, T.H., Modlin, R.L., et al. (1999) CD1 expression by dendritic cells in human leprosy lesions: Correlation with effective host immunity. *J. Immunol.* **162**, 1851–1858.
91. Cooper, A.M., D'Souza, C.D., Frank, A.A., and Orme, I.M. (1997) The course of *Mycobacterium tuberculosis* infection in the lungs of mice lacking expression of either perforin- or granzyme-mediated cytolytic mechanisms. *Infect. Immun.* **65**, 1317–1320.
92. Sousa, A.O., Mazzaccaro, R.J., and Russel, R.G. (2000) Relative contribution of distinct MHC class I-dependent cell populations in protection to tuberculosis infection in mice. *Proc. Natl. Acad. Sci. USA* **97**, 4204–4208.
93. Tascon, R.E., Stavropoulos, E., Lukacs, V., and Colston, M.J. (1998) Protection against *Mycobacterium tuberculosis* infection by CD8⁺ T cells requires the production of gamma interferon. *Infect. Immun.* **66**, 830–834.
94. Rosat, J.P., Grant, E.P., Beckman, E.M., Dascher, C.C., Sieling, P.A., Frederique, D., et al. (1999) CD1-Restricted microbial lipid antigen-specific recognition found in the CD8⁺ αβ T cell pool. *J. Immunol.* **162**, 366–371.
95. Benlagh, K., Weiss, A., Beavis, A., Teyton, L., and Bendelac, A. (2000) In vivo identification of glycolipid antigen-specific T cells using fluorescent CD1d tetramers. *J. Exp. Med.* **191**, 1895–1903.
96. Geluk, A., van Meijgaarden, K.E., Franken, K.L.M.C., Drijfhout, J.W., D'Souza, S., Neckers, A., et al. (2000) Identification of a major epitope of Mycobacterium tuberculosis Ag85B that is recognized by HLA-A*0201-restricted CD8⁺ T cells in HLA-transgenic mice and humans. *J. Immunol.* **165**, 6463–6471.
97. Sarno, E.N., Espinosa, M., Sampaio, E.P., Vieira, L.M.M., Figueiredo, A.A., Miranda, C.F., et al. (1988) Immunological responsivenes to *M. leprae* and BCG antigens in 98 leprosy patients and their household contacts. *Braz. J. Med. Biol. Res.* **21**, 461–470.
98. Mehra V., Convit, J., Rubinstein, A., and Bloom, B.R. (1982) Activated suppressor T cells in leprosy. *J. Immunol.* **129**, 1946–1950.
99. Modlin, R., Mehra, V., Wong, L., Fujimiya, Y., Chang, W.C., Horwitz, D.A., et al. (1986) Suppressor T lymphocytes from lepromatous leprosy skin lesions. *J. Immunol.* **137**, 2831–2834.
100. Seder, R.A. and Paul, W.E. (1994) Acquisition of lymphokine-producing phenotype by CD4⁺ T cells. *Annu. Rev. Immunol.* **12**, 635–673.
101. Eden, W.V. and De Vries, R.R.P. (1984) Occasional review—HLA and leprosy: a re-evaluation. *Lepr. Rev.* **55**, 89–109.
102. Kaplan, G., Weinstein, D.E., Steinman, R.M., Levis, W.R., Elvers, V., Patarroyo, M.E., et al. (1985) An analysis of in vitro T cell responsiveness in lepromatous leprosy. *J. Exp. Med.* **159**, 917–929.
103. Mohagheghpour, N., Gelber, R.R., and Engleman, E.G. (1987) T cell defect in lepromatous leprosy is reversible in vitro in the absence of exogenous growth factors. *J. Immunol.* **138**, 570–574.
104. Laal, S., Bhutani, L.K., and Nath, I. (1985) Natural emergence of antigen-reactive T cells in lepromatous leprosy patients during erythema nodosum leprosum. *Infect. Immun.* **50**, 887–892.
105. Laal, S., Mishra, R.S., and Nath, I. (1987) Type I reactions in leprosy: Heterogeneity in T-cell functions related to the background leprosy type. *Int. J. Lepr.* **55**, 481–487.
106. Kaplan, G., Nusrat, A,, Sarno, E.N., Job, C.K., McElrath, J., Porto, J.A., et al. (1987) Cellular responses to the intradermal injection of recombinant human γ-interferon in lepromatous leprosy patients. *Am. J. Pathol.* **128**, 345–353.
107. Esquenazi, D.A., Sampaio, E.P., Moreira, A.L., Gallo, M.E.N., Almeida, S.M.R., and Sarno, E.N. (1990) Effect of treatment on immune responsivenes in lepromatous leprosy patients. *Lepr. Rev.* **61**, 251–257.
108. Ottenhoff, T.H.M., Converse, P.J., Gebre, N., Wondimu, A., Ehrenberg, J.P., and Kiessling, R. (1989) T cell responses to fractionated *Mycobacterium leprae* antigens in leprosy. The lepromatous nonresponder defect can be overcome in vitro by stimulation with fractionated *M. leprae* components. *Eur. J. Immunol.* **19**, 707–713.

109. Hammerling, G.J., Schonrich, G., Ferber, I., and Arnold, B. (1993) Peripheral tolerance as a multi-step mechanism. *Immunol. Rev.* **133,** 93–104.
110. Cope, A.P., Liblau, R.S., and Yang, X.D. (1997) Chronic tumor necrosis factor alters T cell responses by attenuating T cell receptor signaling. *J. Exp. Med.* **185,** 1573–1584.
111. The, H.S., Seebaran, A., and The, S.J. (2000) TNF receptor 2-deficient CD8 T cells are resistant to Fas/Fas ligand-induced cell death. *J. Immunol.* **165,** 4814–4821.
112. Gupta, A., Sharma, V.K., Vohra, H., and Ganguly, N.K. (1999) Inhibition of apoptosis by ionomycin and zinc in peripheral blood mononuclear cells (PBMC) of leprosy patients. *Clin. Exp. Immunol.* **117,** 56–62.
113. Hirsch, C.S., Toossi, Z., Vanham, G., Johnson, L. J., Peters, P., Okwere, A., et al. (1999) Apoptosis and T cell hyporesponsiveness in pulmonary tuberculosis. *J. Infect. Dis,* **179,** 945–953.
114. Lopes, M.F., Nunes, M.P., Henriques Pons, A., Giese, N., Morse. H.C., Davidson, W.F., et al. (1999) Increased susceptibility of Fas ligand deficient gld mice to Trypanosoma cruzi infection due to a Th2 biased host immune response. *Eur. J. Immunol.* **29,** 81–89.
115. Enk, A.H., Angeloni, V.L., Udey, M.C., and Katz, S.I. (1993) Inhibition of Langerhans' cell antigen-presenting function by IL-10: a role for IL-10 in induction of tolerance. *J. Immunol.* **151,** 2390–2398.
116. Salgame, P.R., Birdi, T.J., Mahadevan, P.R., and Antia, N.H. (1980) Role of macrophages in defective cell-mediated immunity in lepromatous leprosy. I. Factors from macrophage affecting protein synthesis and lymphocyte transformation. *Int. J. Lepr.* **48,** 172–177.
117. Misra, N., Selvakumar, M., Singh, S., Bharadwaj, M., Ramesh, V., Misra, R.S., et al. (1995) Monocyte derived IL-10 and PGE2 are associated with the absence of Th1 cells and in vivo T cell suppression in lepromatous leprosy. *Immunol. Lett.* **48,** 123–128.
118. Zea, A.H., Ochoa, M.T., Ghosh, P., Longo, D.L., Alvord, W.G., Valderrama. L., et al. (1998) Changes in expression of signal transduction proteins in T lymphocytes of patients with leprosy. *Infect. Immun.* **66,** 499–504.
119. Agrewala, J.N., Kumar, B., and Vohra, H. (1998) Potential role of B7-1 and CD28 molecules in immunosuppression in leprosy. *Clin. Exp. Immunol.* **111,** 56–63.
120. Fafitas-Morris, M., Guillen-Vargas, C.M., Navarro-Fierros, S., Alfaro-Bustamante, F., Zaitzeva-Petrovna, G., Daneri-Navarro, A., et al. (1999) Addition of anti-CD28 antibodies restores PBMC proliferation and IFN-gamma production in lepromatous leprosy patients. *J. Interferon Cytokine Res.* **19,** 1237–1243.
121. Greewald, R.J., Boussiotis, V.A., Lorsbach, R.B., Abbas, A.K., and Sharpe, A.H. (2001) CTLA-4 regulates induction of anergy in vivo. *Immunity* **14,** 145–155.
122. Fiorentino, D.F., Bond, M.W., and Mosmann, T.R. (1989) Two types of mouse T helper cell. IV. Th2 clones secrete a factor that inhibits cytokine production by Th1 clones. *J. Exp. Med.* **170,** 2081–2095.
123. de Waal Malefyt, R., Abrams, J., Bennett, B., Figdor, C., and de Vries, J.E. (1991) Interleukin 10 (IL-10) inhibits cytokine synthesis by human monocytes: an autoregulatory role of IL-10 produced by monocytes. *J. Exp. Med.* **174,** 1209–1220.
124. Barnes, P.F., Abrams, J.S., Lu, S., Sieling, P.A., Rea, T.H., and Modlin, R.L. (1993) Patterns of cytokine production by mycobacterium-reactive human T-cell clones. *Infect. Immun.* **61,** 197–201.
125. Inobe, J., Slavin A.J., Komagata, Y., Chen, Y., Liu, L., and Weiner, H.L. (1998) IL-4 is a differentiation factor for transforming growth factor beta secreting Th3 cells and oral administration of IL-4 enhances oral tolerance in experimental allergic encephalomyelitis. *Eur. J. Immunol.* **28,** 2780–2790.
126. MacDonald, T.T. (1999) Effector and regulatory lymphoid cells and cytokines in mucosal sites. *Curr. Top. Microbiol. Immunol.* **236,** 113–135.
127. Ludviksson, B.R., Seegers, D., Resnick, A.S., and Strober, W. (2000) The effect of TGF beta1 on immune responses of naive versus memory CD4+ Th1/Th2 T cells. *Eur J. Immunol.* **30,** 2101–2111.
128. Trinchieri, G. (1995) Interleukin-12: a proinflammatory cytokine with immunoregulatory functions that bridge innate resistance and antigen-specific adaptative immunity. *Annu. Rev. Immunol.* **15,** 251–276.
129. Libraty, D.H., Airan, L.E., Uyemura, K., Jullien, D., Spellberg, B., Rea, T.H., et al. (1997) Interferon-γ differentially regulates interleukin-12 and interleukin-10 production in leprosy. *J. Clin. Invest.* **99,** 336–341.
130. De Jong, R., Janson, A.A., Faber, W.R., Naafs, B., and Ottenhoff, T.H.M. (1997) IL-2 and IL-12 act in synergy to overcome antigen-specific T cell unresponsiveness in mycobacterial disease. *J. Immunol.* **159,** 786–793.
131. Garcia, V.E., Uyemura, K., Sieling, P.A., Ochoa, M.T., Morita, C.T., Okamura, H., et al. (1999) IL-18 promotes type 1 cytokine production from NK cells and T cells in human intracellular infection. *J. Immunol.* **162,** 6114–6121.
132. Sieling, P.A., Wang, X.H., Gately, M.K., Oliveros, J.L., McHugh, T., Barnes, P.F., et al. (1994) IL-12 regulates T helper type 1 cytokine responses in human infectious disease. *J. Immunol.* **153,** 3639–3647.
133. Xu, D., Chan, W.L., Leung, B.P., Hunter, D., Schulz, K., Carter, R.W., et al. (1998) Selective expression and functions of interleukin 18 receptor on T helper (Th) type 1 but not Th2 cells. *J. Exp. Med.* **188,** 1485–1492.
134. Kelso, A. (1995) Th1 and Th2 subsets: Paradigms lost? *Immunol. Today* **16,** 374–379.
135. Callard, R., George, A.J.T., and Stark, J. (1999) Cytokines, chaos, and complexity. *Immunity* **11,** 597–513.
136. Molvig, J., Baek, L., and Christensen, P. (1988) Endotoxin-stimulated human monocyte secretion of interleukin 1, tumor necrosis factor alpha, and prostaglandin E2 shows stable interindividuals differences. *Scand. J. Immunol.* **27,** 705–716.
137. Abel, L., Sanchez, F.O., Oberti, J., Alcais, A., Sanchez, F.O., and Hill, A.V. (1998) Susceptibility to leprosy is linked to the human NRAMP1 gene. *J. Infect. Dis.* **177,** 133–145.
138. Alcais, A., Sanchez, F.O., Thue, N.V., Lap, V.D., Oberti, J., Lagrange, P.H., et al. (2000) Granulomatous reaction to intradermal injection of lepromin (Mitsuda reaction) is linked to human NRAMP1 gene in Vietnamese leprosy sibships. *J. Infect. Dis.* **181,** 302–308.

139. Krooger, K.M., Carville, K.S., and Abraham, L.J. (1997) The −308 tumor necrosis factor- promoter polymorphism effects transcription. *Mol. Immunol.* **34,** 391–399.
140. Skoog, T., Hooft, F.M.V., Kallin, B., Jovinge, S., Boquist, S., Nilsson, J., et al. (1999) A common functional polymorphism (CA substitution at position -863) in the promoter region of the tumour necrosis factor-α (TNF-α) gene associated with reduced circulating levels of TNF-α. *Hum. Mol. Genet.* **8,** 1443–1449.
141. Allen, R.D. (1999) Polymorphism on the human TNFα promoter—random variation or functional diversity? *Mol. Immunol.* **36,** 1017–1027.
142. Stuber, F., Udalova, I.A., Book, M., Drutskaya, L.N., Kuprash, D.V., Turetskaya, R.L., et al. (1996) −308 tumor necrosis factor (TNF) polymorphism is not associated with survival in severe sepsis and is unrelated to lipopolysaccharide inducibility of the human TNF promoter. *J. Inflamm.* **46,** 42–50.
143. Mycko, M., Kowalski, W., Kwinkowski, M., Buenafe, A.C., Szymanska B., Tronczynska, E., et al. (1998) Multiple sclerosis: The frequency of allelic forms of tumor necrosis factor and lymphotoxin-alpha. *J. Neuroimmunol.* **84,** 198–206.
144. McGuire, W., Hill, A.V.S., Allsopp, C.E.M., Greenwood, B.M., and Kwiatkowski, K. (1994) Variation in the TNF-α promoter region associated with susceptibility to cerebral malaria. *Nature* **371,** 508–511.
145. Westendorp, R.G.J., Langermans, J.A.M., Huizinga, T.W.J., Elouali, A.H., Verweij, C.L., Boomsma, D.I., et al. (1997) Genetic influence of cytokine production and fatal meningococcal disease. *Lancet* **349,** 170–173.
146. Roy, S., McGuire, W., Mascie Taylor, C.G., Saha, B., Hazra, S.K., Hill, A.V.S., et al. (1997) Tumor necrosis factor promoter polymorphism and susceptibility to lepromatous leprosy. *J. Infect. Dis.* **176,** 530–532.
147. Santos, A.R., Almeida, A.S., Suffys, P.N., Moraes, M.O., Filho, V.F., Mattos, H.J., et al. (2000) Tumor necrosis factor promoter polymorphism (TNF2) seems to protect against development of severe forms of leprosy in a pilot study in Brazilian patients. *Int. J. Lepr.* **68,** 325–327.
148. Moraes, M.O., Duppre, N.C., Suffys, P.N., Santos, A.R., Almeida, A.S., Nery, J.A.C., et al. (2001) Tumor necrosis factor-α promoter polymorphism TNF2 is associated with a stronger delayed-type hypersensitivity reaction in the skin of borderline tuberculoid leprosy patients. *Immunogenetics* **53,** 45–47.
149. Kumar, A., Short, J., and Parrillo, J.E. (1999) Genetic factors in septic shock. *JAMA* **282,** 579–581.
150. Louis, E., Franchimont, D., Piron, A., Gevart, Y., Schaaf-Lafontaine, N., Roland, S., et al. (1998) Tumor necrosis factor (TNF) gene polymorphism influences TNF production in lipopolysaccharide (LPS)-stimulated whole blood cell culture in healthy humans. *Clin. Exp. Immunol.* **113,** 401–406.
151. Sehgal, V.N. (1987) Reactions in leprosy. Clinical aspects. *Int. J. Dermatol.* **26,** 278–285.
152. Vasquez-Botet, M. and Sanchez, J.L. (1987) Erythema nodosum leprosum. *Int. J. Lepr.* **26,** 436–437.
153. Ridley, D.S. (1969) Reactions in leprosy. *Int. J. Lepr.* **40,** 77–81.
154. Modlin, R.L., Gebhard, J.F., and Taylor, C.R. (1983) In situ characterization of T lymphocytes in the reactional states of leprosy. *Clin. Exp. Immunol.* **53,** 17–23.
155. Arnoldi, J., Gerdes, J., and Flad, H-D. (1990) Immunohistologic assessment of cytokine production of infiltrating cells in various forms of leprosy. *Am. J. Pathol.* **137,** 749–753.
156. Sullivan, L., Sano, S., Pirmez, C., Salgame, P., Muller, C., Hofman, F., et al. (1991) Expression of adhesion molecules in leprosy lesions. *Infect. Immun.* **59,** 4154–4160.
157. Jollife, D.S. (1977) Leprosy reactional states and their treatment. *Br. J. Dermatol.* **97,** 345–352.
158. Sheskin, J. (1975) Thalidomide in lepra reaction. *Int. J. Dermatol.* **14,** 575–576.
159. Nitton, W.J. and Lockwood, D.N.J. (1997) Leprosy reactions: current and future approaches to management. *Baillière's Clin. Infect. Dis.* **4,** 1–23.
160. Fabro, S., Schumacher, H., Smith, R.L., and Williams, R.T. (1964) Teratogenic activity of thalidomide and related compounds. *Life Sci.* **3,** 987–992.
161. Nery, J.A.C., Vieira, L.M.M., Matos, H.J., Gallo, M.E.N., and Sarno, E.N. (1998) Reactional states in multibacillary Hansen disease patients during multidrug therapy. *Rev. Inst. Med. Trop. São Paulo* **40,** 363–370.
162. Cooper, C.L., Mueller, C., Sinchaisri, T-A., Pirmez, C., Chan, J., Kaplan, G., et al. (1989) Analysis of naturally occurring delayed-type hypersensitivity reactions in leprosy by in situ hybridization. *J. Exp. Med.* **169,** 1565–1581.
163. Yamamura, M., Wang, X., Ohmen, J.D., Uyemura, K., Rea, T.H., Bloom, B.R., et al. (1992) Cytokine patterns of immunologically mediated tissue damage. *J. Immunol.* **149,** 1470–1475.
164. Verhagen, C.E., Wierenga, E.A., Buffing, A.A.M., Chand, M.A., Faber, W.R., and Das, P.K. (1997) Reversal reaction in borderline leprosy is associated with a polarized shift to type 1-like *Mycobacterium leprae* T cell reactivity in the lesional skin: a follow up study. *J. Immunol.* **159,** 4474–4483.
165. Linhares, U.C. (2001) Emergence of cell-mediated immune response in multibacillary leprosy patients with reversal reaction effects patients' systemic bacillary load. Master thesis, FIOCRUZ, Rio de Janeiro, Brazil.
166. Wemambu, S.N.C., Turk, J.L., Waters, M.F.R., and Rees, R.J.W. (1969) Erythema nodosum leprosum: a clinical manifestation of the Arthus phenomenon. *Lancet* **2,** 933–935.
167. Waters, M.F.R., Turk, J.L., and Wemambu, S.N.C. (1971) Mechanisms of reactions in leprosy. *Int. J. Lepr.* **39,** 417–428.
168. Rao, R.D. and Rao, P.R. (1987) Enhanced cell-mediated immune response in erythema nodosum leprosum reactions of leprosy. *Int. J. Lepr.* **55,** 36–41.
169. Sreenivasan, P., Misra, M.S., Wilfred, D., and Nath, I. (1998) Lepromatous leprosy patients show T helper 1-like profile with differential expression of interleukin-10 during type 1 and type 2 reactions. *Immunology* **76,** 357–362.
170. Trao, V.T., Huong, P.L.T., Thuang, A.T., Anh, D.D., Trach, D.D., Rook, G.A.W., et al. (1998) Changes in cellular response to mycobacterial antigens and cytokine production patterns in leprosy patients during multiple drug therapy. *Immunology* **94,** 197–206.

171. Nath, I., Vemuri, N., Reddi, A.L., Bharadwaj, M., Abrooks, P., Colston, M.J., et al. (2000) Dysregulation of IL-4 expression in lepromatous leprosy patients with and without erythema nodosum leprosum. *Lepr. Rev.* **40**(*Suppl.*), S130–S137.
172. Sarno, E.N., Grau, G.E., Vieira, L.M.M., and Nery, J.A.C. (1991) Serum levels of tumor necrosis factor-alpha and interleukin-1β during leprosy reactional states. *Clin. Exp. Immunol.* **84**, 103–108.
173. Parida, S.K., Grau, G.E., Zahfer, S.A., and Mukherjee, R. (1992) Serum tumor necrosis factor and interleukin 1 in leprosy and during lepra reactions. *Clin. Immunol. Immunopathol.* **62**, 23–27.
174. Sampaio, E.P., Moraes, M.O., Nery, J.A.C., Santos, A.R., Matos, H.J., and Sarno, E.N. (1998) Pentoxifylline decreases in vivo and in vitro tumor necrosis factor (TNFα) production in lepromatous leprosy patients with erythema nodosum leprosum (ENL). *Clin. Exp. Immunol.* **111**, 300–308.
175. Khanolkar-Young, S., Rayment, N., Brickell, P.M., Katz, D.R., Vinayakumar, S., Colston, M.J., et al. (1995) Tumor necrosis factor-alpha (TNFα) synthesis is associated with the skin and peripheral nerve pathology of leprosy reversal reactions. *Clin. Exp. Immunol.* **99**, 196–202.
176. Sampaio, E.P., Sarno, E.N., Galilly, R., Cohn, Z.A., and Kaplan, G. (1991) Thalidomide selectively inhibits tumor necrosis factor-alpha production by stimulated human monocytes. *J. Exp. Med.* **173**, 699–703.
177. Sampaio, E.P., Moreira, A.L., Sarno, E.N., Malta, A.M., and Kaplan, G. (1992) Prolonged treatment with recombinant interferon induces erythema nodosum leprosum in lepromatous leprosy patients. *J. Exp. Med.* **175**, 1729–1737.
178. Sampaio, E.P., Duppre, N.C., Moreira, A.L., Nery, J.A.C., and Sarno, E.N. (1993) Development of giant reaction in response to PPD skin test in lepromatous leprosy patients. *Int. J. Lepr.* **61**, 205–213.
179. Sampaio, E.P., Kaplan, G., Miranda, A., Nery, J.A.C., Miguel, C.P., Viana, S., et al. (1993) The influence of thalidomide on the clinical and immunological manifestation of erythema nodosum leprosum. *J. Infect. Dis.* **168**, 408–414.
180. Doherty, G.M., Jensen, C., Alexander, R., Buresh, C.M., and Norton, J.A. (1991) Pentoxifylline suppression of tumor necrosis factor gene transcription. *Surgery* **110**, 192–198.
181. Sarno, E.N., Nery, J.A.C., Garcia, C.C., and Sampaio, E.P. (1995) Is pentoxifylline a viable alternative in the treatment of ENL? *Int. J. Lepr.* **63**, 570–571.
182. Nery, J.A.C., Périssé, A.R.S., Sales, A.M., Vieira, L.M.M., Souza, R.V., Sampaio, E.P., et al. (2000) The use of pentoxifylline in the treatment of type II reactional episodes in leprosy. *Indian J. Lepr.* **72**, 457–467.
183. Moraes, M.O., Sarno, E.N., Teles, R.M.B., Almeida, A.S., Saraiva, B.C.C., Nery, J.A.C., et al. (2000) Anti-inflammatory drugs block cytokine mRNA accumulation in the skin and improve the clinical condition of reactional leprosy patients. *J. Invest. Dermatol.* **115**, 1–7.
184. Damasco, M.H.S., Sarno, E.N., Lobno, A.S., Alvarenga, F.B.F., Porto, J.A., Rosankaimir, T., et al. (1992) Effect of cutaneous cell-mediated immune response to rIFN-γ on *M. leprae* viability in the lesions of lepromatous leprosy. *Braz. J. Med. Biol. Res.* **25**, 457–465.
185. Sampaio, E.P., Malta, A.M., Sarno, E.N., and Kaplan, G. (1996) Effect of rhuIFNγ treatment in multibacillary leprosy patients. *Int. J. Lepr.* **64**, 268–273.
186. Sampaio, E.P., Oliveira, R.B., Warwick-Davies, J., Faria Neto, R.B., Griffin, G.E., and Shattock, R.J. (2000) T cell-monocyte contact enhances TNFα production in response to *M. leprae* in vitro. *J. Infect. Dis.* **182**, 1463–1472.
187. Billiau, A. (1996) Interferon-γ biology and role in pathogenesis. *Adv. Immunol.* **62**, 61–129.
188. Balashov, K.E., Smith, D.R., Khoury, S., Hafler, D.A., and Weiner, H.L. (1997) Increased interleukin 12 production in progressive multiple sclerosis: induction by activated CD4+ T cells via CD40 ligand. *Proc. Natl. Acad. Sci. USA* **94**, 599–603.
189. Verhagen, C.E., Van der Pouw Kraan, T.C.T.M., Buffing, A.A.M., Chand, M.A., Faber, W.R., Aarden, L.A., et al. (1998) Type 1- and Type 2-like lesional skin-derived *Mycobacterium leprae*-responsive T cell clones are characterized by co-expression of IFNγ/TNFα and IL-4/IL-5/IL-13 respectively. *J. Immunol.* **160**, 2380–2387.
190. Rogge, L., Barberis-Maino, L., Biffi, M., Passini, N., Presky, D.H., Gubler, U., et al. (1997) Selective expression of an interleukin-12 receptor component by human helper 1 cells. *J. Exp. Med.* **185**, 825–831.
191. Manetti, R., Gerosa, F., Giudizi, M.G., Biagiotti, R., Parronchi, P., Piccinni, M.P., et al. (1994) Interleukin 12 induces stable priming for interferonγ (IFNγ) production during differentiation of human T helper (Th) cells and transient IFN-γ production in established Th2 cell clones. *J. Exp. Med.* **179**, 1273–1283.
192. Moraes, M.O., Sampaio, E.P., Nery, J.A.C., Saraiva, B.C.C., Alvarenga, F.B.F., and Sarno, E.N. (2001) Sequential erythema nodosum leprosum and reversal reaction with similar lesional cytokine mRNA patterns in a borderline leprosy patient. *Br. J. Dermatol.* **144**, 175–181.
193. Van Brakel, W.H. and Khawas, I.B. (1996) Nerve function impairment in leprosy: a epidemiological and clinical study—Part 2: results of steroid treatment. *Lepr. Rev.* **67**, 104–118.
194. Roche, P.W., Theuhnet, J., Le Master, J.W., and Bultin, C.R. (1998) Contribution of type 1 reactions sensory and motor function loss in borderline leprosy patients and the efficacy of treatment with prednisone. *Int. J. Lepr.* **66**, 340–347.
195. Martini, R. (1994) Expression and functional roles of neural cell surface moleculaes and extracellular matrix components during development and regeneration of peripheral nerves. *J. Neurocytol.* **23**, 1–28.
196. Ferguson, T.A. and Muir, D. (2000) MMP-2 and MMP-9 increase the neurite-promoting potential of Schwann cell basal laminae and are upregulated in degenerated nerve. *Mol. Cel. Neurosci.* **16**, 157–167.
197. Sampaio, E.P. and Sarno, E.N. (1996) Role of inflammatory cytokines in tissue injury in leprosy. *Int. J. Lepr.* **64**, S69–S74.
198. Liu, J., Marino, M. W., Wong, G., Grail, D., Dunn, A., Bettadapura, J., et al. (1998) TNF is a potent anti-inflammatory cytokine in autoimmune-mediated demyelination. *Nat. Med.* **4**, 78–83.
199. Selmaj, K.W. and Raine, C.S. (1988) Tumor necrosis factor mediates myelin and oligodendrocyte damage in vitro. *Annu. Neurol.* **23**, 339–346.

200. Ledeen, R.W. and Chakraborty, G. (1998) Cytokines, signal transduction, and inflammatory demyelination: review and hypothesis. *Neurochem. Rev.* **23,** 277–289.
201. Skoff, A.M., Lisak, R.P., Bealmear, B., and Benjamins, J.A. (1998) TNFα and TGFβ act sinergistically to kill Schwann cells. *J. Neurosci. Res.* **53,** 747–756.
202. Steinhoff, U., Wurttenberger, A.W., Bremerich, A., and Kaufmann, S.H.E. (1991) *Mycobacterium leprae* renders Schwann cells and mononuclear phagocytes susceptible or resistant to killer cells. *Infect. Immun* **59,** 684–688.
203. Mitchell, G.W., Williams, G.S., Bosh, E.P., and Hart, M.N. (1991) Class II antigen expression in peripheral neuropaties. *J. Neurol. Sci.* **102,** 170–176.
204. Gold, R., Tokia, K.V., and Hartung, H.P. (1995) Synergistic effect of IFN-gamma and TNF-alpha on expression of immune molecules and antigen presentation by Schwann cells. *Cell. Immunol.* **165,** 65–70.
205. Vergelli, M., Le, H., van Noort, J.M., Dhib-Jalbut, S., McFarland, H., and Martin, R. (1996) A novel population of CD4⁺CD56⁺ myelin-reactive T cells lyses target cells expressing CD56/neural cell adhesion molecule. *J. Immunol.* **157,** 679–685.
206. Antel, J.P., McCrea, E., Ladiwala, U., Qin, Y., and Beche, B. (1998) Non-MHC-restricted cell-mediated lysis of human oligodendrocytes in vitro: relation with CD56 expression. *J. Immunol.* **160,** 1606–1611.
207. Spierings, E. (2000) Immunopathogenesis of leprosy neuritis. Ph.D. thesis, Leiden University, Leiden, The Netherlands.
208. Amiot, F., Boussadia, O., Cases, S., Fitting, C., Lebastard, M., Cavaillon, J-M., et al. (1997) Mice heterozygous for a deletion of the tumor necrosis factor-α and lymphotoxin-α genes: biological importance of a nonlinear response of tumor necrosis factor-α to gene dosage. *Eur. J. Immunol.* **27,** 1035–1042.

V
Cytokines in Other Bacterial Infections

13

Possible Role of Molecular Mimicry in Lyme Arthritis

Abbie L. Meyer and Brigitte T. Huber

1. MOLECULAR MIMICRY

1.1. Introduction to Molecular Mimicry

Molecular mimicry has been raised as an important hypothesis to explain the onset of inappropriate responses to self-antigens in some autoimmune diseases. This mechanism is defined by the presence of shared amino acid (aa) regions between foreign and self-proteins. Examples of presumed mimicry have been reported for epitopes recognized by both T- and B-cells. In the mimicry model, the initiation of autoimmune symptoms is believed to be the result of the persistence of immune cells generated by the host in response to an infectious agent (see Fig. 1A). These cells then recognize similar or identical epitopes within host tissue (see Fig. 1B). True molecular mimicry is marked by the cross-reactivity of a strong microbial antigen with a tissue-specific or ubiquitous host epitope. Once an immune response is generated, the persistence of the microbial antigen is not necessary for the maintenance of the immune response.

Several lines of evidence suggest that cross-reactive T-cell epitopes must be identical or nearly identical in linear amino acid sequence to the initiating microbial region. The length of the linear sequence, usually at least 12–14 amino acids for major histocompatibility complex (MHC) class II (1,2), is limited by the size of peptide that can be processed and presented by the MHC molecule and recognized by the T-cell receptor (TCR). Certain amino acids within the peptide epitope are necessary for binding to the MHC in the binding groove through their side-chain interactions (see Fig. 2, dark ovals). Because of conformational constraints, the side chains from alternate amino acids extend away from the MHC molecule. These amino acids form the surface that the TCRs on the reactive T-cell recognizes (see Fig. 2, gray ovals). As illustrated, there are amino acids that are necessary for binding to the MHC, and others for binding to the TCR (3). The side chains of these amino acids must fit into pockets of the receptors. Some amino acids do not appear to be specific for binding either TCR or MHC, which suggests that some variability in linear amino acid sequence can be tolerated (see Fig. 2, white ovals). Additional MHC-binding flexibility may occur, as long as the side-chain characteristics of the peptide (i.e., acidic, basic, hydrophobic, etc.) remain the same (4). For B-cell or antibody epitopes, on the other hand, similar three-dimensional motifs are required and amino acids that make up the mimicry confirmation may be spaced many amino acids apart.

Lyme arthritis is caused by infection with *Borrelia burgdorferi* (*Bb*) transmitted through the bite of an infected *Ixodes* tick. In some individuals, the symptoms of arthritis persist despite long courses of antibiotics given to eradicate the spirochetes. These individuals have treatment-resistant Lyme arthritis (TRLA) and often have MHC class II alleles that are also associated with an other inflammatory disease, rheumatoid arthritis (5). Furthermore, these patients develop detectable antibody and T-cell proliferative responses to outer surface protein A (OspA) of *Bb* that correlate with the onset of

From: *Cytokines and Chemokines in Infectious Diseases Handbook*
Edited by: M. Kotb and T. Calandra © Humana Press Inc., Totowa, NJ

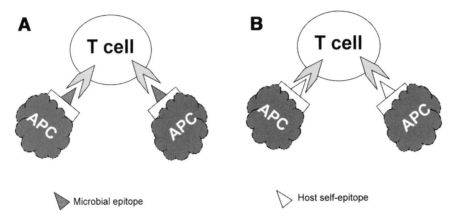

Fig. 1. Mimicry epitopes. **(A)** During microbial infection, the host antigen-presenting cells (APCs) process microbial proteins and present epitopes that have been selected by their ability to bind to major histocompatibility complex (MHC) molecules on the cell surface. T-Cells with T-cell receptors specific for the microbial antigenic epitope recognize the specific peptide/MHC complex, become activated, and expand. **(B)** Expanded population of T-cells specific for the microbial epitope recognize homologous host-specific epitopes, remain activated, and mediate further inflammation or tissue damage.

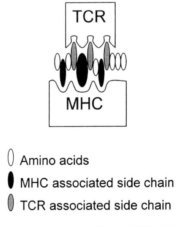

Fig. 2. A 12-amino-acid peptide interacts with the MHC and TCR. Side chains from selected amino acids fit into binding pockets of the MHC molecule, leaving other amino acid side chains exposed to TCRs. When the TCR recognizes and binds the peptide presented in this manner and other costimulatory molecules are bound by their ligands on the antigen-presenting cell, a signal is transmitted to the T-cell to become activated.

the chronic phase of disease *(6,7)*. Fine epitope mapping experiments revealed that T-cells from affected individuals respond to specific regions of the OspA molecule. Given these observations, we propose a mechanism of molecular mimicry to explain the phenomenon of TRLA in genetically susceptible individuals. To test the significance of the molecular mimicry hypothesis, we compared the amino acid sequence of the immunodominant *Bb* epitope to protein database information to determine if there were homologous human peptides. Gross et al. from our laboratory reported a striking correlation between the T-cell response to $OspA_{164-175}$ and the human protein $LFA-1\alpha L_{332-340}$ *(8)*, thereby defining $LFA-1\alpha L_{332-340}$ as a crossreactive epitope. Further experiments with synovial fluid cells from affected joints of patients with TRLA confirmed the cross-reactive response *(8)*. Leukocyte function antigen (LFA)-1 is a protein that is abundantly expressed on T- and B-cells, with the highest expression on T-cell blasts. Also, LFA-1 is upregulated by interferon (IFN)-γ an inflammatory cytokine *(9)*. Consequently, LFA-1 is an excellent crossreactive candidate because it is found at high levels in the inflammatory milieu of the Lyme-diseased joint *(10)*. Thus, a link is established between the generation of an immune response to *Bb* antigens during infection and the possible misdirection of that response to other epitopes, including one that is highly homologous to a self-protein found at the site of disease.

1.2. Models of Molecular Mimicry

Molecular mimicry was first described in the early 1980s in the context of antibody responses to viruses and self *(11,12)*. The first observations included the identification of viruses containing antigenic epitopes with similar or identical host determinants. Virus-specific monoclonal antibodies were identified that crossreacted with host epitopes, implicating crossreactive epitopes in the development of autoimmunity. Remarkably, once the immune response to the crossreactive epitope was initiated, the microbe did not need to be present for the persistence of the immune response. T-Cell-mediated molecular mimicry was first reported when homology between hepatitis B virus polymerase and myelin basic protein (MBP) was identified *(13)*. This six-amino-acid region of homology was found within a known encephalitogenic region of the MBP molecule. Interestingly, upon immunization of rabbits with a peptide containing the homologous region, rabbits developed T-cell responses to MBP and evidence of central nervous system (CNS) infiltration with mononuclear cells resulting in subclinical experimental autoimmune encephalitis (EAE) *(13)*. Today, molecular mimicry has been implicated in several other animal models of autoimmune disease, including autoimmune uveitis *(14)* and heart disease *(15)*, among others reviewed in refs. *16–18*.

The role of mimicry in disease pathogenesis can only be tested experimentally in animal models. Unfortunately, animal models are unavailable for many diseases for which possible microbial mimics have been identified. Still, many cases of mimicry have been demonstrated in vitro following the identification of crossreactive epitopes *(17)*. However, there are only a few instances in which there is convincing in vivo evidence for mimicry as the causative factor for disease, such as in murine herpes keratitis. In humans, herpes keratitis is a major cause of blindness. A model of disease can be induced in genetically susceptible mice by infection with herpes simplex virus-1 (HSV-1) containing the wild-type herpes virion-associated protein, UL6. Destruction of the cornea is the result of the induction of T-cell-mediated inflammation *(19)*. Researchers proceeded to develop keratitis-inducing T-cell lines by which they determined the identity of the keratin-specific protein involved. A database search for homologous microbial peptides revealed UL6, a HSV-1 peptide with strong homology to the keratitis-inducing host epitope *(see* Table 1*)*. When the viral UL6 protein was mutated, altering the mimicry epitope, infection with mutated virus no longer induced keratitis, presumably because T-cells specific for corneal antigens are not expanded upon infection. Meanwhile, the possible epidemiological connection between chlamydia infection and human heart disease was explored in another mouse model of autoimmune disease elicited by microbial mimicry *(15)*. In this model, immunization of mice with a peptide from the *Chlamydia* cysteine-rich outer membrane protein (ChTR1) with strong homology to heart muscle-specific α-myosin heavy chain, results in damage to heart tissue and activation of self-reactive T-cells. Thus, it is possible to experimentally induce destructive self-reactive responses using microbial mimics *(see* Table 1*)*.

1.3. Searching for Mimics

Conventionally, the TCR of the T-helper cell identifies a peptide of approximately 12 amino acids presented in the peptide-binding groove of MHC class II molecules. Along the length of the peptide, certain amino acids are necessary for anchoring the peptide to the MHC molecule; these are essentially invisible to the TCR *(see* Fig. 2*)*. Alternate amino acids are oriented such that they are pre-

Table 1
Mimicry Peptide Identified

Diseases association	Organism	Peptide	Homology	aa sequence
Herpes stromal keratitis *(19)*	Human	IgG2a^b/cornea	Linear	**RKSDSERG**
	HSV-1	UL6$_{299-314}$	Linear	**RKSDXERG**
Treatment-resistant Lyme arthritis *(8)*	Human	LFA-1αL$_{332-340}$	Linear	**YVIEGTSKQ**
	B. burgdorferi	OspA$_{165-173}$	Linear	**YVLEGTLTA**
Heart disease *(15)*	Human	Myosin$_{614-629}$	Linear	SLKLMATLFSTYASAD
	Clamydia	ChTR1$_{25-40}$	Linear	VLETSMAEFTSTNVIS
Multiple sclerosis *(20)*	Human	MBP$_{85-99}$	Consensus	ENPVVHFFKNIVTPR
	Epstein–Barr virus	DNA polymerase		TGGVYHFVKKHVHES
	Influenza type A	Hemagglutinin		YRNLVWFIKKNTRYP
	HSV	DNA polymerase		GGRRLFFVKAHVRES

sented to the TCR, forming a surface that is shaped by the way the peptide lies in the groove of the MHC molecule. How a peptide binds MHC is determined by the amino acid side chain–MHC binding pocket interaction, which is determined by the characteristics of the amino acid side chains. Thus, homologous peptides can be identified in at least two ways. In the first method, databases are searched for highly homologous host peptides using linear amino acid sequences of immunodominant microbial peptides *(8,19)*. In the second method, large numbers of peptides are screened using various peptide-screening methods. In one example, a peptide library is synthesized that contains a pool of peptides that may retain amino acids required for binding to MHC, and other amino acids are substituted at all other positions. Following a screen of the library using peptide-specific T-cell lines, a consensus peptide can be identified and used to search protein databases *(20,21)*. The latter method often identifies the minimal peptide requirements. Then, proteins containing the consensus peptides are tested for cross-reactivity with the peptide-specific T-cell line (*see* Table 1).

Often, multiple sclerosis (MS) patients report symptoms of microbial infection just prior to the onset of a relapse. However, no single virus or bacteria has been identified as the responsible agent. Given the association of relapses with infectious disease, molecular mimicry has been implicated in the context of multiple sclerosis. To test this hypothesis, Wucherpfennig and his collaborators generated MBP$_{85-99}$ specific T-cell clones from an HLA DRB1*1501$^+$ individual with multiple sclerosis *(20)*. The authors characterized the peptide binding the MHC molecule and developed a set of peptide structural criteria with which they could search protein databases. They synthesized candidate peptides and then tested their ability to stimulate MS T-cell clones. After screening more than 70 microbial peptides restricted by minimal sequence requirements, they determined that the T-cell clones could respond to minimally similar peptides from a variety of microbes, including HSV, adenovirus, Epstein–Barr virus (EBV), influenza type A virus, and *Pseudomonas aeruginosa* (*see* Table 1). They determined that despite minimal sequence similarity between them, these peptides may efficiently stimulate MBP$_{85-99}$-specific T-cell clones. These peptides, derived from many different organisms, could stimulate self-specific clones, even though the peptides lack significant linear sequence homology to the human self-epitope. Furthermore, Quaratino et al. *(23)* argue that it is the "antigenic surface" that determines a T-cell's recognition of a peptide. They reported that this surface could be made up of as few as three amino acids and is created when the peptide binds to the MHC to be presented to the T-cell. They used a 12-amino-acid peptide derived from thyroid peroxidase to stimulate a T-cell clone generated from an individual with Grave's disease. When other peptides were presented to the same T-cells, only those that form a similar antigenic surface were stimulatory, even when 8 of 12 of the other amino acids were identical to the original peptide.

Alternatively, molecular mimicry has been defined by homology at the linear sequence level. First, as mentioned earlier, we have identified peptides with strong linear homology to a *Bb* OspA. When GenBank was searched using one of the immunodominant epitopes of OspA, relatively few human proteins with a linear sequence homology of six aa were identified, including the LFA-1αL chain *(8)*. In vitro experiments confirmed that the LFA-derived sequence was stimulatory to OspA T-cell lines. Second, in heart disease, infection with *Chlamydia* species has been linked to cardiovascular disease in humans through an unknown mechanism *(24,25)*. In an experimental model of heart disease, injection of chlamydia-derived peptides with linear homology to murine heart muscle-specific α-myosin causes mice to develop inflammatory heart disease *(15)*. Third, in an other example of linear homology, Zhao et al. *(19)* identified the peptide mimic of the corneal self-antigen epitope (and coincidentally an epitope also found in a variant of the mouse IgG2a molecule), using linear sequence homology comparisons. T-Cell clones generated to recognize corneal antigens also respond to the HSV-1-associated highly homologous peptide (in which seven or eight amino acids are identical) *(19)*. It is not clear if results from experiments using the minimal TCR surface or the full linear epitope reveal truly different mechanisms of mimicry or are simply different approaches attempting to answer the same question: What causes autoimmunity?

2. LYME DISEASE

2.1. Natural History of the Causative Organism

In the United States, Lyme disease is caused by infection with the tick-borne spirochete *B. burgdorferi (Bb)*. In Europe, disease may be caused by *B. afzelii* and *B. garinii*, in addition to *B. burgdorferi (26)*. The spirochete is transmitted to human hosts via ticks of the *Ixodes* species during feeding. In the eastern United States, the larval tick becomes infected during its earliest feed from *Bb*-infected white-footed mice, *Peromyscus leucopus (27)*. In some regions, this leads to high rates of infection among ixodes ticks *(28)*. Ticks feed at each stage of their life cycle: larval, nymphal, and adult. Although during the fall, adult ticks preferentially feed and mate on deer, *Odocoileus virginianus*; during the early summer, nymphal ticks may feed on humans, making them inadvertent hosts *(27)*.

Following attachment of the tick to the host and the initiation of the blood meal, the number of *Bb* within the tick's midgut expressing OspA, an outer surface lipoprotein found on the surface of the spirochete as well as in the periplasmic space between the outer membrane and cell wall *(29)*, begins to decline. Meanwhile, OspC expression increases and the spirochete migrates to the tick's salivary glands, where it is poised to be transmitted to the host *(30)*. These, as well as other variably expressed outer surface proteins (A–E), are thought to help the spirochete adapt to its different host environments *(31)*. Further, once in the human host, the spirochete may use other surface-expressed proteins to home to target tissues. For example, decorin-binding proteins A and B allow disseminated *Bb* to bind to collagen fibrils in the extracellular matrix of heart, nervous system, or joints *(32)*, where it may cause symptoms associated with infection.

2.2. Disease Symptoms

Once *Bb* spirochete has entered the host, infection may cause Lyme disease. Erythema migrans rash, the pathognemonic for *Bb* infection, is observed in about 80% of patients. It is marked by concentric rings of erythema and clearing surrounded by an expanding ring, giving it a bull's-eye like appearance. *Bb* can be isolated from the outer ring and, eventually, the infection is spread to target tissues hematogenously *(33)*. Additionally, infected individuals may complain of flulike symptoms, including fever, aches, and fatigue. If the infection is left untreated, then symptoms may include severe headache, mild neck stiffness, atrioventricular block, oligoarticular arthritis, intense joint inflammation, encephalopathy, and cognitive disturbance *(34,35)*. In the United States, if the infection proceeds without treatment, then approx 60% of infected individuals develop symptoms of arthritis

(36). Patients with symptoms of Lyme disease are treated with antibiotics that presumably clear *Bb* from the host.

In about 10% of individuals with Lyme arthritis, symptoms are not alleviated by one or more courses of antibiotics *(5).* These individuals have TRLA. When synovium or synovial fluid from these patients is tested for *Bb* DNA by polymerase chain reaction (PCR) analysis, results are almost always negative *(37,38),* indicating that *Bb* has been eliminated. Kalish et al. *(6)* reported that patients with TRLA are more likely to have antibodies specific for OspA than patients whose arthritis is responsive to antibiotic treatment. Likewise, Kamrandt et al. *(39)* reported that T-cells specific for OspA can be preferentially found in patients with TRLA compared with responsive disease. Furthermore, these OspA-reactive T-cells are of the Th1 phenotype, making IFN-γ and not IL-4 *(40).* Thus, an interesting question remains as to why individuals infected with *Bb* generate antibody and T-cell responses to OspA during the later course of infection, and continue to produce such antibodies after therapeutic antibiotic treatment is completed and the *Bb* are presumably eradicated.

2.3. Association of TRLA With HLA Class II and the Immune Response

One of the first indications that TRLA was associated with a possible autoimmune response was the strong correlation of treatment-resistant disease with limited HLA haplotypes often associated with severe rheumatoid arthritis *(41,42).* Specifically, the alleles HLA-DRB1*0401, *0404, *0101, and *0102 are associated with the majority of patients with treatment resistant Lyme arthritis *(5).* These alleles share hypervariable region 3 (HVR3), found in the membrane distal domain *(43),* but are otherwise quite distinct. The HVR3 constitutes precisely the region that forms the peptide-binding pocket of the molecule *(41).* Thus, the common HVR3 predicts a similarity in the peptides bound by this group of MHC molecules. Because the main function of MHC molecules is to present peptides to T-cells, this is an indication that T-cells are important in the generation of disease.

The association of a particular MHC class II molecule with TRLA suggests that T-cell stimulation by presented peptides is likely to be important in the persistence of arthritis. Bulk proliferative responses to the protein and various fragments and peptides derived from whole OspA have been identified in Lyme arthritis *(44–46).* These responding T-cells were found to be of the Th1 type, secreting the proinflammatory T-helper cytokine IFN-γ *(47,48),* and could be easily recovered from the synovial fluid of individuals with TRLA *(8).* Recently, Chen et al. showed that Th1 responses to OspA correlate with the severity and duration of Lyme arthritis *(49).* These T-cells can be identified in the synovial fluid of patients with TRLA months to years after antibiotic treatment, but not in other chronic arthritides *(8).*

3. MOLECULAR MIMICRY IN TRLA

3.1. Identification of an OspA-Homologous Protein, LFA-1

Observations suggested that the persistent symptoms of TRLA were the result of an ongoing immune response because of the following reasons. First, patients with TRLA developed T-and B-cell responses to *Bb* OspA correlating well with the occurrence of the treatment-resistant phase of arthritis. Second, because there was a limited HLA class II association in individuals with TRLA, there was the possibility for T-cell involvement in the persistence of arthritis symptoms. Once the immunodominant epitopes of OspA were determined for a subset of patients with the HLA DRB1*0401 haplotype (DR4), the OspA peptide 165–173 emerged as a promising candidate for searching human peptide databases for possible crossreactive epitopes *(8).* Early GenBank searches revealed an epitope within human LFA-1αL, amino acids 332–340 as a homolog *(see* Table 1). Analysis of the peptide using a HLA-binding algorithm predicted that the peptide would be bound by DR4 and thus could be presented to T-cells in a DR4 host. Testing of the epitope and whole LFA-1 molecules confirmed that bulk populations of T-cells responsive to OspA were also responsive to the human homolog, LFA-1αL *(8).*

We wanted to demonstrate at the single-cell level that a single TCR could recognize and respond to both the human LFA-1αL peptide and the bacterial mimic, OspA. We set out to clone T-cells using recently developed MHC class II tetrameric molecules *(50)*. The reagents we used consisted of approximately four biotinylated recombinant HLA DRB1*0401 molecules with covalently attached OspA peptides. Approximately four DR4-peptide molecules were bound together by a fluorescently labeled streptavidin molecule *(50)*. Using these reagents, we could identify and clone T-cells from patient samples that were specific for OspA 165–184 and sort them for cloning by fluorescence-activated cell sorting (FACS) *(51)*. When the OspA-specific clones were tested for their ability to respond to the crossreactive LFA-1αL epitope more than half of the clones responded to the self-peptide over a wide range *(see* Fig. 3) *(51)*. Thus, clones generated from a single T-cell with presumably a single TCR are able to respond to both *Bb* and human peptides.

3.2. Differential Cytokine Secretion

In autoimmune models, the nature of a T-cell response can be categorized in different ways. T-helper 1 (Th1) responses are often associated with T-cell-mediated inflammatory disease models such as experimental autoimmune encephalomyelitis, a model of multiple sclerosis *(53,54)*, and various models of diabetes *(55,56)*. Th1-associated cytokines include, most notably, IFN-γ and IL-2. On the other hand, Th2 responses are usually associated with T-cell regulatory responses because Th2 cytokines often counteract proinflammatory cytokines *(57)*, which results in downmodulating Th1-mediated responses. Th2 cytokines include IL-4, IL-5, IL-10, and, possibly, IL-13. Th2 cell products are also important for the generation and maintenance of B-cell responses to foreign antigens and influence the quality of antibodies secreted and thus are associated with antibody-based models of autoimmunity such as systemic lupus erythematosus *(58)*.

We compared characteristics of OspA/LFA-1αL-reactive versus OspA-only-reactive T-cell clones, measuring the amount of cytokines secreted in response to the stimulating antigen. In these dual-reactive clones, the response to OspA differs quantitatively and qualitatively from the response to LFA-1αL, as measured by proliferation and cytokine production *(see* Fig. 4). Interestingly, stimulation with OspA$_{165-184}$, a 20-aa peptide containing the possible mimicry epitope, induced vigorous proliferation and led to the secretion of large amounts of the Th1-type inflammatory cytokine IFN-γ *(see* Fig. 4A,B, open circles). However OspA stimulation also induced secretion of the likely Th2-type cytokines IL-4, IL-5, and IL-13 in almost all clones tested *(see* Fig. 4A,B, open circles). This OspA-induced cytokine-secretion profile is not easily categorized as Th1 or Th2 and may reflect a common characteristic of human antigen-specific T-cell lines. This is in contrast with the polarized pattern seen in murine T-cell lines *(59)* and models of autoimmunity. Alternately, when the stimulating antigen was LFA-1αL$_{326-345}$, containing the possible mimicry epitope, proliferation was reduced and dual reactive clones produced proportionally more IL-13 than IFN-γ *(see* Fig. 4A,B, filled circles). Although IL-13 has not been characterized yet as a Th2 or Th1 cytokine, it is closely associated with many Th2-associated functions *(60)*, along with a strong association with allergic reactions. In other studies, IL-13 has been shown to play a role in the deposition of fibrin following *Schistosoma* infection *(61)*. Thus, it is possible that LFA-1αL$_{326-345}$-stimulated, IL-13-secreting T-cells could be contributing to the persistent joint inflammation in chronic treatment-resistant Lyme patients.

Clearly, minor differences in the peptide *(see* Table 1) affect the quality and quantity of response to the signal delivered through the TCR. We found that the OspA peptide is strongly agonistic and induces a vigorous T-cell response, even at low concentrations of antigen, indicative of high-affinity TCR recognition. In contrast, the LFA-1αL peptide induces a less efficient interaction with TCR and produces different downstream effects, reminiscent of a partial agonist. Hemmer et al. *(62)* developed a mathematical algorithm that predicts how well a peptide will bind to a given MHC molecule based on its linear sequence of amino acids. In this case, the algorithm predicted that both the OspA$_{165-184}$ and LFA-1αL$_{326-345}$ peptides bind to the HLA-DRB1*0401 molecule with similar affinities *(62,63)*, suggesting that the two peptides are presented to the T-cell with equal efficiency.

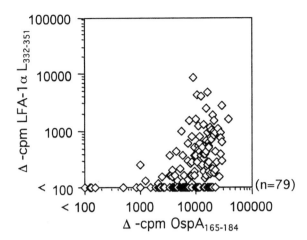

Fig. 3. T-cell clones generated from OspA-tetramer-sorted cells proliferate in response to OspA$_{165-184}$ and LFA-1αL$_{326-345}$. Cloned T-cells from a DRB1*0401$^+$ homozygous patient were cultured with OspA$_{165-184}$, LFA-1αL$_{326-345}$, or media alone plus autologous EBV-transformed B-cells. Data, OspA versus LFA response (open diamond), are expressed in D-cpm (cpm of wells with antigen–cpm of wells with media). From [Trollmo, C., Meyer, A.L., Steere, A.C., Hafler, D.A., and Huber, B.T. (2001) Molecular mimicry in Lyme arthritis demonstrated at the single cell level: LFA-1 alpha L is a partial agonist for outer surface protein A-reactive T cells. *J. Immunol.* **166**, 5286–5291]. Copyright 2001. The American Association of Immunologists.

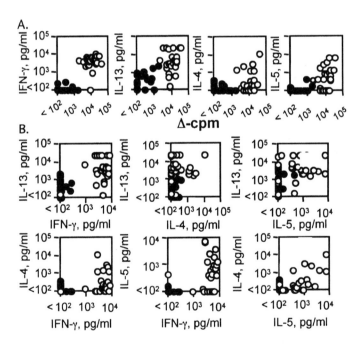

Fig. 4. Differential cytokine production profile of T-cell clones stimulated with Osp$_{165-184}$ (open cirlces), versus LFA-1αL$_{326-345}$ (closed circles). OspA-specific clones were cultured with antigen plus APC and tested for Th1 and Th2 cytokine production 48 h after stimulation, using standard capture enzyme-linked immunosorbent assay. Mean OD$_{450}$ values were calculated, and concentrations were determined from a standard curve. Data are expressed as a comparison (**A**) between D-cpm versus cytokines; and (**B**), Th1 and Th2 cytokines. From [Trollmo, C., Meyer, A.L., Steere, A.C., Hafler, D.A., and Huber, B.T. (2001) Molecular mimicry in Lyme arthritis demonstrated at the single cell level: LFA-1 alpha L is a partial agonist for outer surface protein A-reactive T cells. *J. Immunol.* **166,** 5286–5291]. Copyright 2001. The American Association of Immunologists.

Yet, despite this similarity in antigen presentation, the three-dimensional interaction of each peptide–MHC complex with the TCR differs. Perhaps IL-13 is a cytokine that characterizes weak but stable TCR–antigen interactions. How much T-cell-mediated inflammation in the joint is required to maintain chronic stimulation there is unknown. The question remains: Can LFA-induced T-cell stimulation in the joint maintain inflammatory arthritis?

3.3. The Possibility of Other Significant Molecular Mimicry Epitopes in TRLA

Molecular mimicry in the context of Lyme disease has been of great interest to several groups *(8,20,21,62)*. Experiments using T-cells isolated from patient populations *(8,20)* and T-cell hybridomas from two different HLA DR4 transgenic mouse models have generated varied results *(21,52)*. After mimicry, self-peptides were identified using database homology search and synthesized for in vitro analysis, many microbially specific T-cell lines have been shown to crossreact with human epitopes. In fact, experiments designed to explore the degeneracy of the TCR recognition requirements illustrate that TCRs are flexible and can recognize a surprisingly large collection of peptides in the context of MHC *(20,21)*. One group has identified at least 28 different amino acid sequences that could stimulate 1 or more of a panel of mouse T-cell hybridomas that were first shown to be specific for one specific epitope of OspA *(21)*. Meanwhile, the question remains: Are crossreactive T-cells generated in response to microbial antigen, responsible for the perpetuation of arthritis in the absence of *Bb*? These questions can only be more thoroughly studied once a mouse model of TRLA is developed. In such a model, crossreactive epitopes can be tested for their significance to disease. Given the large number of possible mimicry epitopes reported in studies of mimicry in Lyme arthritis and other disease models, it is surprising that autoimmunity is not more prevalent. The fact that we are not consumed by the effect of molecular mimicry induced autoimmunity raises interesting questions about the power of immune regulation.

4. SUMMARY AND DISEASE MODEL

Molecular mimicry in treatment-resistant Lyme arthritis is suggested by the presence of T-cells that respond both to microbial antigen OspA and to at least one human homolog, including LFA-1. Arthritis may persist in the joint by the following mechanism: In the *Bb*-induced inflammatory joint, OspA is presented to T-cells in the context of class II expressed on the surface of macrophages and dendritic cells (*see* Fig. 1A). T-Cells responding to OspA produce high levels of IFN-γ, which leads to upregulation of LFA-1 on macrophages and T-cells in the joint. Once OspA-specific T-cells have expanded and a critical threshold is reached, these T-cells crossreact with the homologous LFA-1αL epitope presented by antigen-presenting cells (*see* Fig. 1B) in the joint. Responses to LFA-1αL are characterized by IL-13 production, which may contribute to the pathology of the inflamed joint. In this way, inflammation can continue in the joint after eradication of the spirochete once the response to self-epitope has been initiated as a result of the mechanism of molecular mimicry.

REFERENCES

1. Rudensky, A., Preston-Hurlburt, P., Hong, S.C., Barlow, A., and Janeway, C.A., Jr. 1991. Sequence analysis of peptides bound to MHC class II molecules. *Nature* **353,** 622–627.
2. Hemmer, B., Kondo, T., Gran, B., Pinilla, C., Cortese, I., Pascal, J., et al. (2000) Minimal peptide length requirements for CD4(+) T cell clones—implications for molecular mimicry and T cell survival. *Int. Immunol.* **12,** 375–383.
3. Vergelli, M., Hemmer, B., Kalbus, M., Vogt,A.B., Ling, N., Conlon, P., et al. (1997) Modifications of peptide ligands enhancing T cell responsiveness imply large numbers of stimulatory ligands for autoreactive T cells. *J Immunol* **158,** 3746–3752.
4. Murthy, V.L. and Stern, L.J. (1997) The class II MHC protein HLA-DR1 in complex with an endogenous peptide: implications for the structural basis of the specificity of peptide binding. *Structure* **5,**1385–1396.
5. Steere, A.C. and Baxter-Lowe, L.A. (1998) Association of chronic, treatment-resistant Lyme arthritis with rheumatoid arthritis (RA) alleles. *Arthritis Rheum.* **41,** S81.
6. Kalish, R.A., Leong, J.M., and Steere, A.C. (1995) Early and late antibody responses to full-length and truncated constructs of outer surface protein A of *Borrelia burgdorferi* in Lyme disease. *Infect. Immun.* **63,** 2228–2235.

7. Kamradt, T., Lengl-Janssen, B., Strauss, A.F., Bansal, G., and Steere, A.C. (1996) Dominant recognition of a Borrelia burgdorferi outer surface protein A peptide by T helper cells in patients with treatment-resistant Lyme arthritis. *Infect. Immun.* **64,** 1284–1289.

8. Gross, D.M., Forsthuber, T., Tary-Lehmann, M., Etling, C., Ito, K., Nagy, Z.A., et al. (1998) Identification of LFA-1 as a candidate autoantigen in treatment-resistant Lyme arthritis. *Science* **281,** 703–706.

9. Yokota, A., Murata, N., Saiki, O., Shimizu, M., Springer, T.A., and Kishimoto, T. (1995) High avidity state of leukocyte function-associated antigen-1 on rheumatoid synovial fluid T lymphocytes. *J. Immunol.* **155,** 4118–4124.

10. Akin, E., Aversa, J., and Steere, A.C. (2001) Expression of adhesion molecules in synovia of patients with treatment-resistant lyme arthritis. *Infect. Immun.* **69,** 1774–1780.

11. Fujinami, R.S., Oldstone, M.B., Wroblewska, Z., Frankel, M.E., and Koprowski, H. (1983) Molecular mimicry in virus infection: crossreaction of measles virus phosphoprotein or of herpes simplex virus protein with human intermediate filaments. *Proc. Natl. Acad. Sci. USA* **80,** 2346–2350.

12. Haynes, B.F., Robert-Guroff, M., Metzgar, R.S., Franchini, G., Kalyanaraman, V.S., Palker, T.J., et al. (1983) Monoclonal antibody against human T cell leukemia virus p19 defines a human thymic epithelial antigen acquired during ontogeny. *J. Exp. Med.* **157,** 907–920.

13. Fujinami, R.S. and Oldstone, M.B. (1985) Amino acid homology between the encephalitogenic site of myelin basic protein and virus: mechanism for autoimmunity. *Science* **230,** 1043–1045.

14. Singh, V.K., Yamaki, K., Abe, T., and Shinohara, T. (1989) Molecular mimicry between uveitopathogenic site of retinal S-antigen and *Escherichia coli* protein: induction of experimental autoimmune uveitis and lymphocyte cross-reaction. *Cell Immunol.* **122,** 262–273.

15. Bachmaier, K., Neu, N., de la Maza, L.M., Pal, S., Hessel, A., and Penninger, J.M. (1999) Chlamydia infections and heart disease linked through antigenic mimicry. *Science* **283,** 1335–1339.

16. Barnaba, V. and Sinigaglia, F. (1997) Molecular mimicry and T cell-mediated autoimmune disease. *J. Exp. Med.* **185,** 1529–1531.

17. Albert, L.J. and Inman, R.D. (1999) Molecular mimicry and autoimmunity. *N. Engl. J. Med.* **341,** 2068–2074.

18. Maverakis, E., van den Elzen, P., and Sercarz, E.E. (2001) Self-reactive T cells and degeneracy of T cell recognition: evolving concepts-from sequence homology to shape mimicry and TCR flexibility. *J. Autoimmun.* **16,** 201–209.

19. Zhao, Z.S., Granucci, F., Yeh, L., Schaffer, P.A., and Cantor, H. (1998) Molecular mimicry by herpes simplex virus-type 1: autoimmunie disease after viral infection. *Science* **279,** 1344–1347.

20. Wucherpfennig, K.W. and Strominger, J.L. (1995) Molecular mimicry in T cell-mediated autoimmunity: viral peptides activate human T cell clones specific for myelin basic protein. *Cell* **80,** 695–705.

21. Martin, R., Gran, B., Zhao, Y., Markovic-Plese, S., Bielekova, B., Marques, A., et al. (2001) Molecular mimicry and antigen-specific T cell responses in multiple sclerosis and chronic CNS Lyme disease. *J. Autoimmun.* **16,** 187–192.

22. Maier, B., Molinger, M., Cope, A.P., Fugger, L., Schneider-Mergener, J., Sonderstrup, G., et al. (2000) Multiple crossreactive self-ligands for *Borrelia burgdorferi*-specific HLA-DR4-restricted T cells. *Eur. J. Immunol.* **30,** 448–457.

23. Quaratino, S., Thorpe, C.J., Travers, P.J., and Londei, M. (1995) Similar antigenic surfaces, rather than sequence homology, dictate T-cell epitope molecular mimicry. *Proc. Nat. Acad. Sci. USA* **92,** 10,398–10,402.

24. Libby, P., Egan, D., and Skarlatos, S. (1997) Roles of infectious agents in atherosclerosis and restenosis: an assessment of the evidence and need for future research. *Circulation* **96,** 4095–4103.

25. Ridker, P.M., Kundsin, R.B., Stampfer, M.J., Poulin, S., and Hennekens, C.H. (1999) Prospective study of Chlamydia pneumoniae IgG seropositivity and risks of future myocardial infarction. *Circulation* **99,** 1161–1164.

26. Boerlin, P., Peter, O., Bretz, A.G., Postic, D., Baranton, G., and Piffaretti, J.C. (1992) Population genetic analysis of *Borrelia burgdorferi* isolates by multilocus enzyme electrophoresis. *Infect. Immun.* **60,** 1677–1683.

27. Lane, R.S., Piesman, J., and Burgdorfer, W. (1991) Lyme borreliosis: relation of its causitive agent to its tick vectors and hosts in North America and Europe. *Ann. Rev. Entomol.* **36,** 587–609.

28. Brunet, L.R., Spielman, A., and Telford, S.R., III. (1995) Short Report: Density of Lyme disease spirochetes within deer ticks collected from zoonotic sites. *Am. J. Trop. med. Hyg.* **53,** 300–302.

29. Schaible, U.E., Kramer, M.D., Eichmann, K., Modolell, M., Museteanu, C., and Simon, M.M. (1990) Monoclonal antibodies specific for the outer surface protein A (OspA) of *Borrelia burgdorferi* prevent Lyme borreliosis in severe combined immunodeficiency (scid) mice. *Proc. Nat. Acad Sci. USA* **87,** 3768–3772.

30. Schwan, T.G., Piesman, J., Golde, W.T., Dolan, M.C., and Rosa, P.A. (1995) Induction of an outer surface protein on Borrelia burgdorferi during tick feeding. *Proc. Nat. Acad Sci. USA* **92,** 2909–2913.

31. de Silva, A.M. and Fikrig, E. (1997) Arthropod- and host-specific gene expression by *Borrelia burgdorferi. J. Clin. Invest.* **99,** 377.

32. Guo, B.P., Brown, E.L., Dorward, D.W., Rosenberg, L.C., and Hook, M. (1998) Decorin-binding adhesins from *Borrelia burgdorferi. Mol. Microbiol.* **30,** 711–723.

33. Sigal, L.H. (1997) Lyme disease: a review of aspects of its immunology and immunopathogenesis. *Ann. Rev Immunol.* **15,** 63–92.

34. Steere, A.C. (2001) Lyme disease. *N. Engl. J. Med.* **345,** 115–125.

35. Steere, A.C., Levin, R.E., Molloy, P.J., Kalish, R.A., Abraham, J.H.R., Liu, N.Y., et al. (1994) Treatment of Lyme arthritis. *Arthritis Rheum* **37,** 878–888.

36. Steere, A.C. (1989) Lyme disease. *N. Engl. J. Med.* **321,** 586–596.

37. Nocton, J.J., Dressler, F., Rutledge, B.J., Rys, P.N., Persing, D.H., and Steere, A.C. (1994) Detection of *Borrelia burgdorferi* DNA by polymerase chain reaction in synovial fluid from patients with Lyme arthritis. *N. Engl. J. Med.* **330,** 229.

38. Carlson, D., Hernandez, J., Bloom, B.J., Coburn, J. Aversa, J.M., and Steere, A.C. (1999) Lack of *Borrelia burgdorferi* DNA in synovial samples from patients with antibiotic treatment-resistant Lyme arthritis. *Arthritis Rheum.* **42,** 2705–2709.

39. Kamradt, T., Krause, A., and Burmester, G.R. (1995) A role for T cells in the pathogenesis of treatment-resistant Lyme arthritis. *Mol. Med.* **1,** 486–490.

40. Gross, D. M., Steere, A.C., and Huber, B.T. (1998) T helper 1 response is dominant and localized to the synovial fluid in patients with Lyme arthritis. *J. Immunol.* **160,** 1022–1028.

41. Gregersen, P.K. (1992) T-cell receptor-major histocompatibility complex genetic interactions in rheumatoid arthritis. *Rheum. Dis. Clin. North Am.* **18,** 793–807.

42. Weyand, C. M. and Goronzy, J.J. (1999) HLA polymorphisms and T cells in rheumatoid arthritis. *Int. Rev. Immunol.* **18,** 37–59.

43. Sherritt, M.A., Tait, B., Varney, M., Kanaan, C., Stockman, A., Mackay, I.R., et al. (1996) Immunosusceptibility genes in rheumatoid arthritis. *Hum. Immunol.* **51,** 32–40.

44. Sigal, L.H., Steere, A.C., Freeman, D.H., and Dwyer, J.M. (1986) Proliferative responses of mononuclear cells in Lyme disease. Reactivity to *Borrelia burgdorferi* antigens is greater in joint fluid than in blood. *Arthritis Rheum.* **29,** 761–769.

45. Yoshinari, N.H., Reinhardt, B.N., and Steere, A.C. (1991) T cell responses to polypeptide fractions of *Borrelia burgdorferi* in patients with Lyme arthritis. *Arthritis Rheum.* **34,** 707–713.

46. Krause, A., Burmester, G.R., Rensing, A., Schoerner, C., Schaible, U.E., Simon, M.M., et al. (1992) Cellular immune reactivity to recombinant OspA and flagellin from *Borrelia burgdorferi* in patients with Lyme borreliosis. Complexity of humoral and cellular immune responses. *J. Clin. Invest.* **90,** 1077–1084.

47. Oksi, J., Savolainen, J., Pene, J., Bousquet, J., Laippala, B., and Viljanen, M.K. (1996) Decreased interleukin-4 and increased gamma interferon production by peripheral blood mononuclear cells of patients with Lyme borreliosis. *Infect. Immun.* **64,** 3620–3623.

48. Yssel, H., Shanafelt, M.C., Soderberg, C., Schneider, P.V., Anzola, J., and Peltz, G. (1991) *Borrelia burgdorferi* activates a T helper type 1-like T cell subset in Lyme arthritis. *J. Exp. Med.* **174,** 593–601.

49. Chen, J., Field, J.A., Glickstein, L., Molloy, P.J., Huber, B.T., and Steere, A.C. (1999) Association of antibiotic treatment-resistant Lyme arthritis with T cell responses to dominant epitopes of outer surface protein A of *Borrelia burgdorferi. Arthritis Rheum.* **42,** 1813–1822.

50. Crawford, F., Kozono, H., White, J., Marrack, P., and Kappler, J. (1998) Detection of antigen-specific T cells with multivalent soluble class II MHC covalent peptide complexes. *Immunity* **8,** 675–682.

51. Meyer, A.L., Trollmo, C., Crawford, F., Marrack, P., Steere, A., Huber, B.T., et al. (2000) Direct enumeration of Borrelia reactive CD4 T cells ex vivo using MHC class II tetramers. *P.N.A.S.* **97,** 11,433–11,438.

52. Trollmo, C., Meyer, A.L., Steere, A.C., Hafler, D.A., and Huber, B.T. (2001) Molecular mimicry in Lyme arthritis demonstrated at the single cell level: LFA-1 alpha L is a partial agonist for outer surface protein A-reactive T cells. *J. Immunol.* **166,** 5286–5291.

53. Hemmer, B., Vergelli, M., Calabresi, P., Huang, T., McFarland, H.F., and Martin, R. (1996) Cytokine phenotype of human autoreactive T cell clones specific for the immunodominant myelin basic protein peptide (83–99). *J. Neurosci. Res.* **45,** 852–862.

54. Voskuhl, R.R., Martin, R., Bergman, C., Dalal, M., Ruddle, N.H., and McFarland, H.F. (1993) T Helper 1 (Th1) functional phenotype of human myelin basic protein-specific T lymphocytes. *Autoimmunity* **15,** 137–143.

55. Katz, J.D., Benoist, C., and Mathis, D. (1995) T Helper cell subsets in insulin-dependent diabetes. *Science* **268,** 1185–1188.

56. Liblau, R.S., Singer, S.M., and McDevitt, H.O. (1995) Th1 and Th2 CD4+ T cells in the pathogenesis of organ-specific autoimmune diseases. *Immunol. Today* **16,** 34–38.

57. Romagnani, S. (1999) Th1/Th2 cells. *Inflamm. Bowel Dis.* **5,** 285–294.

58. Amel-Kashipaz, M.R., Huggins, M.L., Lanyon, P., Robins, A., Todd, I., and Powell, R.J. (2001) Quantitative and qualitative analysis of the balance between type 1 and type 2 cytokine-producing cd8(-)and cd8(+)t cells in systemic lupus erythematosus. *J. Autoimmun.* **17,** 155–163.

59. Cherwinski, H.M., Schumacher, J.M., Brown, K.D., and Mosmann, T.R. (1987) Two types of mouse helper T cell clone. III. Further differences in lymphokine synthesis between Th1 and Th2 clones revealed by RNA hybridization, functionally monospecific bioassays, and monoclonal antibodies. *J. Exp. Med.* **166,** 1229–1244.

60. Chomarat, P. and Banchereau, J. (1998) Interleukin-4 and interleukin-13: their similarities and discrepancies. *Int. Rev. Immunol.* **17,** 1–52.

61. Fallon, P.G., Richardson, E.J., McKenzie, G.J., and McKenzie, A.N.J. (2000) Schistosome infection of transgenic mice defines distinct and contrasting pathogenic roles for IL-4 and Il-13: IL-13 is a profibrotic agent.*J. Immunol.* **164,** 2585–2591.

62. Hemmer, B., Gran, B., Zhao, Y., Marques, A., Pascal, J., Tzou, A., et al. (1999) Identification of candidate T-cell epitopes and molecular mimics in chronic Lyme disease. *Nat. Med.* **5,** 1375–.

63. Hammer, J., Gallazzi, F., Bono, E., Karr, R.W., Guenot, J., Valsasnini, P., et al. (1995) Peptide binding specificity of HLA-DR4 molecules: correlation with rheumatoid arthritis association. *J. Exp. Med.* **181,** 1847–1855.

14

Cytokine Responses in Patients with Pneumonia

Peter Kragsbjerg and Hans Holmberg

1. INTRODUCTION

The importance of proinflammatory cytokines was first appreciated in studies of patients with sepsis or septic shock, but during the 1990s, the research expanded to include a wide range of infectious and other inflammatory conditions. The first investigations of the role of cytokines in lower-respiratory-tract infections were published in 1992. Since then, clinical studies have been performed on different aspects of inflammation in pneumonia. One group of studies focuses on the pathogenesis of bacterial pneumonia. A second group studies the relation between the microbial etiology of pneumonia and the ensuing inflammatory response. A third group relates the cytokine response in bacterial pneumonia to severity [i.e., SIRS (1), APACHE II (2), or other clinical scoring systems]. A fourth group of studies investigates the role of age in relation to the inflammatory response caused by an acute bacterial pneumonia. Finally, in a few studies, the impact of immunomodulating therapy has been investigated.

The methods for the detection and quantification of cytokine levels vary considerably between different studies, which makes the comparison of results difficult. As sample preparation and storage also influence cytokine measurements, uniform handling of samples is of major importance. In the present chapter, we review the findings presented thus far describing the cytokine responses in adult human subjects with pneumonia. The results are discussed from a clinical point of view.

2. CYTOKINE RESPONSES AND PATHOGENESIS OF BACTERIAL PNEUMONIA

The role of cytokines in the pathogenesis of bacterial infection was primarily studied in patients with septic conditions. As cytokines were found to be central mediators of inflammation, research was soon broadened to include focal infections as well as other inflammatory conditions.

Interleukin (IL)-8 was first demonstrated in bronchial secretions from 105 of 151 patients undergoing mechanical ventilation in the intensive care unit (ICU) (3). When patients with severe pneumonia were compared to patients with acute respiratory distress syndrome (ARDS), elevated broncho-alveolar lavage (BAL) fluid levels of IL-8 were correlated to severity (4). Patients with pneumonia had lower levels of BAL IL-8 than patients with ARDS, but plasma IL-8 concentrations were similar in the two groups. In 42 patients with community-acquired pneumonia (CAP), blood levels of tumor necrosis factor (TNF)-α, IL-6, and soluble IL-2R were compared to polymorpho-nuclear leukocyte and monocyte chemiluminescence response showing elevated levels of cytokines and activated phagocytes in most patients compared to controls (5). The inflammatory response to pneumonia is compartmentalized to the affected lung, as shown by Dehoux et al. (6). In 15 patients

From: *Cytokines and Chemokines in Infectious Diseases Handbook*
Edited by: M. Kotb and T. Calandra © Humana Press Inc., Totowa, NJ

with unilateral pneumonia, the BAL fluid levels of TNF-α, IL-1β, and IL-6 were determined in the affected lung and compared with the levels in the nonaffected lung. BAL fluid levels of all three cytokines were higher in the involved lung compared to the noninvolved lung (*see* Fig. 1). In a later study, a similar result was obtained for IL-8 *(7)* (*see* Fig. 2). The concentrations of IL-8 and another CXC chemokine, growth-related oncogene (GRO)-α were measured in BAL fluid from patients with bacterial pneumonia (*n* = 12), ARDS (*n* = 13), or *Pneumocystis carinii* pneumonia (*n* = 48) *(8)*. Patients with bacterial pneumonia and patients with ARDS had comparable levels of IL-8 and GRO-α suggesting a role also for GRO-α as a chemoattractant in inflammatory conditions in the lung. BAL fluid concentrations and blood concentrations of TNF-α IL-6 and IL-8 were compared in a study of 74 mechanically ventilated patients *(9)*. Patients with bacterial pneumonia and/or ARDS had comparable high levels of IL-6 and IL-8 but no consistently detectable TNF-α in BAL fluid. In blood, the levels of IL-6 and TNF-α were elevated in the group of patients with bacterial pneumonia and/or ARDS. Elevated concentrations of IL-8 in BAL fluid from 31 patients with CAP were also found by Bohnet et al. *(10)* and the levels of IL-8 in BAL fluid were higher in patients with positive microbiological results. Comparison of TNF-α, IL-6, and IL-8 mRNA levels in alveolar macrophages from patients with CAP and BAL fluid levels of the same three cytokines showed elevated mRNA content only for IL-8, but increased concentrations of IL-6 and IL-8 *(11)*. Another potent neutrophil chemoattractant, transforming growth factor (TGF)-β, was studied in 35 patients with pneumonia *(12)*. The BAL fluid concentrations of TGF-β and IL-8 were measured within 12 h from admission to hospital. The levels of TGF-β1, TGF-β2, and IL-8 were found to be elevated in patients with a defined microbiological etiology to the pneumonia. In patients with CAP (*n* = 8) or nosocomial pneumonia (*n* = 12) treated with mechanical ventilation in the ICU, serum levels of TNF-α and IL-6 were higher than the concentrations in the ventilated noninfectious controls *(13)*. BAL fluid levels of IL-6 were also higher in the pneumonia group, but there was no correlation between lung bacterial burden and BAL fluid cytokine levels. All patients with pneumonia in this study had received antibiotic treatment prior to inclusion into the study.

In summary, the studies presented so far have demonstrated the presence of several proinflammatory cytokines in secretions from the respiratory tract of patients with bacterial pneumonia. In most cases, this compartmentalized response is accompanied by a systemic response, primarily of IL-6.

3. CYTOKINE RESPONSES RELATED TO ETIOLOGY

3.1. Streptococcus pneumoniae

The patients included in studies of the cytokine responses in pneumonia vary considerably. In the studies with a well-documented etiology of the pneumonia *Streptococcus pneumoniae* is the most frequent isolated bacteria. In the studies of unilateral bacterial pneumonia, it was demonstrated that the cytokine response to *S. pneumoniae* is local *(6,7)*. BAL fluid concentrations of TNF-α, IL-1β, IL-6, and IL-8 were significantly higher in the involved lung compared to the noninvolved lung. None of the patients were bacteremic and serum TNF-α, IL-1β, and IL-8 levels were not different from those of the control groups. The absence of measurable levels of TNF-α, IL-1β, and IL-8 in the circulation in patients with pneumonia on admission to the hospital is in accordance with the results of other studies and most probably reflects an early brief appearance after onset of disease. However, serum concentrations of IL-6 were elevated in the patients with nonbacteremic pneumonia. The demonstration of elevated IL-6 in serum is in accordance with our studies of patients with pneumonia caused by specific microbial pathogens. In those studies, infections with *S. pneumoniae* were found to cause the highest levels of circulating IL-6 and the patients with bacteremic pneumococcal infection had the highest levels *(14)* (*see* Fig. 3). Most patients with bacterial pneumonia treated in the hospital have elevated serum IL-6, as shown by Örtqvist et al *(15)*. In that study, high levels of IL-6 were associated with longer duration of fever, longer stay in the hospital, and slower recovery, both clinically and radiographically. The finding of the highest levels of IL-6 among patients with pneumococcal

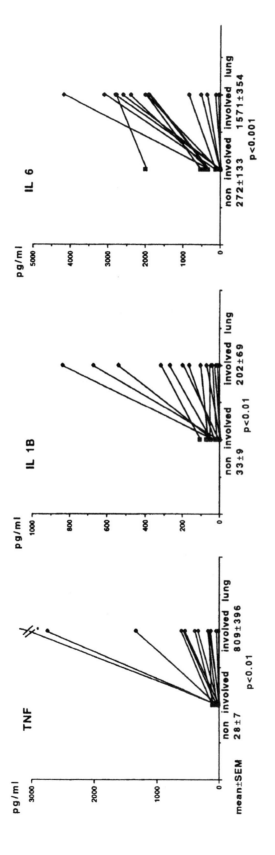

Fig. 1. IL-1β, TNF-α, and IL-6 concentrations in BAL fluids. Cytokines were measured by enzyme-linked immunosorbent assay in BAL fluids recovered from the involved lung and contralateral, noninvolved lung of patients with unilateral pneumonia ($n = 15$) prior to antibiotic therapy. (Reproduced from ref. 6 with permission.)

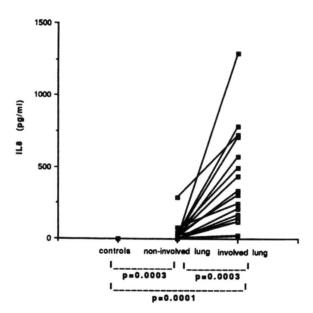

Fig. 2. IL-8 concentrations in BAL fluid recovered from the involved lungs and the contralateral, noninvolved lungs of patients with unilateral pneumonia (*n* = 17) prior to antibiotic therapy and from healthy controls (*n* = 8). (Reproduced from ref. *7* with permission.)

infection was confirmed in this study *(15)* and in a study of 20 patients with bacteremic pneumococcal pneumonia and 20 patients with pneumonia caused by *Mycoplasma (16)*. Bacteremic pneumococcal pneumonia was also found to be associated with high levels of IL-8 and granulocyte colony-stimulating factor (G-CSF) in serum in comparison to patients with pneumonia caused by atypical agents or influenza A infection *(17)* (*see* Fig 4). Patients with bacteremic pneumococcal pneumonia had high levels of IL-6 and G-CSF on admission to the hospital and the serum concentrations decreased within 24 h when appropriate antibiotic treatment was started promptly *(18)* (*see* Fig. 5). The levels of IL-6 were not significantly different from the serum concentrations in patients with bacteremic infections caused by β-hemolytic streptococci, *S. aureus*, or *Escherichia coli*. In bacteremic pneumococcal pneumonia the serum concentrations of G-CSF were higher than those in patients with bacteremic infections caused by other Gram-positive bacteria such as β-hemolytic streptococci and *S. aureus (18)*. Although the concentrations of TNF-α in serum were elevated also in patients with Gram-positive bacteremia including *S. pneumoniae*, the levels were significantly lower than those in patients with Gram-negative bacteremic infection *(18)*. The serum levels of TNF-α, IL-1β, IL-6, macrophage inflammatory protein (MIP)-1β, sTNF-R, IL-1RA, and IL-10 were measured on admission to the hospital and d 3 and 7 in 22 patients with pneumococcal pneumonia *(19)*. IL-6 decreased from high levels on admission to low levels on day 3 thus supporting previous findings. The levels of TNF-α, sTNF-R, IL-1RA, IL-6, and IL-10 showed sustained elevation on d 7 compared to the control group, indicating prolonged inflammatory activity. Thus, in patients with pneumonia, pneumococcal infections elicit the highest levels of IL-6 and G-CSF, which may have a potential for clinical use as markers of a pneumococcal etiology of the pneumonia.

3.2. Chlamydia pneumoniae, Mycoplasma pneumoniae, *and* Legionella

Few studies are performed on the cytokine responses in adult patients with atypical pneumonia. The first study comparing bacterial and atypical or viral agents was performed in 1993 *(14)*. In that study, it was shown that patients with pneumonia caused by *Chlamydia*, *Mycoplasma*, influenza A virus and respiratory syncytial (RS) virus, had lower serum concentrations of IL-6 compared to

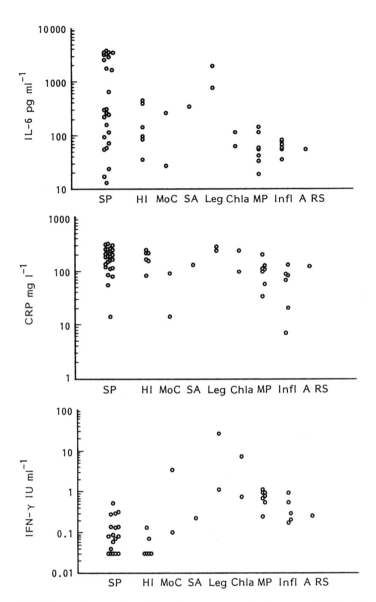

Fig. 3. Serum IL-6, C-reactive protein and interferon-γ_concentrations on admission in patients with pneumonia of different etiologies. SP: *S. pneumoniae* ($n = 27$), HI: *H. influenzae* ($n = 6$), MoC: *M. catarrhalis* ($n = 2$), SA: *S.aureus* ($n = 1$), Leg: *Legionella spp.* ($n = 2$), Chla: *Chlamydia spp.* ($n = 2$), MP: M. *pneumoniae* ($n = 7$), Infl A: influenza A ($n = 6$), RS: respiratory syncytial virus ($n = 1$). (Reproduced from ref. *14* with permission from Elsevier Science.)

patients with pneumonia caused by common bacterial pathogens such as *S. pneumoniae* and *H. influenzae*. In contrast, IFN-γ was shown to be elevated in the group with viral or atypical microorganisms. The finding of lower IL-6 levels in patients with atypical pneumonia such as *Mycoplasma* was supported by the three following studies. In a study of 203 patients with CAP, 16 patients with *Mycoplasma* and 13 patients with viral pneumonia were found to have lower levels compared to patients with pneumococcal pneumonia or other bacteremic pneumonia on admission to hospital *(15)*. Lieberman et al. compared 20 patients with bacteremic pneumococcal pneumonia with 20 patients with pneumonia caused by *Mycoplasma (16)*. Inversely, IL-1β was found to be higher in

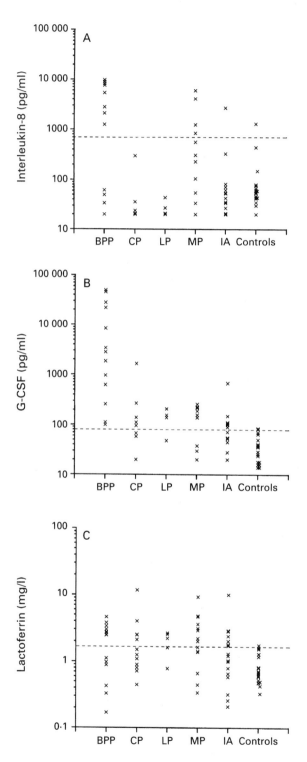

Fig. 4. Distribution of serum concentrations of IL-8 (**A**), G-CSF (**B**), and lactoferrin (**C**) in 63 patients with bacteremic pneumococcal pneumonia (BPP), *Chlamydia* pneumonia (CP), *Legionella* pneumonia(LP), *Mycoplasma* pneumonia (MP), influenza A infection (IA), and in 20 blood donors (controls). (Reproduced from ref. *(17)* with permission from the BMJ Publishing Group.)

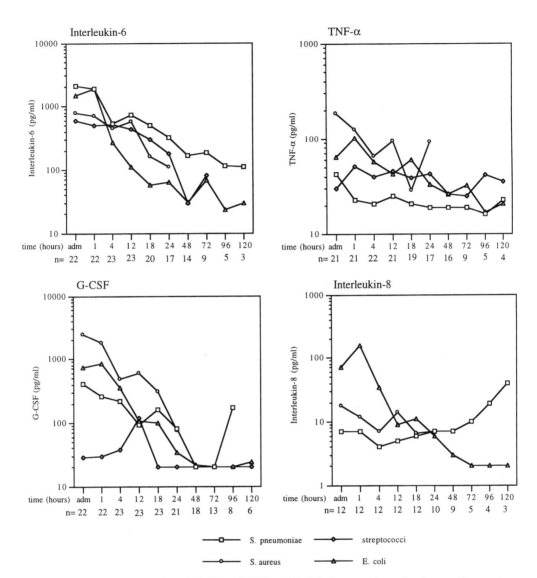

Fig. 5. Median serum levels of IL-6, TNF-α, G-CSF and IL-8 in bacteremic nonfatal cases. Time-points on the *x*-axis are admission (adm), 1 h later (*t* = 1), and 4, 12, 18, 24, 48, 72, 96, and 129 h from admission. *n* is the number of patients sampled at each time-point. (Reproduced from ref. *18* with permission from Taylor & Francis, Stockholm, Sweden.)

patients with *Mycoplasma pneumonia* on admission to the hospital compared to the patients with bacteremic pneumococcal pneumonia. In a study of patients with *Chlamydia* pneumonia (*n* = 13) and *Mycoplasma* pneumonia (*n* = 14), serum concentrations of TNF-α, IL-6, and IFN-γ were found to be elevated on admission *(20)* (*see* Fig. 6). No significant differences between the etiological groups were found, but the levels of IL-6 were in the low range in accordance with our previous study *(14)* and most patients had elevated IFN-γ. The serum concentrations of G-CSF was investigated in eight patients with *Mycoplasma* pneumonia and compared with levels in patients with diverse bacterial infections *(21)*. Serum concentrations were found to be low in the group of patients with *Mycoplasma* pneumonia, a result which is in agreement with the findings in our study *(17)*. Patients with pneumonia caused by *Mycoplasma* (*n* = 14), *Chlamydia* (*n* = 12), and *Legionella* (*n* = 6) had lower levels of

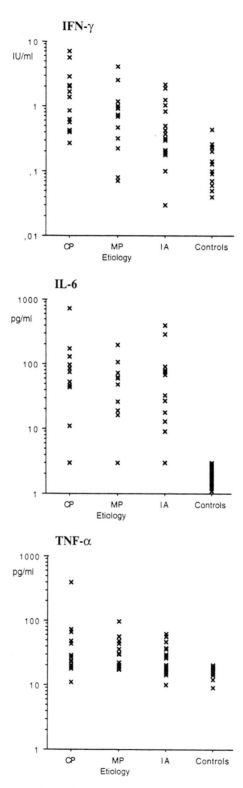

Fig. 6. Scatter of the concentrations of IFN-γ, IL-6 and TNF-α in serum of patients with CP (*Chlamydia pneumoniae*) or MP (*Mycoplasma pneumonia*) or IA (influenza A infection) and in 20 controls. (Reproduced from ref. *20* with permission from S. Karger AG, Basel.

G-CSF in comparison with patients with bacteremic pneumococcal pneumonia. Only three studies include patients with *Legionella* pneumonia *(14,17,22)*. In our previous studies we found elevated levels of IL-6 and IFN-γ but low concentrations of IL-8 and G-CSF on admission to the hospital *(14,17)*. In a study, of 14 patients with *Legionella* pneumonia using bloodsamples taken at variable time-points during the hospital stay, Tateda et al. found elevated levels of the cytokines IFN-γ and IL-12, low levels of proinflammatory cytokines such as TNF-α, IL-1β, IL-6, and no IL-4 or IL-10 *(22)*. The results from these three studies show that in infections caused by intracellular micro-organisms such as *Legionella*, the cytokine response is associated with elevated circulating levels of Th1 cytokines such as IFN-γ and IL-12.

Thus, studies of clinically less severely ill patients with pneumonia have shown that differences do exist in the blood concentrations between different etiologies of the pneumonia. Based on the results presented here determination of blood IL-6 and IFN-γ/IL-12 might have a differential diagnostic potential.

4. CYTOKINE RESPONSES AND SEVERITY

Studies of the systemic inflammatory host response in the critically ill have demonstrated the pathophysiological role of cytokines. It has been shown that the levels of most cytokines reflect that the severity of the condition may be the cause of inflammation becoming infectious, traumatic, or other. In the case of bacterial pneumonia, few studies examine clinical severity grading in relation to systemic cytokine levels. Plasma levels of IL-1β, TNF-α, and IL-6 were measured in critically ill patients with pneumonia, less severely ill patients with pneumonia, severely ill postoperative patients without infection, and a group of patients with nonpneumonic infection *(23)*. In this study, TNF-α was found to be a marker of severity of pneumonia, IL-1β to mark severity of infection, and IL-6 to reflect infectious or noninfectious severity. Using SIRS as the severity classification, bacteremic pneumococcal pneumonia was found to be comparable to other bacteremic infections *(18)* and the serum levels of IL-6, TNF-α, and G-CSF reflected clinical severity. De Werra et al. compared patients with septic shock, cardiogenic shock, and bacterial pneumonia and found plasma levels of TNF-α to reflect severity in patients with infection, whereas plasma IL-6 was highest in septic shock patients, normal in seven patients with pneumonia, and elevated in cardiogenic shock *(24)*. The finding of normal IL-6 levels in patients with bacterial pneumonia is unusual, as most other studies demonstrate high levels of IL-6 even in nonbacteremic patients cared for in a common infectious disease department. Serum IL-10 was studied in 38 patients with CAP divided into a SIRS group and a non-SIRS group and correlated with APACHE II scores *(25)*. IL-6 and IL-10 were found to correlate with severity of illness. Comparing patients with severe pneumonia and ARDS, Bauer et al. found serum TNF-α and IL-1/β to reflect the severity of the lung injury *(26)*. In the studies presented so far, IL-6 consistently emerges as a marker of severity. In individual studies, other cytokines such as IL-10, G-CSF, and TNF-α were also found to mark the severity of the illness.

5. CYTOKINE RESPONSES AND AGE

Previous investigations have shown that increasing age confers increasing impairment of the immune system. In the case of bacterial pneumonia, studies have focused on the ability of elderly patients to mount an inflammatory response to infection. Gon et al. demonstrated lower serum values of G-CSF, GM-CSF, TNF-α, IL-1β, IL-8, and MIP-1α in elderly patients in the acute stage, and the levels in both young and older patients declined on recovery *(27)*. The definition of recovery was set to a span of 5–14 d, which makes comparison with the following study difficult. The inflammatory response during pneumococcal infection was studied in 22 patients divided into groups of young and elderly patients. The circulating concentrations of IL-1β, TNF-α, IL-6, MIP-1β, IL-1RA, IL-10, and sTNFR-I were measured on admission and after 3 and 7 d in the hospital *(19)*. In this study, aging was shown to be associated with prolonged inflammatory activity, but levels of cytokines in young and old patients were similar on admission. Glynn et al. found no difference in serum IL-10 levels in patients divided into groups younger than 60 or older than 70 yr of age, but serum IL-6 concentrations were higher in the patients older than 70 yr of age *(25)*. In that same study, IL-6 and IL-10 were correlated to severity, which raises the question of whether the elderly patients were more severely ill than the younger. Although older age is associated with impaired immune functions, elderly patients may respond with high cytokine levels, but the response may be dysregulated and prolonged.

6. CYTOKINE RESPONSES AND IMMUNEMODULATION

Immunomodulating therapies have been tried in several studies of patients with sepsis or septic shock with disappointing results. Few investigations have been performed on the effect of modulating the cytokine response during acute bacterial pneumonia. Thirty patients with severe CAP were randomized to receive either a single dose of hydrocortisone (10 mg/kg body wt) or placebo before the administration of antibiotics in addition to standard treatment for pneumonia *(28)*. TNF-α was measured on admission and after 2, 6, and 12 h after antibiotic therapy was started. In this study, hydrocortisone had no effect on the serum levels of TNF-α or on the clinical course. A recent study investigated the effect of daily methylprednisolone given after the administration of antibiotics on the inflammatory response in pneumonia in patients treated with mechanical ventilation in the intensive care unit *(29)*. Patients receiving methylprednisolone had lower serum levels of IL-6 and C-reactive protein (CRP) and a lower neutrophil count in BAL fluid. However, the dosage and treatment period varied considerably. Recombinant human (rh) G-CSF for the treatment of CAP was studied in a prospective, double-blind, randomized, placebo-controlled study *(30)*. In all, 756 patients were studied, 376 received placebo and 380 rh G-CSF. The study showed that treatment with rh G-CSF was not harmful but gave no important benefit compared to placebo. In view of the disappointing results of immunomodulation in septic conditions and the complexity of the cytokine response to infection, a better characterization, of an appropriate and a dysregulated cytokine response is needed. Specific markers have to be established and related to the timing of treatment at specific stages during disease.

7. CONCLUSION

The role of cytokines as mediators of inflammation in pneumonia is being defined. The results from studies investigating bacterial pneumonia point to the following:
- In nonbacteremic pneumonia, the inflammatory response is mainly local and the cytokines demonstrated in BAL fluid so far are IL-8, IL-6, TNF-α GRO-α and TGF-β.
- The systemic response in nonbacteremic pneumonia is characterized mainly by elevated levels of IL-6.
- In pneumonia, blood levels of IL-6, IL-8, and G-CSF correlate with severity and prognosis and high levels may suggest *S. pneumoniae* as a probable causative agent.
- In bacteremic pneumonia, the cytokine response is comparable to that of other bacteremic infections.
- Patients with pneumonia caused by intracellular micro-organisms such as *Legionella* have circulating levels of Th1 cytokines such as IFN-γ and IL-12.
- In elderly patients, the cytokine response may be dysregulated and prolonged.
- Immunomodulation in pneumonia by way of suppressing the inflammatory host response using corticosteroids or by stimulating production of phagocytes and phagocytic activity has demonstrated no positive effects so far.

In summary, the cytokine response in human pneumonia is being characterized. Use of single cytokines or groups of cytokines as prognostic or etiological markers in individual cases is made difficult by the large variation in the immune response of individual patients at specific time-points.

REFERENCES

1. Rangel-Frausto, M.S., Pittet, D., Costigan, M., Hwang, T., Davis, C.S., and Wenzel, R.P. (1995) The natural history of the systemic inflammatory response syndrome (SIRS). A prospective study. *JAMA* **273**, 117–123.
2. Knaus, W.A., Draper, E.A., Wagner, D.P., and Zimmerman, J.E. (1985) APACHE II: a severity of disease classification system. *Crit. Care Med.* **13**, 818–829.

3. Rodriguez, J.L., Miller, C.G., DeForge, L.E., Kelty, L., Shanley, C.J., Bartlett, R.H., et al. (1992) Local production of interleukin-8 is associated with nosocomial pneumonia. *J. Trauma* **33**, 74–81.
4. Chollet-Martin, S., Montravers, P., Gibert, C., Elbim, C., Desmonts, J.M., Fagon, J.Y., et al. (1993). High levels of interleukin-8 in the blood and alveolar spaces of patients with pneumonia and adult respiratory distress syndrome. *Infect Immun.* **61**, 4553–4559.
5. Moussa, K., Michie, H.J., Cree, I.A., McCafferty, A.C., Winter, J.H., Dhillon, D.P., et al. (1994) Phagocyte function and cytokine production in community acquired pneumonia. *Thorax* **49**, 107–111.
6. Dehoux, M.S., Boutten, A., Ostinelli, J., Seta, N., Dombret, M.C., Crestani, B., et al. (1994). Compartmentalized cytokine production within the human lung in unilateral pneumonia. *Am. J. Respir. Crit. Care Med.* **150**, 710–716.
7. Boutten, A., Dehoux, M.S., Seta, N., Ostinelli, J., Venembre, P., Crestani, B., et al. (1996) Compartmentalized IL-8 and elastase release within the human lung in unilateral pneumonia. *Am. J. Respir. Crit. Care Med.* **153**, 336–342.
8. Villard, J., Dayer-Pastore, F., Hamacher, J., Aubert, J. D., Schlegel-Haueter, S., et al. (1995). GRO alpha and interleukin-8 in Pneumocystis carinii or bacterial pneumonia and adult respiratory distress syndrome. *Am. J. Respir. Crit. Care Med.* **152**, 1549–1554.
9. Schutte, H., Lohmeyer, J., Rosseau, S., Ziegler, S., Siebert, C., Kielisch, H., et al. (1996). Bronchoalveolar and systemic cytokine profiles in patients with ARDS, severe pneumonia and cardiogenic pulmonary oedema. *Eur. Respir. J.* **9**, 1858–1867.
10. Bohnet, S., Kotschau, U., Braun, J., and Dalhoff, K. (1997). Role of interleukin-8 in community-acquired pneumonia: relation to microbial load and pulmonary function. *Infection* **25**, 95–100.
11. Maus, U., Rosseau, S., Knies, U., Seeger, W., and Lohmeyer, J. (1998) Expression of pro-inflammatory cytokines by flow-sorted alveolar macrophages in severe pneumonia. *Eur. Respir. J.* **11**, 534–541.
12. Buhling, F., Tholert, G., Kaiser, D., Hoffmann, B., Reinhold, D., Ansorge, S., et al. (1999) Increased release of transforming growth factor (TGF)-beta1, TGF-beta2, and chemoattractant mediators in pneumonia. *J. Interferon Cytokine Res.* **19**, 271–278.
13. Monton, C., Torres, A., El-Ebiary, M., Filella, X., Xaubet, A., and de la Bellacasa, J.P. (1999) Cytokine expression in severe pneumonia: a bronchoalveolar lavage study. *Crit. Care Med.* **27**, 1745–1753.
14. Kragsbjerg, P., Vikerfors, T., and Holmberg, H. (1993) Serum levels of interleukin-6, tumour necrosis factor-α, interferon-γ and C-reactive protein in adults with community-acquired pneumonia. *Serodiagn. Immunother. Infect. Dis.* **5**, 156–160.
15. Örtqvist, A., Hedlund, J., Wretlind, B., Carlstrom, A., and Kalin, M. (1995) Diagnostic and prognostic value of interleukin-6 and C-reactive protein in community-acquired pneumonia. *Scand. J. Infect. Dis.* **27**, 457–462.
16. Lieberman, D., Livnat, S., Schlaeffer, F., Porath, A., Horowitz, S., and Levy, R. (1997) IL-1beta and IL-6 in community-acquired pneumonia: bacteremic pneumococcal pneumonia versus *Mycoplasma pneumoniae* pneumonia. *Infection* **25**, 90–94.
17. Kragsbjerg, P., Jones, I., Vikerfors, T., and Holmberg, H. (1995) Diagnostic value of blood cytokine concentrations in acute pneumonia. *Thorax* **50**, 1253–1257.
18. Kragsbjerg, P., Holmberg, H., and Vikerfors, T. (1996) Dynamics of blood cytokine concentrations in patients with bacteremic infections. *Scand. J. Infect. Dis.* **28**, 391–398.
19. Bruunsgaard, H., Skinhoj, P., Qvist, J., and Pedersen, B.K. (1999) Elderly humans show prolonged in vivo inflammatory activity during pneumococcal infections. *J. Infect. Dis.* **180**, 551–554.
20. Kragsbjerg, P., Vikerfors, T., and Holmberg, H. (1998) Cytokine responses in patients with pneumonia caused by *Chlamydia* or *Mycoplasma*. *Respiration* **65**, 299–303.
21. Pauksen, K., Elfman, L., Ulfgren, A.K., and Venge, P. (1994) Serum levels of granulocyte-colony stimulating factor (G-CSF) in bacterial and viral infections, and in atypical pneumonia. *Br. J. Haematol.* **88**, 256–260.
22. Tateda, K., Matsumoto, T., Ishii, Y., Furuya, N., Ohno, A., Miyazaki, S., et al. (1998) Serum cytokines in patients with Legionella pneumonia: relative predominance of Th1-type cytokines. *Clin. Diagn. Lab. Immunol.* **5**, 401–403.
23. Puren, A.J., Feldman, C., Savage, N., Becker, P.J., and Smith, C. (1995) Patterns of cytokine expression in community-acquired pneumonia. *Chest* **107**, 1342–1349.
24. de Werra, I., Jaccard, C., Corradin, S.B., Chiolero, R., Yersin, B., Gallati, H., et al. (1997) Cytokines, nitrite/nitrate, soluble tumor necrosis factor receptors, and procalcitonin concentrations: comparisons in patients with septic shock, cardiogenic shock, and bacterial pneumonia. *Crit. Care Med.* **25**, 607–613.
25. Glynn, P., Coakley, R., Kilgallen, I., Murphy, N., and O'Neill, S. (1999) Circulating interleukin 6 and interleukin 10 in community acquired pneumonia. *Thorax* **54**, 51–55.
26. Bauer, T.T., Monton, C., Torres, A., Cabello, H., Fillela, X., Maldonado, A., et al. (2000) Comparison of systemic cytokine levels in patients with acute respiratory distress syndrome, severe pneumonia, and controls. *Thorax* **55**, 46–52.
27. Gon, Y., Hashimoto, S., Hayashi, S., Koura, T., Matsumoto, K., and Horie, T. (1996) Lower serum concentrations of cytokines in elderly patients with pneumonia and the impaired production of cytokines by peripheral blood monocytes in the elderly. *Clin. Exp. Immunol.* **106**, 120–126.
28. Marik, P., Kraus, P., Sribante, J., Havlik, I., Lipman, J., and Johnson, D.W. (1993) Hydrocortisone and tumor necrosis factor in severe community-acquired pneumonia. A randomized controlled study. *Chest* **104**, 389–392.
29. Monton, C., Ewig, S., Torres, A., El-Ebiary, M., Filella, X., Rano, A., et al. (1999) Role of glucocorticoids on inflammatory response in nonimmunosuppressed patients with pneumonia: a pilot study. *Eur. Respir. J.* **14**, 218–220.
30. Nelson, S., Belknap, S.M., Carlson, R.W., Dale, D., DeBoisblanc, B., Farkas, S., et al. (1998) A randomized controlled trial of filgrastim as an adjunct to antibiotics for treatment of hospitalized patients with community- acquired pneumonia. CAP Study Group. *J. Infect. Dis.* **178**, 1075–1080.

VI
Cytokines in Fungal Infections

15

Cytokines and the Host Defense Against *Aspergillus fumigatus*

Emmanuel Roilides, Joanna Filioti, and Cristina Gil-Lamaignere

1. INTRODUCTION

Among opportunistic mycoses, invasive aspergillosis (IA) is the second most frequent infection and an important cause of morbidity and mortality in susceptible hosts. Such hosts are premature neonates *(1)*, patients undergoing transplantation of bone marrow *(2)* or solid organ *(3)*, patients with hematologic disorders *(4,5)*, chronic granulomatous disease (CGD) *(6)*, human immunodeficiency virus (HIV) infection *(7)*, corticosteroid treatment *(8)*, and a variety of other quantitative and qualitative phagocytic defects. Invasive aspergillosis is now the most frequent opportunistic mold infection worldwide *(8)* and *Aspergillus fumigatus* is the most common species accounting for more than 70% of IA *(8,9)*. Although the mortality of IA is very high and in some cases approaches 100% *(9)*, prevention, early diagnosis and treatment remain quite difficult. These challenges have intensified efforts to better understand host response against *A. fumigatus*, with the ultimate goal to improve its dismal outcome.

Advances in the development of a number of cytokines have suggested new therapeutic options. The critical role of phagocytic defense has become evident and numerical as well as functional reconstitution of effector cells by treatment with cytokines has been attempted. Cytokines that are of most interest because of their ability to upregulate the number and/or the function of phagocytes are the hemopoietic growth factors granulocyte colony-stimulating factor (G-CSF), granulocyte–macrophage colony-stimulating factor (GM-CSF), and macrophage colony-stimulating factor (M-CSF). Cytokines of Th1 response pattern such as interferon-γ (IFN-γ), interleukin-12 (IL-12), and tumor necrosis factor-α (TNF-α) are also of great interest. On the other hand, cytokines of Th2 pattern, such as IL-4 and IL-10, exert an overall suppressive effect or have variable or no effects on the antifungal function of phagocytes.

2. PHAGOCYTIC FUNCTION AGAINST *A. FUMIGATUS*

Pulmonary alveolar macrophages (PAMs) are the first line of defense against *A. fumigatus*. They ingest and destroy inhaled conidia intracellularly, hence preventing their germination to hyphae and, subsequently, their invasion to tissues (recently reviewed in refs. *8, 10, and 11*). Although the elimination of conidia takes place even when their number reaching alveoli is large, there is a direct relationship between intrapulmonary inoculum challenge and tissue injury as well as mortality in animal models *(12,13)*. In order to evade phagocytosis by PAMs or to cross membranes and anatomical barriers, *A. fumigatus* conidia produce enzymes such as elastase and other proteases. The elabo-

From: *Cytokines and Chemokines in Infectious Diseases Handbook*
Edited by: M. Kotb and T. Calandra © Humana Press Inc., Totowa, NJ

rated proteases are not only capable of crossing barriers but also of hydrolyzing endogenous antimicrobial peptides *(14)*, resulting in survival and germination to hyphae.

Pulmonary alveolar macrophages can recognize and bind conidia through ligand–receptor interaction *(15)* even when complement and immunoglobulins are not available, as this happens in the terminal airways. Murine PAMs have been shown to recognize and attach to *A. fumigatus* conidia through lectinlike attachment sites in the absence of opsonins. In addition, human monocytes (MNCs) bind conidia by a glucoside inhibitable receptor *(16)*. The effects of cytokines on these receptors are not well understood yet.

Resting conidia are relatively resistant to both oxygen-dependent and nonoxidative antimicrobial products of phagocytes *(17,18)*. To the contrary, swollen conidia are more susceptible to oxygen-dependent metabolites and trigger a more potent oxidative burst. Killing of conidia starts 4–6 hr after phagocytosis (i.e., when conidia start to swell and become metabolically active). Rat PAMs produce nitric oxide (NO) in response to *A. fumigatus* conidia. Increased NO production by IFN-γ-activated PAMs has been found, together with increased attachment of *A. fumigatus* conidia *(19)*.

As second line of defense, polymorphonuclear leukocytes (PMNs) and MNCs are collected at the site of infection trying to destroy the escaping hyphae—opsonized or not—by secreting microbicidal oxidative myeloperoxidase-dependent and myloperoxidase-independent as well as nonoxidative metabolites. PMNs are the most numerous circulating phagocytes. They can damage hyphae by attachment to their cell wall through glycoprotein ligands even without opsonization. Their antifungal function is dependent on the stimulation of phagocytes by hyphal surface ligands and on functional NADPH oxidase and oxygen-dependent antifungal metabolites (i.e., H_2O_2 and HClO). These conclusions are based on the findings that PMNs of patients with CGD exhibit impaired hyphal damage *(120)* and that mice with X-linked CGD are prone to infections as a result of *A. fumigatus (21)*. Nonoxidative killing systems such as cationic proteins have also been found to be important components of antihyphal machinery *(17)*. Mice deficient in the PMN granule serine proteases elastase and/or cathepsin G are susceptible to IA, despite normal PMN development and recruitment *(22)*.

Human monocytes have similar antifungal activities against *A. fumigatus*, but their oxygen-dependent antifungal activity appears to be less potent than that of PMNs *(23)*. MNCs also produce NO, which has been found to be a potent antifungal mechanism in mice, although its antifungal role has not been established in humans *(24,25)*. When PMN defenses are defective, MNCs can substitute for some of PMN function, even though MNC oxygen-dependent antifungal activity is less potent than that of PMNs.

Among other cells, Kupffer and splenic adherent cells also possess anti-*Aspergillus* conidia capacity; however, this is inferior to that against *Candida albicans* (Roilides et al., unpublished data). Platelets attach to cell walls of *A. fumigatus* hyphae and are stimulated, causing some damage to the hyphae by loss of fungal cell wall integrity and release of fungal surface glycoproteins *(26)*. Whether this mechanism is affected by cytokines is unclear.

Lymphocytes comprise up to 30% of the cells present in human broncho-alveolar lavage fluid and thus may be important in early host response to *A. fumigatus*. When incubated with *A. fumigatus* conidia for 20 h, highly purified 5-d-old IL-2- and phytohemagglutinin-activated lymphocytes exhibit a contact-dependent ability to reduce adherence of germinating conidia of *A. fumigatus* but not hyphal damage *(27)*.

Impaired macrophage function (i.e., by the effect of corticosteroids) combined with quantitative or qualitative PMN defects result in invasion of tissues and vessels and these appear to be the main reasons for the development of invasive pulmonary aspergillosis (IPA). Decreased capacity against hyphae and conidia of *A. fumigatus* by PMNs and MNCs, as happens in HIV-infected patients *(28,29)*, may be related to the well-described CD4[+] T-helper lymphocyte dysfunction of these patients and the Th1/Th2 cytokine dysregulation that follows *(30)*.

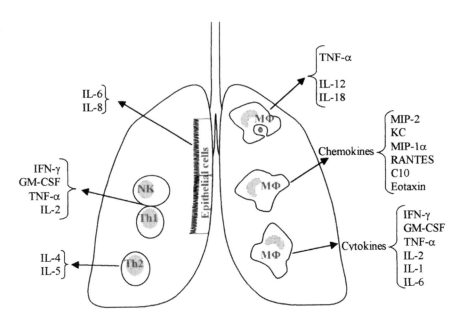

Fig. 1. Network of cytokines and chemokines induced in response to inhaled conidia of *A. fumigatus*.

3. CYTOKINE AND CHEMOKINE PRODUCTION IN RESPONSE TO *A. FUMIGATUS* (FIG. 1)

3.1. Cytokine Production

Immune system responds to challenges by *A. fumigatus* with secretion of a number of cytokines. Although lymphocytes do not have significant antifungal effector activity, cocultures of *A. fumigatus* conidia with mononuclear leukocytes result in the secretion of high levels of IFN-γ, GM-CSF, TNF-α and IL-2, but not of IL-4 or IL-10 *(31)*. IL-1 is also produced by macrophages as a result of stimulation by conidia, hyphae, and even fungal cell wall components *(32,33)* such as mannoproteins. Aflatoxin B1, a mycotoxin produced by *Aspergillus*, causes the production of important cytokines, such as IL-1α, IL-6, and TNF-α, by human MNCs *(34)*.

Activated Th cells secrete IL-4 in response to *Aspergillus* antigens *(35)*. Dendritic cells also produce Th1 cytokines, suggesting a positive role for these cells in host response *(36)*. Proteases secreted by *A. fumigatus* induce cytokine production by lung epithelial cells. A recent study focusing on the mechanism(s) by which these proteases elicit especially IL-6 and IL-8 production in epithelial cells demonstrated that IL-6 and IL-8 gene expressions are upregulated by transcriptional mechanisms *(37)*.

Cytokine networking in the lungs in response to inhaled conidia of *A. fumigatus* has been comprehensively studied in immunocompetent as well as immunosuppressed mice. In an initial phase, the challenge of immunocompetent mice with inhaled conidia of *A. fumigatus* is followed by an intense clearance of the fungus, possibly through PAMs and recruited PMNs, accompanied by the rapid release of TNF-α, IL-6, and IL-1β. As a final phase, cellular and fungal debris are cleaned by recruited MNCs, cytokine production rapidly decreases, and pneumonia self-heals *(38)*.

Inhalation of conidia also results in the production of IL-18, IL-12 and IFN-γ, which play a protective role in IPA, as proven by the fact that neutralization of these cytokines alone or in combination results in a significant increase of *A. fumigatus* burden in the lungs *(39)*. Moreover, treatment of mice with neutralizing anti-TNF-α as well as anti-GM-CSF antibodies reduces the PMN influx into the lungs and delays fungal clearance, showing the central role that both TNF-α and GM-CSF play in the recruitment of PMNs into the lungs *(32)*.

In contrast, cortisone-treated mice have a distorted clearance of conidia, delayed cytokine production, delayed inflammatory cell recruitment, as well as sustained release of IL-6 and IL-1β; in addition, they exhibit widespread tissue necrosis, further increases in PMN trafficking but no MNC recruitment, respiratory failure, and 100% mortality within 5 d *(38)*.

3.2. Chemokine Production

Challenge with *A. fumigatus* conidia provokes the production of a number of chemokines in the lungs, resulting in augmented recruitment and activation of MNCs and PMNs.

ELR$^+$ CXC chemokines are a subfamily of chemokines that play a critical role in PMN chemotaxis and activation both in vitro and in vivo. ELR$^+$ CXC chemokines macrophage inflammatory protein-2 (MIP-2) and cytokine-induced neutrophil chemoattractant (KC) are induced in response to intratracheal administration of conidia. Neutralization of the common ELR$^+$ CXC chemokine receptor, CXCR2, by antibody results in reduced PMN influx to the lungs, development of invasive disease indistinguishable from the disease in neutropenic animals, and a markedly increased mortality. In contrast, animals with constitutive lung-specific transgenic expression of KC had a low fungal burden in the lungs and reduced mortality *(40)*.

Macrophage inflammatory protein-1α belongs to the CC chemokine subfamily with potent chemotactic activity for various subsets of mononuclear leukocytes. Studies with neutropenic mice challenged with inhaled conidia and antibody-mediated depletion of MIP-1α showed a sixfold increase in mortality, associated with a 12-fold increase in lung fungal burden. Flow cytometry on whole-lung suspensions revealed a 41% reduction in lung monocytes/macrophages, but no difference in other lung leukocyte subsets *(41)*. During the peak of infection in mice with aspergillosis, MIP-1α, monocyte chemoattractant protein-1 (MCP-1), and MIP-2 are induced within the lung *(32)*.

Intrapulmonary challenge with *A. fumigatus* conidia elevates lung concentrations of RANTES in addition to MIP-1α significantly. When the role of their receptor, CC chemokine receptor 1 (CCR1), was investigated in a model of *A. fumigatus*-sensitized CCR1 wild-type (+/+) and CCR1 knockout (–/–) mice, it was found that both groups of mice exhibited similar increases in serum IgE and leukocytes in the broncho-alveolar lavage. Whole-lung levels of IFN-α were significantly higher, whereas IL-4, IL-13, and Th2-inducible chemokines such as C10, eotaxin, and macrophage-derived chemokine, were significantly lower in whole-lung samples from CCR1–/– mice compared with CCR1+/+ mice at 30 d after the conidial challenge *(42)*.

Monocyte chemoattractant protein-1 receptor, CCR2, is another essential mediator of host defense against *A. fumigatus*. Mice lacking CCR2 because of targeted deletion have been shown to exhibit a major defect in the recruitment of PMNs. In addition, these animals have significantly more eosinophils and lymphocytes in broncho-alveolar lavage samples and significant increases in serum levels of total IgE, IL-5, IL-13, eotaxin, and RANTES. They are also markedly susceptible to the injurious effects of an intrapulmonary challenge with live conidia, as compared with mice that express CCR2 *(43)*.

Taken together, the above studies indicate that chemokine receptors are critical mediators of host defense against *A. fumigatus*, especially in the setting of neutropenia, and may be important targets in devising future therapeutic strategies against IA.

4. CYTOKINES WITH ENHANCING EFFECTS ON HOST DEFENSE AGAINST *A. FUMIGATUS* (TABLE 1)

4.1. G-CSF

In vitro studies have demonstrated that this cytokine regulates both the number and the function of intact PMNs against *A. fumigatus* hyphae. It increases PMN-mediated damage of hyphae (opsonized or not) mainly by enhancement of PMN O_2^- production *(44,45)*. It activates PMN function even when it is suppressed. Thus, it enhances the antifungal activity of PMNs from HIV-infected patients *(46)* and

Table 1
Cytokines with Enhancing Effects on Phagocytes and the Specific Antifungal Functions Against A. fumigatus That They Enhance

Cytokines/functions	PMN	MNC/macrophages
G-CSF		
O_2^- production	↑	—
Hyphal damage	↑	—
Corticosteroid immunosuppression	Restoration	—
GM-CSF		
O_2- production	↑	↑
Hyphal damage	↑	↑
Corticosteroid immunosuppression		
(O_2- and hyphal damage)	Restoration	Restoration
Differentiation and proliferation		↑
M-CSF		
Phagocytosis	—	↑
O_2- production	—	↑
Conidial damage	—	↑
Hyphal damage	—	↑
IFN-γ		
Oxidative burst	↑	↑
Hyphal damage	↑	↑
Corticosteroid immunosuppression	Restoration	Restoration
TNF-α		
Phagocytosis		↑
O_2- production	↑	↑
Conidial damage		No effect
Hyphal damage	↑	↑
IL-12		
O_2^- production		↑
Hyphal damage		↑

restores the suppression of antifungal activity against *A. fumigatus* as a result of corticosteroids *(47)* with mechanism(s) that still remain unclear. Additionally, it protects PMNs from the catastrophic effects of isolation and irradiation leading to a promising PMN transfusion therapy *(48)*.

This upregulation of human PMNs by G-CSF has also been observed in studies with normal and immunosuppressed mice *(49)*. However, these data suggest that the protection that G-CSF may offer IA differs depending on the cause of suppression. Thus, G-CSF did not protect IA mice that had been immunosuppressed by corticosteroid treatment *(49)*. By comparison, when mice became neutropenic by 5-fluorouracil and were given either G-CSF or the antifungal triazole posaconazole, they benefited from both agents separately, and the effect of the combination was additive. In contrast, when the mice were immunosuppressed by hydrocortisone, G-CSF strongly antagonized the antifungal activity of posaconazole in its action against IA. These variable findings suggest that perhaps the outcome of cytokine therapy in IA depends on host factors in different pathways *(50)*.

The additive effect between G-CSF and voriconazole has been demonstrated in vitro when the two compounds were combined with PMNs against *A. fumigatus (51)*. A similar effect has been demonstrated in the neutropenic murine model of IA with G-CSF and posaconazole *(50)*.

The effects of G-CSF on PMN-mediated fungicidal activity were also evaluated in humans by the administration of G-CSF (300 µg/d subcutaneously) to five healthy volunteers for 6 d. Although G-CSF significantly enhanced PMN-mediated damage of *C. albicans* hyphae by 33% on d 2 and by 44% on d 6, it did not significantly change the ability of PMNs to induce damage of hyphae of either *A. fumigatus* or *Fusarium solani (52)*.

4.2. GM-CSF

This cytokine stimulates both the number and the function of PMNs, but less potently than G-CSF *(53)*. Additionally, it promotes the differentiation and proliferation of MNCs and enhances their function *(54)*. Like G-CSF, it upregulates intact phagocytes and restores the antifungal activity of phagocytes that have become immunosuppressed by corticosteroids against hyphae of *A. fumigatus (55,56)*. Of note, GM-CSF-treated human MNCs exhibit enhanced O_2^- production and hyphal damage of unopsonized hyphae of this fungus *(32)*. Additionally, it plays a central role in the recruitment of PMNs into the lung in response to *A. fumigatus (51)*.

In vitro studies have shown additive effects of GM-CSF and voriconazole when added to PMNs or MNCs against *A. fumigatus (51)*.

4.3. M-CSF

This cytokine affects the number and the function of mononuclear phagocytes and not the function of PMNs. It upregulates oxidation-dependent mechanisms resulting in enhanced damage of both conidia and hyphae of *A. fumigatus (57)*. In addition, it increases secondary production of other cytokines such as IL-1, IFN-γ and TNF-α *(58)*. When M-CSF-treated PAMs combine with amphotericin β lipid complex, the damage of *A. fumigatus* is even higher *(59)*.

However, when the ex vivo effects of M-CSF on MNCs from cancer patients who received prolonged courses of the cytokine were evaluated, an enhanced antifungal activity against blastoconidia of *C. albicans* but not against hyphae of *A. fumigatus* was found *(60)*.

Consistent with the beneficial effects of M-CSF on host macrophage defenses in vitro, M-CSF (100–600 µg/kg/d) treatment of neutropenic rabbits with IPA was associated with increased survival and decreased pulmonary injury (decreased pulmonary infarction score). These findings were associated with improved pulmonary computerized tomographic scanning scores and a better outcome than the control rabbits *(61)*. In addition, when PAMs from lungs of the M-CSF group of rabbits were studied microscopically, it was found that they exhibited significantly greater phagocytosis of *A. fumigatus* conidia.

4.4. IFN-γ

This broad spectrum cytokine enhances PMN- and MNC-induced hyphal damage of *A. fumigatus* and restores the phagocytic activity of immunosuppressed cells against this fungus *(44,47,56)*. IFN-γ treated PMNs exhibited enhanced oxidative burst and damaging capacity to both serum-opsonized and unopsonized hyphae of *A. fumigatus (44)*. PMNs from IFN-γ -treated CGD patients damaged *A. fumigatus* hyphae more than did PMNs from the control group *(62)*. IFN-γ has been also shown to reverse mononuclear phagocyte dysfunction caused by corticosteroids in mice with IA immunocompromised with corticosteroids *(63)*.

Compared to G-CSF and GM-CSF, IFN-γ induces the strongest hyphal damage, recorded in a study where the in vitro effects of the three cytokines on PMNs and MNCs of healthy volunteers were evaluated *(64)*. Nevertheless, the combination of IFN-γ with either G-CSF or GM-CSF exhibited an additive effect on anti-*Aspergillus* activities of human PMNs and MNCs compared to each cytokine alone *(44,55)*.

The combination of IFN-γ with TNF-α exhibits an additive effect. Indeed, when the two cytokines were administered to mice immunosuppressed by corticosteroids with IA, the mortality was minimized (from 40–60% to 0%). This finding was associated with a low fungal burden in organs as evidenced by culture and histology *(63)*, suggesting a protective role of these cytokines against IA.

The immunoenhancing role of IFN-γ against aspergilli has been shown in a prospective random-ized placebo-controlled study in patients with CGD. In this study, the incidence of serious infections in the IFN-γ group was considerably reduced and the frequency of pneumonia as a result of aspergil-lus was somewhat decreased *(65)*. In agreement with the above study, several case reports of CGD patients with IA showed a better outcome after adjunctive IFN-γ treatment *(66–69)*.

4.5. TNF-α

This cytokine increases the O_2^- and H_2O_2 release in response to soluble and particulate stimuli. Moreover, TNF-α augments the production of other cytokines, such as GM-CSF (reviewed in ref. *70*).

In vitro studies have demonstrated that TNF-α enhances the antifungal activities of all the phago-cytes against *A. fumigatus*. For example, it stimulates PMNs for damaging hyphae and it enhances PAM phagocytosis of conidia, although the intracellular killing of conidia remains the same. It also increases O_2^- production by MNCs, but, generally, the effects on MNC functions are moderate *(71)*.

Studies in both neutropenic and nonneutropenic mice infected by *A. fumigatus* conidia intratracheally showed increased lung TNF-α levels and peribronchial infiltration of PMNs and MNCs. In addition, neutralization of TNF-α resulted in reduced levels of the CXC chemokine MIP-2, the CC chemokines MIP-1α and JE (mouse homolog of human MCP-1), as well as the PMN influx in the lungs. These results of TNF-α neutralization were associated with increased mortality of both neutropenic and non-neutropenic animals. When a TNF-α agonist peptide was given to cyclophos-phamide-treated animals before challenge with conidia, the survival improved, which supports the prophylactic use of this cytokine *(40)*. In another study, neutralization of TNF-α as well as of GM-CSF reduced lung influx of PMNs and fungal clearance *(32)*. Additionally, when TNF-α with IFN-γ were used therapeutically in corticosteroid-treated mice with IA, there was no mortality and a lower fungal burden in organs, as demonstrated by culture and histology *(63)*.

4.6. IL-12

This cytokine appears to predominantly exert its anti-*Aspergillus* activity by stimulating IFN-γ secretion from Th1 cells in vivo *(35)*. However, incubation of peripheral blood mononuclear cells from healthy adults with recombinant human IL-12 appears to also directly enhance the capacity of human MNCs to elicit oxidative burst and damage hyphae of *A. fumigatus* via an IFN-γ-independent route *(72)*.

Resistance in leukopenic mice was associated with unimpaired innate antifungal activity of pul-monary phagocytic cells, concomitant with a high-level production of TNF-α and IL-12 and the presence of interstitial lymphocytes producing IFN-γ and IL-2 *(73)*.

Treatment of immunocompetent mice with *Aspergillus* crude culture filtrate resulted in the devel-opment of local and peripheral protective Th1 memory responses, mediated by antigen-specific CD4+ T-cells producing IFN-γ and IL-2 capable of conferring protection upon adoptive transfer to naive recipients *(74)*.

5. CYTOKINES WITH SUPPRESSIVE OR VARIABLE EFFECTS ON HOST DEFENSE AGAINST *A. FUMIGATUS* (TABLE 2)

5.1. IL-4

This is a Th2 cytokine with predominant suppressive effects on a variety of immune cells. It suppresses antifungal activity of mononuclear phagocytes against *A. fumigatus* hyphae but does not affect phagocytosis of conidia, findings suggesting a lack of a pathogenic role of IL-4 on early phase and a suppressive role on late phase of development of IA *(75)*.

Studies on murine IA demonstrated impaired PMN antifungal activity, concomitant with a pre-dominant production of IL-4 by CD4+ splenocytes. In contrast, treatment with soluble IL-4 receptor resulted in acquired resistance to the lethal infection and cured more than 70% of the mice *(35)*. In the same murine model of IA, resistance to *A. fumigatus* was correlated with intact functions of conidial

Table 2
Cytokines with Suppressive or Variable Effects on MNCs and the
Specific Antifungal Functions Against A. fumigatus That They Affect

MNC function	IL-4	IL-10
Phagocytosis	No	↑
Inhibition of germination	No	↑
Conidial killing	No	No
O_2- production	↓	↓
Hyphal damage	↓	↓

killing and hyphal damage by lung phagocytes. In these mice, resistance could be augmented by gene knockout-achieved IL-4 deficiency or by neutralization of either IL-4 or IL-10 (73,76). Conversely, susceptibility to IA was correlated with impaired conidial killing and hyphal damage, as well as with increased IL-4 and IL-10 production. Furthermore, when IL-4–/– mice were studied, they were more resistant than wild type (WT) mice to infection caused by multiple intranasal injections of viable *A. fumigatus* conidia. These results suggested that IL-4 renders mice susceptible to infection with *A. fumigatus* by inhibition of protective Th1 responses (76).

In a murine model of IPA, resistance was associated with a decreased inflammatory lung pathology and the occurrence of an IL-12-dependent Th1-type reactivity that are both impaired by IL-4 (74).

5.2. IL-10

This pluripotent Th2 cytokine has multiple effects on both PMNs and MNCs. Although it increases the early host response evidenced as phagocytic activity of mononuclear phagocytes against *A. fumigatus* conidia, it suppresses their oxidative burst and antifungal activity against hyphae of the organism, both of which are late host response events (77).

Although beneficial in some bacterial infections, exogenous IL-10 has been shown to be deleterious in models of fungal infection. Administration of IL-10 to mice increases susceptibility to the challenging fungus and reduces survival after infectious challenge (78). IL-10–/– mice survived significantly longer than did WT mice during IA (79). Additionally, determination of fungal burdens in the kidneys and brain showed that IL-10–/– mice carried significantly lower burdens in both organs than did WT mice on d 3. Semiquantitative histological analyses showed fewer inflammatory foci in the brain and kidneys of IL-10–/– mice than WT mice and that the extent of infection and associated tissue injury were greater in WT mice. These data indicate that IL-10 increases the host susceptibility to lethal infection and the fungal burden in the kidneys and brain, facts that may be related to greater Th2 or lesser Th1 responses or downregulation of macrophage responses (79).

In IL-10-deficient mice, *A. fumigatus* infection did not induce significant acute toxicity. To the contrary, the mice showed reduced fungal burden and fungus-associated inflammatory response. This fact was associated with upregulation of innate and acquired antifungal Th1 responses, such as a dramatically higher production of IL-12, NO, and TNF-α as well as IFN-γ by CD4+ T-cells (78). The suppressive role of IL-10 in host defenses against IA may be associated with the finding that non-neutropenic patients with IA have higher serum IL-10 levels, and IL-10 levels correlate with a poor outcome of IA, leading to death (80).

6. CONCLUDING REMARKS

The increasing incidence of IA is of alarming importance in the management of immunocompromised patients. Stimulation of host defense normalization combined with antifungal therapy is the cornerstone of successful treatment. Much has been recently learned about phagocytic cell function and cytokine involvement in immunopathogenesis of IA by a number of in vitro studies.

The roles of phagocytes and of each cytokine against *A. fumigatus* have been better understood. Reconstitution of immune response by either exogenous administration of enhancing cytokines or transfusion of allogeneic phagocytes treated with enhancing cytokines appears to be a promising adjunct to antifungal chemotherapy for this difficult-to-treat and frequently fatal disease. Moreover, caution needs to be exerted during therapy with anti-inflammatory cytokines, which also have suppressive effects on host defenses against *A. fumigatus (81)*. On the other hand, potential inhibition of suppressive effects exerted by anti-inflammatory cytokines may improve the outcome of IA and this can serve as a model of immunotherapy for difficult-to-treat infections.

REFERENCES

1. Groll, A.H., Jaeger, G., Allendorf, A., Herrmann, G., Schloesser, R., and von Loewenich, V. (1998) Invasive pulmonary aspergillosis in a critically ill neonate: case report and review of invasive aspergillosis during the first 3 months of life. *Clin. Infect. Dis.* **27**, 437–452.
2. Wald, A., Leisenring, W., van Burik, J.A., and Bowden, R.A. (1997) Epidemiology of Aspergillus infections in a large cohort of patients undergoing bone marrow transplantation. *J. Infect. Dis.* **175**, 1459–1466.
3. Brown, R.S., Lake, J.R., Katzman, B.A., Ascher, N.L., Somberg, K.A., Emond, J.C., et al. (1996) Incidence and significance of Aspergillus cultures following liver and kidney transplantation. *Transplantation* **61**, 666–669.
4. Denning, D.W., Marinus, A., Cohen, J., Spence, D., Herbrecht, R., Pagano, L., et al. (1998) An EORTC multicentre prospective survey of invasive aspergillosis in haematological patients: diagnosis and therapeutic outcome. EORTC Invasive Fungal Infections Cooperative Group. *J. Infect.* **37**, 173–80.
5. Weinberger, M., Elattar, I., Marshall, D., Steinberg, S.M., Redner, R.L., Young, N.S., et al. (1992) Patterns of infection in patients with aplastic anemia and the emergence of *Aspergillus* as a major cause of death. *Medicine (Balt.)* **71**, 24–43.
6. Winkelstein, J.A., Marino, M.C., Johnston, R.B., Boyle, J., Curnutte, J., Gallin, J.I., et al. (2000) Chronic granulomatous disease. Report on a national registry of 368 patients. *Medicine (Balt.)* **79**, 155–169.
7. Mylonakis, E., Barlam, T.F., Flanigan, T., and Rich, J.D. (1998) Pulmonary aspergillosis and invasive disease in AIDS: review of 342 cases. *Chest* **114**, 251–262.
8. Latge, J.P. (1999) *Aspergillus fumigatus* and aspergillosis. *Clin. Microbiol. Rev.* **12**, 310–350.
9. Denning, D.W. (1998) Invasive aspergillosis. *Clin. Infect. Dis.* **26**, 781–803.
10. Roilides, E., Katsifa, H., and Walsh, T.J. (1998) Pulmonary host defences against *Aspergillus fumigatus*. *Res. Immunol.* **149**, 454–465.
11. Schneemann, M. and Schaffner, A. (1999) Host defense mechanism in *Aspergillus fumigatus* infections. *Contrib. Microbiol.* **2**, 57–68.
12. Francis, P., Lee, J.W., Hoffman, A., Peter, J., Francesconi, A., Bacher, J., et al. (1994) Efficacy of unilamellar liposomal amphotericin B in treatment of pulmonary aspergillosis in persistently granulocytopenic rabbits: the potential role of bronchoalveolar lavage D-mannitol and galactomannan as markers of infection. *J. Infect. Dis.* **169**, 356–368.
13. Dixon, D.M., Polak, A., and Walsh, T.J. (1989) Fungus dose-dependent primary pulmonary aspergillosis in immunosuppressed mice. *Infect. Immun.* **57**, 1452–1426.
14. De Lucca, A.J., Bland, J.M., Jacks, T.J., Grimm, C., Cleveland, T.E., and Walsh, T.J. (1997) Fungicidal activity of cecropin A. *Antimicrob. Agents Chemother.* **41**, 481–483.
15. Elstad, A., Douglas, H., and Braude, E. (1991) Aspergillosis and lung defenses. *Semin. Resp. Infect.* **6**, 27–36
16. Kan, V.L. and Bennett, J.E. (1991) Beta 1,4-oligoglucosides inhibit the binding of *Aspergillus fumigatus* conidia to human monocytes. *J. Infect. Dis.* **163**, 1154–1156.
17. Levitz, S., Selsted, M.E., Ganz, T., Lehrer, R.I., and Diamond, R.D. (1986) In vitro killing of spores and hyphae of *Aspergillus fumigatus* and *Rhizopus oryzae* by rabbit neutrophil cationic peptides and bronchoalveolar macrophages. *J. Infect. Dis.* **154**, 483–489.
18. de Repentigny, L., Petitbois, S., Boushira, M., Michaliszyn, E., Senechal, S., Gendron, N., et al. (1993) Aquired immunity in experimental murine aspergillosis is mediated by macrophages. *Infect. Immun.* **61**, 3791–3802.
19. Gross, N.T., Nessa, K., Camner, P., and Jarstrand, C. (1999) Production of nitric oxide by rat alveolar macrophages stimulated by Cryptococcus neoformans or *Aspergillus fumigatus*. *Med. Mycol.* **37**, 151–157.
20. Rex, J.H., Bennett, J.E., Gallin, J.I., Malech, H.L., and Melnick, D.A. (1990) Normal and deficient neutrophils can cooperate to damage *Aspergillus fumigatus* hyphae. *J. Infect. Dis.* **162**, 523–528.
21. Morgenstern, D.E., Gifford, M.A., Li, L.L., Doerschuk, C.M., and Dinauer, M.C. (1997) Absence of respiratory burst in X-linked chronic granulomatous disease mice leads to abnormalities in both host defense and inflammatory response to *Aspergillus fumigatus*. *J. Exp. Med.* **185**, 207–218.
22. Tkalcevic, J., Novelli, M., Phylactides, M., Iredale, J.P., Segal, A.W., and Roes, J. (2000) Impaired immunity and enhanced resistance to endotoxin in the absence of neutrophil elastase and cathepsin G. *Immunity* **12**, 201–210.
23. Schaffner, A., Douglas, H., and Braude, A. (1982) Selective protection against conidia by mononuclear and against mycelia by polymorphonuclear phagocytes in resistance to *Aspergillus:* observations on these two lines of defense in vivo and in vitro with human and mouse phagocytes. *J. Clin. Invest.* **69**, 617–631.
24. Michaliszyn, E., Senechal, S., Martel, P., and de Repentigny, L. (1995) Lack of involvement of nitric oxide in killing of *Aspergillus fumigatus* conidia by pulmonary alveolar macrophages. *Infect. Immun.* **63**, 2075–2078.

25. Schneemann, M., Schoedon, G., Hofer, S., Blau, N., Guerrero, L., and Schaffner, A. (1993) Nitric oxide synthase is not a constituent of the antimicrobial armature of human mononuclear phagocytes. *J. Infect. Dis.* **167**, 1358–1363.
26. Christin, L., Wysong, D.R., Meshulam, T., Hastey, R., Simons, E.R., and Diamond, R.D. (1998) Human platelets damage *Aspergillus fumigatus* hyphae and may supplement killing by neutrophils. *Infect. Immun.* **66**, 1181–1189.
27. Martins, M.D., Rodriguez, L.J., Savary, C.A., Grazziutti, M.L., Deshpande, D., Cohen, D.M., et al. (1998) Activated lymphocytes reduce adherence of Aspergillus fumigatus. *Med. Mycol.* **36**, 281–289.
28. Roilides, E., Holmes, A., Blake, C., Pizzo, P.A., and Walsh, T.J. (1993) Impairment of neutrophil fungicidal activity in HIV-infected children against *Aspergillus fumigatus* hyphae. *J. Infect. Dis.* **167**, 905–911.
29. Roilides, E., Holmes, A., Blake, C., Pizzo, P.A., and Walsh, T.J. (1993) Defective antifungal activity of monocyte-derived macrophages from HIV-infected children against *Aspergillus fumigatus. J. Infect. Dis.* **168**, 1562–1565.
30. Shearer, G.M. and Clerici, M. (1992) T helper cell immune dysfunction in asymptomatic, HIV-1-seropositive individuals: The role of TH1-TH2 cross-regulation. *Chem. Immunol.* **54**, 21–43.
31. Grazziutti, M.L., Savary, C.A., Ford, A., Anaissie, E.J., Cowart, R.E., and Rex, J.H. (1997) *Aspergillus fumigatus* conidia induce a Th1-type cytokine response. *J. Infect. Dis.* **176**, 1579–1583.
32. Schelenz, S., Smith, D.A., and Bancroft, G.J. (1999) Cytokine and chemokine responses following pulmonarry challenge with *Aspergillus fumigatus:* obligatory role of TNF-α and GM-CSF in neutrophil recruitment. *Med. Mycol.* **37**, 183–194.
33. Taramelli, D., Cocuzza, G., Basilico, N., Sala, G., and Malabarba, M.G. (1996) Production of cytokines by alveolar and peritoneal macrophages stimulated by *Aspergillus fumigatus* conidia or hyphae. *J. Med. Vet. Mycol.* **34**, 49–56.
34. Rossano, F., Ortega, D.L., Buommino, E., Cusumano, V., Losi, E., and Catania, M.R. (1999) Secondary metabolites of *Aspergillus* exert immunobiological effects on human monocytes. *Res. Microbiol.* **150**, 13–19.
35. Cenci, E., Perito, S., Enssle, K.-H., Mosci, P., Latge, J.-P., Romani, L., et al. (1997) Th1 and Th2 cytokines in mice with invasive aspergillosis. *Infect. Immun.* **65**, 564–570.
36. Clemons, K.V., Calich, V.L., Burger, E., Filler, S.G., Grazziutti, M., Murphy, J., et al. (2000) Pathogenesis I: interactions of host cells and fungi. *Med. Mycol.* **38**,*(Suppl 1)*, 99–111.
37. Borger, P., Koeter, G. H., Timmerman, J.A., Vellenga, E., Tomee, J.F., and Kauffman, H.F. (1999) Proteases from *Aspergillus fumigatus* induce interleukin (IL)-6 and IL-8 production in airway epithelial cell lines by transcriptional mechanisms. *J. Infect. Dis.* **180**, 1267–1274.
38. Duong, M., Ouellet, N., Simard, M., Bergeron, Y., Olivier, M., and Bergeron, M.G. (1998) Kinetic study of host defense and inflammatory response to *Aspergillus fumigatus* in steroid-induced immunosuppressed mice. *J. Infect. Dis.* **178**, 1472–1482.
39. Brieland, J.K., Jackson, C., Menzel, F., Loebenberg, D., Cacciapuoti, A., Halpern, J., et al. (2001) Cytokine networking in lungs of immunocompetent mice in response to inhaled *Aspergillus fumigatus. Infect. Immun.* **69**, 1554–1560.
40. Mehrad, B., Strieter, R.M., and Standiford, T.J. (1999) Role of TNF-alpha in pulmonary host defense in murine invasive aspergillosis. *J. Immunol.* **162**, 1633–1640.
41. Mehrad, B., Moore, T.A., and Standiford, T.J. (2000) Macrophage inflammatory protein-1 alpha is a critical mediator of host defense against invasive pulmonary aspergillosis in neutropenic hosts. *J. Immunol.* **165**, 962–968.
42. Blease, K., Mehrad, B., Standiford, T. J., Lukacs, N. W., Kunkel, S. L., Chensue, S. W., et al. (2000) Airway remodeling is absent in CCR1–/– mice during chronic fungal allergic airway disease. *J. Immunol.* **165**, 1564–1572.
43. Blease, K., Mehrad, B., Standiford, T. J., Lukacs, N. W., Gosling, J., Boring, L., et al. (2000) Enhanced pulmonary allergic responses to *Aspergillus* in CCR2–/– mice. *J. Immunol.* **165**, 2603–2611.
44. Roilides, E., Uhlig, K., Venzon, D., Pizzo, P.A., and Walsh, T.J. (1993) Enhancement of oxidative response and damage caused by human neutrophils to *Aspergillus fumigatus* hyphae by granulocyte colony-stimulating factor and gamma interferon. *Infect. Immun.* **61**, 1185–1193.
45. Liles, W.C., Huang, J.E., van Burik, J.A., Bowden, R.A., and Dale, D.C. (1997) Granulocyte colony-stimulating factor administered in vivo augments neutrophil-mediated activity against opportunistic fungal pathogens. *J. Infect. Dis.* **175**, 1012–1015.
46. Vecchiarelli, A., Monari, C., Baldelli, F., Pietrella, D., Retini, C., Tascini, C., et al. (1995) Beneficial effect of recombinant human granulocyte colony-stimulating factor on fungicidal activity of polymorphonuclear leukocytes from patients with AIDS. *J. Infect. Dis.* **171**, 1448–1454.
47. Roilides, E., Uhlig, K., Venzon, D., Pizzo, P.A., and Walsh, T.J. (1993) Prevention of corticosteroid-induced suppression of human polymorphonuclear leukocyte-induced damage of *Aspergillus fumigatus* hyphae by granulocyte colony-stimulating factor and interferon-γ. *Infect. Immun.* **61**, 4870–4807.
48. Rex, J.H., Bhalla, S.C., Cohen, D.M., Hester, J.P., Vartivarian, S.E., and Anaissie, E.J. (1995) Protection of human polymorphonuclear leukocyte function from the deleterious effects of isolation, irradiation, and storage by interferon-γ and granulocyte colony-stimulating factor. *Transfusion* **35**, 605–611.
49. Polak-Wyss, A. (1991) Protective effect of human granulocyte colony-stimulating factor on *Cryptococcus* and *Aspergillus* infections in normal and immunosuppressed mice. *Mycoses* **34**, 205–215.
50. Graybill, J.R., Bocanegra, R., Najvar, L.K., Loebenberg, D., and Luther, M.F. (1998) Granulocyte colony-stimulating factor and azole antifungal therapy in murine aspergillosis: role of immune suppression. *Antimicrob. Agents Chemother.* **42**, 2467–2673.
51. Vora, S., Chauhan, S., Brummer, E., and Stevens, D.A. (1998) Activity of voriconazole combined with neutrophils or monocytes against *Aspergillus fumigatus:* effects of granulocyte colony-stimulating factor and granulocyte-macrophage colony-stimulating factor. *Antimicrob. Agents Chemother.* **42**, 2299–2303.

52. Gaviria, J.M., van Burik, J.A., Dale, D.C., Root, R.K., and Liles, W.C. (1999) Modulation of neutrophil-mediated activity against the pseudohyphal form of Candida albicans by granulocyte colony-stimulating factor (G-CSF) administered in vivo. *J. Infect. Dis.* **179,** 1301–1304.

53. Lieschke, G.J. and Burgess, A.W. (1992) Granulocyte colony-stimulating factor and granulocyte-macrophage colony-stimulating factor (1). *N. Engl. J. Med.* **327,** 28–35.

54. Morrissey, P.J., Grabstein, K.H., and Reed, S.G. (1989) Granulocyte-macrophage colony-stimulating factor: a potent activation signal for mature macrophages and monocytes. *Int. Arch. Allergy Immunol.* **88,** 40–45.

55. Roilides, E., Holmes, A., Blake, C., Venzon, D., Pizzo, P.A., and Walsh, T.J. (1994) Antifungal activity of elutriated human monocytes against *Aspergillus fumigatus* hyphae: Enhancement by granulocyte–macrophage colony-stimulating factor and interferon-γ. *J. Infect. Dis.* **170,** 894–849.

56. Roilides, E., Blake, C., Holmes, A., Pizzo, P.A., and Walsh, T.J. (1996) Granulocyte–macrophage colony-stimulating factor and interferon-γ prevent dexamethasone-induced imunosuppression of antifungal monocyte activity against *Aspergillus fumigatus* hyphae. *J. Med. Vet. Mycol.* **34,** 63–69.

57. Roilides, E., Sein, T., Holmes, A., Blake, C., Pizzo, P.A., and Walsh, T.J. (1995) Effects of macrophage colony-stimulating factor on antifungal activity of mononuclear phagocytes against *Aspergillus fumigatus. J. Infect. Dis.* **172,** 1028–1034.

58. Roilides, E. and Pizzo, P.A. (1992) Modulation of host defenses by cytokines: evolving adjuncts in prevention and treatment of serious infections in immunocompromised hosts. *Clin. Infect. Dis.* **15,** 508–524.

59. Roilides, E., Lyman, C.A., Filioti, J., Akpogheneta, O., Sein, T., Gil-Lamaignere, C., et al. (2002) Amphotericin B formulations exert additive antifungal activity in combination with pulmonary alveolar macrophages and polymorphonuclear leukocytes against *Aspergillus fumigatus. Antimicrob. Agents Chemother.* **46,** 1974–1976.

60. Roilides, E., Lyman, C.A., Mertins, S.D., Cole, D.J., Venzon, D., Pizzo, P.A., et al. (1996) Ex vivo effects of macrophage colony-stimulating factor on human monocyte activity against fungal and bacterial pathogens. *Cytokine* **8,** 42–48.

61. Gonzalez, C., Lyman, C.A, Lee, S., Del Guercio, C., Roilides, E., Bacher, J., et al. Recombinant human macrophage colony-stimulating factor augments pulmonary host defences against *Aspergillus fumigatus. Cytokine* **21,** 87–95.

62. Rex, J.H., Bennett, J.E., Gallin, J.I., Malech, H.L., Decarlo, E.S., and Melnick, D.A. (1991) In vivo interferon-γ therapy augments the in vitro ability of chronic granulomatous disease neutrophils to damage *Aspergillus hyphae. J. Infect. Dis.* **163,** 849–852.

63. Nagai, H., Guo, J., Choi, H., and Kurup, V. (1995) Interferon-γ and tumor necrosis factor-α protect mice from invasive aspergillosis. *J. Infect. Dis.* **172,** 1554–1560.

64. Gaviria, J.M., van Burik, J.A., Dale, D.C., Root, R.K., and Liles, W.C. (1999) Comparison of interferon-gamma, granulocyte colony-stimulating factor, and granulocyte–macrophage colony-stimulating factor for priming leukocyte-mediated hyphal damage of opportunistic fungal pathogens. *J. Infect. Dis.* **179,** 1038–1041.

65. The International Chronic Granulomatous Disease Cooperative Study Group (1991) A controlled trial of interferon gamma to prevent infection in chronic granulomatous disease. *N. Engl. J. Med.* **324,** 509–516.

66. Touza Rey, F., Martinez Vazquez, C., Alonso, J., Mendez Pineiro, M.J., Rubianes Gonzalez, M., and Crespo Casal, M. (2000) The clinical response to interferon-gamma in a patient with chronic granulomatous disease and brain abcesses due to *Aspergillus fumigatus. Ann. Med. Int.* **17,** 86–87.

67. Pasic, S., Abinun, M., Pistignjat, B., Vlajic, B., Rakic, J., Sarjanovic, L., et al. (1996) Aspergillus osteomyelitis in chronic granulomatous disease: treatment with recombinant gamma-interferon and itraconazole. *Pediatr. Infect. Dis. J.* **15,** 833–834.

68. Bernhisel-Broadbent, J., Camargo, E.E., Jaffe, H.S., and Lederman, H.M. (1991) Recombinant human interferon-γ as adjunct therapy for *Aspergillus* infection in a patient with chronic granulomatous disease. *J. Infect. Dis.* **163,** 908–911.

69. Tsumura, N., Akasu, Y., Yamane, H., Ikezawa, S., Hirata, T., Oda, K., et al. (1999) *Aspergillus* osteomyelitis in a child who has p67-phox-deficient chronic granulomatous disease. *Kurume Med. J.* **46,** 87–90.

70. Roilides, E., Farmaki, E., Lyman, CA. (2002) Immune reconstitution against human mycoses. in *Fungal Pathogenesis: Principles and Clinical Applications* (Calderone, R. and Cihlar, R., eds.) Marcel Dekker, New York, pp. 433–460.

71. Roilides, E., Dimitriadou-Georgiadou, A., Sein, T., Kadiltzoglou, I., and Walsh, T.J. (1998) Tumor necrosis factor alpha enhances antifungal activities of polymorphonuclear and mononuclear phagocytes against *Aspergillus fumigatus. Infect. Immun.* **66,** 5999–6003.

72. Roilides, E., Tsaparidou, S., Kadiltsoglou, I., Sein, T., and Walsh, T.J. (1999) Interleukin-12 enhances antifungal activity of human mononuclear phagocytes against *Aspergillus fumigatus:* implications for a gamma interferon-independent pathway. *Infect. Immun.* **67,** 3047–3050.

73. Cenci, E., Mencacci, A., Fe d' Ostiani, C., Del Sero, G., Mosci, P., Montagnoli, C., et al. (1998) Cytokine- and T helper-dependent lung mucosal immunity in mice with invasive pulmonary aspergillosis. *J. Infect. Dis.* **178,** 1750–1760.

74. Cenci, E., Mencacci, A., Bacci, A., Bistoni, F., Kurup, V.P., and Romani, L. (2000) T Cell vaccination in mice with invasive pulmonary aspergillosis. *J. Immunol.* **165,** 381–388.

75. Roilides, E., Dimitriadou, A., Kadiltsoglou, I., Pizzo, P.A., Karpouzas, J., and Walsh, T.J. (1995) Effects of interleukin-4 on antifungal activity of mononuclear phagocytes against hyphae and conidia of *Aspergillus fumigatus, 7th European Congress of Clinical Microbiology and Infectious Diseases* (abstract).

76. Cenci, E., Mencacci, A., Del Sero, G., Bacci, A., Montagnoli, C., Fe d' Ostiani, C., et al. (1999) Interleukin-4 causes susceptibility to invasive pulmonary aspergillosis through suppression of protective type 1 responses. *J. Infect. Dis.* **180,** 1957–1968.

77. Roilides, E., Dimitriadou, A., Kadiltsoglou, I., Sein, T., Karpouzas, J., Pizzo, P. A., et al. (1997) IL-10 exerts suppressive and enhancing effects on antifungal activity of mononuclear phagocytes against *Aspergillus fumigatus. J. Immunol.* **158,** 322–329.

78. Del Sero, G., Mencacci, A., Cenci, E., Fe d' Ostiani, C., Montagnoli, C., Bacci, A., et al. (1999) Antifungal type 1 responses are upregulated in IL-10-deficient mice. *Microbes Infect.* **1,** 1169–1180.
79. Clemons, K.V., Grunig, G., Sobel, R.A., Mirels, L.F., Rennick, D.M., and Stevens, D.A. (2000) Role of IL-10 in invasive aspergillosis: increased resistance of IL-10 gene knockout mice to lethal systemic aspergillosis. *Clin. Exp. Immunol.* **122,** 186–191.
80. Roilides, E., Sein, T., Roden, M., Schaufele, R.L., and Walsh, T. J. (2001) Elevated serum concentrations of interleukin-10 in nonneutropenic patients with invasive aspergillosis. *J. Infect. Dis.* **183,** 518–520.
81. Warris, A., Bjorneklett, A., and Gaustad, P. (2001) Invasive pulmonary aspergillosis associated with infliximab therapy. *N. Engl. J. Med.* **344,** 1099–1100.

16
Cytokines of Innate and Adaptive Immunity
to *Candida albicans*

Luigina Romani

1. INTRODUCTION

Host defense mechanisms against fungi are numerous and range from relatively primitive and constitutively expressed, nonspecific defenses to sophisticated adaptive mechanisms that are specifically induced during infection *(1,2)*. Although the role of innate immunity was originally considered to be a process for defense of the host early in infection, it is now clear that there is an important reciprocal relationship between innate and adaptive immune responses *(2)*. Cytokines and other mediators play an essential role in this process and, indeed, may not only activate the innate cell population but also drive the adaptive immune response down different pathways of differentiation, ultimately determining the type of effector response that is generated toward pathogens *(2–4)*. Cytokines (including interleukin [IL]-12 and interferon [IFN]-γ) are known to act to stimulate either Th1-type immune responses, which mainly protect against intracellular pathogens, or Th2 responses involved in protection against extracellular pathogens, such as helminths (including IL-4, IL-5, IL-6, IL-10, and IL-13) *(5)*. The cytokine microenvironment also influences innate cell populations, including macrophages, polymorphonuclear neutrophils (PMNs), natural killer (NK) cells, and, particularly, stimulating the differentiation of dendritic cells (DCs) with distinct immunoregulatory properties that may promote Th1- or Th2-type adaptive immune responses *(6)*. To limit the pathologic consequences of an excessive inflammatory cell-mediated immune reaction, the immune system resorts to a number of protective mechanisms, including the reciprocal cross-regulatory effects of Th1- and Th2-type effector cytokines, such as IFN-γ and IL-4 *(5)*. However, Th2-type cytokines may also have strong down regulatory effects on the Th1-promoting properties of innate cells. Thus, innate and adaptive immune responses are intimately linked and controlled by sets of molecules and receptors that act to generate the most effective form of immunity for protection against pathogens.

Cytokines act in a highly complex coordinated network in which they induce or repress their own synthesis as well as that of other cytokines and cytokine receptors *(7)*. In addition, many cytokines appear to be pleiotropic, with the corollary that the cytokine network is highly flexible, because there is considerable overlap and redundancy between the function of individual cytokines. Therefore, improved understanding of the function of each individual cytokine may facilitate their use as immunological adjuvants in a variety of vaccination and therapeutic strategies.

In this chapter, I will outline current concepts of cytokine regulation of the development and expression of protective and nonprotective immune responses to *Candida albicans*.

From: *Cytokines and Chemokines in Infectious Diseases Handbook*
Edited by: M. Kotb and T. Calandra © Humana Press Inc., Totowa, NJ

2. HOST IMMUNE RESPONSE TO *C. ALBICANS* INFECTION: AN INTEGRATED VIEW

Candida albicans is associated with a wide spectrum of diseases in humans, ranging from allergy, severe intractable mucocutaneous diseases to life-threatening bloodstream infections *(8)*. Candidal infections are a significant clinical problem for a variety of immunocompetent and immuno-compromised patients *(9,10)*. In the latter group, neutropenia and acquired immunodeficiency syndrome (AIDS) epitomize the two major conditions (i.e., the defect in antifungal effector function and the defect in T-cell directive immunity, which predispose to invasive and superficial infections, respectively) *(3)*. The beneficial effect of immunomodulators in clinical and preclinical models of the infection *(11–13)* suggests that maneuvers aimed at restoring the host defective antifungal immune responsiveness can be exploited for prophylaxis and therapy.

Innate and acquired cell-mediated immunity have been acknowledged as the primary mediators of host resistance to *C. albicans (1–3)*. With the recognition of the reciprocal influences between the innate and the adaptive Th immunity *(14)*, it appears that an integrated immune response determines the lifelong commensalism of the fungus at the mucosal level, as well as the transition from mucosal saprophyte to pathogen.

Innate immunity plays an essential role in orchestrating the subsequent adaptive immunity to *C. albicans (15, 16)*. Through the involvement of a set of germline-encoded receptors (referred to as pattern recognition receptors [PRRs]) *(17–20)*, cells of the innate immune system not only discriminate between different forms of *C. albicans*, but also contribute to discrimination between self and pathogens at the level of the adaptive Th immunity *(19,21,22)* (*see* Fig. 1). As the different Th cell subsets are endowed with the ability to release a distinct panel of cytokines, capable of activating and deactivating signals to effector phagocytes, the activation of an appropriate Th subset may be instrumental in the generation of a successful immune response to the fungal pathogen *(15,22–26)* (*see* Fig. 2). In its basic conception, the paradigm calls for (1) an association between Th1 responses and the onset/maintenance of phagocyte-dependent immunity, critical for opposing infectivity of the commensal or clearing pathogenic fungi from infected tissues, (2) the occurrence of Th2 responses in infections and diseases, and (3) the reciprocal regulation of Th1 and Th2 cells, occurring either directly or through regulatory T-cells, resulting in a dynamic balance between these two types of reactivity, that may operate from commensalism to infection and may contribute to the induction and maintenance of protective memory antifungal responses with minimum immunopathology.

2.1. The Innate Immunity

2.1.1. The Antifungal Effector Mechanisms

The observation that invasive candidiasis occurs in concomitance with defects in PMN number and functions *(27)*, together with the detection of cells and mediators of the innate immune system with antifungal effector activities *(3)*, has led to the central dogma of resistance to invasive candidiasis [i.e., that resistance is mediated by the innate immune system, which includes circulating PMNs and monocytes, tissue macrophages, natural killer cells, and soluble molecules, including opsonins (specific antibodies, and components of classical and alternative complement pathways), mannose-binding proteins, collectins, and defensins *(2, 3, 21, 22)*]. Although freshly isolated phagocytic cells clearly express intrinsic anti-*Candida* activity, numerous studies have demonstrated that expression of the full candidacidal function of both neutrophils and monocyte/macrophages requires activation by colony-stimulating factors (CSFs) *(3,11)*. However, optimal expression of the antifungal effector activity of cells of the innate immune system is attained in association with antigen-driven immune responses *(2, 3)*. This may occur through the release of cytokines with activating (IFN-γ/tumor necrosis factor [TNF]-α) and deactivating IL-4/IL-10 signals to effector phagocytes *(28)*.

It is becoming clear that the engagement of distinct receptors and PRRs on phagocytic cells may result in profoundly different downstream intracellular events that have important consequences in

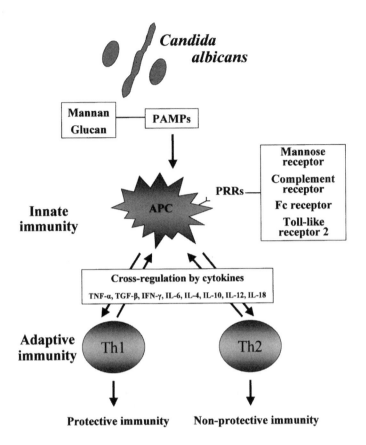

Fig. 1. Immunological determination of self and non-self in candidiasis. Pathogen-associated molecular patterns (PAMPs) of *C. albicans* are recognized by innate immune cells (including dendritic cells, macrophages, and neutrophils) via PRRs. This process signals to innate cells the presence of the foreign organism and activates the secretion of a battery of effector cytokines that play a variety of roles in directing the immune response.

the expression of the overall antifungal immune defense. Thus, although binding and internalization of fungal cells by PMNs may occur through mannose receptors (MR), complement receptor 3 (CR3), and receptors for immunoglobulins (FcR), effective phagocytosis and killing of *C. albicans* occurs via targeting FcγRI (CD64) and FCαRI (CD89) receptors (reviewed in *ref. 21*). As with PMNs, internalization via constitutively competent MR does not represent an effective way of clearing the yeasts by macrophages. Actually, the enhancement of phagocytosis and killing of *C. albicans* by macrophages correlated with a decreased number of mannose receptors *(29)*. The most efficient uptake is dependent on CR3-mediated phagocytosis of both serum opsonized and unopsonized yeasts, a process inhibitable by cell wall components of the fungus (reviewed in *ref. 21*). However, interaction with macrophage CR3 leads to suppression of the immune response to the microorganism (further discussed in Subheading 2.1.2.). Thus, phagocytes use different receptors to phagocytose opsonized and unopsonized *Candida* cells *(21,22)*.

Recent studies indicated that DCs also behave as potent antifungal effector cells in *C. albicans* infection *(19)*. These cells may be of particular importance in candidiasis, considering that the fungus behaves as a commensal as well as a true pathogen of skin and mucosal surfaces *(8)*, known to be highly enriched with DCs. DCs phagocytose both yeast and hyphal forms of the fungus through different receptors and phagocytic mechanisms. After phagocytosis of yeasts or hyphae, the downstream cellular events are clearly different. Ingestion of yeasts, but not hyphae, activates DCs for candidacidal

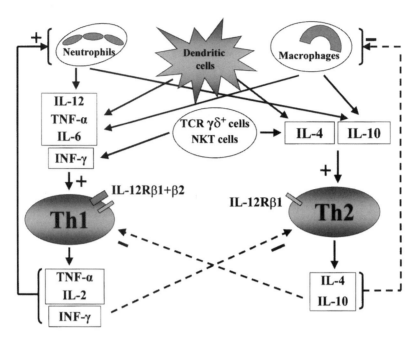

Fig. 2. Cytokine regulation of the innate and adaptive immunity to *C. albicans*. Cells of the innate immune system, by discriminating between different forms of the fungus, produce sets of cytokines and costimulatory molecules through which signals to the adaptive T-helper (Th) immune system. Effector cytokines produced by Th1 or Th2 cells may, in turn, feed back on the innate immune system, affecting both its antifungal effector and immunomodulatory functions. Solid and dotted lines refer to positive and negative regulatory pathways, respectively.

activity, including nitric oxide production. Thus, these results indicate that DCs may fulfill the requirement of a cell uniquely capable of sensing the different forms of fungi in terms of antifungal effector functions and type of Th immune responses elicited (further discussed in Subheading 2.1.2.).

Although the effectiveness of this effector system is undoubtedly acknowledged, it has also been recognized that invasive infections may occur in the presence of an adequate effector count, a finding emphasizing the concepts that optimal antifungal immune resistance is achieved through the combined and interdependent effort of innate and adaptive immune mechanisms and that the innate immune system functions as both a guide and instructor of the subsequent adaptive immunity.

2.1.2. The Instructive Role

The instructive role of the innate immune system in the adaptive immune responses to *C. albicans* occurs at different levels (30). Qualitative or quantitative defects of antifungal effector phagocytes results in the development of anticandidal Th2, rather than Th1, cell responses (30, 31). As CD4⁺ Th cell differentiation in vivo was found to be critically affected by the tissue fungal load (30), an important role of phagocytic cells relies on their ability to control the fungal growth through their antifungal effector mechanisms. In addition to this, however, the instructive role of the innate immune system in the adaptive immune response to the fungus is operative at the levels of discriminative productions of cytokine and expression of costimulatory molecules (30). Discrimination occurs though the involvement of PRRs, including the Toll-like receptors (TLRs), recognizing invariant molecular structures shared by fungi [also known as PAMPs (pathogen-associated molecular patterns) (18,19,21,22)]. PRRs and TRLs now appear to be involved in the recognition of PAMPs on different classes of pathogens: lipopolysaccharide (LPS) of Gram-negative bacteria, lipoteichoic acid and peptidoglycan of Gram-positive bacteria, mannan and glucan of fungi, phosphoglycan of parasites and unmethylated CpG motifs from procaryotic DNA *(18)*.

In candidiasis, the engagement of PRRs and TLRs with PAMPS creates signals that (1) induce opsonization for phagocytosis and/or the activation of the lectin pathways of complement, (2) promote phagocytosis, and (3) induce effector functions that initiate the expression of inflammatory cytokines and the adaptive immunity *(32)*.

The PAMP/PRR interactions are important for stimulating cellular secretion of effector cytokines. The types of effector cytokine that are produced by cells of the innate immune system, particularly DCs, are induced by the types of antigen that bind particular PRRs on innate cells. For example, the mannose receptor induced expression of some cytokines, such as IL-1α, IL-6, IL-12 and granulocyte–macrophage-CSF (GM-CSF) in response to the fungus, whereas some chemokine responses were mediated by other receptors *(33)*. The engagement of another PRR, the FcγR, down regulated the production of IL-12 by DCs, thereby favoring the development of a Th2-type adaptive immune response *(32)*. It is interesting to note that the engagement of FcγR mainly occurs with the hyphal form of the fungus, a finding linking fungal virulence to the development of a nonprotective Th response. From this scenario, it follows that if the entry of fungal cells occurs through a phagocyte receptor other than the MRs, this may result in a failure to activate IL-12-dependent protective Th1 responses. Thus, not only are different PRRs involved in the recognition of the different forms of the fungus, but also the engagement of different PRRs is involved in different cellular responses. Alternatively, the use of different PRRs by the different forms may represent one important strategy of immune evasion and parasitism of the fungus. This seems to be the case. CR3 engagement is one of the most efficient receptors for the uptake of opsonized yeasts *(21)*. However, as already stated, for effective killing and cytokine release to occur, the concomitant engagement of the FcγRI or FCαRI receptors is required *(21)*. Thus, signaling through CR3 may not lead to phagocyte activation. It has recently been shown that signaling via CR3 down-regulates IL-12 production in response to *Histoplasma capsulatum (34)*. In the case of *C. albicans*, the interaction with macrophage CR3 led to suppression of the immune response to the fungus. Interestingly, CR3 has binding sites for *Candida* hyphae more than *Candida* yeasts *(35)* and therefore may represent one of the most important binding sites for the hyphal form. This may result in a failure to induce IL-12 and protective Th1 immunity in response to *Candida* hyphae. Chiani has recently reported that human monocytes fail to induce IL-12 in response to the hyphal form of the fungus *(36)*. As discussed next, effector cytokines are, in turn, important for regulating expression and functions of PRRs.

All together, these observations suggest that the use of the different PRRs, either alone or simultaneously, may result in the coupling or uncoupling phagocytosis with inflammatory and immunological responseΔ Hence, the innate immune system appears to have the ability to autonomously decide whether or not to implicate the adaptive immune system.

2.2. The Adaptive Immunity: The Th Paradigm

The clinical circumstances in which recurrent *Candida* infections occur definitely suggest an association with impaired cell-mediated immunity, yet only in the last decade has direct evidence of this relationship been obtained in experimental models of mucosal or invasive candidiasis *(3,15,23–26,37,38)*. The general thrust of these studies is that the major function of the T-lymphocytes in *Candida* infections is the production of cytokines with activating and deactivating signals to fungicidal effector phagocytes. Therefore, host resistance to the fungus appears to be dependent on the induction of cellular immunity, mediated by T-lymphocytes and nonspecific effector phagocytes *(2,3,22)*. The qualitative pattern of cytokines secreted by T-cells will ultimately determine the efficacy of the effector response mediated by phagocytes.

The discovery that subsets of CD4+ Th cells could be distinguished according to their ability to produce discrete patterns of cytokines *(5)* offered the conceptual framework of the adaptive immunity in *C. albicans (15,23–26)*. Th1 cells, by their production of IFN-γ and TNF-α, are responsible for directing cell-mediated immune responses to the fungus. By producing IL-4 and IL-10, Th2 cells have been strongly implicated in dampening the protective antifungal Th1 immunity and mediating fungal allergy. That acquired immunity to *C. albicans* correlates with the expression of local or peripheral Th1 reactivity has also been confirmed by studies in adult healthy humans *(38,39)*. Underlying acquired immunity to the fungus, such as the expression of delayed-type hypersensitivity, the fungus is demonstrable in adult immunocompetent individuals and is presumed to prevent mucosal colonization from progression to symptomatic infection *(23–26)*. The expression of this cutaneous reactivity is often defective in neonates, in immunocompromised individuals, as well as in patients, with recurrent or persistent infection with the fungus or immunopathology associated with it *(23–25)*. Human lymphocytes show strong proliferative responses after stimulation with *Candida* antigens *(40)* and produce a number of different cytokines *(41)*. Because of their action on circulating leukocytes, the cytokines produced by *Candida*-specific T-cells may be instrumental in mobilizing and activating anticandidal effectors *(28)*, thus providing prompt and effective control of infectivity once *Candida* has established itself in mucosal tissues or spread to internal organs. A Th1-type reactivity may characterize the saprophytic yeast carriage of healthy subjects, whereas Th2-type responses would be mostly associated with susceptibility to recurrent or persistent infection *(42)* and allergy *(25)*. For example, in patients with a defective IL-12/IFN-γ pathway, such as those with hyperimmunoglobulinemia E syndrome, both an impaired IL-12 response to the fungus *(43)* and visceral candidiasis *(44)* are observed. Of interest, suppression of cell-mediated immunity may be a consequence of *C. albicans* infection, as demonstrated by much experimental and clinical evidence. Polysaccharide antigens of the fungus generate a complex series of interactions resulting in the suppression of both T- and B-cell responses to the homologous antigen. These effects are mediated by antigen-nonspecific inhibitory factors that are able to block the synthesis of cytokines by human monocytes and T-cells (reviewed in *ref. 26*).

It is important to note that experimental and clinical evidence indicate that differences may exist in cell and cytokine requirement for antifungal resistance at mucosal or peripheral levels *(26,37)*, a notion exemplified by the long-recognized association between disseminated candidiasis and qualitative and quantitative defects of neutrophils and between chronic mucosal infections and T-cell abnormalities *(8)*. The concept of a reciprocal regulation between the phagocyte system and the T-cell compartment may provide a unifying thread between the systemic immune responses and events occurring at the mucosal surface. The expression of acquired resistance at both mucosal and nonmucosal effector sites may involve common mechanisms in humans who develop systemic immunity as a consequence of their mucosal colonization. These mechanisms likely operate through the action of Th1 lymphocytes, the cytokines they release, and nonspecifically activated effector cells. The unitary role for cell-mediated immunity in anticandidal resistance would predict that, for example, eradication of an established infection, whether superficial or deep-seated, could be accelerated by recruitment of antigen-specific cells that would provide the locally high cytokine concentrations needed for optimal activation of the anticandidal effector phagocytes.

3. CYTOKINES IN RESPONSE TO *C. ALBICANS* INFECTION

Upon contact with *C. albicans*, cells of the innate immune system release a battery of chemokines and cytokines that have profound effects on the functional activity of the innate response and on subsequent events of adaptive immunity. The local release of these effector molecules serve to regulate cell trafficking of various types of leukocyte, thus initiating the inflammatory response, and to activate phagocytic cells to a microbicidal state. The role of chemokines in candidiasis is relatively unknown. It has been shown that this organism can induce the production of chemokines (reviewed in *ref. 4*). In vitro studies have shown that peripheral blood mononuclear cells produce some chemokines upon exposure to the fungus. Interestingly, the production of chemokines appears to occur differently in response to the yeast or hyphal forms of the fungus *(45)* and to be dependent on the engagement of selective PRRs *(33)*. A prominent role for macrophage chemoattractant protein (MCP)-1 in the local control of the infection was observed in experimental vaginal candidiasis, where MCP-1 neutralization resulted in an increased infectivity of the fungus *(46)*. Instead, truncated CXC chemokines might aid in the clearance of disseminated *C. albicans* infection, as administration of truncated KC increased survival of mice to the infection *(47)*.

Tumor necrosis factor-α, IL-1β, IL-6, IL-8, and CSFs are proinflammatory cytokines readily produced upon interaction of phagocytes and fibroblasts with fungal cells and are detected in *Candida* sepsis *(21, 22, 48, 49)*. TNF-α is essential in the innate control of disseminated infection caused by *C. albicans (30,50)*. It is produced by PMN in an opsonic-dependent manner *(51)* and by macrophages in response to β-1,2 linked mannooligosaccharides *(51)* and in a Fas–FasL-dependent interaction *(53)*. TNF-α is also produced by endothelial cells in response to the fungus and mediates the secretion of IL-8 by these cells *(54)*. The cytokine regulates the recruitment of inflammatory cells, triggers the respiratory burst and induces expression of costimulatory molecules. Although IL-1 shares many properties with TNF-α, both IL-1β and IL-6, which mainly act through recruitment of PMNs, do not seem to be as essential as TNF-α in the innate antifungal response. Administration of IL-1β has been beneficial in mice with candidiasis; nevertheless, IL-1 deficiency does not increase the susceptibility of mice to the infection as does IL-6 deficiency *(30)*. IL-8 is implicated in the recruitment and functional activation of PMN against the fungus *(55,56)*.

Interferon-γ is a key cytokine in the innate control of the infection *(57,58)*. It stimulates migration, adherence, phagocytosis, and oxidative killing of PMNs and activates macrophages and endothelial cells for fungicidal activity. Studies in mice and humans have clearly shown the importance of IFN-γ as one major determinant of innate resistant to candidiasis *(57, 58)*. However, other studies have revealed the dispensability of IFN-γ as an effector molecule *(59, 60)*, thus revealing the complex role of IFN-γ in the intimate intricacy between the innate and the adaptive immunity to the fungus (further discussed in Subheading 5).

Interleukin-12 is recognized as essential for the induction of protective Th1 responses to the fungus *(61)*. Upon phagocytosis of the fungus, IL-12 is produced by different cells, including PMNs *(61)*, monocytes (36) and DCs *(19)*. IL-12 shares with IL-18, both produced during infection, the ability to induce IFN-γ *(61,62)*. For PMNs and DCs, IL-12 appears to be released in response to a *Candida* strain that initiates Th1 development in vivo and inhibited in response to a virulent strain *(19,31)*. Human PMNs also produce bioactive IL-12 in response to a mannoprotein fraction of *C. albicans*, capable of inducing Th1 cytokine expression in peripheral blood mononuclear cells *(61)*. Because of the large number of neutrophils present in the blood or inflammatory tissues in infection *(31)*, it is likely that neutrophil production of cytokines may influence the development and/or maintenance of the Th repertoire to *C. albicans*.

Interleukin-2 is detected in mice with candidiasis, and its production, early in infection, correlates with disease progression *(63)*. However, IL-2 also have a critical role in the activation of innate effector cells, because of the selective presence of IL-2Rβ on effector phagocytes *(64)*.

One most important cytokine produced in the course of the infection is IL-10. It is readily produced by macrophages *(65)* and PMNs *(31)* upon phagocytosis of the fungus and plays a crucial role in determining susceptibility to the infection *(30)*. High levels of IL-10 are seen in patients with chronic disseminated candidiasis *(66)*. IL-10 acts by impairing the antifungal effector functions of phagocytes, including secretion of inflammatory cytokines and IL-12, and by inhibiting the development of protective cell-mediated immunity *(30,67,68)*. It also acts as one major cytokine discriminating between virulent and less virulent forms of the fungus *(31,69)*.

Similar to IL-10, transforming growth factor (TGF)-β is produced by macrophages and appears to discriminate between virulent and less virulent forms of the fungus in mice with candidiasis *(70)*. In addition, TGF-β is a pivotal cytokine in regulating the levels of local cell-mediated immune reactivity in vaginal candidiasis *(71)*.

In addition to IL-10, IL-4 may act as one major discriminative factor of susceptibility and resistance in disseminated candidiasis *(30)*. Ablation of IL-4 renders susceptible mice resistant to candidiasis. Although IL-4 may inhibit the fungicidal activity of phagocytes *(28,72)*, it also activates phagocytes *(73–75)*. Thus, one likely mechanism of the inhibitory activity of IL-4 in infection relies on its ability to promote Th2 reactivity, thus dampening protective Th1 responses. It has been found that DCs produce IL-4 upon phagocytosis of hyphae but not yeasts of *C. albicans (19)*, thus sensing the different forms of the fungus in terms of cytokine production. Ingestion of yeasts activated DCs for IL-12 and nitric oxide production and priming of Th1 cells, whereas ingestion of hyphae inhibited IL-12, nitric oxide, and Th1 priming, and induced IL-4 *(19)*. These results indicate that DCs fulfill the requirement of a cell uniquely capable of sensing the virulent and nonvirulent forms of the fungus in terms of type of immune response elicited. Considering that the morphogenesis of *C. albicans* is activated in vivo by a wide range of signals *(76)* and that human DCs also phagocytose *C. albicans (77)* and activate T-cell responses to the fungus, DCs appear to meet the challenge of Th priming and education in *C. albicans* saprophytism and infections. Figure 3 illustrates the most important cytokines and their functions in candidiasis.

4. CROSS-REGULATION OF ADAPTIVE AND INNATE IMMUNITY BY CYTOKINES

Th1 and Th2 CD4[+] T-cells develop from a common naive CD4[+] T-cell precursor and several parameters have been reported to influence the pathway of differentiation of CD4[+] T-cell precursors *(5)*. Among these, cytokines appear to play a major role, acting not only as modulators of antifungal effector functions but also as key regulators in the development of the different Th subsets from precursor Th cells. Development of protective anticandidal Th1 responses requires the concerted actions of several cytokines such as IFN-γ, TGF-β, IL-6, TNF-α and IL-12 in the relative absence of inhibitory Th2 cytokines, such as IL-4 and IL-10, which inhibit the induction of Th1 responses *(15,26)*. Early in infection, neutralization of Th1 cytokines (IFN-γ and IL-12) leads to the onset of Th2 rather than Th1 responses, whereas neutralization of Th2 cytokines (IL-4 and IL-10) allows for the development of Th1 rather than Th2 cell responses. These evidence illustrate that the profiles of cytokines that are induced early in infection are of critical importance for the subsequent immuno-logical control of the infection. The initial encounter with the fungus elicits an innate response that will, to a large extent by means of cytokines, determine the nature of the ensuing adaptive response.

As already emphasized, cytokines expressed during the adaptive immune response may, in addition to regulating the expression and maintenance of Th cell phenotypes, also act on innate cells as a feedback mechanism for the purpose of controlling the infection and the maintenance or amplification of immunity. The feedback control by cytokines is operative at both the levels of effector function and instructive activity. Thus, TNF-α, IFN-γ, and IL-2 are all endowed with the ability to activate effector phagocytes to a fungicidal state *(28,64)*. In contrast, both IL-4 and IL-10 are potent inhibitors of the effector activity of monomorphonuclear and polymorphonuclear cells against the fungus *(28,67,72)*. Both the oxidative- and nonoxidative-dependent mechanisms of fungal killing are oppositely regulated by Th1 and Th2 cytokines *(78–80)*. Cytokines also regulate the expression levels of costimulatory molecules on innate cells, thus directly affecting the crosstalk between cells of the innate and the adaptive immunity. In this regard, both TNF-α and IL-10 were found to be required for optimal expression of costimulatory molecules on phagocytes *(30)*.

Effector cytokines are also important for regulating expression and functions of PRRs. The mannose-receptor-mediated uptake of unopsonized *Candida* yeasts may lead to phagocyte abuse if not accompanied by the coordinate activation of the cell cytotoxic machinery *(29)*. Increased expression of the receptor with no induced cytotoxicity was induced upon exposure of macrophages to IL-4 *(74)*. In contrast, IFN-γ downregulated the expression of macrophage mannose receptors and, nevertheless, results in effective killing, presumably via increased coupling of the receptor to cytotoxic functions *(29)*. Thus, Th1 and Th2 cytokines may cooperate to stimulate mannose-receptor-mediated phagocytosis of the fungus *(73)*.

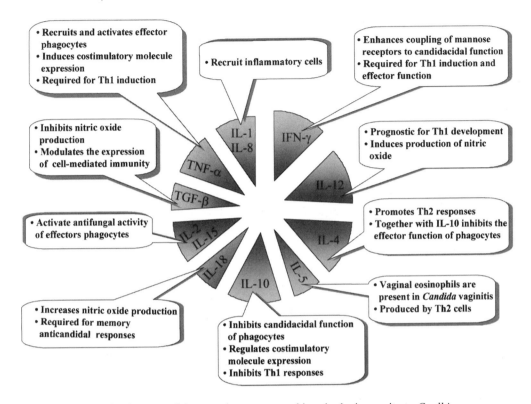

Fig. 3. Major features of the most important cytokines in the immunity to *C. albicans.*

5. THE CYTOKINE PARADOXES IN CANDIDIASIS: RULES AND EXCEPTIONS

Further studies have clearly revealed that individual cytokines can produce opposing effects depending on dose and timing of their participation in the immune response and that some cytokines exert their effects on both the innate and adaptive immunity. For instance, both qualitative and quantitative changes in antifungal effector functions of phagocytic cells, particularly neutrophils, and the activation of nonprotective Th2 responses are observed in the absence of TNF-α or IL-6 *(30)*. One likely mechanism of Th2 development in mice with candidiasis is the increased fungal burden in the organs, as the production of IL-4, and hence Th2 activation, is strictly dependent on the fungal dose *(31)*. Therefore, the defective antifungal effector functions of phagocytes and, consequently, the unopposed fungal growth may account for the failure to mount a protective Th1 response in the absence of TNF-α or IL-6. However, TNF-α was also found to be required for optimal expression of costimulatory molecules on phagocytic cells and for IL-12 responsiveness in CD4+ Th1 cells, whereas decreased production of IL-12 and increased production of IL-10 occurred in the absence of IL-6 *(30)*. Therefore, a cytokine may exert disparate and multiple activities in the immune response to the fungus.

Interferon-γ, like TNF-α, is one major activating signal for effector phagocytes *(28,57)*. However, the absence of IFN-γ can be compensated for by other activating signals for the prompt and efficient activation of the innate immune system *(59)*. Instead, the absence of IFN-γ correlated with the failure to mount protective anticandidal Th1 responses because of an impaired IL-12 responsiveness rather than IL-12 production *(59)*. The activities of IL-12 are mediated through a high-affinity receptor composed of two subunits, designated β1 and β2. Of these two subunits, β2 is more restricted in its distribution, and regulation of its expression is likely a central mechanisms by which IL-12 responsiveness is controlled *(81)*. Indeed, the IL-12Rβ2 subunit expression on activated CD4+ Th1 cells is known to correspond to loss of IL-12 responsiveness and represents an early step in the commitment of T-cells to the Th2 pathway *(82)*. Because IFN-γ is necessary to override the IL-4-induced inhibition of IL-12β2 receptor expression in Th1 cells *(82)*, it is likely that in murine candidiasis, the Th1-promoting activity of IFN-γ may rely on its ability to maintain IL-12 responsiveness on CD4+ cells, by sustaining the IL-12Rβ2 expression.

Interleukin-2 belongs to the Th1 effector cytokines, with activating activity for effector phagocytes *(64)*. However, high levels production of IL-2, early in infection, correlated with disease progression in susceptible mice *(63)*. Thus, the positive activating signal for cells of the innate system is counteracted by the Th2-promoting activity of the cytokine. Therefore, IL-2 may have opposite effects in cells of the innate and adaptive immune systems.

Although IL-4 impaired the antifungal function of effector cells, induced anticandidal Th2 development and exogenous IL-4 exacerbated candidiasis in mice, IL-4 also primed neutrophils for IL-12 synthesis *(75)*. This may account for the requirement for IL-4 in the generation of memory anticandidal Th1 response. Paradoxically, the induction and maintenance of memory Th1 resistance also requires IL-10 and TGF-β *(15)*. Thus, cytokines with inhibitory activity in developing Th1 cell responses are indeed required for sustained Th1 reactivity to the fungus. The possible regulatory cells and mechanisms underlying the expression of immunological memory to *C. albicans* are not yet understood. However, it is intriguing that different Th cells and cytokines are produced in response to different fungal antigens *(83)*. It is possible that the temporally distinct expressions of different antigens during fungal growth in vivo have a role in the expression of immunological memory responses to *C. albicans*, through the induction of regulatory T-cells.

Interleukin-10 impaired the development of protective Th1 responses through inhibition of the nitric oxide-dependent mechanism of antifungal activity of effector phagocytes *(67,78–80)*. However, IL-10 was also required for optimal development of Th1 cells by regulating the expression of costimulatory molecules on innate cells *(84)*. Thus, IL-10 had opposite effects on infection, largely dependent on its concentration *(78)*.

Altogether, the data indicate that (1) the cytokine requirement for the expression of innate antifungal defense may be different from that required for the expression of Th1-mediated protection, (2) a single cytokine may participate in both the innate and the adaptive phase of the response to the fungus, sometimes exhibiting opposite effects, (3) the effect of cytokines may depend on the dose, and (4) a hierarchic pattern exists of cytokine-mediated regulation of antifungal Th cell development and effector function. Early in infection, production of some proinflammatory cytokines (TNF-α and IL-6) appears to be essential for the successful control of infection and the resulting protective Th1-dependent immunity. Both IL-12 production and IL-12 responsiveness are required for the development of Th1 cell responses, which are maintained in the presence of physiological levels of IL-4, IL-10, TGF-β, and IL-18. Thus, a finely regulated balance of directive cytokines, rather than the relative absence of opposing cytokines, appears to be required for optimal development and maintenance of Th1 reactivity in mice with candidiasis. Figure 4 summarizes some cytokine paradoxes in candidiasis.

6. CYTOKINES AS ADJUVANT THERAPY

As clinical resistance represents a significant component of the overall drug resistance of the antifungals *(87)*, one major strategy to prevent antifungal drug resistance is to improve the immune functions of the immunocompromised host. A variety of cytokines *(57,58)*, chemokines *(47)* and growth factors *(88,89)* proved to be beneficial in experimental fungal infections. However, establishing the clinical utility of cytokines as therapy for fungal infections in patients has been difficult *(12)*. The basic strategies pursued include the increase of number, function, and mobility of phagocytic effector cells, as cytokines, effector cells, and antifungals work synergistically to oppose fungal growth. The CSFs have been the target of most investigations *(11,90,91)*.

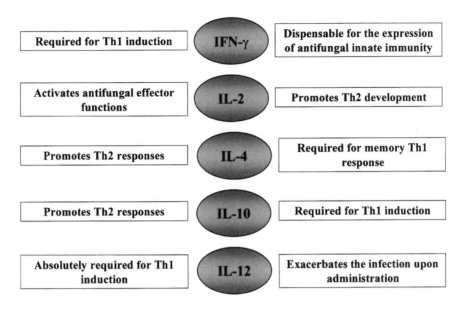

Fig. 4. The cytokine paradoxes in candidiasis: rules and exceptions.

Recently, the Th1/Th2 balance itself was found to be the target of immunotherapy *(89–92)*. Readdressing the Th balance by combination therapy with cytokines or cytokine antagonists represented an effective strategy for the treatment of candidiasis in immunocompromised and nonimmunocompromised hosts. Indeed, the therapeutic efficacy of antifungals in experimental candidiasis was significantly increased by the concomitant inhibition of Th2 cytokines, or the addition of Th1 cytokines and depended on host immune reactivity *(92,93)*. Moreover, the efficacy of antifungals relied on the concomitant cytokine milieu, as, for instance, the efficacy of amphotericin B was increased in the absence of IL-4 and decreased in the absence of IFN-γ. Also, the requirement for cytokines was different among antifungal drugs. Thus, in experimental protocols of therapy, amphotericin B, more than fluconazole, synergized with IL-4 inhibitors in the accomplishment of antifungal activity, whereas fluconazole, more than amphotericin B, synergized with IL-12 *(93)*. All together, these experimental evidence indicate that potentiating the Th1 pathway or dampening the Th2 pathway are possible strategies of immune intervention in combination with antifungals.

7. CONCLUSIONS

A large body of evidence supports the model of specific immunity to *C. albicans* infections as being highly susceptible to cytokine influences and reciprocally regulated by cells of the innate immune system *(94,95)*. Unfortunately, despite encouraging studies in both preclinical and experimental settings, there has been only a small series of studies using immune modulators in treatment of human fungal infections *(96)*. The Th1/Th2 paradigm, although somewhat simplistic, appears to be useful in the identification of cytokines suitable for clinical intervention. The identification of PRRs as a critical component of the innate recognition system is a fundamental breakthrough in immunology, which may have important clinical implications. The understanding of those PRR functions and dysfunctions that are suitable for cytokine manipulation in candidal infections remains a future challenge.

ACKNOWLEDGMENTS

Many thanks are owed to numerous collaborators over the years in different sections of the work described. This work was supported by grants from the AIDS 50C.27 project.

REFERENCES

1. Romani, L. and Howard, D. H. (1995) Mechanisms of resistance to fungal infections. *Curr. Opin. Immunol.* **7**, 517–523.
2. Romani, L and Kaufmann, S. H. E. (1998) Immunity to fungi. *Res. Immunol.* **149**, 277–493.
3. Ashman, R.B., and Papadimitriou, J. M. (1995) Production and function of cytokines in natural and acquired immunity to *Candida albicans* infection. *Microbiol. Rev.* **59**, 646–672.
4. Traynor, T. R. and Huffnagle, G. B. (2001) The role of chemokines in fungal infections. *Med. Mycol.* **39**, 41–50.
5. O' Garra, A. (1998) Cytokines induce the development of functionally heterogeneous T helper cell subsets. *Immunity* **8**, 275–283.
6. Banyer, J. L., Hamilton, N. H. R., Ramshaw, I. A. and Ramsay, A. J. (2000) Cytokines in innate and adaptive immunity. *Rev. Immunogenet* **2**, 359–373.
7. Callard, R., George, A. J. T., and Stark, J. (1999) Cytokines, chaos, and complexity. *Immunity* **11**, 507–5513.
8. Calderone, R.A. (2002) *Candida* and candidiasis, 1st ed., ASM Press.
9. Pfaller, M. A. (1996) Nosocomial candidiasis. Emerging species, reservoirs and models of transmission. *Clin. Infect. Dis.* **22 (Suppl. 2)**, S89–S94.
10. Jarvis, W. R. (1995) Epidemiology of nosocomial fungal infections, with emphasis on *Candida* species. *Clin. Infect. Dis.* **20**, 1526–1530.
11. Kullberg, B. J. and Anaissie, E. J. (1998) Cytokines as therapy for opportunistic fungal infections. *Res. Immunol.* **149**, 478–488.
12. Stevens, D. A. (1998) Combination immunotherapy and antifungal chemotherapy. *Clin. Infect. Dis.* **26**, 1266–1269.
13. Rodriguez-Adrian, L. J., Grazziutti , M. L., Rex, H. J, and Anaissie, E. J. (1998) The potential role of cytokine for fungal infections in patients with cancer: Is recovery from neutropenia all that is needed? *Clin. Infect. Dis.* **26**, 1270–1278.
14. Fearon, J. D. and Locksley, R. M. (1996) The instructive role of innate immunity in the acquired immune response. *Science* **272**, 50–54.
15. Romani, L. (1999) Immunity to *Candida albicans*: Th1, Th2 cells and beyond. *Curr. Opin. Microbiol.* **2**, 363–367.
16. Romani, L. (2000) Innate and adaptive immunity in *Candida albicans* infections and saprophytism. *J. Leukocyte Biol.* **68**, 175–179.
17. Medzihitov, R. and Janeway, C. A. Jr. (1997) Innate immunity: impact on the adaptive immune response. *Curr. Opin. Immunol.* **12**, 13–19.
18. Aderem, A. and Ulevitch, R. J. (2000) Toll-like receptors in the induction of the innate immune response. *Nature* **406**, 782–787.
19. Fè d'Ostiani, C., Del Sero, G., Bacci, A., Montagnoli, C., Spreca, A., Mencacci, et al. (2000) Dendritic cells discriminate between yeasts and hyphae of the fungus *Candida albicans*: implications for initiation of Th immunity in vitro and in vivo. *J. Exp. Med.* **191**, 1661–1674.
20. Mcknight, A. and Gordon, S. (2000) Forum in Immunology: innate recognition systems. *Microbes Infect.* **2**, 239–336.
21. Romani, L. (2002) Innate immunity against fungal pathogens, in *Fungal Pathogenesis: Principles and Clinical Applications* (Chilar, R. and Calderone, R., eds.), Marcel Dekker, New York, pp. 401–432.
22. Romani, L. and Bistoni, F. (2002) Systemic immunity in candidiasis, in *Fungal Pathogenesis: Principles and Clinical Applications* (Chilar, R. and Calderone, R., eds.), Marcel Dekker, New York, pp. 483–514.
23. Fidel, P. L., Jr., and Sobel, J. D. (1994) The role of cell-mediated immunity in candidiasis. *Trends Microbiol.* **6**, 202–206.
24. Puccetti, P., Romani, L., and Bistoni, F. (1995) A Th1-Th2-like switch in candidiasis: new perspectives for therapy. *Trends Microbiol.* **3**, 237–240.
25. Romani, L. (1997) The T-cell response to fungi. *Curr. Opin. Immunol.* **9**, 484–490.
26. Romani, L., Puccetti, P., and Bistoni, F. (1996) Biological role of helper T-cell subsets in candidiasis. *Chem. Immunol.* **63**, 113–137.
27. Bodey, G. P., Buckley, M., Sathe, Y. S., and Freireich, E. J. (1986) Quantitative relationship between circulating leukocytes and infection in patients with acute leukemia. *Ann. Inter. Med.* **64**, 328–340.
28. Djeu, J. Y. (1993) Modulators of immune response to fungi. in *Fungal infections and immune responses* (Murphy, J. W., Friedman, H. and Bendinelli, M., eds.), Plenum Press, New York, pp. 521–532.
29. Marodi, L., Schreiber, S., Anderson, D. C., MacDermott, R. P., Korchak, H. M. and Johnston, R. B. Jr. (1993) Enhancement of macrophage candidacidal activity by interferon-γ increased phagocytosis, killing and calcium signal mediated by a decreased number of mannose receptors. *J. Clin. Invest.* **91**, 2596–2601.
30. Mencacci , A., Cenci, E., Bistoni, F., Del Sero, G., Bacci, A., Montagnoli, C., et al. (1998) Specific and nonspecific immunity to *Candida albicans*: a lesson from genetically modified animals. *Res. Immunol.* **149**, 352–361.
31. Montagnoli, C., Bacci, A., Bozza, S., Gaziano, R. Spreca, A., and Romani, L. (2002) The interaction of fungi with dendritic cells: implications for Th immunity and vaccination. *Curr. Mol. Med.*, **2**, 507–524.
32. Romani, L., Montagnoli, C., Bacci, A., Bozza, A., Spreca, A., Allavena, P., et al. The exploitation of distinct recognition receptor in dendritic cellsdetermines the full range of host's immune relationships with *Candida albicans,* submitted.
33. Yamamoto, Y., Klein, T. W. and Friedman, H. (1997) Involvement of mannose receptor incytokine interleukin-1β (IL-1β), IL-6, and granulocyte-macrophage colony stimulating factor responses, but not chemokine macrophage inflammatory protein 1α_(MIP-1α), MIP-2, and KC responses, caused by attachment of *Candida albicans* to macrophages. *Infect. Immun.* **65**, 1877–1882.

34. Marth, T., and Kelsall, B. L. (1997) Regulation of interleukin-12 by complement receptor 3 signaling. *J. Exp. Med.* **185,** 1987–1995.

35. Forsyth, C. B., Plow, E. F., and Zang, L. (1998) Interaction of the fungal pathogen *Candida albicans* with integrin CD11b/CD18: recognition by the I domain is modulated by the lectin-like domain and the CD18 subunit. *J. Immunol.* **161,** 6198–6205.

36. Chiani, P., Bromuro, C., and Torosantucci, A. (2000) Defective induction of interleukin-12 in human monocytes by germ-tube forms of *Candida albicans. Infect. Immun.* **68,** 5628–5634.

37. Fidel, P. L., Jr. (1999) Host defense against oropharyngeal and vaginal candidiasis: Site-specific differences. *Rev. Iberoam. Mycol.* **16,** 8–15.

38. Fidel, P. L., Ginsburg, K. A., Cutright, J. L., Wolf, N. A., Leaman, D., Dunlap, K., et al. (1997) Vaginal-associated immunity in women with recurrent vulvovaginal candidiasis: evidence for vaginal Th1-type responses following intra-vaginal challenge with *Candida* antigen. *J. Infect. Dis.* **176,** 728–739.

39. La Sala, A., Urbani, F., Torosantucci, A., Cassone, A., and Ausiello, C. (1996) Mannoproteins from *Candida albicans* elicit a Th1-type-1 cytokine profile in human *Candida* specific long-term T cell cultures. *J. Biol. Regul. Homeost. Agents* **10,** 8–12.

40. Ausiello, C. M., Spagnoli, G. C., Boccanera, M., Casalinuovo, I., Malavasi, F., Casciani, C. U., et al. (1986) Proliferation of human peripheral blood mononuclear cells induced by *Candida albicans* and its cell wall fractions. *J. Med. Microbiol.* **22,** 195–202.

41. Ausiello, C. M., Urbani, F., Gessani, S., Spagnoli, G. C., Gomez, M. J. and Cassone, A. (1986) Cytokine gene expression in human peripheral blood mononuclear cells stimulated by mannoprotein constituents from *Candida albicans. Infect. Immun.* **61,** 4105–4111.

42. Talluri, G., Marella, V. K., Shirazian, D., and Wise, G. J. (1999) Immune response in patients with persistent candiduria and occult candidemia. *J. Urol.* **162,** 1361–1364.

43. Borges W. G., Augustine, N. H., and Hill, H. R. (2000) Defective interleukin-12/interferon-gamma pathway in patients with hyperimmunoglobulinemia E syndrome. *J. Pediatr.* **136,** 176–180.

44. Yates A.B., Mehrotra, D., and Moffitt, J. E. (1997) *Candida* endocarditis in a child with hyperimmuneglobulinemia E syndrome. *J. Allergy Clin. Immunol.* **99,** 770–702.

45. Torosantucci, A., Chiani, P., and Cassone, A. (2000) Differential chemokine response of human monocytes to yeast and hyphal forms of *Candida albicans* and its relation to the beta-1,6 glucan of the fungal cell wall. *J. Leukocyte Biol.* **68,** 923–932.

46. Saavedra, M., Taylor, B., Lukacs, N., and Fidel, P. Jr. (1999) Local production of chemokines during experimental vaginal candidiasis. *Infect. Immun.* **67,** 5820–5826.

47. King, A. G., Johanson, K., Frey, C. L., deMarssh, P. L., White, J. R., McDevitt, J. P., et al. (2000) Identification of unique truncated KC/GRO beta chemokines with potent hematopoietic and anti-infective activities. *J. Immunol.* **164,** 3774–3782.

48. Presterl, E, Lassnigg, A., Mueller-Uri, P., El-Menyaw, I., and Graninger, W. (1999) Cytokines in sepsis due to *Candida albicans* and in bacterial sepsis. *Eur. Cytokine Netw.* **10,** 423–430.

49. Dongari-Bagtzoglou, A., Wen, K., And Lamster I. B. (1999) *Candida albicans* triggers interleukin-6 and interleukin-8 responses by oral fibroblasts in vitro. *Oral Microbiol. Immunol.* **14,** 364–370.

50. Netea, M. G., van Tits, L. J., Curfs, J. H., Amiot, F. F., Meis, J. F., van der Meer, J. W. et al. (1999) Increased susceptibility of TNF-alpha lymphotoxin-alpha double knockout mice to systemic candidiasis through impaired recruitment of neutrophils and phagocytosis of *Candida albicans. J. Immunol.* **163,** 1498–1505.

51. Bazzoni, F., Cassatella, M. A., Laudanna, C., and Rossi, F. (1991) Phagocytosis of opsonized yeast induces tumor necrosis factor-alpha mRNA accumulation and protein release by human polymorphonuclear leukocytes. *J. Leukocyte Biol.* **50,** 223–228.

52. Jouault, T., Fradin, C., Trinel, P .A., Bernigaud, A., and Poulain, D. (1998) Early signal transduction induced by *Candida albicans* in macrophages through shedding of a glycolipid. *J. Infect. Dis.* **178,** 792–802.

53. Netea, M. G., van Der Meer, J. W., Meis, J. F., and Kullberg, B. J. (1999) Fas–FasL interactions modulate host defense against systemic *Candida albicans* infection. *J. Infect. Dis.* **180,** 1648–1655.

54. Orozco, A. S., Zhou, X., and Filler, S. G. (2000). Mechanisms of the proinflammatory response of endothelial cells to *Candida albicans* infection. *Infect. Immun.* **68,** 1134–1141.

55. Balish, E., Wagner, R. D., Vasquez-Torres, A., Jones-Carson, J., Pierson, C. and Warner, T. (1999) Mucosal and systemic candidiasis in IL-8R/h–/– BALB/c mice. *J. Leukocyte Biol.* **66,** 144–150.

56. Kimeny, L., Szolnoky, G., Kenderessy, A. S., Gyulai, R., Kiss, M., Michel, G., et al. (1998) Identification of a soluble interleukin-8 inhibitor in the supernatant of polymorphonuclear cells. *Immunol. Lett.* **64,** 23–29.

57. Murphy, J. W., Bistoni, F., Deepe, G. S, Blackstock, R. A., Buchanan, K., Ashman, R. B., et al. (1998) Type 1 and type 2 cytokines: from basic science to fungal infections. *Med. Mycol.* **36** (S1):109–118.

58. Stevens D. A., Walsh, T. J., Bistoni, F., Cenci, E., Clemons, K. V., Del Sero, G., et al. (1998) Cytokines and mycoses. *Med. Mycol.* **36** (S1), 171–182.

59. Cenci, E., Mencacci , A., Del Sero, G., Fè d'Ostiani, C., Mosci , P., Kopf, et al. (1998) IFN-γ is required for IL-12 responsiveness in mice with *Candida albicans* infection. *J. Immunol.* **161,** 3543–3550.

60. Qian, Q., and Cutler, J. E. (1997) γ-Interferon is not essential in host defense against disseminated candidiasis in mice. *Infect. Immun.* **65,** 1748–1756.

61. Romani, L., Puccetti, P., and Bistoni, F. (1997) Interleukin-12 in infectious diseases. *Clin. Microbiol. Rev.* **10,** 611–636.

62. Mencacci, A., Bacci, A., Cenci, E., Montagnoli, C., Fiorucci, S., Casagrande, A., et al. (2000) Interleukin 18 restores defective Th1 immunity to *Candida albicans* in caspase 1-deficient mice. *Infect. Immun.* **68,** 5126–5131.

63. Spaccapelo, R., Del Sero, G., Mosci, P., Bistoni, F., and Romani, L. (1997) Early T cell unresponsiveness in mice with candidiasis and reversal by IL-2. Effect on T helper cell development. *J. Immunol.* **158,** 2294–2302.
64. Djeu, J. Y., Liu, J. H., Wei, S., Rui, H., Pearson, C. A., Leonard, M. J, et al. (1993) Function associated with IL-2 receptor-beta on human neutrophils. Mechanism of activation of antifungal activity against *Candida albicans* by IL-2. *J. Immunol.* **150,** 960–970.
65. Del Sero, G., Mencacci, A., Cenci, E., Fè d'Ostiani, C., Montagnoli, C., Bacci, A., et al. (1999) Antifungal type 1 responses are upregulated in IL-10-deficient mice. *Microbes Infect.* **1,** 1169–1180.
66. Roilides, E., Sein, T., Schaufele, R., Chanock, S. J., and Walsh, T. J. (1998) Increased serum concentrations of interleukin-10 in patients with hepatosplenic candidiasis. *J. Infect. Dis.* **178,** 589–592.
67. Roilides, E., Anastasiou-Katsiardani, A., Dimitriadou-Georgiadou, A., Kadiltsoglou, I., Tsaparidou, S., Panteliadis, C. and Wash, T. J. (1998) Suppressive effects of interleukin-10 on human mononuclear phagocyte function against *Candida albicans* and *Staphylococcus aureus. J. Infect. Dis.* **178,** 1734–1742.
68. Roilides, E., Katsifa, H., Tsaparidou, S., Stergiopoulos, T., Panteliadis, C, et al. (2000) Interleukin-10 suppresses phagocytic and antihyphal activities of human neutrophils. *Cytokine* **12,** 370–387.
69. Xiong, J., Kang, K., Liu, L., Yoshida, Y., Cooper, K., and Ghannoum, M. (2000) *Candida albicans* and *Candida krusei* differentially induce human blood mononuclear cell interleukin-12 and gamma interferon production. *Infect. Immun.* **68,** 2464–2469.
70. Spaccapelo, R., Romani, L., et al. (1995) TGF-β is important in determining the in vivo patterns of susceptibility or resistance in mice infected with *Candida albicans. J. Immunol.* **155,** 1349–1360.
71. Taylor, B. N., Saavedra, M. and Fidel, P. Jr. (2000) Local Th1/Th2 cytokine production during experimental vaginal candidiasis: potential importance of transforming growth factor-beta. *Med. Mycol.* **38,** 419–431.
72. Roilides, E., Kadiltsoglou, I., Dimitriadou, A., Hatzistilianou, M., Manitsa, A., Karpouzas, et al. (1997) Interleukin-4 suppresses antifungal activity of human mononuclear phagocytes against *Candida albicans* in association with decreased uptake of bastoconidia. *FEMS Immunol. Med. Microbiol.* **19,** 169–180.
73. Raveh, D., Kruskal, B. A., Farland, J., and Ezekowitz, R. A. (1998) Th1 and Th2 cytokines cooperate to stimulate mannose-receptor-mediated phagocytosis. *J. Leuk. Biol.* **64,** 108–13.
74. Stein, M., Keshav, S., Harris, N., and Gordon, S. (1992) Interleukin 4 potently enhances murine macrophages mannose receptor activity: a marker of alternative immunologic macrophage activation. *J. Exp. Med.* **176,** 287–292.
75. Mencacci, A., Del Sero, G., Cenci, E., Fè d'Ostiani, C., Bacci, A., Montagnoli, C., et al. (1998) IL-4 is required for development of protective CD4+ T helper type 1 cellresponses to *Candida albicans. J. Exp. Med.* **187,** 307–317.
76. Brown, A. J. P., and Gow, N. A. R. (1999) Regulatory networks controlling *Candida albicans* morphogenesis. *Trends Microbiol.* **7,** 333–338.
77. Chen, B-G., Shi, Y., Smith, J. D., Choi, D., Geiger, J. D., and Mulè, J. J. (1998) The role of tumor necrosis factor-α in modulating the quantity of peripheral blood-derived, cytokine-driven human dendritic cells and its role in enhancing the quality of dendritic cell function in presenting soluble antigens to CD4+ T-cells in vitro. *Blood* **91,** 4652–4661.
78. Tonnetti. L., Spaccapelo, R., Cenci, E., Mencacci, A., Puccetti, P., Coffman, R. L., et al. (1995) Interleukin-4 and -10 exacerbate candidiasis in mice. *Eur. J. Immunol.* **25,** 1559–1565.
79. Cenci, E., Romani, L., Mencacci, A., Spaccapelo, R., Schiaffella, E., Puccetti, P., et al. (1993) Interleukin-4 and interleukin-10 inhibit nitric oxide-dependent macrophage killing of *Candida albicans. Eur. J. Immunol.* **23,** 1034–1038.
80. Romani, L., Puccetti, P., Mencacci, A., Cenci, E., Spaccapelo, R., Tonnetti, L., et al. (1993) Neutralization of IL10 upregulates nitric oxide production and protects susceptible mice from challenge with *Candida albicans. J. Immunol.* **152,** 3514–3521.
81. Gately, M. K., Renzetti, L. M., Magram, J., Stern, A. S., Adorini, L., Gubler, U, et al. (1998) The interleukin-12/interleukin-12-receptor system: role in normal and pathologic immune responses. *Annu. Rev. Immunol.* 16, 495–521.
82. Szabo, S. J., Dighe, A. S., Gubler, U., and Murphy, K. M. (1997) Regulation of the interleukin (IL)-12Rβ2 subunit expression in developing T helper 1(Th1) and Th2 cells. *J. Exp. Med.* **185,** 817–824.
83. Cassone, A., De Bernardis, F., Ausiello, C. M., Gomez, M. J., Boccanera, M., La Valle, R., et al. (1998) Immunogenic and protective *Candida albicans* constituents. *Res. Immunol.* **149,** 289–289.
84. Mencacci, A., Cenci, E., Del Sero, G., Fè d'Ostiani, C., Mosci, P., Bistoni, F., Trinchieri, G., Adorini, L., Romani, L. (1998) IL-10 is required for development of protective CD4+ T helper type 1 cell responses to *Candida albicans. J. Immunol.* **161,** 6228–6237.
85. Musso, T., Calosso, L., Zucca, M., Millesimo, M., Puliti, M., Bulfone-Paus, S., et al. (1998) Interleukin-15 activates proinflammatory and antimicrobial functions in polymorphonuclear cells. *Infect. Immun.* **66,** 2640–2607.
86. Vazquez, N., Walsh, T. J., Friedman, D., Chanock, S. J., and Lyman, C. A. (1998) Interleukin-15 augments superoxide production and microbicidal activity of human monocytes against *Candida albicans. Infect. Immun.* **66,** 145–150.
87. Alexander, B. D., and Perfect, J. R. (1997) Antifungal resistance trends towards the year 2000. Implications for therapy and new approaches. *Drugs* **54,** 657–678.
88. Kullberg, B. J., Netea, M. G., Curfs, J. H., Keuter, M., Meis, J. F., and van der Meer, J. W. (1998) Recombinant murine granulocyte colony-stimulating factor protects against acute disseminated *Candida albicans* infection in nonneutropenic mice. J. Infect. Dis. **177,** 175–181.
89. van Spriel, A. B., van den Herik-Oudijk, I. E., and van den Winkel, J. D. (2000) A single injection of polyethylene–glycol granulocyte colony-stimulating factor strongly prolongs survival of mice with systemic candidiasis. *Cytokine* **12,** 666–670.
90. Roilides, E., Dignani, M. C., Anaissie, E. J. and Rex, J. H. (1998) The role of immunoreconstitution in the management of refractory opportunistic fungal infections. *Med. Mycol.* **1,** 12–25.

91. Roilides, E. and Farmaki, E. (2001) Granulocyte colony-stimulating factor and other cytokines in antifungal therapy. *Clin. Microbiol. Infect.* **7**, 62–67.
92. Cenci, E, Mencacci, A., Del Sero, G., Bistoni, F., and Romani, L. (1997) Induction of protective Th1 responses to *Candida albicans* by antifungal therapy alone or in combination with an interleukin-4 antagonist. *J. Infect. Dis.* **176**, 217–226.
93. Mencacci, A., Cenci, E., Bacci, A., Bistoni, F., and Romani, L. (2000) Host immune reactivity determine the efficacy of combination immunotherapy and antifungal chemotherapy in candidiasis. *J. Infect. Dis.* **181**, 686–694.
94. Poynton, C. H., Barnes, R. A., and Rees, J. (1998) Interferon-γ and granulocyte-macrophage colony-stimulating factor for the treatment of hepatosplenic candidosis in patients with acute leukemia. *Clin. Infect. Dis.* **26**, 239–240.
95. Polonelli, L. and Cassone, A. (1999) Novel strategies for treating candidiasis. *Curr. Opin. Infect. Dis.* **12**, 61–69.
96. Farmaki, E. and Roilides, E. (2001) Immunotherapy in patients with systemic mycoses: a promising adjunct. *Biodrugs* **15**, 207–214.

VII
Cytokines in Parasitic Infections

17

Th1 and Th2 Cytokines in Leishmaniasis

Fabienne Tacchini-Cottier, Geneviève Milon, and Jacques A. Louis

1. INTRODUCTION

The intracellular protozoan *Leishmania* are obligate parasites of macrophages that can infect various mammalian hosts such as rodents, dogs, and humans *(1)*. At least 20 *Leishmania* species can trigger pathogenic processes in humans. The host-to-host transmission of the parasite occurs through the bite of its hematophagous vector, the female sandfly, which is of the genus *Phlebotomus* in the Old World and *Lutzomyia* in the New World.

In humans, a large spectrum of clinical manifestations characterize the long-term parasitism driven by *Leishmania* spp, ranging from asymptomatic, mild, self-curing to fatal diseases. Cutaneous leishmaniasis (CLs) is mainly due to *Leishmania major* in the Old World. It is self-limiting and self-curing but may leave disfiguring scars. CL resulting from *L. tropica* is more chronic and its most severe form is difficult to cure. In both cases, spontaneous cure and long-standing immunity are the most common outcome. In the New World, *L. mexicana* usually causes benign self-healing lesions. Leishmaniasis recidivans (LR) and diffuse cutaneous leishmaniasis (DCLs) may follow simple cutaneous cases in rare conditions involving immune and nonimmune contexts.

Mucocutaneous leishmaniasis (MCLs) can lead to partial or total destruction of the mucosal epithelia of the mouth, nose, throat, and surrounding tissues. It is mostly related to *Leishmania* species of the New World. Its initial phase starts at the site of parasite delivery, namely the skin; Metastatic spread of the parasite to mucosal tissues arises years later after healing of the initial lesion.

Parasites of the *L. donovani* complex are the causal agents of visceral leishmaniasis. Most human infections with this visceralizing strain remain subclinical and are not diagnosed. In visceral leishmaniasis (kala-azar), which is potentially lethal if not treated, uncontrolled parasite burden is observed in organs such as the spleen, liver, and bone marrow, which are distant from the cutaneous sites of parasites delivery. It is characterized by anemia, splenomegaly, hepatomegaly, irregular fever, and loss of weight. The most severe form is fatal if untreated. Post-kala-azar dermal leishmaniasis (PDKL) may occur at the end of chemotherapy.

2. EXPERIMENTAL MODELS OF LEISHMANIASIS

Mice have been widely used as experimental hosts of leishmania to decipher some of the features of human leishmaniasis. The outcome of this experimental infection may differ according to the strain of parasites used, the genetic background of the host, the site(s) of parasite inoculation, the developmental stage of the *Leishmania* inoculum, and the reactivity of the host immune system.

From: *Cytokines and Chemokines in Infectious Diseases Handbook*
Edited by: M. Kotb and T. Calandra © Humana Press Inc., Totowa, NJ

2.1. Experimental Models of Cutaneous Leishamaniasis

2.1.1. Mouse Models of Cutaneous Leishmaniasis Following Infection with L. major

Subcutaneous injections of *L. major* stationary-phase promastigotes in mice of most inbred strains such as C57BL/6, 129/SV, and C3H/He lead to self-healing cutaneous lesions. Following parasite inoculation (millions of stationary-phase promastigotes), the surviving/invasive parasites establish themselves at the site of *L. major* inoculation and within the draining lymph node, with no further parasite spreading during the first 3 d following parasite inoculation *(2,3)*. A small lesion develops that heals slowly, and the site of inoculation (most often the footpad) is back to normal size by 5–6 wk after *L. major* inoculation. In addition, these mice will not develop any lesion if they receive a second inoculum of *L. major*. These mice are referred to as mice "resistant to infection with *L. major.*"

In susceptible strains such as BALB/c mice, subcutaneous delivery of *L. major* stationary-phase promastigotes induces the development of a lesion that does not heal. The surviving/invasive parasites establish themselves not only within the site of inoculation and the draining lymph node but also in the spleen and liver (visceralization). This spreading is associated with progressive disease. If BALB/c mice receive a second inoculum of *L. major*, a lesion will develop: these mice are referred to as "mice susceptible to infection with *L. major.*"

This extensively studied model of infection has contributed to the unraveling of some of the complex interactions occurring between the *Leishmania* parasite and the immune system of its mammalian host (reviewed in refs. *3* and *4*).

In most of the instances, relatively high doses of stationary-phase parasites (10^6–10^7) were injected within the footpads of mice. Delivery within the ear dermis of a low dose of *L. major* metacyclic promastigotes has also been used in an attempt to mimic more closely the natural conditions of *L. major* delivery *(5)*. Although relevant, the data obtained with this model will not be reviewed within the present chapter.

2.1.2. Other Models of Cutaneous Leishmaniasis

Experimental murine infections with *Leishmania* of the mexicana complex, *L. mexicana mexicana*, and *L. mexicana amazonensis*, induce nonhealing lesions in mice of the same strains known to be "resistant to *L. major* infection," such as C57BL/6 and C3H *(6,7)*. Subcutaneous infection of BALB/c mice with high numbers of *L. mexicana mexicana* promastigotes induces slowly progressive primary lesions that do not heal, although they ulcerate less rapidly than the lesions of BALB/c mice infected with *L. major* promastigotes *(8)*.

Hamsters have also been reported to be susceptible to infections by *L. b. brazilensis*, *L. mexicana*, and *L. amazonensis* *(9,10)*. Differences in lesion progression have been observed according to the site of inoculation chosen. Such differences have also been reported following infections with *L. major (11)*.

2.1.3. Relevance of the Mouse Model to Human Leishmaniasis

So-called resistant mice healing subcutaneous infections with *L. major* develop a self-limiting cutaneous ulcer sharing many features with the human lesion.

Nonhealer ("susceptible") animals differ in some aspects from human skin infections that do not heal, such as DCL. For example, after *L. major* infection, no visceralization is observed in humans, whereas it is observed in nonhealing BALB/C mice infected with this parasite. The immune processes developing in these mice may, however, constitute an interesting model for deciphering the chronic features of cutaneous leishmaniasis.

2.2. Murine Models of Visceral Leishmaniasis

There exist several murine models of so-called visceral leishmaniasis that share some pathologic features such as hepatosplenomegaly and granuloma formation, with human kala-azar *(12)*.

Considerable work has been performed using *L. donovani* in mice. In this experimental model, parasitism is initiated by the intravenous injection of parasites. Resident macrophages of the liver, spleen, and bone marrow become rapidly parasitized. According to their genetic backgrounds, mice differ in their early and late reactivity to the parasitic processes driven by *L. donovani*. Most often, the parasite load increases generally in the liver, spleen, and within the bone marrow. Recently, the subsets of mononuclear phagocytes parasitized by *L. donovani* were described *(13)*. Less frequently, hepatosplenomegaly is also noticed as a very late feature.

Mice resistant to *L. donovani* contain the infection and their spleen and liver revert to normal size. In mice of susceptible phenotype, the infection is not contained, especially within the spleen, leading to the death of the animal.

The *L. infantum* and *L. chagasi* parasite subspecies of the *L. donovani* complex have also been delivered intravenously to mice of different genetic backgrounds. Similar to infection with *L. donovani*, intracellular amastigotes multiply rapidly and an efficient granulomatous tissue response occurs in the liver of infected BALB/c mice, resulting in the reduction of the parasite load. In the spleen however, chronic infection develops with parasite survival, and destruction of the splenic architecture occurs *(14–16)*.

Infection of hamsters with *L. donovani* has been recently described, reproducing most of the clinicopathological features of human visceral *leishmaniasis*. Their pathogenic mechanisms are currently deciphered *(17)*.

3. IMPORTANCE OF T-HELPER SUBSETS AND RELATED CYTOKINES IN THE MURINE MODEL OF CUTANEOUS LEISHMANIASIS

3.1. Definition of T-Helper Subsets and Their Effector Mechanisms of Action In Vivo

Two functionally distinct subsets of CD4$^+$ T-helper cells have been described first in the mouse *(18)* and then in humans *(19)* on the basis of their secretion of distinct cytokines with specific immunomodulatory effects (reviewed in refs. *20* and *21*). Some of these cytokines act either in secondary lymphoid organs or in peripheral tissues, where they are recruited at the site of an inflammatory process. Once reactivated within the inflammatory tissues and according to their secretion of cytokines, CD4$^+$ T-helper lymphocytes will exert regulatory and/or effector functions, including (1) clearance of the micro-organism inoculated, (2) control of its proliferation (reduction or increase), and (3) remodeling/repair of the tissue containing the micro-organism. The outcome of infection will depend on these tightly controlled processes.

CD4$^+$ Th1 lymphocytes secrete cytokines such as interferon (IFN)-γ (signature cytokine), interleukin (IL)-2, IL-3, tumor necrosis factor (TNF)β, granulocyte–macrophage colony stimulating factor (GM-CSF), and TNF-α. Within peripheral nonlymphoid tissues loaded with intracellular micro-organisms, Th1 cells have been associated with cell-mediated immunity, more specifically in the complete or partial clearance of these intracellular micro-organisms. CD4$^+$ Th1 cells contribute, through the IFN-γ they secrete and in synergy with TNF-α to the clearance of the invading micro-organisms or at least in the reduction of their number. Within the secondary lymphoid organs, B-lymphocytes received the early signals switching on their entry into the cell cycle and their differentiation program; signals provided by CD4$^+$ T-helper lymphocytes will trigger these activated B-lymphocytes to become memory B cells or plasmocytes. In the mouse, IFN-γ induces mainly the IgG2a and IgG3 isotypes *(22)*, whereas in humans, it induces more IgG1 and IgG3 *(23)*.

CD4$^+$ Th2 lymphocytes produce mainly IL-4, IL-5 (signature cytokines), IL-13, IL-3, IL-6, transforming growth factor (TGF)-β and IL-10. Th2 cells promote the proliferation and differentiation of antigen-binding B-cells. IL-4 is the major inducer of B-cell switching signal for IgE production as well as for the production of noncomplement-fixing IgG such as IgG1 in mice and IgG4 in humans *(22)*. In addition, in nonperipheral tissues, Th2 lymphocytes, after their reactivation may (1), through their secretion of IL-4, prevent macrophage activation, favoring growth of intracellular micro-organisms and (2), through their production of IL-5, allow the survival of eosinophils that may favor the destruction of cell lineages other than the surrounding leukocytes.

Interestingly, the two Th1/Th2 subsets produce cytokines that can cross-regulate each other's development and effector functions, so that once the development toward a restricted cytokine profile (Th1 or Th2) is set up, it has a tendency to stay polarized in that direction (reviewed in ref. 20). The essential role of these two T-cell subsets in the outcome of pathological processes has fostered great interest in the understanding of the mechanisms driving the development toward Th1 or Th2 type of cell in various disease processes.

A common CD4+ T-cell precursor can differentiate into either Th1 or Th2 cells. Th1 cells were shown (1) to mediate delayed-type hypersensitivity, (2) to promote the elimination of intracellular parasites, and (3) to be important in mediating pathogenic autoreactivity and allograft rejection. Th2 cells have been associated with protective responses following parasitic infections with helminths as well as in the pathology of allergic responses (20,21,24,25).

In addition to cytokines, different factors have also been reported to influence differentiation into Th1 or Th2 phenotypes such as the dose of antigen used (reviewed in ref. 26). The role of antigen-presenting cells (APCs) in shaping the T-helper cells differentiation pathway is also of importance as they provide, at the initiation of CD4+ T-cell responses, early activation signals mediated by cytokines involved in differentiation and costimulatory molecules. In vitro and in vivo studies have shown that CD28 was important for Th2 differentiation in the presence of IL-2 (27), whereas in the absence of IL-2, interactions between CD28/CTLA4 seemed to be essential for the priming of both subsets of T-helper cells. The CD40 molecule on the surface of T-cells and its T-cell ligand (CD40L) on the surface of APCs, also play a role in Th differentiation by fostering macrophages and dendritic cells to produce the IL-12 required for early production of IFN-γ by T-cells.

3.2. Importance of the Murine Model of L. major Infection in Deciphering the Events Leading to CD4+ Th Polarization In Vivo

Studies with the protozoan parasite L. major were instrumental in establishing the functional relevance of the two CD4+ Th cell subsets, showing that "resistance" and "susceptibility" to infection correlated with the development of Th1 and Th2 responses, respectively. The development of Th1 responses in mice of most inbred strains (such as C57BL/6 and C3H) is associated with healing, whereas the development of Th2 responses in susceptible strains such as BALB/c is associated with nonhealing lesions and its inability to control parasite growth (reviewed in ref. 4).

3.2.1. Effector Functions of Cytokines Produced by Th1 and Th2 Cells in the L. major Model

Interferon-γ, the major effector cytokine produced by Th1 cells plays a key function in activating macrophages, enhancing their leishmanicidal and leihmaniastatic properties. Indeed, IFN-γ was shown to be critical for the cure of leishmaniasis in mice. Other cytokines produced by Th1 cells are involved in the recruitment (IL-3, GM-CSF), diapedesis, and activation (TNF-α, TNF-β) of inflammatory leukocytes and macrophages.

Several cytokines secreted by Th2 cells have anti-inflammatory properties. Thus, IL-4 and IL-13 antagonize the macrophage-activating effect of IFN-γ, IL-10 downregulates many macrophage responses, and TGF-β has antiproliferative effects and blocks the IFN-γ-induced macrophage activation (28). Furthermore, treatment with mAb against TGF-β in CB6F1 mice that normally display intermediate susceptibility to L. major promoted rapid healing by enhancing in vivo nitric oxide production (29). Thus, Th2 cells play both effector and regulatory roles in immune responses.

In an other mouse model of infection, using subcutaneous injection of L. amazonensis, local injection of rTGF-β in resistant mice at the site of parasite inoculation resulted in nonhealing of the lesions. Susceptible BALB/c mice treated with a neutralizing anti-TGF-β antibody during the course of infection with *L. amazonensis* decreased markedly the lesion size within 5 wk after infection. IFN-γ mRNA was observed in the draining lymph node of these mice, whereas no IFN-γ, but IL-4, was detected in the draining lymph nodes of infected mice treated with a control antibody *(30)*. Thus, TGF-β production may prevent *Leishmania* destruction by host macrophages.

4. NON-T-LEUKOCYTES AS A SOURCE OF TH1/TH2 DIFFERENTIATION SIGNALS

The major population acting as host for *Leishmania* parasites are nonactivated/deactivated mononuclear phagocytes that either reside in the extravascular compartment of cutaneous tissues or that differentiate from monocytes that extravasated from the vascular bed as a result of inflammatory processes. Generally, in tissues in which inflammatory processes are taking place, rapidly released mediators by perivascular mast cells act on endothelial cells of postcapillary venules. As a result, their adhesive properties are modified, allowing recruitment of blood leukocytes, a process also under the control of chemokines. Effector memory T-lymphocytes recirculate in peripheral tissues. If they are not reactivated, their effector functions within the tissues will depend on the factors triggered by the presence of the micro-organism, and the network of cytokines/chemokines secreted by these non-T-cells as well as by tissue cells of nonhematopoietic lineages.

Dendritic leukocytes (DLs) reside in most peripheral tissues of the body. They can capture micro-organisms, bind and phagocyte apoptotic cells, and reach the draining lymph node through the afferent lymphatic vessels. It is not clear yet at which time following the subcutaneous inoculation of stationary-phase *L. major* promastigotes that these processes occur. Depending on the presence on their membrane of costimulatory molecules, DLs are thought to act as a source of T-helper differentiation signals. Neutrophils and mastocytes may also have a potential role as a source of differentiation signals. In all cases, the potential role of these non-T-leukocytes will depend on many parameters, including the status of the parasite within these cells (alive of dead), their migrating properties, and their final localization within the draining lymph node.

5. FACTORS INVOLVED IN T-HELPER DIFFERENTIATION IN THE MOUSE MODEL OF CUTANEOUS INFECTION WITH *L. MAJOR*

5.1. The Role of Costimulatory Molecules in T-Helper Differentiation

The importance of CD28/B7 interactions in Th development has also been reported in the murine model of infection with *L. major*, showing that the B7 molecules are important in Th2 responses *(31)*, whereas mice genetically deficient in the CD28 gene have failed to show a role for this molecule, in either Th1 or Th2 development *(32)*.

The role of the CD40/CD40L interaction in the development of Th1 cells in the murine model of infection with *L. major* has been demonstrated by several approaches: Mice with a resistant genetic background, made deficient in CD40 or CD40L, infected with *L. major*, developed progressive lesions, failed to mount a Th1 response *(33)*, and produced high levels of the Th2 cytokine IL-4 *(34)*.

CD40-activated dendritic cells (DCs) express the ligand for the CD4 activation antigen, OX40 (CD134) *(35,36)*. In vitro activation of OX40 and CD28 was reported to promote IL-4 expression [OX40 expression is CD28-dependent *(37,38)*], suggesting a role for OX40/OX40L interactions in Th2 differentiation. Evidences for such a role were provided by experiments where administration of blocking antibodies against OX40 ligand (OX40L) in BALB/c mice abrogated progression of disease and reduced the production of Th2 cytokines *(39)*.

5.2. The Role of Cytokines in Th1 Differentiation Following Infection with *L.* **major**

Cytokines, among several other T-cell-polarizing signals, are considered to be crucial in influencing the pathway of differentiation of CD4[+] T-lymphocytes precursors.

5.2.1. Role of IL-12 in the Differentiation of CD4+ T-Cells Toward the Th1 Phenotype

The cytokine IL-12 is a heterodimer composed of a 35-kDA subunit that associates covalently with a 42-kDA subunit to form the biologically active IL-12 p70 heterodimer. The p35 and p40 genes are located on separated genes that are regulated independently. IL-12 is produced by many cells, including macrophages, dendritic cells, polymorphonuclear cells, and B-cells (reviewed in ref. *40*).

Interleukin-12 has multiple biological functions, including the induction of IFN-γ by T-cells and natural killer (NK) cells *(41,42)* and thereby NK cells were thought to play a critical role in the development of protective Th1 cellular responses. The role of IL-12 in Th differentiation has been extensively studied in vitro, mainly using naïve T-cells obtained from T cell receptor αβ transgenic mice (TCRαβ). In these studies, it was demonstrated that the addition of IL-12 p70 during CD4+ T-cell differentiation was necessary and sufficient to induce differentiation of CD4+ Th1 cells *(43–45)*.

In the murine model of infection with *L. major*, IL-12 was also shown to direct the development of CD4+ Th1 cells within the draining lymph node of mice with a resistant genetic background. Thus, resistant mice treated with anti-IL-12 mAb showed a transient Th2 response. Similarly, resistant mice whose p35 or p40 IL-12 gene was disrupted developed a Th2 response *(46–48)*.

Injection of rIL-12 to BALB/c mice during the first week of infection could induce the development of Th1 responses and resistance to *L. major* in these otherwise highly susceptible mice *(46,49)*.

Interleukin-12 signaling occurs through the IL-12 receptor (IL-12R) composed of two subunits, the IL-12Rβ1 and IL-12 Rβ2 chains, which are expressed selectively on T-cells that have engaged their TCR and on NK cells *(50)*. Loss of IL-12Rβ2 chain may result in extinction of IL-12 signaling during in vitro priming. In the model of infection with *L. major*, a correlation between the maintenance of expression of the IL-12Rβ2 chain in CD4+ T-cells and the development of Th1 response was observed. Furthermore, during Th2 differentiation, within the draining lymph node of BALB/c mice infected with *L. major*, T cells lost expression of the IL-12Rβ2 chain and became unresponsive to IL-12 both in vitro and in vivo *(51–53)*.

Genetic differences have been reported to influence the regulation of the IL-12 receptor both in vitro and in vivo. BALB/c TCR transgenic T-cells cultured under nonpolarizing conditions lost expression of IL-12Rβ2 chain, whereas T-cells from the B10.D2 strain did not. However, in the presence of IL-4, T-cells from both strains became unresponsive to IL-12 *(54)*.

In the murine model of infection with *L. major*, resistant C3H mice treated with a mAb against IL-12 could mount a Th1 response after the development of a transient Th2 response. This was explained by the maintenance of a population of CD4+ T-cells in these mice that expressed both the IL-12Rβ1 and the IL-12Rβ2 chains during the initial Th2 response *(55)*.

Interestingly, in the murine model of infection with *L. amazonensis*, C3H mice that are susceptible to infection were reported to be unresponsive to IL-12 and its Th1-promoting effects. This was demonstrated to result from a defective induction of the IL-12Rβ2 chain expression in CD4+ T-cells that was observed only in mice infected with *L. amazonensis* but not in mice injected with *L. major (56)*.

These results indicate that induction and maintenance of IL-12 responsiveness is critical for the development of a functional Th1 response.

5.2.2. The Role of IL-18 in Th1 Differentiation

Interleukin-18 was originally described as IFN-γ-inducing factor constitutively secreted by T-cells and NK cells *(57)*. IL-18 was reported to synergize with IL-12 to induce Th1 development in vivo, but it does not appear to be able to induce Th1 development on its own *(58)*. To assess the role of IL-18 in Th1 polarization and resistance to infection with *L. major*, mice lacking the IL-18 gene were infected with *L. major*.

In a first study, IL-18$^{-/-}$ mice on a CD1 "resistant" genetic background were shown to be susceptible to infection with decreased Th1 and increased Th2 cytokines within their draining lymph node *(59)*. However, in a similar study using IL-18$^{-/-}$ mice on a C57BL/6 genetic background, larger lesions were observed early after infection, but eventually the mice resolved their lesions and developed a Th1 response, showing that, in this experimental context, IL-18 did not play a critical role in the development of protective Th1 responses following infection with *L. major (60)*.

Recent in vitro experiments demonstrated that CD4$^+$ T-lymphocytes from different genetic backgrounds could differentiate along a Th1 or Th2 profile when stimulated with IL-18 *(61)*. These results may explain the discrepancies observed in the two studies involving IL-18$^{-/-}$ mice on different genetic backgrounds. Xu et al. also showed that although IL-18 by itself could not induce Th1 differentiation of naïve CD4$^+$ T-lymphocytes in vitro, it could, by itself induce Th2 differentiation of CD4$^+$ T-lymphocytes from BALB/c strains but not from C57BL/6 or CBA mice *(61)*.

5.2.3. The Role of IFN-γ in the Differentiation of CD4$^+$ T-Cells Toward the Th1 Phenotype

The role of IFN-γ in the differentiation of Th1 cells is not as clear as that of IL-12. Neutralization of IFN-γ in vitro was reported to inhibit Th1 differentiation *(44,62)*, whereas in another study, IFN-γ appeared to play no role in the differentiation of Th1 cells *(45)*. A role for IFN-γ in priming Th1 cell differentiation was demonstrated using transgenic T-cells in vitro *(63)*. When IL-4 was not produced, the IL-12Rβ2 chain was maintained on activated CD4$^+$ T-cells, allowing IL-12 to induce Th1 development independently of IFN-γ. Thus, it is likely that, in vivo, activated CD4$^+$ T-cells may not require IFN-γ signaling for the maintenance of IL-12Rβ2 chain expression and IL-12 signaling. IFN-γ may, thus, be required for Th1 differentiation only when some IL-4 is produced.

In the model of infection with *L. major*, the presence of IFN-γ was reported to favor the maturation of Th1 cell differentiation in mice of the resistant C3H/HeN strain. Neutralization of IFN-γ during the first days of infection with *L. major* prevented the differentiation of Th1 cells and favored, instead, Th2 cell differentiation *(64,65)*. Furthermore, C57BL/6 mice made genetically deficient in IFN-γ failed to develop Th1 responses and developed an aberrant Th2 response. Administration of exogenous rIL-12 at the onset of infection in these mice suppressed the IL-4 mRNA expression otherwise observed in their draining lymph node 5 d after infection with *L. major* and allowed Th1 differentiation *(66)*. However, resistant mice on another genetic background (SV129) made deficient for the IFN-γ receptor developed a normal Th1 response following infection with *L. major (67)*, suggesting genetic differences in the requirement for IFN-γ in Th1 maturation following infection with *L. major*.

5.3. Production of T-Helper 1-Polarizing Cytokines by Non-T-Leukocytes After Infection with L. major

In the murine model of infection with *L. major*, non-T-leukocytes, namely neutrophils, NK cells, and mononuclear phagocytes, are recruited very rapidly to the site of parasite inoculation, especially when non-metacyclic promastigotes are dominant in the inoculum. Polymorphonuclear neutrophils are recruited within 1 h of subcutaneous injection of *Leishmania* in mice of both susceptible and resistant strains. However, their number drop dramatically to less than 10% of the cutaneous cellular infiltrate 3 d later in resistant mice when macrophage infiltrate gradually predominates. In susceptible BALB/c mice, the number of neutrophils at the site of parasite inoculation remains elevated (at least 50% of the cellular infiltrate) *(68–69)*. Polymorphonuclear neutrophils (PMNs) could contribute to the development of adaptive effector T-cells through production of cytokines involved in T-helper polarization, such as IL-12 and TGF-β, both reported to be secreted by neutrophils *(70,71)*. The importance of neutrophils in influencing T-helper differentiation in the model of infection with *L. major* was suggested by experiments showing that transient neutrophil depletion contributed to the marked reduction of lesion development and decreased production of IL-4 in otherwise susceptible mice. Interestingly, neutrophil depletion did not alter significantly the resolution of lesions in resistant mice, in which macrophages activated to the microbicidal/microbistatic mode are considered as the major effector cells, nor did it alter the development of Th1 polarization.

Thus, whereas neutrophils may play minor contribution to the removal of *L. major* in mice from resistant strains, they appear to contribute to the inability to heal lesions in susceptible mice by an as yet unknown mechanism, contributing to Th2 differentiation *(69)*.

An early protective role for NK cells, other leukocytes expected to be rapidly recruited to a site loaded with micro-organisms has been suggested by experiments in which resistant C57BL/6 mice, depleted of NK cells, showed rapid dissemination of parasites to sites distant from the site of parasite delivery (footpads). The effect of NK cells resulted from their secretion of IFN-γ *(2)*. Early production of IFN-γ following infection with *L. major* was reported to originate predominantly from NK cells *(72–75)*. These observations suggested that the IFN-γ produced by NK cells could contribute to Th1 cell differentiation. However, several studies showed that the IFN-γ produced early by NK cells was neither required for Th1 differentiation nor for the inhibition of parasite replication. Using mice with selective deficiency in IFN-γ gene in either the T-cell or the NK-cell compartment, it was shown that mice with selective disruption of the IFN-γ-producing NK cells were fully able to develop Th1 response *(76)*. This conclusion was confirmed using mice lacking NK cells, which were able to develop an efficient Th1 response and to control the *L. major* infection *(77)*. In an other study, depletion of NK cells using mAb against NK1.1 and AsGM-1 mAb also failed to alter the T-helper balance developing following infection with *L. major (78)*. It remains that NK cells, together with other factors such as IFN-α and IFN-β *(79)*, may still have a functional role in the early inhibition of parasite growth that is independent of the effector function of Th1 cells.

5.4. Role of IL-4 as a Th2 Polarizing Cytokine Promoting a Stable Th2 Phenotype After Infection with L. major

Using naive CD4+ T-cells from mice transgenic for αβ TCR chains, IL-4 has been demonstrated to be a key cytokine promoting Th2 cell differentiation in vitro *(45,80)*. In the murine model of infection with *L. major*, analysis of IL-4 mRNA expression revealed that the levels of IL-4 mRNA were high a few days after infection and remained elevated over the infection in the draining lymph nodes of mice of susceptible strains, whereas it was very low in mice of strains resistant to *L. major* infections *(81,82)* Draining lymph node cells from infected mice obtained a few days after infections produced high levels of IL-4 when restimulated in vitro with the parasite, whereas cell-resistant mice did not produce any detectable IL-4 upon restimulation *(83)*. A single injection of anti-IL-4 mAb given early in infection in susceptible mice was sufficient to redirect Th1 cell maturation, allowing these otherwise susceptible mice to resolve their lesions. Furthermore, these mice became immune to reinfection with *L. major (84,85)*. The expression of an IL-4 transgene in mice of healer phenotype was sufficient to render them susceptible to infection *(86)*.

More recently, the role of IL-4 in the development of polarized Th2 cells following infection of BALB/c mice with *L. major* has been studied in mice with a deleted IL-4 gene. Results obtained by different groups differed markedly. One study revealed that mice genetically deficient in IL-4 were resistant to infections with *L. major* and developed impaired Th2 responses *(87)*, confirming an essential role for IL-4 in Th2 differentiation. In another study, mice deficient in IL-4 production remained susceptible to infection with *L. major* and developed polarized Th1 responses, suggesting that in the absence of IL-4, other molecules may drive Th2 cell maturation following infection with *L. major (88)*. To clarify this issue and to investigate whether another Th2 cytokine, IL-13, could, in the absence of IL-4, play a compensatory role in Th2 cell differentiation, susceptible BALB/c mice deficient for the IL-4 receptor-α chain (IL-4Rα) were used. IL-13 also uses the IL-4Rα chain for signaling along with the IL-13Rα1 ligand specific chain *(89–91)*; and therefore, mice deficient in the IL-4Rα chain are deficient for both IL-4 and IL-13 signaling. These mice were resistant to infection with the IR173 *L. major* strain but remained susceptible to the LV39 *L. major* strain *(92)*. In another study, BALB/c mice genetically deficient for the IL-4Rα chain contained the infection with the LV39

L. major strain during the first 80 d of infection, developing a Th1 type of immune response, however, after 3 mo, these mice developed nonhealing lesions *(93)*.

Although confusing, these results suggest that in the artificial absence of IL-4, IL-13, and/or other IL-4-independent mechanisms may also be involved in driving Th2 differentiation and its associated susceptibility to *L. major* in BALB/c mice.

5.5. Role of Early IL-4 in the Differentiation of CD4⁺ T-Cells Toward the Th2 Phenotype During Infection with L. major

Interventions that modulate Th differentiation in susceptible BALB/c mice infected with *L. major* are successful only when performed during a short period of time (i.e., during the first few days preceding and/or following *L. major* inoculation). A burst of IL-4 mRNA expression rapidly induced in the draining lymph node of BALB/c mice was reported during the first day following parasite inoculation *(94)*. Although returning to a basal level of transcription 48 h after *L. major* injection, increased levels of IL-4 mRNA were again observed in the draining lymph nodes 5 d after infection, reflecting the development of Th2 responses in these mice. The early peak of IL-4 mRNA expression was only observed in mice of susceptible strains and, in our hands, was never observed in resistant mice such as C57BL/6, C3H, and 129 mice. This early increase in IL-4 mRNA transcripts could be downregulated by the exogenous addition of IL-12 and/or IFN-γ. Treatment of resistant C57BL/6 mice with mAb against IFN-γ or IL-12 at the initiation of infection allowed the expression of the peak of IL-4 mRNA transcripts to a level similar to that observed in susceptible BALB/c mice *(94)*.

CD4⁺ T-cells have been shown to be necessary for the expression of the early IL-4 mRNA burst observed only in susceptible BALB/c mice during the first day following infection with *L. major* *(94)*. Further studies revealed that the IL-4 mRNA increase observed at that time was restricted to a subpopulation of CD4⁺ T-cells expressing the Vβ4Vα8 TCR chains *(95)*. The second wave of IL-mRNA increase starting 5 d after infection with *L. major* was, however, not restricted to the single population of T-cells expressing the Vβ4Vα8 TCR, but IL-4 transcription occurred in a broader range of CD4⁺ T-cells with diverse TCR *(96)*.

The CD4⁺ T-cells responsible for the early burst of IL-4 mRNA expression in response to *L. major* with restricted TCRs are reactive to the Leishmania homolog of mammalian RACK-1 (LACK) *(97)*. Indeed, subcutaneous injection of the recombinant LACK protein of *L. major* in BALB/c mice also induced an increase in IL-4 mRNA only within the CD4⁺ Vβ4Vα population of T-cells 16 h later *(95)*. Injection of the LACK recombinant protein in resistant mice did not induce any increase in IL-4 mRNA expression at any time-point after injection *(95)*.

These results suggest that the early IL-4 response observed during the first day following infection with *L. major* is triggered by the interaction of a LACK-derived peptide presented by I-A^d to a restricted CD4⁺ population expressing the Vβ4Vα8 TCR. The subsequent development of Th2 response occurring a few days later is, however, not restricted to this single CD4⁺ T-cell subpopulation.

The importance of this early production of IL-4 by CD4⁺ Vβ4Vα8 T-cells in the development of a Th2 phenotype and in the susceptibility to *L. major* was further demonstrated by results showing that Vβ4 CD4⁺-deficient BALB/c mice developed a Th1 response and were resistant to infection. Administration of IL-4 during the first 2 d after infection with *L. major* in Vβ4-deficient mice could substitute for the absence of Vβ4Vα8 CD4⁺ T-cells and restored Th2 cell development, resulting in progressive disease *(98)*.

The importance of the LACK antigen in driving Th2 differentiation was also demonstrated under different experimental conditions. BALB/c mice with the transgenic expression of LACK under the control of the major histocompatibility complex (MHC) class II promoter are tolerant to LACK. These mice were shown to have a diminished Th2 response and were resistant to infection with *L. major (99)*.

5.6. Production of the Early IL-4 by Vα8Vβ4 CD4⁺ T-Cells Renders CD4⁺ T-Cells Specific for L. major Antigens Unresponsive to IL-12

The susceptibility of BALB/c mice to infection with *L. major* can be reverted by continuous injection of rIL-12 during the first days after infection *(46)*. Noteworthy, IL-12 given to BALB/c mice 1 d before parasite inoculation could suppress the early IL-4 mRNA response to *L. major* by the Vβ4Vα8 CD4⁺ T-cell, resulting in Th1 differentiation *(94)*. However, if IL-12 was injected later than 48 h after infection with *L. major* (i.e., after the early IL-4 mRNA burst in response to *L. major* had occurred), no effect was observed and Th2 differentiation occurred normally. The inability of IL-12, given at that time, to drive Th1 cell development was the result of the downregulation of the IL-12Rβ2 chain expression on primed CD4⁺ T-lymphocytes. Further experiments showed that the early IL-4 produced by the LACK-specific Vβ4Vα8 CD4⁺ T-cells was responsible for the downregulation of the IL-12Rβ2 expression on CD4⁺ T-cells from BALB/c mice, resulting in a state of IL-12 unresponsiveness *(52)*.

These data confirmed results obtained in vitro, showing that naive CD4⁺ T-cells from BALB/c mice, which have a tendency to differentiate toward Th2 cells, are unresponsive to IL-12 because of the downregulation of the IL-12 receptor chain (IL-12Rβ2) on these cells *(50)*.

These results suggest that following infection with *L. major* in BALB/c mice, Th2 cell differentiation and the associated susceptible phenotype are the result of an early burst of IL-4 production. This early IL-4 is responsible for the downregulation of the IL-12Rβ2 chain expression, leading to IL-12 unresponsiveness in CD4⁺ T-cells.

5.7. Does TCR Affinity Dictate the Th1/Th2 Effector Choice?

The importance of Vβ4Vα8 TCR was discussed in the previous subsection. Recently, two studies showed TCR-dependent signaling triggered by LACK-derived peptides. One study relied on LACK-derived altered peptide ligands that differed from a single amino acid. CD4⁺ T-cells from TCR transgenic mice expressing the Vβ4Vα8 receptor were used to characterize how altered peptide ligands could activate the IL-4 secretion in transgenic LACK-specific T-cells and in vivo in BALB/c mice. Altered LACK peptides antagonized the production of IL-4 by transgenic T-cells cocultured with LACK in vitro. Pretreatment of BALB/c mice with altered LACK peptides conferred a healer phenotype on these normally susceptible mice *(100)*. These results suggested that the endogenous T-cell repertoire recognizing the LACK antigen has limited diversity.

In a second study, susceptible (BALB/c) and resistant (B10.D2) mice bearing the same I-Aᵈ MHC class II gene were made transgenic for the β-chain of a LACK-specific TCR *(101)*. The fate of LACK-specific CD4⁺ T-lymphocytes was compared in these mice using LACK-peptide/I-Aᵈ multimers upon subcutaneous inoculation of stationary promastigotes. Upon incubation with syngenic APCs and LACK peptide, transgenic T-cells from resistant mice were shown to produce more IFN-γ and less IL-4 and IL-5 than those from susceptible BALB/c mice. Furthermore, I-Aᵈ/LACK T-cells from infected BALB/c mice were shown to express low-affinity TCR, whereas I-Aᵈ LACK T lymphocytes from B10.D2 resistant mice expressed a high-affinity TCR *(101)*.

Thus, upon infection with *L. major* stationary-phase promastigotes, the Th1-dominated protective response that developed in B10.D2 mice was associated with the selective activation and transient expansion of CD4⁺ T-lymphocytes, recognizing LACK with a high affinity. These results suggest that there may exist differences in the TCR usage between mice of similar MHC haplotypes and that these differences could influence the development of *Leishmania*-specific immune responses.

More experiments exploring the interactions between TCR affinity and T-helper differentiation are needed to establish whether a causal relationship between these two parameters exist.

6. CONCLUSIONS AND PERSPECTIVES

The murine model of infection with *L. major* has contributed to unraveling the important role of functionally distinct CD4[+] Th1 and Th2 cells on the outcome of the long-term parasitism initiated by these intracellular parasites, and on the resulting healing or nonhealing pathogenic processes they drive through the complex crosstalk they establish with the immune system. Furthermore, this model was crucial in understanding the mechanisms leading to selective differentiation of Th1 or Th2 CD4[+] T-lymphocytes. Events occurring during the first 3 d following subcutaneous inoculation of millions of stationary-phase promastigotes appeared essential in determining the outcome of the infection in mice of susceptible and resistant phenotypes.

Nevertheless, it is important to consider that the issue of Th1/Th2 effector choice needs further studies in humans before being translated in any immunopreventive or immunotherapeutic measures. Indeed, the extent of human genetic polymorphism and the fact that *Leishmania* species known to initiate human cutaneous lesions did coevolve more closely with wild-type rodents than with humans *(1)* have to be taken into consideration.

REFERENCES

1. Ashford, R.W. (2000) The Leishmaniases as emerging and reemerging zoonoses. *Int. J. Parasitol.* **30**, 1269–1281.
2. Laskay, T., Diefenbach, A., Rollinghoff, M., and Solbach, W. (1995) Early parasite containment is decisive for resistance to *Leishmania major* infection. *Eur. J. Immunol.* **25**, 2220–2227.
3. Solbach, W. and Laskay, T. (2000) The host response to *Leishmania* infection. *Adv. Immunol.* **74**, 275–317.
4. Reiner, S.L. and Locksley, R.M. (1995) The regulation of immunity to *Leishmania major. Ann. Rev. Immunol.* **13**, 151–177.
5. Belkaid, Y., Mendez, S., Lira, R., Kadambi, N., Milon, G., and Sacks, D. (2000) A natural model of *Leishmania major* infection reveals a prolonged "silent" phase of parasite amplification in the skin before the onset of lesion formation and immunity. *J. Immunol.* **165**, 969–977.
6. Afonso, L.C. and Scott, P. (1993) Immune responses associated with susceptibility of C57BL/10 mice to *Leishmania amazonensis. Infect. Immun.* **61**, 2952–2959.
7. Soong, L., Chang, C.H., Sun, J., Longley, B.J., Jr., Ruddle, N.H., Flavell, R.A., et al. (1997) Role of CD4[+] T cells in pathogenesis associated with *Leishmania amazonensis* infection. *J. Immunol.* **158**, 5374–5383.
8. Torrentera, F.A., Glaichenhaus, N., Laman, J.D., and Carlier, Y. (2001) T-cell responses to immunodominant LACK antigen do not play a critical role in determining susceptibility of BALB/c mice to *Leishmania mexicana. Infect. Immun.* **69**, 617–621.
9. Hommel, M., Jaffe, C.L., Travi, B., and Milon, G. (1995) Experimental models for leishmaniasis and for testing antileishmanial vaccines. *Ann. Trop. Med. Parasitol.* **89**, 55–73.
10. Wilson, H.R., Dieckmann, B.S., and Childs, G.E. (1979) *Leishmania braziliensis* and *Leishmania mexicana:* experimental cutaneous infections in golden hamsters. *Exp. Parasitol.* **47**, 270–283.
11. Nabors, G.S. and Farrell, J.P. (1994) Site-specific immunity to *Leishmania major* in SWR mice: the site of infection influences susceptibility and expression of the antileishmanial immune response. *Infect. Immun.* **62**, 3655–3662.
12. Bradley, D.J. and Kirkley, J. (1977) Regulation of *Leishmania* populations within the host. I. the variable course of *Leishmania donovani* infections in mice. *Clin. Exp. Immunol.* **30**, 119–129.
13. Lang, T., Ave, P., Huerre, M., Milon, G., and Antoine, J.C. (2000) Macrophage subsets harbouring *Leishmania donovani* in spleens of infected BALB/c mice: localization and characterization. *Cell Microbiol.* **2**, 415–430.
14. Leclercq, V., Lebastard, M., Belkaid, Y., Louis, J., and Milon, G. (1996) The outcome of the parasitic process initiated by *Leishmania infantum* in laboratory mice: a tissue-dependent pattern controlled by the Lsh and MHC loci. *J. Immunol.* **157**, 4537–4545.
15. Kaye, P.M., Cooke, A., Lund, T., Wattie, M., and Blackwell, J.M. (1992) Altered course of visceral leishmaniasis in mice expressing transgenic I-E molecules. *Eur. J. Immunol.* **22**, 357–364.
16. Wilson, M.E. and Weinstock, J.V. (1996) Hepatic granulomas in murine visceral leishmaniasis caused by *Leishmania chagasi. Methods* **9**, 248–254.
17. Melby, P.C., Chandrasekar, B., Zhao, W., and Coe, J.E. (2001) The hamster as a model of human visceral leishmaniasis: progressive disease and impaired generation of nitric oxide in the face of a prominent Th1-like cytokine response. *J. Immunol.* **166**, 1912–1920.
18. Mosmann, T.R. and Coffman, R.L. (1989) TH1 and TJ2 cells: different patterns of lymphokine secretion lead to different functional properties. *Ann. Rev. Immunol.* **7**, 145–173.
19. Romagnani, S. (1991) Human TH1 and TH2 subsets: doubt no more. *Immunol. Today* **12**, 256–257.
20. Abbas, A., Murphy, K.M., and Sher, A. (1996) Functional diversity of helper T lymphocytes. *Nature* **383**, 787–793.

21. Romagnani, S. (1996) Th1 and Th2 in human diseases. *Clin. Immunol. Immunopathol.* **80,** 225–235.
22. Coffman, R.L., Lebman, D. A., and Rothman, P. (1993) Mechanism and regulation of immunoglobulin isotype switching. *Adv. Immunol.* **54,** 229–270.
23. Kawano, Y., Noma, T., Kou, K., Yoshizawa, I., and Yata, J. (1995) Regulation of human IgG subclass production by cytokines: human IgG subclass production enhanced differentially by interleukin-6. *Immunology* **84,** 278–284.
24. Paul, W.E. and Seder, R.A. (1994) Lymphocyte responses and cytokines. *Cell* **76,** 241–251.
25. Seder, R.A. (1994) Acquisition of lymphokine-producing phenotype by CD4⁺ T cells. *J. Allergy Clin. Immunol.* **94,** 1195–1202.
26. Constant, S.L. and Bottomly, K. (1997) Induction of Th1 and Th2 CD4⁺ T cell responses: the alternative approaches. *Ann. Rev. Immunol.* **15,** 297–322.
27. Seder, R.A., Germain, R.N, Linsley, P.S., and Paul, W.E. (1994) CD28-mediated costimulation of interleukin 2 (IL-2) production plays a critical role in T cell priming for Il-4 and interferon g production. *J. Exp. Med.* **179,** 299–304.
28. Ding, A., Nathan, C.F., Graycar, J., Derynck, R., Stuehr, D.J., and Srimal, S. (1990) Macrophage deactivating factor and transforming growth factors-beta 1, - beta 2 and -beta 3 inhibit induction of macrophage nitrogen oxide synthesis by IFN-gamma. *J. Immunol.* **145,** 940–944.
29. Li, J., Hunter, C.A., and Farrell, J.P. (1999) Anti-TGF-beta treatment promotes rapid healing of *Leishmania major* infection in mice by enhancing in vivo nitric oxide production. *J Immunol.* **162,** 974–979.
30. Barral-Netto, M., Barral, A., Brownell, C.E., Skeiky, Y.A.W., Ellingsworth, L.R., Twardzik, D.R., et al. (1992) Transforming growth factor-β in leishmanial infection: a parasite escape mechanism. *Science* **257,** 545–548.
31. Brown, J.A., Titus, R.G., Nabavi, N., and Glimcher, L.H. (1996) Blockade of CD86 ameliorates *Leishmania major* infection by down regulating the Th2 response. *J. Inf. Dis.* **147,** 1303–1308.
32. Brown, D.R., Green, J.M., Moskowitz, N.H., Davis, M., Thompson, C.B., and Reiner, S.L. (1996) Limited role of CD28-mediated signals in T helper subset differenciation. *J. Exp. Med.* **184,** 803–810.
33. Campbell, K.A., Ovendale, P.J., Kennedy, M.K., Fanslow, W.C., Reed, S.G., and Maliszewski, C.R. (1996) CD40 ligand is required for protective cell-mediated immunity to *Leishmania major. Immunity* **4,** 283–289.
34. Kamanaka, M., Yu, P., Yasui, T., Yoshida, K., Kawabe, T., Horii, T., et al. (1996) Protective role of CD40 in *Leishmania major* infection at two distinct phases of cell-mediated immunity. *Immunity* **4,** 275–281.
35. Ohshima, Y., Tanaka, Y., Tozawa, H., Takahashi, Y., Maliszewski, C., and Delespesse, G. (1997) Expression and function of OX40 ligand on human dendritic cells. *J Immunol.* **159,** 3838–3848.
36. Brocker, T. (1999) The role of dendritic cells in T cell selection and survival. *J. Leukocyte Biol.* **66,** 331–335.
37. Flynn, S., Toellner, K.M, Raykundalia, C., Goodall, M., and Lane, P. (1998) CD4 T cell cytokine differentiation: the B cell activation molecule, OX40 ligand, instructs CD4 T cells to express interleukin 4 and upregulates expression of the chemokine receptor, Blr-1. *J. Exp. Med.* **188,** 297–304.
38. Ohshima, Y., Yang, L.P., Uchiyama, T., Tanaka, Y., Baum, P., Sergerie, M., et al. (1998) OX40 costimulation enhances interleukin-4 (IL-4) expression at priming and promotes the differentiation of naive human CD4(+) T cells into high IL-4-producing effectors. *Blood* **92,** 3338–3345.
39. Akiba, H., Miyahira, Y., Atsuta, M., Takeda, K., Nohara, C., Futagawa, T., et al. (2000) Critical contribution of OX40 ligand to T helper cell type 2 differentiation in experimental leishmaniasis. *J. Exp. Med.* **191,** 375–380.
40. Trinchieri, G. (1998) Interleukin-12: a cytokine at the interface of inflammation and immunity. *Adv. Immunol.* **70,** 83–243.
41. Chan, S.H., Perussia, B., Gupta, J.W., Kobayashi, M., Pospisil, M., Young, H.A., et al. (1991) Induction of IFN-γ production by NK cell stimulatory factor (NKSF): characterization of the responder cells and synergy with other inducers. *J. Exp. Med.* **173,** 869–879.
42. D'Andrea, A., Rengaraju, M., Valiante, N.M., Chehimi, J., Kubin, M., Aste, M., et al. (1992) Production of natural killer cell stimulatory factor (interleukin-12) by peripheral blood mononuclear cells. *J. Exp. Med.* **176,** 1387–1398.
43. Hsieh, C.S., Macatonia, S.E., O'Garra, A., and Murphy,M K.M. (1995) T cell genetic background determines default T helper phenotype development in vitro. *J. Exp. Med.* **181,** 713–721.
44. Macatonia, S.E., Hsieh, C.-S., Murphy, k.m., and O'Garra, A. (1993) Dendritic cells and macrophages are required for Th1 development of CD4⁺ T cells from αβ TCR transgenic mice: IL-12 substitution for macrophages to stimulate IFN-γ production is IFN-γ dependent. *Int. Immunol.* **5,** 1119–1128.
45. Seder, R.A., Gazzinelli, R., Sher, A., and Paul, W.E. (1993) Interleukin 12 acts directly on CD4⁺ T cells to enhance priming for inteferon-γ production and diminishes interleukin 4 inhibition of such priming. *Proc. Natl. Acad. Sci. USA* **90,** 10,188–10,192.
46. Sypek, J.P., Chung, C.L., Mayor, S.E.H., Subramanyam, S.J., Goldman, S.J., Sieburth, D.S., et al. (1993) Resolution of cutaneous leishmanialsis: interleukin 12 iniates a protective T helper type 1 immune response. *J. Exp. Med.* **177,** 1797–1802.
47. Heinzel, F.P., Rerko, R.M., Ahmed, F., and Pearlman, E. (1995) Endogenous IL-12 is required for control of Th2 cytokine responses capable of exacerbating Leishmaniasis in normally resistant mice. *J. Immunol.* **155,** 730–739.
48. Mattner, F., Magram, J., Ferrante, J., Launois, P., Di Padova, K., Behin, R., et al. (1996) Genetically resistant mice lacking interleukin-12 are susceptible to infection with *Leishmania major* and mount a polarized Th2 cell response. *Eur. J. Immunol.* **26,** 1553–1559.
49. Heinzel, F.P., Schoenhaut, D.S., Rerko, R.M., Rosser, L.E., and Gately, M.K. (1993) Recombinant interleukin 12 cures mice infected with *Leishmania major. J. Exp. Med.* **177,** 1505–1509.
50. Szabo, S.J., Dighe, A.S., Gübler, U., and Murphy, K.M. (1997) Regulation of the interleukin (IL)-12Rβ2 subunit expression in developping T helper (Th1) and Th2 cells. *J. Exp. Med.* **185,** 817–824.
51. Guler, M.L., Gorham, J.D., Hsieh, C.S., Mackey, A.J., Steen, R.G., Dietrich, W.F., and Murphy, K.M. (1996) Genetic susceptibility to *Leishmania:* IL-12 responsiveness in TH1 cell development. *Science* **271,** 984–987.

52. Himmelrich, H., Parra-Lopez, C., Tacchini-Cottier, F., Louis, J.A., and Launois, P. (1998) The IL-4 rapidly produced in BALB/c mice after infection with *Leishmania major* downregulates the IL-12 receptor β2 chain expression on CD4⁺ T cells resulting in a state of unresponsiveness to IL-12. *J. Immunol.* **161**, 6156–6163.
53. Jones, D., Elloso, M.M., Showe, L., Williams, D., Trinchieri, G., and Scott, P. (1998) Differential regulation of the interleukin-12 receptor during the innate immune response to *Leishmania major*. *Infect. Immun.* **66**, 3818–3824.
54. Jacobson, N.G., Szabo, S.J., Guler, M.L., Gorham, J.D., and Murphy, K.M. (1996) Regulation of interleukin-12 signalling during T helper phenotype development. *Adv. Exp. Med. Biol.* **409**, 61–73.
55. Hondowicz, B.D., Park, A.Y., Elloso, M.M., and Scott, P. (2000) Maintenance of IL-12-responsive CD4⁺ T cells during a Th2 response in *Leishmania major*-infected mice. *Eur. J. Immunol.* **30**, 2007–2014.
56. Jones, D.E., Buxbaum, L.U., and Scott, P. (2000) IL-4-independent inhibition of IL-12 responsiveness during *Leishmania amazonensis* infection. *J. Immunol.* **165**, 364–372.
57. Okamura, H., Tsutsi, H., Komatsu, T., Yutsudo, M., Hakura, A., Tanimoto, T., et al. (1995) Cloning of a new cytokine that induces IFN-gamma production by T cells. *Nature* **378**, 88–91.
58. Robinson, D., Shibuya, K., Mui, A., Zonin, F., Murphy, E., Sana, T., et al. (1997) IGIF does not drive Th1 development but synergizes with IL-12 for interferon-gamma production and activates IRAK and NFkappaB. *Immunity* **7**, 571–581.
59. Wei, X.Q., Leung, B.P., Niedbala, W., Piedrafita, D., Feng, G.J., Sweet, M., et al. (1999) Altered immune responses and susceptibility to *Leishmania major* and Staphylococcus aureus infection in IL-18-deficient mice. *J. Immunol.* **163**, 2821–2828.
60. Monteforte, G.M., Takeda, K., Rodriguez-Sosa, M., Akira, S., David, J.R., and Satoskar, A.R. (2000) Genetically resistant mice lacking IL-18 gene develop Th1 response and control cutaneous *Leishmania major* infection. *J. Immunol.* **164**, 5890–5893.
61. Xu, D., Trajkovic, V., Hunter, D., Leung, B.P., Schulz, K., Gracie, J.A., et al. (2000) IL-18 induces the differentiation of Th1 or Th2 cells depending upon cytokine milieu and genetic background. *Eur. J. Immunol.* **30**, 3147–3156.
62. Hsieh, C.-S., Macatonia, S.E., Tripp, C.S., Wolf, S.F., O'Garra, A., and Murphy, K.M. (1993) Development of TH1 CD4⁺ T cells through IL-12 produced by *Listeria*-induced macrophages. *Science* **260**, 547–549.
63. Wenner, C.A., Güler, M.L., Macatonia, S.E., O'Garra, A., and Murphy, K.M. (1996) Roles of IFN-γ and IFN-α in IL-12-induced T helper cell-1 development. *J. Immunol.* **156**, 1442–1447.
64. Scott, P.A. (1991) IFN-γ modulates the early development of Th1 and Th2 responses in a murine model of cutaneous leishmaniasis. *J. Immunol.* **147**, 3149–3155.
65. Belosevic, M., Finbloom, D.S., van der Meide, P.H., Slayter, M.V., and Nacy, C.A. (1989) Administration of monoclonal anti-IFN-γ antibodies in vivo abrogates natural resistance of C3H/HeN mice to infection wih *Leishmania major*. *J. Immunol.* **143**, 266–274.
66. Wang, Z.E., Zheng, S., Corry, D.B., Dalton, D.K., Seder, R.A., Reiner, S.L., et al. (1994) Interferon gamma-independent effects of interleukin 12 administered during acute or established infection due to *Leishmania major*. *Proc. Nat. Acad. Sci USA* **91**, 12,932–12,936.
67. Swihart, K., Fruth, U., Messmer, N., Hug, K., Behin, R., Huang, S., et al. (1995) Mice from a genetically resistant background lacking the interferon gamma receptor are susceptible to infection with *Leishmania major* but mount a polarized T helper cell 1-type CD4⁺ T cell response. *J. Exp. Med.* **181**, 961–971.
68. Beil, W.J., Meinardus-Hager, G., Neugebauer, D.C., and Sorg, C. (1992) Differences in the onset of the inflammatory response to cutaneous leishmaniasis in resistant and susceptible mice. *J. Leukocyte Biol.* **52**, 135–142.
69. Tacchini-Cottier, F., Zweifel, C., Belkaid, Y., Mukankundiye, C., Vasei, M., Launois, P., et al. (2000) An immunomodulatory function for neutrophils during the induction of a CD4⁺ Th2 response in BALB/c mice infected with *Leishmania major*. *J. Immunol.* **165**, 2628–2636.
70. Fava, R.A., Olsen, N.J., Postlethwaite, A.E., Broadley, K.N., Davidson, J.M., Nanney, L.B., et al. (1991) Transforming growth factor beta 1 (TGF-beta 1) induced neutrophil recruitment to synovial tissues: implications for TGF-beta-driven synovial inflammation and hyperplasia. *J. Exp. Med.* **173**, 1121–1132.
71. Cassatella, M.A., Meda, L., Gasperini, S., D'Andrea, A., Ma, X., and Trinchieri, G. (1995) Interleukin-12 production by human polymorphonuclear leukocytes. *Eur. J. Immunol.* **25**, 1–5.
72. Laskay, T., Rollinghoff, M., and Solbach, W. (1993) Natural killer cells participate in the early defense against *Leishmania major* infection in mice. *Eur. J. Immunol.* **23**, 2237–2241.
73. Reiner, S.L., Zheng, S., Wang, Z.-E., Stowring, L., and Locksley, R.M. (1994) *Leishmania* promastigotes evade interleukin 12 (IL-12) induction by macrophages and stimulate a broad range of cytokines from CD4⁺ T cells during initiation of infection. *J. Exp. Med.* **179**, 447–456.
74. Scharton, T.M. and Scott, P. (1993) Natural killer cells are a source of interferon gamma that drives differentiation of CD4⁺ T cell subsets and induces early resistance to *Leishmania major* in mice. *J. Exp. Med.* **178**, 567–577.
75. Scharton-Kersten, T., Afonso, L.C.C., Wysocka, M., Trinchieri, G., and Scott, P. (1995) IL-12 is required for natural killer cell activation and subsequent T helper 1 cell development in experimental leishmaniasis. *J. Immunol.* **154**, 5320–5330.
76. Wakil, A.E., Wang, Z.E., Ryan, J.C., Fowell, D.J., and Locksley, R.M. (1998) Interferon gamma derived from CD4(+) T cells is sufficient to mediate T helper cell type 1 development. *J. Exp. Med.* **188**, 1651–1656.
77. Satoskar, A.R., Stamm, L.M., Zhang, X., Satoskar, A.A., Okano, M., Terhorst, C., et al. (1999) Mice lacking NK cells develop an efficient Th1 response and control cutaneous *Leishmania major* infection. *J. Immunol* **162**, 6747–6754.
78. Wang, M., Ellison, C.A., Gartner, J.G., and HayGlass, K.T. (1998) Natural killer cell depletion fails to influence initial CD4 T cell commitment in vivo in exogenous antigen-stimulated cytokine and antibody responses. *J. Immunol.* **160**, 1098–1105.

79. Mattner, J., Schindler, H., Diefenbach, A., Rollinghoff, M., Gresser, I., and Bogdan, C. (2000) Regulation of type 2 nitric oxide synthase by type 1 interferons in macrophages infected with *Leishmania major*. *Eur. J. Immunol.* **30,** 2257–2267.

80. Hsieh, C.-S., Heimberger, A.B., Gold, J.S., O'Garra, A., and Murphy, K.M. (1992) Differential regulation of T helper phenotype development by interleukins 4 and 10 in an αβ T-cell-receptor transgenic system. *Proc. Natl. Acad. Sci. USA* **89,** 6065–6069.

81. Locksley, R.M., Heinzel, F.P., Sadick, M.D., Holaday, B.J., and Gardner, K.D. (1987) Murine cutaneous leishmaniasis: susceptibility correlates with differential expansion of helper T cell subset. *Ann. Inst. Pasteur/Immunol* **138,** 744–749.

82. Heinzel, F.P., Sadick, M.D., Holaday, B.J., Coffman, R.L., and Locksley, R.M. (1989) Reciprocal expression of interferon γ or interleukin 4 during the resolution or progression of murine leishmaniasis. *J. Exp. Med. 169,* 59–72.

83. Coffman, R.L., Varkila, K., Scott, P., and Chatelain, R. (1991) Role of cytokines in the differentiation of CD4+ T cell subsets in vivo. *Immunol. Rev.* **123,** 189–205.

84. Chatelain, R., Varkila, K., and Coffman, R.L. (1992) IL-4 induces a Th2 response in *Leishmania major*-infected mice. *J. Immunol.* **148,** 1182–1187.

85. Sadick, M.D., Heinzel, F.P., Holaday, B.J., Pu, R.T., Dawkins, R.S., and Locksley, R.M. (1990) Cure of murine leishmaniasis with anti-interleukin 4 monoclonal antibody. Evidence for a T cell-dependent, interferon-γ independent mechanism. *J. Exp. Med.* **171,** 115–127.

86. Leal, L.M.C.C., Moss, D.W., Kuhn, R., Muller, W., and Liew, F.Y. (1993) Interleukin-4 transgenic mice of resistant background are susceptible to *Leishmania major* infection. *Eur. J. Immunol.* **23,** 566–569.

87. Kopf, M., Brombacher, F., Kölher, G., Kienzle, G., Widmann, K.-H., Lefrang, K., et al. (1996) IL-4 deficient Balb/c mice resist infection with *Leishmania major*. *J. Exp. Med.* **184,** 1127–1136.

88. Noben-Trauth, N., Kropf, P., and Muller, I. (1996) Susceptibility to *Leishmania major* infection in IL-4 deficient mice. *Science* **271,** 912–913.

89. Aman, M.J., Tayebi, N., Obiri, N.I., Puri, R.K., Modi, W.S., and Leonard, W.J. (1996) cDNA cloning and characterization of the human interleukin 13 receptor alpha chain. *J. Biol. Chem.* **271,** 29,265–29,270.

90. Hilton, D.J., Zhang, J.G., Metcalf, D., Alexander, W.S., Nicola, N.A., and Willson, T.A. (1996) Cloning and characterization of a binding subunit of the interleukin 13 receptor that is also a component of the interleukin 4 receptor. *Proc. Natl. Acad. Sci. USA* **93,** 497–501.

91. Gauchat, J.F., Schlagenhauf, E., Feng, N.P., Moser, R., Yamage, M., Jeannin, P., et al. (1997) A novel 4-kb interleukin-13 receptor alpha mRNA expressed in human B, T, and endothelial cells encoding an alternate type-II interleukin- 4/interleukin-13 receptor. *Eur. J. Immunol.* **27,** 971–978.

92. Noben-Trauth, N., Paul, W.E., and Sacks, D.L. (1999) IL-4- and IL-4 receptor-deficient BALB/c mice reveal differences in susceptibility to *Leishmania major* parasite substrains. *J. Immunol.* **162,** 6132–6140.

93. Mohrs, M., Ledermann, B., Kohler, G., Dorfmuller, A. Gessner, A., and Brombacher, F. (1999) Differences between IL-4- and IL-4 receptor alpha-deficient mice in chronic Llishmaniasis reveal a protective role for IL-13 receptor signaling. *J. Immunol.* **162,** 7302–7308.

94. Launois, P., Ohteki, T., Swihart, K., MacDonald, H.R., and Louis, J.A. (1995) In susceptible mice, *Leishmania major* induceS very rapid interleukin-4 production by CD4+ T cells which are NK1.1-. *Eur. J. Immunol.* **25,** 3298–3307.

95. Launois, P., Maillard, I., Pingel, S., Swihart, K., Xenarios, I., Acha-Orbea, H., et al. (1997) IL-4 rapidly produced by Vβ4 Vα8 CD4+ T cells in BALB/c mice infected with *Leishmania* major instructsTh2 cell development and susceptibility to infection. *Immunity* **16,** 541–549.

96. Launois, P., Tacchini-Cottier, F., Parra-Lopez, C., and Louis, J.A. (1998) Cytokines in parasitic diseases: the example of cutaneous leishmaniasis. *Int. Rev. Immunol* **17,** 157–180.

97. Mougneau, E., Altare, F., Wakil, A.E., Zheng, S., Coppola, T., Wang, Z.E., et al. (1995) Expression cloning of a protective Leishmania antigen. *Science* **268,** 563–536.

98. Himmelrich, H., Launois, P., Maillard, I., Biedermann, T., Tacchini-Cottier, F., Locksley, R.M., et al. (2000) In BALB/c mice, IL-4 production during the initial phase of infection with *Leishmaniai major* is necessary and sufficient to instruct Th2 cell development resulting in progressive disease. *J. Immunol.* **164,** 4819–4825.

99. Julia, V., Rassoulzadegan, M., and Glaichenhaus, N. (1996) Resistance to *Leishmania major* induced by tolerance to a single antigen. *Science* **274,** 421–423.

100. Pingel, S., Launois, P., Fowell, D.J., Turck, C.W., Southwood, S., Sette, A., et al. (1999) Altered ligands reveal limited plasticity in the T cell response to a pathogenic epitope. *J. Exp. Med.* **189,** 1111–1120.

101. Malherbe, L., Filippi, C., Julia, V., Foucras, G., Moro, M., Appel, H., et al. (2000) Selective activation and expansion of high-affinity CD4+ T cells in resistant mice upon infection with *Leishmania major*. *Immunity* **13,** 771–782.

18

Cytokines in the Regulation of Innate and Adaptive Immunity to *Toxoplasma gondii*

Ulrike Wille and Christopher A. Hunter

1. INTRODUCTION

The obligate intracellular protozoan parasite *Toxoplasma gondii* (*T. gondii*) was first identified in 1908 by Nicolle and Manceaux *(1)* in the rodent *Ctenodactylus gundi* and derived the genus name from the crescent shape of the organism (Greek: toxon = arc) observed in this host. In 1939, Wolf et al. *(2)* provided the first description of congenital disease caused by *T. gondii* and so identified this parasite as a pathogen of humans. It is now recognized that *T. gondii* is present in industrialized and developing countries and serology studies indicate that 10–70% of human populations, depending on geographic region and ethnicity, are infected. In addition, this is a common infection in animals and represents an important cause of abortion in farm animals. Thus, *T. gondii* represents one of the most common parasitic pathogens of man and is of considerable economic importance.

In terms of public health, most adults infected with *T. gondii* are asymptomatic, but it has long been recognized that when primary infection occurs during pregnancy, there is a risk of vertical transmission of *T. gondii* to the fetus and the development of congenital toxoplasmosis *(3)*. *T. gondii* is also an important opportunistic parasite in patients with primary and acquired immune deficiencies. This was first recognized in patients with cancers associated with decreased immune function *(4,5)*, and with the increasing use of immune suppressive therapies to treat cancer and aid transplantation, clinical toxoplasmosis became more common *(6–8)*. During the early 1980s, *T. gondii* was recognized as an important opportunistic infection in patients with AIDS (acquired immunodeficiency syndrome) *(7)*, and as a consequence, increased amounts of research have been performed to understand the mechanisms by which the immune system normally protects against the parasite and how defects in the immune system can lead to clinical toxoplasmosis. These studies have highlighted the important role of cell-mediated immunity in long-term resistance to *T. gondii* and this chapter summarizes the role of cytokines in the regulation of innate and adaptive immunity to this parasite.

2. BIOLOGY OF *T. GONDII*

The life cycle of *T. gondii* is complex with several distinct developmental stages and multiple hosts (*see* Fig. 1). Cats (wild and domestic) are the definitive host of *T. gondii*, whereas all warm-blooded vertebrates can serve as intermediate hosts. The natural life cycle has two infectious cyst-forming stages: oocysts, which contain sporozoites, and tissue cysts, which contain bradyzoites. Ingestion of oocysts or tissue cysts by intermediate hosts results in the activation of the parasites that invade the gut epithelium and differentiate into the tachyzoite form. Tachyzoites have a low tissue specificity and are capable of infecting almost every type of cell in the host. They actively invade

From: *Cytokines and Chemokines in Infectious Diseases Handbook*
Edited by: M. Kotb and T. Calandra © Humana Press Inc., Totowa, NJ

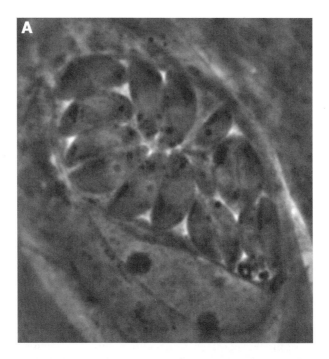

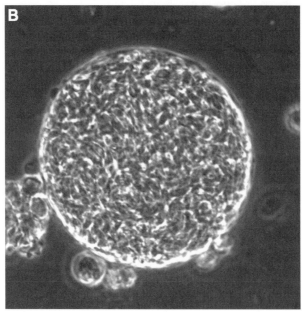

Fig. 1. Infectious stages of *T. gondii* in the intermediate host. A human fibroblast originally infected with a single tachyzoite of *T. gondii* contains, after 4 rounds of parasite replication, 16 tachyzoites (**A**). Tachyzoites actively invade host cells and undergo five to eight rounds of asexual division withing a parsitophorous vacuole. Eventually, this leads to cytolysis of the cell and the released parasites invade new cells. In all hosts, a small percentage of tachyzoites differenciate into bradyzoites, which form tissue cysts (**B**). Cysts contain multiple bradyzoites and are found in various tissues, but most commonly in sites such as the brain, retina, cardiac, and skeletal muscle. Cysts are present for the lifetime of the host and represent a source of persistent infection, but this developmental stage is also infective to new hosts if ingested. (Courtesy of Dr. O. Harb, Dr. F. Dzierszinski, and Dr. D. Roos.)

host cells and undergo five to eight rounds of asexual division within a parasitophorous vacuole. Eventually, this leads to cytolysis of the cell and the released parasites invade new cells. In cats that are infected for the first time, these events are accompanied by the development of sexual forms of *T. gondii* that fuse to form nonsporulated oocysts. Oocysts are shed in the feces for approximately 2 wk but need to undergo the process of sporogony before they become infectious. This is the only developmental stage of *T. gondii* that survives outside the host and represents a source of environmental contamination.

In all hosts, a small percentage of tachyzoites differentiate into bradyzoites, which form tissue cysts found in multiple tissues, but most commonly in sites such as the brain, retina, cardiac, and skeletal muscle. Cysts are present for the lifetime of the host and represent a source of persistent infection, but this developmental stage is also infective to new hosts if ingested. The events that trigger the transition from tachyzoite to bradyzoite are not completely understood, but in vitro studies have shown that bradyzoite formation occurs in response to stress *(9–11)*. In vivo, the switch from tachyzoite to bradyzoite is likely immune mediated and the production of nitric oxide, which inhibits replication of tachyzoites, has been shown to stimulate bradyzoite formation *(12)*. The rupture of cysts occurs periodically and the released bradyzoites can infect new host cells and transform back into tachyzoites. The factors that lead to this reactivation are unclear, but the release of parasites from cysts is likely a continuous process that provides a constant stimulus to the immune system. As a consequence, IgG antibody titers for *T. gondii* remain high for the lifetime of the host and serology is a useful tool for the identification of chronically infected individuals. In addition to oocysts and tissue cysts, the tachyzoite stage can also be infectious. Although this stage is normally killed in the stomach, it can cause infection when introduced by other routes and is the infectious stage for the fetus.

3. CLINICAL TOXOPLASMOSIS

3.1. Congenital Toxoplasmosis

Congenital toxoplasmosis continues to be one of the most serious complications associated with this infection. Normally, immunocompetent women infected with *T. gondii* develop protective immunity, and although they remain chronically infected, transmission of the parasite from mother to fetus during a subsequent pregnancy is rare. However, if infection occurs for the first time during pregnancy, vertical transmission of *T. gondii* to the fetus can occur and result in congenital disease. The severity of congenital toxoplasmosis depends on the developmental stage of the fetus at the time of infection. If infection occurs during the first trimester of pregnancy, when the fetus is poorly developed, it can result in severe congenital defects (hydrocephalus, mental and psychomotor retardation, blindness, retinochoroiditis, epilepsy). Should the parasite be transmitted during the third trimester of pregnancy, when development of the fetus is almost complete, complications caused by the parasite are less severe. Although transmission of *T. gondii* from mother to fetus is rare in chronically infected women, the immune status of the mother plays an important role. Thus, in human immunodeficiency virus (HIV)-positive women, the loss of immune functions can lead to reactivation of the parasite and there is an increased likelihood of congenital transmission. Moreover, the risk as well as the consequences of infection increase if the fetus itself is HIV-positive *(13)*.

3.2. Toxoplasmosis in Immunocompromised Patients

After primary infection with *T. gondii*, immunity to the parasite is maintained for the lifetime of the host as long as the immune system remains intact. However, in patients with acquired defects in T-cell function, reactivation of infection and clinical disease can occur. Historically, this was first recognized in patients with neoplastic diseases, such as leukemia and Hodgkin's and non-Hodgkin's lymphoma *(5,14–19)*. These cancers are associated with suppression of the immune system and chemotherapy can also result in reduced immune function. During the 1970s, transplantation became an established therapy and its success was dependent on the use of immunosuppressive drugs to suppress T-cell function and so prevent rejection of the donor organ. As a result, the use of these treatment regimes in patients infected with *T. gondii* led to the emergence of a new population of patients at risk of developing toxoplasmosis *(4)*. A decade later, with the advent of the AIDS pandemic, a third group of patients susceptible to toxoplasmosis emerged. Infection with HIV leads to a decrease in CD4$^+$ and CD8$^+$ T-cell numbers, and in individuals chronically infected with *T. gondii*, there is a loss of parasite-specific T-cells associated with reactivation of the latent infection *(20,21)*. Although the loss of T-cells is the primary defect in patients with AIDS that predisposes these individuals to reactivation of infection, there appear to be other factors that contribute to the development of disease. For example, infection of macrophages with HIV inhibits the ability of these cells to control parasite replication *(22)*, and monocytes from patients with AIDS have a defect in their ability to control parasite replication *(23,24)*. Thus, there are defects in T-cell and macrophage functions in patients with AIDS that may contribute to the reactivation of infection. In addition, the production of proinflammatory cytokines associated with resistance to *T. gondii* has been shown to enhance HIV replication *(25–29)* and studies using an HIV transgenic mouse showed that infection with *T. gondii* enhanced proviral gene expression *(30)*. These studies suggest that in AIDS patients who develop Toxoplasmic encephalitis (TE), there is a vicious cycle in which the immune response to *T. gondii* leads to enhanced viral replication and a decrease in numbers of T-cells which further predisposes to TE.

In contrast to the above-described patients who have acquired immune deficiencies, toxoplasmosis has recently been recognized as an opportunistic infection in patients with X-linked hyper-IgM syndrome *(31,32)*. This primary immune deficiency is a consequence of deficient signaling through the CD40L molecule and is characterized by low or absent serum IgG and IgA and normal or increased IgM. Although these patients were initially identified because of their gross defects in humoral immunity, it is now recognized that they also have defects in cell-mediated immunity, which correlates with their susceptibility to intracellular infections *(31,33,34)*. Interestingly, patients with AIDS also have defects in their ability to express CD40L *(35,36)*, suggesting that in addition to the overall loss of T-cells, this specific defect in T-cell function may also contribute to the increased susceptibility to *T. gondii*.

3.3. Diagnosis and Treatment of Toxoplasmosis

In chronically infected asymptomatic individuals, circulating antibodies against the parasite can be detected in serum and body fluids for the lifetime of the host, which makes serology a useful tool for the identification of infected individuals. In most of the immunocompromised patients who develop toxoplasmosis, serodiagnosis suggests that disease is normally the result of the reactivation of a pre-existing infection and not primary infection. However, given the high seroprevalence rates for this infection, seropositivity does not necessarily distinguish between asymptomatic individuals and those with active clinical disease. Whereas the use of enzyme-linked immunosorbent assay (ELISA) to detect parasite specific IgM and IgG provides the ability to distinguish the acute phase of infection from the chronic stage, diagnosis of active disease is frequently dependent on the detection of parasites in tissues removed by biopsy or at necropsy.

Clinical toxoplasmosis is treated most commonly with drugs that target the folate metabolism of the parasite. Pyrimethamine is the principle drug for treatment of toxoplasmosis, and when used in combination with sulfadiazine or clindamycin, it is highly effective in preventing tachyzoite replication *(37)*. Similar regimes are used to treat acute infection during pregnancy and have been shown to reduce the incidence of congenital disease by approximately 50% *(38)*. However, there are several problems associated with the use of current treatment regimes. Although these drugs can inhibit the replication of the tachyzoite, they do not target the bradyzoite stage and so fail to eradicate the infection. Thus, treatment may have to be continued for the lifetime of an immunocompromised patient. In addition, the long-term use of these drugs is problematic, as they can cause severe side effects and many immunocompromised patients tolerate these treatments poorly. Therefore, the development of more efficient therapies to treat toxoplasmosis is necessary, and recent research has focused on the identification of new drug targets as well as the use of immunotherapy to manage this opportunistic infection.

4. CELL-MEDIATED IMMUNITY TO *T. GONDII*

In the last two decades, there has been a tremendous growth in our understanding of how immunity to *T. gondii* is initiated and maintained. The recognition that *T. gondii* is an opportunistic pathogen in patients with primary or acquired immune deficiencies that result in suppression or loss of T-cell functions highlights the role of T-cells in the control of this infection. Based on studies with human cells and murine models, it is clear that infection with *T. gondii* induces a strong cell-mediated immune response. The parasite stimulates innate and adaptive resistance to infection and both non-specific and antigen-specific mechanisms are involved in the defense. The response induced in the host after primary infection is distinct from the immune response that is necessary to maintain immunity. During the acute infection, the host has to initiate an immune response to control parasite replication, whereas during the chronic phase of toxoplasmosis, the host has to maintain immunity to prevent reactivation of disease. Although there are various host factors that appear to be more important in one phase than in the other, the production of interferon (IFN)-γ is essential for resistance throughout the course of infection. Early studies to define the role of cytokines in immunity to *T. gondii* demonstrated that IFN-γ could activate macrophages to control parasite replication and that treatment with IFN-γ enhanced resistance to this parasite *(39,40)*. However, it was the critical studies of Suzuki and Remington that showed that neutralization of endogenous IFN-γ resulted in unrestricted parasite replication and identified IFN-γ as the major mediator of resistance to *T. gondii (41)*. Subsequent research has focused on defining the events that lead to the production of this cytokine and how IFN-γ mediates its protective effects.

4.1. Innate Immunity to **T. gondii**

The early immune response to *T. gondii* is characterized by an innate mechanism of resistance and the development of a strong adaptive response, characterized by the selection and expansion of parasite specific T-cells that make IFN-γ (Th1-type response). These innate and adaptive events do not occur in isolation, and it is the innate production of interleukin (IL)-12, which is critical for both mechanisms of resistance *(42–44)*. In murine models, infection with *T. gondii* leads to the rapid production of IL-12 with elevated levels detected within hours *(45–47)*. This, in turn, stimulates natural killer (NK) cells to produce IFN-γ, which initiates the control of parasite replication prior to the development of adaptive T-cell responses *(48)* (*see* Fig. 2). The importance of the innate immune response in defense against *T. gondii* is demonstrated by studies with SCID (severe combined immune deficiency) mice that lack functional B- and T-cells. In these mice, there is no adaptive response and infection with *T. gondii* leads to production of IL-12, which stimulates NK-cell production of IFN-γ. Although these mice survive infection for approximately 20 d, in the absence of IL-12 or IFN-γ, SCID mice are unable to control parasite replication and succumb to infection within 10 d *(48,49)*. Conversely, treatment of SCID mice with IL-12 results in enhanced resistance to *T. gondii* and this effect can be abolished by neutralization of IFN-γ or depletion of NK cells. Together, these results demonstrate that the protective effects of exogenous IL-12 act through the induction of IFN-γ by NK cells *(48)*.

Although IL-12 is central to NK-cell production of IFN-γ, alone it is a poor inducer of this response and other stimuli such as tumor necrosis factor (TNF)-α, IL-1β, IL-18, or costimulation through CD28 are required for optimal IL-12-induced production of IFN-γ *(48–53)*. Infection with *T. gondii* results in increased production of these cytokines, upregulation of B7 expression by macrophages, and increased expression of CD28 by activated NK cells *(53–58)*. The significance of these events has been shown by the increased susceptibility of SCID mice treated with antagonists of TNF-α or the CD28/B7 interaction and by experiments that demonstrated that the protective effects of exog-

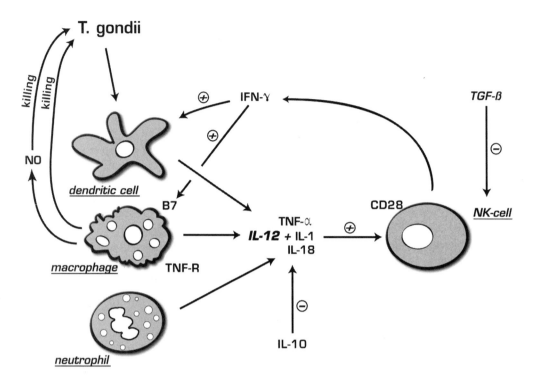

Fig. 2. Innate immunity to *T. gondii*. Infection with *T. gondii* leads to the production of IL-12 by macrophages, dendritic cells (DCs) and neutrophils that initiates production of IFN-γ by NK cells. This IFN-γ stimulates
macrophages and DCs to produce increased levels of IL-12 and, in combination with TNF-α, the production of
nitric oxide (NO) by macrophages. The IL-12-induced activation of NK cells is enhanced by other factors such
as IL-1β, TNF-α, IL-18 and costimulation through the CD28/B7 interaction. In contrast, IL-10 and TGF-β have
inhibitory functions on the innate response and suppress accessory cell functions and NK-cell activity.

enous IL-12 are dependent on endogenous IL-1 *(49,52,59)*. Moreover, although endogenous IL-18
does not appear to be necessary for innate resistance to *T. gondii*, administration of IL-18 to SCID
mice augments NK-cell-mediated immunity to the parasite associated with enhanced production of
IFN-γ and significantly reduced parasite burden *(53)*. In addition to their ability to produce IFN-γ,
NK cells from infected mice have been reported to be cytotoxic for extracellular tachyzoites *(60)* and
IL-2-activated human NK cells are cytotoxic for cells infected with *T. gondii (61)*.

Although there are several factors that lead to NK-cell production of IFN-γ, there are also cytokines
that antagonize this response. Transforming growth factor (TGF)-β has been shown to directly inhibit the ability of NK cells to produce IFN-γ *(59,62)* and TGF-β is produced in vitro and in vivo in
response to *T. gondii (55,59,63)*. The in vivo significance of these findings was shown by studies in
which treatment of SCID mice with neutralizing anti-TGF-β increased the survival time of mice after
infection, whereas administration of TGF-β to infected SCID mice resulted in increased susceptibility of these mice *(59)*. In contrast to the direct effect of TGF-β on NK cells, the ability of IL-10 to
antagonize NK-cell responses is the result of its inhibitory effects on accessory cell production of
proinflammatory cytokines, including IL-12 *(64,65)*. The role of IL-10 in innate immunity to *T. gondii*
is illustrated by the enhanced production of IFN-γ by splenocytes from infected SCID mice when IL-
10 is neutralized in vitro and by the remarkable increase in resistance to *T. gondii* of IL-10-deficient
SCID mice compared with normal SCID mice *(66)*.

Although there is now a good understanding of the role of cytokines in the regulation of innate immunity to *T. gondii*, the initial events that lead to the production of IL-12 and the cells involved in this process are still uncertain. Macrophages *(44)*, dendritic cells (DCs) *(46)*, and neutrophils *(45,67)* have all been described as early IL-12 sources, but the mechanisms that underly these responses are unknown. Parasite extracts can directly stimulate the production of IL-12 by activated macrophages *(44)*, DCs *(46)*, and neutrophils *(45)*, suggesting that there are specific receptors that recognize parasite antigens. In recent years, Toll-like receptors expressed by macrophages and DCs have been shown to be important for the recognition of bacterial and fungal products and for initiating the production of cytokines and upregulation of costimulatory molecules. The evolution of pattern recognition receptors to identify invading micro-organisms seems to be a key feature of innate immunity (*see* recent reviews *68–70*), and a similar mechanism may be used to recognize *T. gondii* and initiate the production of IL-12. In support of this hypothesis are studies that demonstrated that glycosylphosphatidylinositol anchors of *Trypanosoma cruzi* activate Toll-2, which is required for the production of IL-12 *(71)*. However, other mechanisms may alert the immune system to the presence of invading parasites, and cytolysis of infected cells by *T. gondii* may provide a "danger" signal *(72)*. Alternatively, the production of chemokines by infected cells *(73–75)* may stimulate the immune system and recent studies indicate that signaling through the chemokine receptor CCR5 stimulates CD8α^+ DCs to produce IL-12 essential for resistance to *T. gondii (76)*. Defining the pathways and the receptors that are involved in the innate production of IL-12 following infection with *T. gondii* represents a major question in this field that is a key to understanding how the host initiates innate and adaptive responses to this infection.

4.2. Adaptive Immunity to T. gondii

Although NK cells provide an innate mechanism of resistance against *T. gondii*, it is limited and T-cells are essential to provide long-term protection. This is best illustrated by the immunocompromised patients with defects in T-cell function who develop toxoplasmosis and by experimental studies that showed that long-term resistance of SCID mice to *T. gondii* is only possible if they are reconstituted with both CD4$^+$ and CD8$^+$ T-cells *(77,78)*. There is evidence that CD8$^+$ T-cells are the major source of IFN-γ- during chronic infection, but the ability of parasite specific CD4$^+$ T-cells to make IL-2 is required for the production of IFN-γ by CD8$^+$ T-cells *(79–84)*. Thus, several studies have shown that optimal resistance to *T. gondii* is dependent on both CD4$^+$ and CD8$^+$ T-cells albeit either population alone does provide a level of protection *(79,82,85)*. More recently, studies using gene knockout mice have extended these observations. For example, mice that lack the common γ-chain (which is part of the receptors for IL-2, IL-4, IL-7, IL-9, and IL-15) lack NK cells and CD8$^+$ T-cells, but when infected with *T. gondii*, the ability of CD4$^+$ T-cells to produce IFN-γ is sufficient to control the early stage of infection *(86)*. Similarly, β$_2$-microglobulin knockout mice that have reduced levels of major histocompatibility complex (MHC) class I and lack functional CD8$^+$ T-cells survive acute infection with *T. gondii* associated with an increased expansion of a unique NK-like population of cells that produce IFN-γ *(87)*. Nevertheless, both the γ-chain and β$_2$-microglobulin knockout mice succumb to infection during the chronic stage of infection *(86,88)*, indicating that CD4$^+$ T-cells are sufficient for resistance during the acute stage of toxoplasmosis, but both CD4$^+$ and CD8$^+$ T-cells are required for the long-term control of this parasite (*see* Fig. 3).

The innate immune system has an important role in the development of protective T-cell responses, and the early production of IL-12 is critical to direct the development of a strong adaptive immune response dominated by the production of IFN-γ. The requirement of IL-12 for the generation of parasite-specific T-cells to produce IFN-γ is best illustrated by studies that showed that in the absence of IL-12, mice fail to develop protective T-cell responses and die as a consequence of an overwhelming parasitemia *(42,43,48,89)*. However, there are reports of IL-12-independent pathways

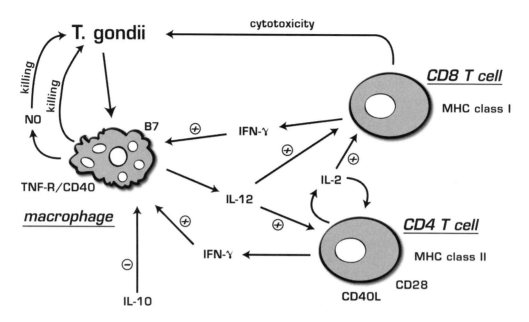

Fig. 3. Adaptive immunity to *T. gondii*. Following infection with *T. gondii*, early production of IL-12 by the innate immune system together with antigen presentation leads to the development and expansion of parasite-specific T-cells that produce IFN-γ. During the chronic phase of infection, the ability of CD4+ T-cells to make IL-2 is required for the production of IFN-γ by CD8+ T-cells. Other factors that are important in T-cell activation are costimulatory signals provided by the CD28/B7 and CD40/CD40L interactions. The ability of IL-10 to inhibit accessory cell functions required for optimal T-cell stimulation is important for preventing the development of infection-induced immune pathology.

that provide a limited mechanism of resistance to *T. gondii (90,91)*. In the absence of IL-12 or IL-12-mediated signaling through STAT-4, mice are highly susceptible to infection with *T. gondii*. However, in the absence of IL-12, mice infected with low doses of a temperature sensitive strain of *T. gondii* make enough IFN-γ to provide a limited mechanism of resistance *(90,92)*. Similarly, STAT-4 knockout mice infected with *T. gondii* can produce low levels of IFN-γ, which can be augmented by treating with the combination of IL-2 plus IL-18 *(91)*. In both of these cases, the IL-12-independent mechanisms of resistance do not provide long-term protection and mice eventually succumb to the parasite. Similar findings have been observed in other experimental systems *(93,94)* and these studies raise questions about which cytokines are involved in stimulating the IL-12-independent pathways that lead to the production of IFN-γ during toxoplasmosis.

The innate production of IL-12 is essential for stimulating the early production of IFN-γ from NK cells and directing the development of T-cell IFN-γ responses. However, the early production of IFN-γ will also prime macrophages and DCs to produce increased levels of IL-12, which, in turn, amplifies innate and adaptive responses. In addition, once T-cells are activated, they upregulate expression of CD40L, which signals through CD40 expressed by macrophages and DCs to enhance IL-12 production. The involvement of this mechanism in adaptive responses to *T. gondii* has been shown by several in vitro and in vivo studies. Thus, CD40L knockout mice produce reduced levels of IL-12 during acute toxoplasmosis, but these levels of IL-12 are sufficient to drive production of normal levels of IFN-γ *(95)*. In studies using human cells in vitro, it has been shown that the CD40/CD40L interaction is essential for the production of IL-12 and IFN-γ by peripheral blood mononuclear cells (PBMCs) stimulated with live parasites *(31)*. Moreover, peripheral blood mononuclear cells (PBMCs) from hyper-IgM patients (which are defective in the CD40/CD40L interaction) make reduced levels of IL-12 and IFN-γ when stimulated with live parasites, but exogenous IL-12 restores their ability to make IFN-γ *(31,96)*. These findings suggest that the susceptibility of patients with deficiencies in CD40L-mediated signaling to toxoplasmosis is caused by the lack of IL-12 and may also explain the susceptibility of these patients to other intracellular opportunistic pathogens *(33)*.

Other factors that are important in T-cell activation include the costimulatory molecule CD28, which is expressed by T-cells, and its ligands B7-1 and B7-2, which are expressed on accessory cells. The interaction of CD28 with B7 provides a second signal that regulates the ability of T-cells to produce cytokines, proliferate, and protect against apoptosis. Infection with *T. gondii* leads to increased expression of B7 by infected cells in vitro *(97,98)*, and uninfected and infected cells isolated from the local sites of infection in mice express increased levels of B7 *(56,57,99)*. In vitro studies using human and mouse cells have demonstrated that the B7/CD28 interaction is required for optimal production of IFN-γ by parasite-specific T-cells *(98,100)*. However, in vivo studies using CD28 knockout mice have shown that these mice develop a T-cell response that is sufficient to protect against infection with *T. gondii*, but CD28 is required for the generation or maintenance of optimal numbers of parasite specific CD4+ T-cells. As a consequence, chronically infected or immunized CD28 knockout mice are susceptible to a secondary challenge with a virulent strain of *T. gondii*, demonstrating an important role for CD28 in the generation/maintenance of a memory response *(100)*.

4.3. Immune Response to T. gondii in the Gut

Many of the above-described studies have used mice that were infected intraperitoneally. Although this allows the analysis of the early events in a localized environment, the natural route of infection with *T. gondii* is oral, and the gut is the initial site of entry for the parasite. This environment has unique populations of T-cells and accessory cells that sample and present antigens from the gut, and there may be fundamental differences in the immune response in the gut versus that in the peritoneum. Nevertheless, the local events that occur in the gut following infection have not been extensively studied, but recent studies have started to address the effects associated with resistance or pathology induced after infection with *T. gondii* in the gut. It is known that within 24 h following oral infection, parasites are found in the mesenteric lymph nodes and dissemination from the gut to other organs via blood or lymphatics starts about 24 h later. By d 4 postinfection, parasites have disseminated through the body and are present in the liver and lungs. The local response induced by the parasite involves both humoral and cellular mechanisms. IgA antibodies can be detected in intestinal fluids 3–4 wk following infection and studies using *Toxoplasma*-specific secretory IgA antibodies suggested that these antibodies may be important in preventing infection of enterocytes by *T. gondii* *(101)*. Infection also results in the expansion of intraepithelial CD8+ T-cells that are cytotoxic for infected cells and produce IFN-γ when stimulated with parasite antigen in vitro *(102)*. Furthermore, adoptive transfer experiments revealed that the transfer of intraepithelial lymphocytes (IELs) from orally infected mice into naive mice provides enhanced resistance against oral infection *(103,104)*, demonstrating the role for IELs as a primary barrier against infection with *T. gondii*.

Most of the studies described so far have focused on the role of CD4+ and CD8+ cells that express αβ T-cell receptor chains, but there are also populations of γδ T-cells that are enriched at mucosal sites, including the gut, and that are involved in resistance to *T. gondii*. Although normal αβ T-cells express T-cell-receptor chains, which are highly variable, γδ T-cells express a more limited repertoire of T-cell-receptor chains and it has been proposed that these cells recognize a narrow range of antigens presented in the context of CD1 *(105–107)*. As a consequence, these cells may represent an evolutionary bridge between the innate and adaptive responses. A role for γδ T-cells after infection with *T. gondii* is indicated by studies in which mice deficient in αβ T-cells and challenged with the parasite had a mechanism of resistance that was dependent on γδ T-cells *(108)*. In humans, the stimulation of PBMCs from naive individuals with *T. gondii* results in an expansion of γδ T-cells *(109)*, and during the acute stage of toxoplasmosis, there is a marked expansion of this T-cell subpopulation

(110,111). Because γδ T-cells are enriched in the gut, their ability to lyse infected cells and produce IFN-γ in response to *T. gondii* may provide an explanation for their role in resistance to *T. gondii* *(108,109,112)*. The events that lead to activation and expansion of γδ T-cells following infection have not been well defined, but it has been shown that γδ T-cells can induce macrophages to express heat-shock proteins (HSPs) through their ability to produce IFN-γ and this is associated with a protective role for these cells during toxoplasmosis *(113)*.

4.4. IFN-γ-Mediated Effector Mechanisms to Control T. gondii

The ability of macrophages to produce cytokines, present antigens and provide costimulatory signals is important in resistance to *T. gondii*, but in addition to their regulatory functions, macrophages are also important effector cells. When activated by IFN-γ plus TNF-α, macrophages are able to inhibit parasite replication *(114,115)*. Although parasite killing in mouse macrophages is nitric oxide (NO)-mediated *(116)*, the ability of human macrophages to control parasite replication is NO independent *(117)*. The mechanisms whereby NO inhibits parasite replication are uncertain, but NO is able to react with various reactive groups in proteins, including thiols, heme groups, iron–sulfur clusters, and phenolic and aromatic amino acid residues that would affect important metabolic pathways. In addition, NO can damage DNA and it is associated with membrane damage and inhibition of cellular proliferation (for review, *see* ref. *118*). However, NO is not only antimicrobial but also contributes to the immune suppression observed during the acute phase of toxoplasmosis. Thus, the high levels of NO produced during the acute phase of infection are partly responsible for the reduced proliferative responses observed in these mice and may be a function of the ability of NO to promote apoptosis through upregulation of p53, activation of caspases, chromatin condensation, and DNA fragmentation *(119–124)*.

Although NO is an important molecule for the ability of mouse macrophages to control parasite replication in vitro, it appears that NO has a relatively minor role in resistance during the acute phase of toxoplasmosis. Mice deficient in inducible nitric oxide synthase (iNOS) survive the acute phase, but succumb to the parasite during the chronic phase of infection *(89,125,126)*. Death of these mice is accompanied by enhanced parasite replication in the brain associated with severe necrotizing encephalitis *(89)*. Taken together with previous studies that have shown that IFN-γ is critical during the acute and chronic stages of infection, these findings indicate the presence of an IFN-γ-dependent iNOS-independent mechanism of resistance that is sufficient to control parasite replication in the periphery. Although this novel mechanism has not yet been identified, recent studies with mice deficient in either IFN-γ-induced GTPase (IGTP) or LRG-47, both members of a family of IFN-γ-regulated genes, have started to provide an insight into the IFN-γ-dependent mechanisms that control parasite replication during the acute stage of infection. Thus, although IGTP and LRG-47 are not required for the production of IL-12, IFN-γ, or NO during infection, in their absence, mice are unable to control parasite replication *(127,128)*. These studies indicate that the protective effects of IFN-γ during the acute phase of disease are mediated through IGTP and LRG-47 and inhibition of parasite replication appears to be NO-independent. Because both of these proteins localize predominantly to the endoplasmic reticulum (ER), the authors hypothesize that IGTP and LRG-47 may regulate vesicular transport within the macrophage, including the transport of IFN-γ-induced toxic mediators to the parasitophorous vacuole.

As mentioned earlier, the ability of human macrophages to control parasite replication is NO independent, but in vitro studies have shown that treatment of human macrophages with exogenous leukotriene B4 (LTB4) induces intracellular killing of *T. gondii*, suggesting a toxoplasmacidal activity for leukotrienes *(129)*. However, the parasite is able to suppress the release of leukotrienes, but this effect is reversed when macrophages are incubated with IFN-γ, supporting the important role of IFN-γ in mediating the toxoplasmacidal activity of macrophages. Although IFN-γ stimulates production of NO and leukotrienes, it also induces tryptophan degradation in human macrophages and fibroblasts *(130,131)*. Tryptophan degradation has been described as an inhibitory factor on parasite replication *(130,131)*, but, so far, its effect has been shown in vitro only and the relevance of this mechanism to the control of *T. gondii* in vivo remains unclear. Similarly, in vitro studies have shown that iron starvation is important in the ability of enterocytes to control the replication of *T. gondii* *(132)*. Together, these studies demonstrate the presence of a variety of antimicrobial effector mechanisms in human and murine systems that inhibit replication of *T. gondii*, and it is important to understand how these mechanisms integrate to control this organism in the different sites that it can affect.

4.5. Pathogenesis of Toxoplasmic Encephalitis

The previous subsections dealt with some of the cytokines involved in the development of parasite-specific T-cell responses necessary for resistance to *T. gondii*. However, because of the persistent nature of this infection, immunity has to be maintained in order to control reactivation of the parasite. This is complicated by the presence of parasites in immune-privileged sites, in particular the brain and the eye. Systemic disease can also occur at other sites, such as the lungs, gut, and heart, and is normally correlated with uncontrolled replication of *T. gondii*, which results in necrosis in the affected tissue. However, in immunocompromised patients who are chronically infected with *T. gondii*, reactivation of infection is frequently manifested by the development of TE. The presence of the blood-brain barrier, the lack of a lymphatic system, low levels of MHC expression, and the ability of glial cells to suppress T-cell responses all contribute to the immune-privileged status of the brain *(133–135)*. Whether this lack of immune reactivity contributes to the persistence of the cyst stage of *T. gondii* at this site or ensures that the effects of reactivation will be more severe than at other sites in the periphery is uncertain. Nevertheless, it is clear that T-cells play an important role in controlling reactivation of disease, as demonstrated by the close correlation of the loss of T-cells during AIDS and the development of TE in these patients. The fact that TE does not develop in chronically infected immune-competent individuals implies that although T-cells have limited access to the brain, they are able to control chronic infection with *T. gondii*. In experimental models, CD4+ and CD8+ T-cells have been shown to infiltrate the brain after infection with this parasite *(136,137)* and many studies have demonstrated that production of IFN-γ by CD4+ and CD8+ T-cells is required to maintain resistance to *T. gondii* in the brain *(80,82)*. In addition to their ability to produce IFN-γ, the ability of CD8+ T-cells to lyse parasite-infected cells *(138,139)* may contribute to the control of parasite replication in the brain. The importance of this pathway in vivo has been shown by studies in which infection of mice that lack perforin-dependent cytolytic activity leads to increased susceptibility of mice to the chronic stage of infection *(140)*. However, it is thought that the main protective effects of CD4+ and CD8+ T-cells in the brain are the result of their ability to produce IFN-γ. Thus, in chronically infected mice, depletion of CD4+ and CD8+ T-cells results in reactivation of disease and the development of severe TE *(80,82)*. Moreover, depletion of endogenous IFN-γ during chronic infection results in reactivation of toxoplasmosis and early mortality of mice *(80,141)*, whereas administration of IFN-γ reduces tachyzoites proliferation and decreases inflammation in murine brains *(142)*. The idea that lymphocytes are the only source of IFN-γ in the brain during TE has recently been challenged. In studies using IFN-γ knockout mice treated with sulfadiazine to allow the mice to progress to the chronic stage of infection, immune cells from wild-type mice were unable to provide protection *(143)*. Based on these data, it has been proposed that a non-T-cell source of IFN-γ, perhaps macrophage, astrocyte, or dendritic cell, may be necessary for the ability of T-cells to protect against TE.

Although the presence of T-cells in the brain is important for resistance to *T. gondii*, it is important to recognize that there is a balance between protective immunity in the brain and the development of immunopathology. This is illustrated by the original observation of Israelski et al., who demonstrated that depletion of CD4+ T-cells decreases the severity of TE *(144)*. Similarly, chronically infected CD28 knockout mice have decreased numbers of CD4+ T-cells in their brains compared with wild-type mice and, as a consequence, have less severe inflammation and are more resistant to the pathological consequences of TE than wild-type mice *(99)*. Thus, CD4+ T-cells appear to have a dual role during chronic infection: While mediating resistance to *T. gondii*, they also contribute to immunopathology in the brain.

The unique nature of the protective T-cell response in the brain is illustrated by comparing the factors that regulate T-cell production of IFN-γ in the periphery versus the brain. Analysis of the peripheral T-cell responses have shown that IL-12 is required to initiate the protective Th1-type response. Furthermore, stimulation through CD28 is required for optimal CD4$^+$ T-cell production of IL-2, which is essential for the ability of CD8$^+$ T-cells to make IFN-γ *(100)*. In contrast, the ability of T-cells isolated from the brains of mice with TE to produce IFN-γ is largely independent of IL-2, IL-12, or CD28 signaling *(99)*. These findings indicate that the protective T-cell responses in the brain are not regulated in a conventional manner and raises the question about the cytokines and costimulatory factors that regulate protective T-cell responses in the brain and whether they are unique to this immune privileged site.

Initial studies on the role of IL-12 in resistance to *T. gondii* demonstrated that this cytokine was only required during the first few days of infection *(43,48)*. However, these conclusions have had to be reassessed and there is now evidence that IL-12 is also required for the maintenance of protective T-cell responses *(42)*. In those studies, IL-12 p40 knockout mice treated with recombinant IL-12 during the first 2 wk postinfection develop Th1-type responses and survive the infection. However, 4–6 wk after cessation of IL-12 treatment, these mice develop severe TE associated with a decrease in IFN-γ mRNA expression in the brain. Splenocytes from these mice stimulated with parasite antigens have a marked reduction in their ability to produce IFN-γ, but when stimulated with STAg (soluble *Toxoplasma* antigen) and IL-12, these cells are able to produce increased levels of IFN-γ *(42)*. There are several interpretations of these data and Yap and colleagues proposed that terminally differentiated T-cells that are recruited from lymphoid organs into the brain are unable to produce IFN-γ when generated in the absence of IL-12. If this is correct, it implies that parasite specific T-cells need to be continually generated to maintain immunity to *T. gondii*. Alternatively, because IL-12 has recently been shown to decrease activation-induced cell death *(145)*, it is possible that it plays a role in the maintenance of memory cells.

In addition to T-cells that infiltrate into the brain during TE, resident glial cells are also likely to be important in controlling TE. For example, both astrocytes and the resident macrophages (microglia) show signs of activation during TE in humans and murine models *(146–150)*. Both cell types produce proinflammatory cytokines when stimulated with *T. gondii* in vitro *(151)* and Schlüter and colleagues *(152)* demonstrated that microglial expression of MHC class II molecules is increased during TE and this upregulation is probably mediated by IFN-γ. Similarly, it has recently been recognized that during TE, there are populations of myeloid DCs in the brain that produce IL-12 and that may contribute to the regulation of the immune response in this immunoprivileged site *(153)*. In addition to regulatory roles, murine and human microglia are able to inhibit parasite replication when activated with IFN-γ and TNF-α *(154–156)*. Although parasite killing in murine microglia is NO mediated, human microglia do not express iNOS and their ability to inhibit parasite replication is independent of NO *(154,155)*. In contrast, human astrocytes affect parasite replication through production of NO *(157)*, whereas murine astrocytes inhibit parasite replication independently of NO and tryptophan degradation *(158)*. Recent studies indicate that this is dependent on IGTP *(159)*, consistent with data that IFN-γ stimulates NO-independent mechanisms of resistance in nonhemopoietic cells in the brain *(160)*.

As mentioned earlier, the use of iNOS knockout mice showed that the production of NO is not required for acute resistance to *T. gondii*, but it is essential to control parasite replication in the brain *(89)*. This is likely a reflection of the role of resident microglia or infiltrating macrophages that can produce NO and so inhibit tachyzoite replication. Studies using bone marrow chimeric mice showed that long-term resistance to *T. gondii* requires expression of the IFN-γ and TNF-α receptors on both hemopoietic and nonhemopoietic cells, whereas expression of iNOS is only critical in hemopoietic cells, and production of NO by nonhemopoietic cells plays little if any role in resistance to *T. gondii* *(160)*. In order to fully activate macrophages to produce NO, IFN-γ requires TNF-α as a second signal *(114,115,161,162)*; however, recent studies using TNF-receptor knockout mice revealed that iNOS activation in macrophages can occur independently of TNF-α-receptor signaling *(163)*. To explain these findings, Yap and colleagues suggested that the parasite itself may provide signals that activate iNOS *(163)*, but other stimuli such as the CD40/CD40L interaction could be involved, because this pathway synergizes with IFN-γ to stimulate macrophages to produce NO and may contribute to the control of parasite replication in the brain *(95)*.

Although the protective immune response to *T. gondii* is dominated by a Th1-type response, several studies have suggested a regulatory role for IL-4, IL-6, and IL-10, cytokines associated with Th2 type responses, in optimal resistance to *T. gondii*. Early studies demonstrated that levels of IL-4 mRNA are upregulated in the brains of mice following infection *(147)* and the presence of gene transcripts in mice with progressive TE suggests a role for IL-4 during chronic infection. Indeed, IL-4-deficient mice survive the acute phase of infection, but succumb during chronic toxoplasmosis *(164)*. In the absence of IL-4, production of IFN-γ is impaired, which subsequently leads to greater numbers of tachyzoites in the brain of these mice *(164)*. These data suggest that IL-4 is involved in preventing the development of TE. In contrast to these reports are studies that suggest a role for IL-4 during acute infection *(165)*. Splenocytes from IL-4-deficient mice show enhanced production of IFN-γ when stimulated ex vivo 7 d postinfection *(165)*. However, the group also reports enhanced mortality in these mice, although cysts numbers and pathology in the brain are decreased *(165)*.

Another cytokine associated with resistance to TE is IL-6. In vitro, IL-6 has been shown to enhance parasite proliferation in macrophages and it antagonizes the IFN-γ-mediated toxoplasmacidal activity in these cells *(166)*. However, in vivo studies support a role for IL-6 in preventing the development of TE. IL-6 mRNA is expressed in brains of mice infected with *T. gondii (55,167,168)*, and IL-6 can be detected in the cerebrospinal fluid following infection *(167)*. Administration of anti-IL-6 antibodies during the chronic phase of infection has been shown to decrease cyst numbers and elevate serum levels of IFN-γ *(169)*. However, because treatment with anti-IL-6 paradoxically enhances IL-6 serum levels, the effects seen after administration of anti-IL-6 might be the result of increased levels of IL-6 rather than the lack of this cytokine. This would suggest a protective role for IL-6 in the response to *T. gondii* and studies using IL-6-deficient mice support these findings. Thus, infection of IL-6 knockout mice with *T. gondii* leads to decreased production of IFN-γ associated with increased cyst numbers and severe inflammation in the brain *(170,171)*. Furthermore, IL-6-deficient mice have lower percentages of CD4$^+$ T-cells and higher percentages of CD8$^+$ T-cells compared to wild-type mice *(170)*, suggesting that IL-6 affects the composition of the T-cell subpopulations in the brain. Together, these data support a role for this cytokine in controlling the development of TE, but these data need to be interpreted with care, as the IL-6 knockout mice have a defect in their neutrophil responses *(172)* and several studies have linked neutrophil function with resistance to *T. gondii* *(45,67,173)*.

Although IL-10 is an antagonist of the innate response during acute infection with *T. gondii*, it also appears to contribute to development of TE during chronic toxoplasmosis. Thus, neutralization of IL-10 in chronically infected mice results in a decreased parasite burden *(174)*. These data are supported by studies comparing the role of IL-10 during chronic toxoplasmosis in genetically susceptible and resistant mice. C57BL/6 mice that are susceptible to the development of TE express increased levels of IL-10 mRNA in their brains during the late stage of infection *(168)*, whereas resistant BALB/c mice fail to express this cytokine in the brain *(175)*. These findings suggest that intracerebral expression of IL-10 by microglia, macrophages, and T-cells interferes with the immune response to *T. gondii*. The ability of IL-10 to antagonize accessory cell functions required for T-cell production of IFN-γ *(176,177)* and its inhibitory effect on macrophage production of NO required to control replication of *T. gondii (178)* suggest a mechanism whereby the local production of IL-10 promotes parasite replication in the brain.

Although we understand the role of many of the cytokines involved in resistance to TE, there are other factors associated with increased susceptibility to TE, including the genetic background of the host. In murine models, there is a genetic basis for susceptibility to TE and the MHC class I gene *Ld* has been shown to confer resistance against TE, indicating the important role of class I-restricted CD8[+] T-cell responses *(179)*. Of interest are studies that provided evidence that additional non-MHC-linked genes also play a role in the pathogenesis of TE *(180)*. Similarly, there appears to be a genetic predisposition to the development of TE in patients with AIDS, associated with a gene or genes in the human leukocyte antigen (HLA) complex *(181)*.

4.6. Role of B-Cells During Infection with T. gondii

The development of cell-mediated immunity induced by *T. gondii* is accompanied by the production of high levels of anti-*Toxoplasma* antibodies. Traditionally, the humoral immune response was thought to play a subordinate role during toxoplasmosis because, as an intracellular parasite, *T. gondii* is relatively inaccessible to antibodies, and initial studies showed that the transfer of serum from infected animals failed to protect mice after challenge with a virulent strain of the parasite *(182)*. However, other studies have demonstrated that treatment of mice with anti-*Toxoplasma* antibodies before infection leads to enhanced resistance *(183,184)*. Studies by Taylor and Frenkel examined the effects of B-cell depletion on infection with *T. gondii*, suggesting that antibodies have little effects during acute infection but may become important during the chronic phase of infection *(185)*. Recently, these data were confirmed by Kang and colleagues, who showed that B-cells are required for long-term resistance to *T. gondii (186)*. Following infection, B-cell-deficient (μMT) mice survive the acute phase but develop severe TE associated with increased numbers of cysts. However, μMT mice that receive anti-*Toxoplasma* IgG antibodies after infection survive infection and have significantly lower cyst numbers and fewer areas of inflammation associated with tachyzoites in the brain *(186)*, suggesting a direct role for antibodies in resistance to *T. gondii*.

There are several possible explanations for the role of antibodies in resistance to *T. gondii*. It has long been recognized that when opsonized with specific *Toxoplasma* antibodies, tachyzoites are actively phagocytosed and killed by macrophages *(187,188)*. Moreover, opsonization can induce complement activation and lead to killing of *T. gondii (189)*. Other studies have shown that serum derived from wild-type mice that were vaccinated with *T. gondii* inhibited the ability of tachyzoites to infect cultured fibroblasts, whereas serum derived from vaccinated μMT mice did not affect invasion. This suggests a direct effect of anti-*Toxoplasma* antibodies in blocking the ability of tachyzoites to infect host cells *(190)*. An alternative explanation for the protective effects of antibodies is provided by the studies of Shimada and colleagues *(191)*, which showed that anti-*Toxoplasma* antibodies induce the switch from tachyzoites to bradyzoites in vitro.

In addition to antibody production, B-cells also present antigen, provide costimulation for T-cells, and Denkers and colleagues have suggested a role for B-cells in the production of protective IL-12 during the chronic phase of toxoplasmosis *(192)*. After infection with *T. gondii*, splenocytes from IL-5 knockout mice showed decreased B-cell numbers in culture when stimulated with STAg. Because the loss of B-cells correlated with a reduced production of IL-12, these researchers suggested that B-cells could be directly involved in the production of IL-12 or they might affect IL-12 levels indirectly either by inducing the expression of CD40L on T-cells *(193)* or by expressing CD40L themselves *(194,195)*.

4.7. Regulation of Immunopathology

Although the studies in the previous subsections illustrate the importance of a strong cell-mediated immune response for resistance to *T. gondii*, it needs to be recognized that this protective response can lead to severe immunopathology. As a consequence, certain cytokines are important in the balance between protective and pathological responses. Probably the best example is provided by the role of IL-10 during toxoplasmosis. IL-10 inhibits accessory cell functions of macrophages by downregulating the production of IL-12, IL-1, and TNF-α, cytokines that are required for optimal stimulation of IFN-γ production by T-cells and NK cells. The suppressive effects of IL-10 are necessary to prevent immune hyperactivity, as shown by studies with IL-10 knockout mice. The lack of IL-

10 during acute toxoplasmosis results in the systemic overproduction of proinflammatory cytokines and a lethal immune-mediated pathology *(66,196)*. However, treatment of infected IL-10 knockout mice with monoclonal antibodies against IL-12 or IFN-γ leads to a delay in time to death *(66)*, demonstrating the important role of IL-10 in balancing the production of cytokines in the host. Studies by Gazzinelli and colleagues *(196)* revealed that the lethal immune hyperactivity in IL-10 knockout mice is mediated by CD4+ T-cells, because in vivo depletion of CD4+ T-cells protected these mice from parasite-induced mortality. As discussed earlier, costimulation is normally associated with protection, but in the absence of IL-10, both the B7/CD28 and CD40/CD40L interactions contribute to the development of immunopathology. Simultaneous blockade of CD28/B7 and CD40/CD40L signaling in IL-10 knockout mice decreases the production of IFN-γ and expression of iNOS in the liver and spleen *(57)*, which prevents the lethal shocklike reaction normally observed in these mice. However, although IL-10 has been shown to reduce macrophage expression of MHC class II, CD40, B7.1, and B7.2 *(197–201)*, it does not regulate expression of these molecules during acute toxoplasmosis *(56,57,202)*.

The local events induced by *T. gondii* in the gut can also result in severe pathology, depending on the genetic background of the mice. Thus, infection of C57BL/6 mice (H-2b haplotype) can lead to a lethal immune-induced pathology in the gut mediated by CD4+ T-cells and IFN-γ *(203)*. Similar to studies described above with the IL-10 knockout mice, blockade of costimulation through CD44 (which enhances CD4+ T-cell production of IFN-γ) reduces the development of pathology in the gut associated with decreased production of IFN-γ *(204)*. Moreover, IFN-γ induces Fas-mediated apoptosis of CD4+ and CD8+ T-cells in Peyer's patches of C57BL/6 mice, which results in a significant decrease of both T-cell subsets in the ileum of the mice *(205)*, and NO has been shown to enhance the development of necrosis in the gut associated with this inflammatory response *(206)*. In contrast to susceptible C57BL/6 mice, most other strains of mice, including BALB/c (H-2d haplotype) mice, fail to develop pathology in the gut following infection with *T. gondii (203)*. Two recent studies have helped to understand how these mice prevent the development of immune pathology in the gut. Buzoni-Gatel et al. demonstrated that the ability of IELs to produce TGF-β prevents the development of pathology, and the protective effect of TGF-β could be the result of its ability to inhibit production of IFN-γ and NO *(207)*. Similarly, in the absence of IL-10, BALB/c mice develop a lethal intestinal pathology similar to that seen in C57BL/6 mice *(208)*. Similar results are described in studies with IL-10 knockout mice that are prone to developing spontaneous enterocolitis. The pathology in these mice is associated with increased production of proinflammatory cytokines by macrophages and CD4+ T-cells when stimulated with Th1-dependent antigens *(209,210)*. Thus, through its ability to decrease production of IFN-γ, IL-10 is an important regulator of immune pathology and this regulatory role is independent of the genetic background of the mice. Together, these studies indicate that, during infection, the production of inflammatory cytokines is balanced by the production of regulatory cytokines such as IL-10 and TGF-β. Both cytokines have suppressive effects on accessory cell functions required for stimulation of cell-mediated immunity after infection with *T. gondii*. However, IL-10 and TGF-β play a critical role in allowing the development of protective responses while minimizing the immune pathology that can accompany these strong cell-mediated responses.

5. CONCLUSIONS

In the last decade, there has been a tremendous growth in the availability of mice that lack various immune molecules, which has allowed researchers to define the complex interactions that regulate the immune response to *T. gondii*. Some of the findings have been unexpected and highlighted new areas of research. For example, the events that lead to the generation of IL-12-independent IFN-γ responses or the identification of iNOS-independent mechanisms of resistance to *T. gondii* have defined new questions that are not just specific to toxoplasmosis but that provide important information on how cell-mediated immunity works. One of the challenges that now faces this field is to determine if this information can be used to promote resistance to *T. gondii* through the design of effective vaccines or by selectively augmenting the immune response in immunocompromised individuals at risk of developing clinical toxoplasmosis. Vaccine-induced immunity to *T. gondii* does wane with time, but it has been shown that exogenous IL-15 helps to maintain vaccine-induced protective CD8[+] T-cell responses *(211)*. Furthermore, a number of cytokines such as IFN-γ, IL-12, TNF-α, IL-1, and IL-2, which have been shown to enhance protective immunity in murine models, have been proposed for trials in patients with TE. For example, administration of IL-1, IL-2, or TNF-α to mice infected with *T. gondii* resulted in a lower number of cysts in the brain and a significant decrease in mortality of these mice *(161,212)*. However, there are many factors to consider before clinical use of these cytokines in immunotherapy, as the use of cytokines may depend on the type of patient to be treated. Thus, many of these cytokines have been reported to enhance replication of HIV *(213)* and may not be suitable for treatment of TE in patients with AIDS. In contrast, other stimuli such as IL-12, IFN-γ, and soluble CD40L have been shown to restore suppressed immune functions in AIDS patients and to have inhibitory effects on parasite replication *(36,48,142,213,214)*. Thus, they are strong candidates for immunotherapy. However, an effect on viral replication would not be a consideration in patients with other primary or acquired immune deficiencies, and many of these stimuli may be appropriate in the context of patients being treated with immune-suppressive therapies or with defects in the CD40/CD40L interaction. In addition, the combination of chemotherapy and immunotherapy can lead to efficient treatment regimes against TE. Administration of IL-12 together with clindamycin and atovaquone has been shown to potentiate the effects of these drugs *(215)*, and studies with IFN-γ and roxithromycin demonstrate a synergistic effect when used in combination *(216)*. Thus, an understanding of the parasite itself together with the immune mechanisms induced after infection represent opportunities to develop new approaches to manage clinical disease.

ACKNOWLEDGMENT

This work was supported by NIH grants AI 41158 and AI 42334.

REFERENCES

1. Nicolle, C. and Manceaux, L. (1908) Sur une infection a corps de Leishman (ou organismes voisins) du gondi. *C. R. Acad. Sci. (Paris)* **147**, 763–766.
2. Wolf, A., Cowen, D., and Paige, B.H. (1939) Human toxoplasmosis. (Occurence in infants as an encephalomyelitis. Verification by transmission to animals). *Science* **89**, 226–227.
3. Wong, S.Y. and Remington, J.S. (1994) Toxoplasmosis in pregnancy. *Clin. Infect. Dis.* **18**, 853–861.
4. Ruskin, J. and Remington, J.S. (1976) Toxoplasmosis in the compromised host. *Ann. Intern. Med.* **84**, 193–199.
5. Israelski, D.M. and Remington, J.S. (1993) Toxoplasmosis in patients with cancer. *Clin. Infect. Dis.* **Suppl 2**, S423–S435.
6. Britt, R.H., Enzmann, D.R., and Remington, J.S. (1981) Intracranial infection in cardiac transplant recipients. *Ann. Neurol.* **9**, 107–119.
7. Israelski, D.M. and Remington, J.S. (1988) Toxoplasmic encephalitis in patients with AIDS. *Infect. Dis. Clin. North. Am.* **2**, 429–445.
8. Slavin, M.A., Meyers, J.D., Remington, J.S., and Hackman, R.C. (1994) Toxoplasma gondii infection in marrow transplant recipients: a 20 year experience. *Bone Marrow Transplant* **13**, 549–557.
9. Weiss, L.M., Ma, Y.F., Takvorian, P.M., Tanowitz, H.B., and Wittner, M. (1998) Bradyzoite development in Toxoplasma gondii and the hsp70 stress response. *Infect. Immun.* **66**, 3295–3302.
10. Weiss, L.M. and Kim, K. (2000) The development and biology of bradyzoites of *Toxoplasma gondii*. *Front. Biosci.* **5**, D391–D405.
11. Bohne, W., Holpert, M., and Gross, U. (1999) Stage differentiation of the protozoan parasite *Toxoplasma gondii*. *Immunobiology* **201**, 248–254.
12. Bohne, W., Heesemann, J., and Gross, U. (1994) Reduced replication of *Toxoplasma gondii* is necessary for induction of bradyzoite-specific antigens: a possible role for nitric oxide in triggering stage conversion. *Infect. Immun.* **62**, 1761–1767.
13. Remington, J.S., Mc Leod, R., and Desmond, G. (1995) Toxoplasmosis, in *Infectious Diseases of the Fetus. Newborn Infant*, 4th ed. (Remington J.S. and Klein, J.O., eds.), W.B. Saunders, Philadelphia, pp. 140–267.
14. Frenkel, J.K., Amare, M., and Larsen, W. (1978) Immune competence in a patient with Hodgkin's disease and relapsing toxoplasmosis. *Infection* **6**, 84–91.

15. Hakes, T.B. and Armstrong, D. (1983) Toxoplasmosis. Problems in diagnosis and treatment. *Cancer* **52**, 1535–1540.
16. Yeo, J.H., Jakobiec, F.A., Iwamoto, T., Richard, G., and Kreissig, I. (1983) Opportunistic toxoplasmic retinochoroiditis following chemotherapy for systemic lymphoma. A light and electron microscopic study. *Ophthalmology* **90**, 885–898.
17. Vietzke, W.M., Gelderman, A.H., Grimley, P.M., and Valsamis, M.P. (1968) Toxoplasmosis complicating malignancy. Experience at the National Cancer Institute. *Cancer* **21**, 816–827.
18. Armstrong, D., Young, L.S., Meyer, R.D., and Blevins, A.H. (1971) Infectious complications of neoplastic disease. *Med. Clin. North. Am.* **55**, 729–745.
19. Carey, R.M., Kimball, A.C., Armstrong, D., and Lieberman, P.H. (1973) Toxoplasmosis. Clinical experiences in a cancer hospital. *Am. J. Med.* **54**, 30–38.
20. Luft, B.J. and Remington, J.S. (1992) Toxoplasmic encephalitis in AIDS. *Clin. Infect. Dis.* **15**, 211–222.
21. Crowe, S.M., Carlin, J.B., Stewart, K.I., Lucas, C.R., and Hoy, J.F. (1991) Predictive value of CD4 lymphocyte numbers for the development of opportunistic infections and malignancies in HIV-infected persons. *Acquired Immune Defic. Syndrome* **4**, 770–776.
22. Biggs, B.A., Hewish, M., Kent, S., Hayes, K., and Crowe, S.M. (1995) HIV-1 infection of human macrophages impairs phagocytosis and killing of *Toxoplasma gondii*. *J. Immunol.* **154**, 6132–6139.
23. Delamarre, F.G., Stevenhagen, A., Kroon, F.P., van Eer, M.Y., Meenhorst, P.L., and van Furth R. (1994) Effect of IFN-gamma on the proliferation of *Toxoplasma gondii* in monocytes and monocyte-derived macrophages from AIDS patients. *Immunology* **83**, 646–650.
24. Delamarre, F.G., Stevenhagen, A., Kroon, F.P., van Eer, M.Y., Meenhorst, P.L., and van Furth, R. (1995) Reduced toxoplasmastatic activity of monocytes and monocyte-derived macrophages from AIDS patients is mediated via prostaglandin E2. *AIDS* **9**, 441–445.
25. Perales, M.A., Skolnik, P. R., and Lieberman, J. (1996) Effect of interleukin 12 on in vitro HIV type 1 replication depends on clinical stage. *AIDS Res. Hum. Retroviruses* **12**, 659–668.
26. Poli, G., Kinter, A.L., and Fauci, A.S. (1994) Interleukin 1 induces expression of the human immunodeficiency virus alone and in synergy with interleukin 6 in chronically infected U1 cells: inhibition of inductive effects by the interleukin 1 receptor antagonist. *Proc. Natl. Acad. Sci. USA* **91**, 108–112.
27. Ito, M., Baba, M., Sato, A., Hirabayashi, K., Tanabe, F., Shigeta, S., and De Clercq, E. (1989) Tumor necrosis factor enhances replication of human immunodeficiency virus (HIV) in vitro. *Biochem. Biophys. Res. Commun.* **158**, 307–312.
28. Butera, S.T. (1993) Cytokine involvement in viral permissiveness and the progression of HIV disease. *J. Cell Biochem.* **53**, 336–342.
29. Valdez, H. and Lederman, M.M. (1997–1998) Cytokines and cytokine therapies in HIV infection. *AIDS Clin. Rev* 187–228.
30. Gazzinelli, R.T., Sher, A., Cheever, A., Gerstberger, S., Martin, M. A., and Dickie, P. (1996) Infection of human immunodeficiency virus 1 transgenic mice with *Toxoplasma gondii* stimulates proviral transcription in macrophages in vivo. *J. Exp. Med.* **183**, 1645–1655.
31. Subauste, C.S., Wessendarp, M., Sorensen, R.U., and Leiva, L.E. (1999) CD40-CD40 ligand interaction is central to cell-mediated immunity against *Toxoplasma gondii:* patients with hyper IgM syndrome have a defective type 1 immune response that can be restored by soluble CD40 ligand trimer. *J. Immunol.* **162**, 6690–6700.
32. Tsuge, I., Matsuoka, H., Nakagawa, A., Kamachi, Y., Aso, K., Negoro, T., et al. (1998) Necrotizing toxoplasmic encephalitis in a child with the X-linked hyper-IgM syndrome. *Eur. J. Pediatr.* **157**, 735–737.
33. Levy, J., Espanol-Boren, T., Thomas, C., Fischer, A., Tovo, P., Bordigoni, P., et al. (1997) Clinical spectrum of X linked hyper-IgM syndrome. *J. Pediatr.* **131**(1 Pt. 1), 47–54.
34. Leiva, L.E., Junprasert, J., Hollenbaugh, D., and Sorensen, R.U. (1998) Central nervous system toxoplasmosis with an increased proportion of circulating gamma delta T cells in a patient with hyper-IgM syndrome. *J. Clin. Immunol.* **18**, 283–290.
35. Vanham, G., Penne, L., Devalck, J., Kestens, L., Colebunders, R., Bosmans, E., et al. (1999) Decreased CD40 ligand induction in CD4 T cells and dysregulated IL-12 production during HIV infection. *Clin. Exp. Immunol.* **117**, 335–342.
36. Subauste, C.S., Wessendarp, M., Smulian, A.G., and Frame, P.T. (2001) Role of CD40 ligand signaling in defective type-1 cytokine responses in HIV infection. *J. Infect. Dis.* **185** Suppl 1: 583–589.
37. Behbahani, R., Moshfeghi, M., and Baxter, J.D. (1995) Therapeutic approaches for AIDS related toxoplasmosis. *Ann. Pharmacother* **29**, 760–768.
38. Desmonts, G. and Courvreur, J. (1974) Congenital toxoplasmosis: a prospective study of 378 pregnancies. *N. Engl. J. Med.* **290**, 1110–1116.
39. Black, C.M., Catterall, J.R., and Remington, J.S. (1987) In vivo and in vitro activation of alveolar macrophages by recombinant interferon-γ. *J. Immunol.* **138**, 491–495.
40. McCabe, R.E., Luft, B.J., and Remington, J.S. (1984) Effect of murine interferon gamma on murine toxoplasmosis. *J. Infect. Dis.* **150**, 961–962.
41. Suzuki, Y., Orellana, M.A., Schreiber, R.D., and Remington, J.S. (1988) Interferon gamma: the major mediator of resistance against *Toxoplasma gondii*. *Science* **240**, 516–518.
42. Yap, G., Pesin, M., and Sher, A. (2000) Cutting edge: IL-12 is required for the maintenance of IFN-γ production in T cells mediating chronic resistance to the intracellular pathogen, *Toxoplasma gondii*. *J. Immunol.* **165**, 628–631.
43. Khan, I.A., Matsuura, T., and Kasper, L.H. (1994) Interleukin-12 enhances murine survival against acute toxoplasmosis. *Infect. Immun.* **62**, 1639–1642.
44. Gazzinelli, R.T., Wysocka, M., Hayashi, S., Denkers, E.Y., Hieny, S., Caspar, P., et al. (1994) Parasite-induced IL-12 stimulates early IFN-gamma synthesis and resistance during acute infection with *Toxoplasma gondii*. *J. Immunol.* **153**, 2533–2543.

45. Bliss, S.K., Zhang, Y., and Denkers, E.Y. (1999) Murine neutrophil stimulation by *Toxoplasma gondii* antigen drives high level production of IFN-gamma-independent IL-12. *J. Immunol.* **163,** 2081–2088.
46. Reis e Sousa, C., Yap, G., Schulz, O., Rogers, N., Schito, M., Aliberti, J., et al. (1999) Paralysis of dendritic cell IL-12 production by microbial products prevents infection-induced immunopathology. *Immunity* **11,** 637–647.
47. Sousa, C.R., Hieny, S., Scharton-Kersten, T., Jankovic, D., Charest, H., Germain, R.N., et al. (1997) In vivo microbial stimulation induces rapid CD40 ligand-independent production of interleukin 12 by dendritic cells and their redistribution to T cell areas. *J. Exp. Med.* **186,** 1819–1829.
48. Gazzinelli, R.T., Hieny, S., Wynn, T.A., Wolf, S., and Sher, A. (1993) Interleukin 12 is required for the T-lymphocyte-independent induction of interferon gamma by an intracellular parasite and induces resistance in T-cell-deficient hosts. *Proc. Natl. Acad. Sci. USA* **90,** 6115–6119.
49. Hunter, C.A., Subauste, C.S., Van Cleave, V.H., and Remington, J.S. (1994) Production of gamma interferon by natural killer cells from *Toxoplasma gondii*-infected SCID mice: regulation by interleukin-10, interleukin-12, and tumor necrosis factor alpha. *Infect. Immun.* **62,** 2818–2824.
50. Sher, A., Oswald, I.P., Hieny, S., and Gazzinelli, R.T. (1993) *Toxoplasma gondii* induces a T-independent IFN-gamma response in natural killer cells that requires both adherent accessory cells and tumor necrosis factor-alpha. *J. Immunol.* **150,** 3982–3989.
51. Hunter, C.A., Chizzonite, R., and Remington, J.S. (1995) Interleukin-1β is required for the ability of IL-12 to induce production of IFN-γ by NK cells: a role for IL-1β in the T cell independent mechanism of resistance against intracellular pathogens. *J. Immunol.* **155,** 4347–4354.
52. Hunter, C.A., Ellis-Neyer, L., Gabriel, K.E., Kennedy, M.K., Grabstein, K.H., Linsley, P.S., et al. (1997) The role of the CD28/B7 interaction in the regulation of NK cell responses during infection with *Toxoplasma gondii*. *J. Immunol.* **158,** 2285–2293.
53. Cai, G., Kastelein, R., and Hunter, C.A. (2000) Interleukin-18 (IL-18) enhances innate IL 12-mediated resistance to *Toxoplasma gondii*. *Infect. Immun.* **68,** 6932–6938.
54. Gazzinelli, R.T., Amichay, D., Scharton-Kersten, T., Grunwald, E., Farber, J.M., and Sher, A. (1996) Role of macrophage-derived cytokines in the induction and regulation of cell mediated immunity to *Toxoplasma gondii*. *Curr. Topics Microbiol. Immunol.* **219,** 127–139.
55. Hunter, C.A., Abrams, J.S., Beaman, M.H., and Remington J.S. (1993) Cytokine mRNA in the central nervous system of SCID mice infected with *Toxoplasma gondii:* importance of T cell-independent regulation of resistance to *T. gondii*. *Infect. Immun.* **61,** 4038–4044.
56. Wille, U., Villegas, E.N., Striepen, B., Roos, D.S., and Hunter, C.A. (2001) Interleukin 10 does not contribute to the pathogenesis of a virulent strain of *Toxoplasma gondii*. *Parasite Immunol.* **23,** 291–296.
57. Villegas, E.N., Wille, U., Craig, L., Linsley, P.S., Rennick, D.M., Peach, R., et al. (2000) Blockade of costimulation prevents infection-induced immunopathology in interleukin-10-deficient mice. *Infect. Immun.* **68,** 2837–2844.
58. Subauste, C.S. and Wessendarp, M. (2000) Human dendritic cells discriminate between viable and killed *Toxoplasma gondii* tachyzoites: dendritic cell activation after infection with viable parasites results in CD28 and CD40 ligand signaling that controls IL-12-dependent and independent T cell production of IFN-gamma. *J. Immunol.* **165,** 1498–1505.
59. Hunter, C.A., Bermudez, L., Beernink, H., Waegell, W., and Remington, J.S. (1995) Transforming growth factor-β inhibits interleukin-12-induced production of interferon-γ by natural killer cells: a role for transforming growth factor-β in the regulation of T-cell independent resistance to *Toxoplasma gondii*. *Eur. J. Immunol.* **25,** 994–1000.
60. Hauser, W.E.J. and Tsai, W. (1986) Acute *toxoplasma* infection of mice induces spleen NK cells that are cytotoxic for *T. gondii* in vitro. *J. Immunol.* **136,** 313–319.
61. Subauste, C.S., Dawson, L., and Remington, J.S. (1992) Human lymphokine-activated killer cells are cytotoxic against cells infected with *Toxoplasma gondii*. *J. Exp. Med.* **176,** 1511–1519.
62. Bellone, G., Aste-Amezaga, M., Trinchieri, G., and Rodeck, U. (1995) Regulation of NK cell functions by TGF-beta 1. *J. Immunol.* **155,** 1066–1073.
63. Bermudez, L.E., Covaro, G., and Remington, J. (1993) Infection of murine macrophages with *Toxoplasma gondii* is associated with release of transforming growth factor beta and downregulation of expression of tumor necrosis factor receptors. *Infect. Immun.* **61,** 4126–4130.
64. D'Andrea, A., Aste-Amezaga, M., Valiante, N.M., Ma, X., Kubin, M., and Trinchieri, G. (1993) Interleukin 10 (IL-10) inhibits human lymphocyte interferon gamma-production by suppressing natural killer cell stimulatory factor/IL-12 synthesis in accessory cells. *J. Exp. Med.* **178,** 1041–1048.
65. Tripp, C.S., Wolf, S.F., and Unanue, E.R. (1993) Interleukin 12 and tumor necrosis factor alpha are costimulators of interferon gamma production by natural killer cells in severe combined immunodeficiency mice with listeriosis, and interleukin 10 is a physiologic antagonist. *Proc. Natl. Acad. Sci. USA* **90,** 3725–3729.
66. Ellis-Neyer, L., Grunig, G., Fort, M., Remington, J.S., Rennick, D., and Hunter, C.A. (1997) Role of IL-10 in regulation of T-cell-dependent and T-cell-independent mechanism of resistance. *Infect. Immun.* **65,** 1675–1682.
67. Bliss, S.K., Butcher, B. A., and Denkers, E. Y. (2000) Rapid recruitment of neutrophils containing prestored IL-12 during microbial infection. *J. Immunol.* **165,** 4515–4521.
68. Kaisho, T., and Akira, S. (2000) Critical roles of Toll-like receptors in host defense. *Crit. Rev. Immunol.* **20,** 393–405.
69. Means, T.K., Golenbock, D.T., and Fenton, M.J. (2000) Structure and function of Toll-like receptor proteins. *Life Sci.* **68,** 241–258.
70. Medzhitov, R. and Janeway, C. Jr. (2000) The Toll receptor family and microbial recognition. *Trends Microbiol.* **8,** 452–456.
71. Campos, M.A., Almeida, I.C., Takeuchi, O., Akira, S., Valente, E.P., Procopio, D.O., et al. (2001) Activation of toll like receptor-2 by glycosylphosphatidylinositol anchors from a protozoan parasite. *J. Immunol.* **167,** 416–423.

72. Matzinger, P. (1998) An innate sense of danger. *Semin. Immunol.* **10**, 399–415.
73. Bliss, S.K., Marshall, A.J., Zhang, Y., Denkers, E.Y. (1999) Human polymorphonuclear leukocytes produce IL-12, TNF-alpha, and the chemokines macrophage-inflammatory protein-1 alpha and -1 beta in response to *Toxoplasma gondii* antigens. *J. Immunol.* **162**, 7369–7375.
74. Denney, C.F., Eckmann, L., and Reed, S.L. (1999) Chemokine secretion of human cells in response to *Toxoplasma gondii* infection. *Infect. Immun.* **67**, 1547–1552.
75. Blader, I.J., Manger, I.D., and Boothroyd, J.C. (2001) Microarray analysis reveals previously unknown changes in *Toxoplasma gondii*-infected human cells. *J. Biol. Chem.* **276**, 24223–24231.
76. Aliberti, J., Reis e Sousa, C., Schito, M., Hieny, S., Wells, T., Huffnagle, G. B., et al. (2000) CCR5 provides a signal for microbial induced production of IL-12 by CD8 α+ dendritic cells. *Nat. Immunol.* **1**, 83–87.
77. Beaman, M.H., Araujo, F.G., and Remington, J.S. (1994) Protective reconstitution of the SCID mouse against reactivation of toxoplasmic encephalitis. *J. Infect. Dis.* **169**, 375–383.
78. Johnson, L.L. (1992) SCID mouse models of acute and relapsing chronic *Toxoplasma gondii* infections. *Infect. Immun.* **60**, 3719–3724.
79. Gazzinelli, R.T., Hakim, F.T., Hieny, S., Shearer, G.M., and Sher, A. (1991) Synergistic role of CD4+ and CD8+ T lymphocytes in IFN-γ production and protective immunity induced by attenuated *Toxoplasma gondii* vaccine. *J. Immunol.* **146**, 286–292.
80. Gazzinelli, R., Xu, Y., Hieny, S., Cheever, A., and Sher, A. (1992) Simultaneous depletion of CD4+ and CD8+ T lymphocytes is required to reactivate chronic infection with *Toxoplasma gondii. J. Immunol.* **149**, 175–180.
81. Kelly, C.D., Welte, K., and Murray, H.W. (1987) Antigen-induced human interferon gamma production. Differential dependence on interleukin 2 and its receptor. *J. Immunol.* **139**, 2325–2358.
82. Suzuki, Y. and Remington, J.S. (1988) Dual regulation of resistance against *Toxoplasma gondii* infection by Lyt-2+ and Lyt-1+, L3T4+ T cells in mice. *J. Immunol.* **140**, 3943–3946.
83. Canessa, A., Pistoia, V., Roncella, S., Merli, A., Melioli, G., Terragna, A., et al. (1988) An in vitro model for *Toxoplasma* infection in man. Interaction between CD4+ monoclonal T cells and macrophages results in killing of trophozoites. *J. Immunol.* **140**, 3580–3588.
84. Denkers, E.Y., Scharton-Kersten, T., Barbieri, S., Caspar, P., and Sher, A. (1996) A role for CD4+ NK1.1+ lymphocytes as major histocompatibility complex class II independent helper cells in the generation of CD8+ effector function against intracellular infection. *J. Exp. Med.* **184**, 131–139.
85. Parker, S.J., Roberts, C.W., and Alexander, J. (1991) CD8+ T cells are the major lymphocyte subpopulation involved in the protective immune response to *Toxoplasma gondii* in mice. *Clin. Exp. Immunol.* **84**, 207–212.
86. Scharton-Kersten, T., Nakajima, H., Yap, G., Sher, A., and Leonard W.J. (1998) Infection of mice lacking the common cytokine receptor gamma-chain (gamma(c)) reveals an unexpected role for CD4+ T lymphocytes in early IFN-gamma-dependent resistance to *Toxoplasma gondii. J. Immunol.* **160**, 2565–2569.
87. Denkers, E.Y., Gazzinelli, R.T., Martin, D., and Sher, A. (1993) Emergence of NK1.1+ cells as effectors of IFNgamma dependent immunity to *Toxoplasma gondii* in MHC class I deficient mice. *J. Exp. Med.* **178**, 1465–1472.
88. Denkers, E.Y. and Gazzinelli, R.T. (1998) Regulation and function of T-cell-mediated immunity during *Toxoplasma gondii* infection. *Clin. Microbiol. Rev.* **11**, 569–588.
89. Scharton-Kersten, T.M., Yap, G., Magram, J., and Sher, A. (1997) Inducible nitric oxide is essential for host control of persistent but not acute infection with the intracellular pathogen *Toxoplasma gondii. J. Exp. Med.* **185**, 1261–1273.
90. Scharton-Kersten, T., Caspar, P., Sher, A., and Denkers, E.Y. (1996) *Toxoplasma gondii*: evidence for interleukin-12-dependent and-independent pathways of interferon-gamma production induced by an attenuated parasite strain. *Exp. Parasitol.* **84**, 102–114.
91. Cai, G., Radzanowski, T., Villegas, E.N., Kastelein, R., and Hunter, C.A. (2000) Identification of STAT4-dependent and independent mechanisms of resistance to *Toxoplasma gondii. J. Immunol.* **165**, 2619–2627.
92. Ely, K.H., Kasper, L.H., and Khan, I.A. (1999) Augmentation of the CD8+ T cell response by IFN-γamma in IL-12-deficient mice during *Toxoplasma gondii* infection. *J. Immunol.* **162**, 5449–54.
93. Schijns, V.E., Haagmans, B.L., Wierda, C.M., Kruithof, B., Heijnen, I.A., Alber, G., et al. (1998) Mice lacking IL-12 develop polarized Th1 cells during viral infection. *J. Immunol.* **160**, 3958–3964.
94. Oxenius, A., Karrer, U., Zinkernagel, R.M., and Hengartner, H. (1999) IL-12 is not required for induction of type 1 cytokine responses in viral infections. *J. Immunol.* **162**, 9659–9673.
95. Reichmann, G., Walker, W., Villegas, E.N., Craig, L., Cai, G., Alexander, J., et al. (2000) The CD40/CD40 ligand interaction is required for resistance to toxoplasmic encephalitis. *Infect. Immun.* **68**, 1312–1318.
96. Seguin, R. and Kasper, L.H. (1999) Sensitized lymphocytes and CD40 ligation augment interleukin-12 production by human dendritic cells in response to *Toxoplasma gondii. J. Infect. Dis.* **179**, 467–474.
97. Fischer, H.G., Dorfler, R., Schade, B., and Hadding, U. (1999) Differential CD86/B7-2 expression and cytokine secretion induced by Toxoplasma gondii in macrophages from resistant or susceptible BALB H-2 congenic mice. *Int. Immunol.* **11**, 341–349.
98. Subauste, C.S., de Waal Malefyt, R., and Fuh, F. (1998) Role of CD80 (B7.1) and CD86 (B7.2) in the immune response to an intracellular pathogen. *J. Immunol.* **160**, 1831–1840.
99. Reichmann, G., Villegas, E.N., Craig, L., Peach, R., and Hunter, C.A. (1999) The CD28/B7 interaction is not required for resistance to *Toxoplasma gondii* in the brain but contributes to the development of immunopathology. *J. Immunol.* **163**, 3354–3362.
100. Villegas, E.N., Elloso, M.M., Reichmann, G., Peach, R., and Hunter, C.A. (1999) Role of CD28 in the generation of effector and memory responses required for resistance to *Toxoplasma gondii. J. Immunol.* **163**, 3344–3353.

101. Mack, D.G. and McLeod, R. (1992) Human *Toxoplasma gondii*-specific secretory immunoglobulin A reduces *T. gondii* infection of enterocytes in vitro. *J. Clin. Invest.* **90**, 2585–2592.

102. Chardes, T., Buzoni-Gatel, D., Lepage, A., Bernard, F., and Bout, D. (1994) *Toxoplasma gondii* oral infection induces specific cytotoxic CD8 α/β+ Thy-1+ gut intraepithelial lymphocytes, lytic for parasite-infected enterocytes. *J. Immunol.* **153**, 4596–4603.

103. Buzoni-Gatel, D., Lepage, A.C., Dimier-Poisson, I.H., Bout, D.T., and Kasper, L.H. (1997) Adoptive transfer of gut intraepithelial lymphocytes protects against murine infection with *Toxoplasma gondii*. *J. Immunol.* **158**, 5883–5889.

104. Buzoni-Gatel, D., Debbabi, H., Moretto, M., Dimier-Poisson, I.H., Lepage, A.C., Bout, D.T., et al. (1999) Intraepithelial lymphocytes traffic to the intestine and enhance resistance to *Toxoplasma gondii* oral infection. *J. Immunol.* **162**, 5846–5852.

105. Sieling, P.A. (2000) CD1-Restricted T cells: T cells with a unique immunological niche. *Clin. Immunol* **96**, 3–10.

106. Jayawardena-Wolf, J. and Bendelac, A. (2001) CD1 and lipid antigens: intracellular pathways for antigen presentation. *Curr. Opin. Immunol.* **13**, 109–113.

107. Sugita, M., Moody, D.B., Jackman, R.M., Grant, E.P., Rosat, J.P., Behar, S.M., et al. (1998) CD1-a new paradigm for antigen presentation and T cell activation. *Clin. Immunol. Immunopathol.* **87**, 8–14.

108. Kasper, L.H., Matsuura, T., Fonseka, S., Arruda, J., Channon, J.Y., and Khan, I.A. (1996) Induction of γδ T cells during acute murine infection with *Toxoplasma gondii*. *J. Immunol.* **157**, 5521–5527.

109. Subauste, C.S., Chung, J.Y., Do, D., Koniaris, A.H., Hunter, C.A., Montoya, J.G., et al. (1995) Preferential activation and expansion of human peripheral blood γδ T cells in response to *Toxoplasma gondii* in vitro and their cytokine production and cytotoxic activity against *T. gondii*-infected cells. *J. Clin. Invest.* **96**, 610–619.

110. Scalise, F., Gerli, R., Castellucci, G., Spinozzi, F., Fabietti, G.M., Crupi, S., et al. (1992) Lymphocytes bearing the gd T-cell receptor in acute toxoplasmosis. *Immunology* **76**, 668–670.

111. De Paoli, P., Basaglia, G., Gennari, D., Crovatto, M., Modolo, M.L., and Santini, G. (1992) Phenotypic profile and functional characteristics of human gamma and delta T cells during acute toxoplasmosis. *J. Clin. Microbiol.* **30**, 729–731.

112. Hisaeda, H., Sakai, T., Maekawa, Y., Ishikawa, H., Yasutomo, K., and Himeno, K. (1996) Mechanisms of HSP65 expression induced by gamma delta T cells in murine *Toxoplasma gondii* infection. *Pathobiology* **64**, 198–203.

113. Hisaeda, H., Sakai, T., Ishikawa, H., Maekawa, Y., Yasutomo, K., Good, R.A., et al. (1997) Heat shock protein 65 induced by gd T cells prevents apoptosis of macrophages and contributes to host defense in mice infected with *Toxoplasma gondii*. *J. Immunol.* **159**, 2375–2381.

114. Sibley, L.D., Adams, L.B., Fukutomi, Y., and Krahenbuhl, J.L. (1991) Tumor necrosis factor-alpha triggers antitoxoplasmal activity of IFN-gamma primed macrophages. *J. Immunol.* **147**, 2340–2345.

115. Langermans, J.A., Van der Hulst, M.E., Nibbering, P.H., Hiemstra, P.S., Fransen, L., and Van Furth, R. (1992) IFNgamma-induced L-arginine-dependent toxoplasmastatic activity in murine peritoneal macrophages is mediated by endogenous tumor necrosis factor-alpha. *J. Immunol.* **148**, 568–574.

116. Adams, L.B., Hibbs, J.B., Jr., Taintor, R.R., and Krahenbuhl, J.L. (1990) Microbiostatic effect of murine-activated macrophages for *Toxoplasma gondii*. Role for synthesis of inorganic nitrogen oxides from L-Arginine. *J. Immunol.* **144**, 2725–2729.

117. Murray, H.W. and Teitelbaum, R.F. (1992) L-Arginine-dependent reactive nitrogen intermediates and the antimicrobial effect of activated human mononuclear phagocytes. *J. Infect. Dis.* **165**, 513–517.

118. Fang, F.C. (1997) Perspectives series: host/pathogen interactions. Mechanisms of nitric oxide-related antimicrobial activity. *J. Clin. Invest.* **99**, 2818–2825.

119. Albina, J.E. and Henry, W.L. (1991) Suppression of lymphocyte proliferation through the nitric oxide synthesizing pathway. *J. Surg. Res.* **50**, 403–409.

120. Albina, J.E. and Reichner, J.S. (1998) Role of nitric oxide in mediation of macrophage cytotoxicity and apoptosis. *Cancer Metastasis Rev.* **17**, 39–53.

121. Candolfi, E., Hunter, C.A., and Remington, J.S. (1994) Mitogen- and antigen-specific proliferation of T cells in murine toxoplasmosis is inhibited by reactive nitrogen intermediates. *Infect. Immun.* **62**, 1995–2001.

122. Gregory, S.H., Wing, E.J., Hoffman, R.A., and Simmons, R.L. (1993) Reactive nitrogen intermediates suppress the primary immunologic response to *Listeria*. *J. Immunol.* **150**, 2901–2109.

123. Chung, H.T., Pae, H.O., Choi, B.M., Billiar, T.R., and Kim, Y.M. (2001) Nitric oxide as a bioregulator of apoptosis. *Biochem. Biophys. Res. Commun.* **282**, 1075–1079.

124. Brune, B., von Knethen, A., and Sandau, K.B. (1998) Nitric oxide and its role in apoptosis. *Eur. J. Pharmacol.* **351**, 261–272.

125. Khan, I.A., Matsuura, T., Fonseka, S., and Kasper, L.H. (1996) Production of nitric oxide (NO) is not essential for protection against acute Toxoplasma gondii infection in IRF-1–/– mice. *J. Immunol.* **156**, 636–643.

126. Khan, I.A., Matsuura, T., and Kasper, L.H. (1998) Inducible nitric oxide synthase is not required for long-term vaccine-based immunity against *Toxoplasma gondii*. *J. Immunol.* **161**, 2994–3000.

127. Taylor, G.A., Collazo, C.M., Yap, G.S., Nguyen, K., Gregorio, T.A., Taylor, L.S., et al. (1999) Pathogen-specific loss of host resistance in mice lacking the IFN-gamma-inducible gene IGTP. *Proc. Natl. Acad. Sci. USA* **97**, 751–755.

128. Collazo, C.M., Yap, G.S., Sempowski, G.D., Lusby, K.C., Tessarollo, L., Woude, G.F., et al. (2001) Inactivation of LRG-47 and IRG-47 reveals a family of interferon gamma-inducible genes with essential, pathogen-specific roles in resistance to infection. *J. Exp. Med.* **194**, 181–188.

129. Yong, E.C., Chi, E.Y., and Henderson, W.R. (1994) Toxoplasma gondii alters eicosanoid release by human mononuclear phagocytes: role of leukotrienes in interferon gamma-induced antitoxoplasma activity. *J. Exp. Med.* **180**, 1637–1648.

130. Pfefferkorn, E.R. (1984) Interferon gamma blocks the growth of *Toxoplasma gondii* in human fibroblasts by inducing the host cells to degrade tryptophan. *Proc. Natl. Acad. Sci. USA* **81**, 908–912.

131. Murray, H.W., Szuro-Sudol, A., Wellner, D., Oca, M.J., Granger, A.M., Libby, D.M., et al. (1989) Role of tryptophan degradation in respiratory burst independent antimicrobial activity of gamma interferon-stimulated human macrophages. *Infect. Immun.* **57**, 845–849.

132. Dimier, I.H. and Bout, D.T. (1998) Interferon-gamma-activated primary enterocytes inhibit *Toxoplasma gondii* replication: a role for intracellular iron. *Immunology* **94**, 488–495.

133. Benveniste, E.N. (1988) Lymphokines and monokines in the neuroendocrine system. *Prog. Allergy* **43**, 84–120.

134. Fontana, A., Frei, K., Bodmer, S., and Hofer, E. (1987) Immune-mediated encephalitis: on the role of antigen-presenting cells in brain tissue. *Immunol. Rev.* **100**, 185–201.

135. Perry, V.H. (1998) A revised view of the central nervous system microenvironment and major histocompatibility complex class II antigen presentation. *J. Neuroimmunol.* **90**, 113–121.

136. Hunter, C.A. and Remington, J.S. (1994) Immunopathogenesis of toxoplasmic encephalitis. *J. Infect. Dis.* **170**, 1057–1067.

137. Schlüter, D., Kaefer, N., Hof, H., Wiestler, O.D., and Deckert-Schlüter, M. (1997) Expression pattern and cellular origin of cytokines in the normal and *Toxoplasma gondii*-infected murine brain. *Am. J. Pathol.* **150**, 1021–1035.

138. Hakim, F.T., Gazzinelli, R.T., Denkers, E., Hieny, S., Shearer, G.M., and Sher, A. (1991) CD8+ T cells from mice vaccinated against *Toxoplasma gondii* are cytotoxic for parasite infected or antigen-pulsed host cells. *J. Immunol.* **147**, 2310–2316.

139. Subauste, C.S., Koniaris, A.H., and Remington, J.S. (1991) Murine CD8+ cytotoxic T lymphocytes lyse *Toxoplasma gondii*-infected cells. *J. Immunol.* **147**, 3955–3559.

140. Denkers, E.Y., Yap, G., Scharton-Kersten, T., Charest, H., Butcher, B.A., Caspar, P., et al. (1997) Perforin-mediated cytolysis plays a limited role in host resistance to *Toxoplasma gondii. J. Immunol.* **159**, 1903–1908.

141. Suzuki, Y., Conley, F.K., and Remington, J.S. (1989) Importance of endogenous IFN gamma for prevention of toxoplasmic encephalitis in mice. *J. Immunol.* **143**, 2045–2050.

142. Suzuki, Y., Conley, F.K., and Remington, J.S. (1990) Treatment of toxoplasmic encephalitis in mice with recombinant gamma interferon. *Infect. Immun.* **58**, 3050–3055.

143. Kang, H. and Suzuki, Y. (2001) Requirement of non-T cells that produce gamma interferon for prevention of reactivation of *Toxoplasma gondii* infection in the brain. *Infect. Immun.* **69**, 2920–2927.

144. Israelski, D.M., Araujo, F.G., Conley, F.K., Suzuki, Y., Sharma, S., and Remington, J.S. (1989) Treatment with anti-L3T4 (CD4) monoclonal antibody reduces the inflammatory response in toxoplasmic encephalitis. *J. Immunol.* **142**, 954–958.

145. Palmer, E.M., Farrokh-Siar, L., Maguire Van Seventer, J., and van Seventer, G.A. (2001) IL-12 decreases activation-induced cell death in human naive th cells costimulated by intercellular adhesion molecule-1. I. IL-12 alters caspase processing and inhibits enzyme function. *J. Immunol.* **167**, 749–758.

146. Hunter, C.A., Roberts, C.W., Murray, M., and Alexander, J. (1992) Detection of cytokine mRNA in the brains of mice with toxoplasmic encephalitis. *Parasite Immunol.* **14**, 405–413.

147. Hunter, C.A., Roberts, C.W., and Alexander, J. (1992) Kinetics of cytokine mRNA production in the brains of mice with progressive toxoplasmic encephalitis. *Eur. J. Immunol* **22**, 2317–2322.

148. Gray, F., Gherardi, R., Wingate, E., Wingate, J., Fenelon, G., Gaston, A., et al. (1989) Diffuse "encephalitic" cerebral toxoplasmosis in AIDS. Report of four cases. *J. Neurol.* **236**, 273–277.

149. Conley, F.K. and Jenkins, K.A. (1981) Immunohistological study of the anatomic relationship of Toxoplasma antigens to the inflammatory response in the brains of mice chronically infected with *Toxoplasma gondii. Infect. Immun.* **31**, 1184–1192.

150. Ferguson, D.J. and Hutchison, W.M. (1987) An ultrastructural study of the early development and tissue cyst formation of Toxoplasma gondii in the brains of mice. *Parasitol. Res.* **73**, 483–491.

151. Fischer, H.G., Nitzgen, B., Reichmann, G., and Hadding, U. (1997) Cytokine responses induced by *Toxoplasma gondii* in astrocytes and microglial cells. *Eur. J. Immunol.* **27**, 1539–1548.

152. Schlüter, D., Deckert-Schlüter, M., Schwendemann, G., Brunner, H., and Hof, H. (1993) Expression of major histocompatibility complex class II antigens and levels of interferon-γ, tumour necrosis factor, and interleukin-6 in cerebrospinal fluid and serum in *Toxoplasma gondii*-infected SCID and immunocompetent C.B-17 mice. *Immunology* **78**, 430–435.

153. Fischer, H.G., Bonifas, U., and Reichmann, G. (2000) Phenotype and functions of brain dendritic cells emerging during chronic infection of mice with *Toxoplasma gondii. J. Immunol.* **164**, 4826–4834.

154. Chao, C.C., Anderson, W.R., Hu, S., Gekker, G., Martella, A., and Peterson, P.K. (1993) Activated microglia inhibit multiplication of *Toxoplasma gondii* via a nitric oxide mechanism. *Clin. Immunol. Immunopathol.* **67**, 178–183.

155. Chao, C.C., Gekker, G., Hu, S., and Peterson, P.K. (1994) Human microglial cell defense against *Toxoplasma gondii*. The role of cytokines. *J. Immunol.* **152**, 1246–1252.

156. Chao, C.C., Hu, S., Gekker, G., Novick, W.J., Jr., Remington, J.S., and Peterson, P.K. (1993) Effects of cytokines on multiplication of *Toxoplasma gondii* in microglial cells. *J. Immunol.* **150**, 3404–3410.

157. Peterson, P.K., Gekker, G., Hu, S., and Chao, C. C. (1995) Human astrocytes inhibit intracellular multiplication of Toxoplasma gondii by a nitric oxide-mediated mechanism. *J. Infect. Dis.* **171**, 516–518.

158. Halonen, S.K., Chiu, F., and Weiss, L.M. (1998) Effect of cytokines on growth of *Toxoplasma gondii* in murine astrocytes. *Infect. Immun.* **66**, 4989–4993.

159. Halonen, S.K., Taylor, G. A., and Weiss, L. M. (2001) Interferon-gamma induced inhibition of *Toxoplasma gondii* in astrocytes is mediated by IGTP. *Inf. Immun.* **69**, 5573–5576.

160. Yap, G.S. and Sher, A. (1999) Effector cells of both nonhemopoietic and hemopoietic origin are required for interferon (IFN)-gamma- and tumor necrosis factor (TNF)-alpha-dependent host resistance to the intracellular pathogen, *Toxoplasma gondii. J. Exp. Med* **189**, 1083–1092.

161. Chang, H.R., Grau, G.E., and Pechere, J.C. (1990) Role of TNF and IL-1 in infections with *Toxoplasma gondii. Immunology* **69**, 33–37.

162. Langermans, J.A., Nibbering, P.H., Van Vuren-Van Der Hulst, M.E., and Van Furth, R. (2001) Transforming growth factor-beta suppresses interferon-gamma-induced toxoplasmastatic activity in murine macrophages by inhibition of tumour necrosis factor-alpha production. *Parasite Immunol.* **23**, 169–175.

163. Yap, G.S., Scharton-Kersten, T., Charest, H., and Sher, A. (1998) Decreased resistance of TNF receptor p55- and p75-deficient mice to chronic toxoplasmosis despite normal activation of inducible nitric oxide synthase in vivo. *J. Immunol.* **160**, 1340–1345.

164. Suzuki, Y., Yang, Q., Yang, S., Nguyen, N., Lim, S., Liesenfeld, O., et al. (1996) IL-4 is protective against development of toxoplasmic encephalitis. *J. Immunol.* **157**, 2564–2569.

165. Roberts, C.W., Ferguson, D.J., Jebbari, H., Satoskar, A., Bluethmann, H., and Alexander, J. (1996) Different roles for interleukin-4 during the course of *Toxoplasma gondii* infection. *Infect. Immun.* **64**, 897–904.

166. Beaman, M.H., Hunter, C. A., and Remington, J. S. (1994) Enhancement of intracellular replication of *Toxoplasma gondii* by IL-6. Interactions with IFN-γ and TNF-α. *J. Immunol.* **153**, 4583–4587.

167. Deckert-Schlüter, M., Albrecht, S., Hof, H., Wiestler, O. D., and Schlüter, D. (1995) Dynamics of the intracerebral and splenic cytokine mRNA production in *Toxoplasma gondii* resistant and -susceptible congenic strains of mice. *Immunology* **85**, 408–418.

168. Gazzinelli, R.T., Eltoum, I., Wynn, T.A., and Sher, A. (1993) Acute cerebral toxoplasmosis is induced by in vivo neutralization of TNF-α and correlates with the down regulated expression of inducible nitric oxide synthase and other markers of macrophage activation. *J. Immunol.* **151**, 3672–3681.

169. Suzuki, Y., Yang, Q., Conley, F.K., Abrams, J.S., and Remington, J.S. (1994) Antibody against interleukin-6 reduces inflammation and numbers of cysts in brains of mice with toxoplasmic encephalitis. *Infect. Immun.* **62**, 2773–2778.

170. Suzuki, Y., Rani, S., Liesenfeld, O., Kojima, T., Lim, S., Nguyen, T.A., et al. (1997) Impaired resistance to the development of toxoplasmic encephalitis in interleukin-6-deficient mice. *Infect. Immun.* **65**, 2339–2345.

171. Jebbari, H., Roberts, C.W., Ferguson, D.J., Bluethmann, H., and Alexander, J. (1998) A protective role for IL-6 during early infection with *Toxoplasma gondii. Parasite Immunol.* **20**, 231–239.

172. Dalrymple, S.A., Lucian, L.A., Slattery, R., McNeil, T., Aud, D.M., Fuchino, S., et al. (1995) Interleukin-6-deficient mice are highly susceptible to *Listeria monocytogenes* infection: correlation with inefficient neutrophilia. *Infect. Immun.* **63**, 2262–2268.

173. Sayles, P.C. Johnson, L.L. (1996-1997) Exacerbation of toxoplasmosis in neutrophil depleted mice. *Nat. Immun.* **15**, 249–258.

174. Deckert-Schlüter, M., Buck, C., Weiner, D., Kaefer, N., Rang, A., Hof, H., et al. (1997) Interleukin-10 downregulates the intracerebral immune response in chronic Toxoplasma encephalitis. *J. Neuroimmunol.* **76**, 167–176.

175. Hunter, C.A., Litton, M.J., Remington, J.S., and Abrams, J.S. (1994) Immunocytochemical detection of cytokines in the lymph nodes and brains of mice resistant or susceptible to toxoplasmic encephalitis. *J. Infect. Dis.* **170**, 939–945.

176. Fiorentino, D.F., Zlotnik, A., Mosmann, T.R., Howard, M., and O'Garra, A. (1991) IL-10 inhibits cytokine production by activated macrophages. *J. Immunol.* **147**, 3815–3822.

177. Moore, K.W., O'Garra, A., de Waal Malefyt, R., Vieira, P., and Mosmann, T.R. (1993) Interleukin-10. *Annu. Rev. Immunol.* **11**, 165–190.

178. Gazzinelli, R.T., Oswald, I.P., James, S.L., and Sher, A. (1992) IL-10 inhibits parasite killing and nitrogen oxide production by IFN-γ-activated macrophages. *J. Immunol.* **148**, 1792–1796.

179. Brown, C.R., Hunter, C.A., Estes, R.G., Beckmann, E., Forman, J., David, C., et al. (1995) Definitive identification of a gene that confers resistance against *Toxoplasma* cyst burden and encephalitis. *Immunology* **85**, 419–428.

180. Deckert-Schlüter, M., Schlüter, D., Schmidt, D., Schwendemann, G., Wiestler, O.D., and Hof, H. (1994) Toxoplasma encephalitis in congenic B10 and BALB mice: impact of genetic factors on the immune response. *Infect. Immun.* **62**, 221–228.

181. Suzuki, Y., Wong, S.Y., Grumet, F.C., Fessel, J., Montoya, J.G., Zolopa, A.R., et al. (1996) Evidence for genetic regulation of susceptibility to toxoplasmic encephalitis in AIDS patients. *J. Infect. Dis.* **173**, 265–268.

182. Nakayama, I. (1965) Effects of immunization procedures in experimental toxoplasmosis. *Keio J. Med.* **14**, 63–72.

183. Pavia, C.S. (1986) Protection against experimental toxoplasmosis by adoptive immunotherapy. *J. Immunol.* **137**, 2985–2990.

184. Johnson, A.M., McDonald, P.J., and Neoh, S.H. (1983) Monoclonal antibodies to *Toxoplasma* cell membrane surface antigens protect mice from toxoplasmosis. *J. Protozool.* **30**, 351–356.

185. Frenkel, J.K. and Taylor, D.W. (1982) Toxoplasmosis in immunoglobulin M-suppressed mice. *Infect. Immun.* **38**, 360–367.

186. Kang, H., Remington, J.S., and Suzuki, Y. (2000) Decreased resistance of B cell-deficient mice to infection with *Toxoplasma gondii* despite unimpaired expression of IFN-γ, TNF-α, and inducible nitric oxide synthase. *J. Immunol.* **164**, 2629–2634.

187. Anderson, S.E.J., Bautista, S.C., and Remington, J.S. (1976) Specific antibody dependent killing of *Toxoplasma gondii* by normal macrophages. *Clin. Exp. Immunol.* **26**, 375–380.

188. Sibley, L.D., Weidner, E., and Krahenbuhl, J.L. (1985) Phagosome acidification blocked by intracellular *Toxoplasma gondii. Nature* **315**, 416–419.

189. Schreiber, R.D. and Feldman, H.A. (1980) Identification of the activator system for antibody to *Toxoplasma* as the classical complement pathway. *J. Infect. Dis* **141**, 366–369.
190. Sayles, P.C., Gibson, G.W., and Johnson, L.L. (2000) B cells are essential for vaccination-induced resistance to virulent *Toxoplasma gondii*. *Infect. Immun.* **68**, 1026–1033.
191. Shimada, K., O'Connor, G.R., and Yoneda, C. (1974) Cyst formation by *Toxoplasma gondii* (RH strain) in vitro. The role of immunologic mechanisms. *Arch. Ophthalmol.* **92**, 496–500.
192. Zhang, Y. and Denkers, E.Y. (1999) Protective role for interleukin-5 during chronic *Toxoplasma gondii* infection. *Infect. Immun.* **67**, 4383–4392.
193. Jaiswal, A.I. and Croft, M. (1997) CD40 ligand induction on T cell subsets by peptide presenting B cells: implications for development of the primary T and B cell response. *J. Immunol.* **159**, 2282–2291.
194. Wykes, M., Poudrier, J., Lindstedt, R., and Gray, D. (1998) Regulation of cytoplasmic, surface and soluble forms of CD40 ligand in mouse B cells. *Eur. J. Immunol.* **28**, 548–559.
195. Grammar, A.C., Bergman, M.C., Miura, Y., Fujita, K., Davis, L.S., and Lipsky, P.E. (1995) The CD40 ligand expressed by human B cells costimulates B cell responses. *J. Immunol.* **154**, 4996–5010.
196. Gazzinelli, R.T., Wysocka, M., Hieny, S., Scharton-Kersten, T., Cheever, A., Kuhn, R., et al. (1996) In the absence of endogenous IL-10, mice acutely infected with *Toxoplasma gondii* succumb to a lethal immune response dependent on CD4+ T cells and accompanied by overproduction of IL-12, IFN-γ and TNF-α. *J. Immunol.* **157**, 798–805.
197. Ding, L., Linsley, P.S., Huang, L.Y., Germain, R.N., and Shevach, E.M. (1993) IL-10 inhibits macrophage costimulatory activity by selectively inhibiting the up-regulation of B7 expression. *J. Immunol.* **151**, 1224–1234.
198. Koch, F., Stanzl, U., Jennewein, P., Janke, K., Heufler, C., Kampgen, E., et al. (1996) High level IL-12 production by murine dendritic cells: upregulation via MHC class II and CD40 molecules and downregulation by IL-4 and IL-10. *J. Exp. Med.* **184**, 741–746.
199. Kubin, M., Kamoun, M., and Trinchieri, G. (1994) Interleukin 12 synergizes with B7/CD28 interaction in inducing efficient proliferation and cytokine production of human T cells. *J. Exp. Med.* **180**, 211–222.
200. Koppelman, B., Neefjes, J.J., de Vries, J.E., and de Waal Malefyt, R. (1997) Interleukin-10 down-regulates MHC class II α/β peptide complexes at the plasma membrane of monocytes by affecting arrival and recycling. *Immunity* **7**, 861–871.
201. Suttles, J., Milhorn, D.M., Miller, R.W., Poe, J.C., Wahl, L.M., and Stout, R.D. (1999) CD40 signaling of monocyte inflammatory cytokine synthesis through an ERK1/2-dependent pathway. A target of interleukin (IL)-4 and (IL)-10 anti-inflammatory action. *J. Biol. Chem.* **274**, 5835–5842.
202. Luder, C.G., Lang, T., Beuerle, B., and Gross, U. (1998) Down-regulation of MHC class II molecules and inability to up-regulate class I molecules in murine macrophages after infection with *Toxoplasma gondii*. *Clin. Exp. Immunology* **112**, 308–316.
203. Liesenfeld, O., Kosek, J., Remington, J.S., and Suzuki, Y. (1996) Association of CD4+ T cell-dependent, interferon-gamma-mediated necrosis of the small intestine with genetic susceptibility of mice to peroral infection with *Toxoplasma gondii*. *J. Exp. Med.* **184**, 597–607.
204. Blass, S.L., Pure, E., and Hunter, C.A. (2001) A role for CD44 in the production of IFN-γ and immunopathology during infection with *Toxoplasma gondii*. *J. Immunol.* **166**, 5726–5732.
205. Liesenfeld, O., Kosek, J.C., and Suzuki, Y. (1997) Gamma interferon induces Fas dependent apoptosis of Peyer's patch T cells in mice following peroral infection with *Toxoplasma gondii*. *Infect. Immun.* **65**, 4682–4689.
206. Liesenfeld, O. (1999) Immune responses to *Toxoplasma gondii* in the gut. *Immunobiology* **201**, 229–239.
207. Buzoni-Gatel, D., Debbabi, H., Mennechet, F.J., Martin, V., Lepage, A.C., Schwartzman, J.D., et al. H. (2001) Murine ileitis after intracellular parasite infection is controlled by TGF-beta-producing intraepithelial lymphocytes. *Gastroenterology* **120**, 914–924.
208. Suzuki, Y., Sher, A., Yap, G., Park, D., Neyer, L.E., Liesenfeld, O., et al. (2000) IL-10 is required for prevention of necrosis in the small intestine and mortality in both genetically resistant BALB/c and susceptible C57BL/6 mice following peroral infection with *Toxoplasma gondii*. *J. Immunol.* **164**, 5375–5382.
209. Kuhn, R., Lohler, J., Rennick, D., Rajewsky, K., and Muller, W. (1993) Interleukin-10 deficient mice develop chronic enterocolitis. *Cell* **75**, 263–274.
210. Berg, D.J., Davidson, N., Kuhn, R., Muller, W., Menon, S., Holland, G., et al. (1996) Enterocolitis and colon cancer in interleukin 10-deficient mice are associated with aberrant cytokine production and CD4+ TH1-like responses. *J. Clin. Invest.* **98**, 1010–1020.
211. Khan, I.A. and Casciotti, L. (1999) IL-15 prolongs the duration of CD8+ T cell-mediated immunity in mice infected with a vaccine strain of *Toxoplasma gondii*. *J. Immunol.* **163**, 4503–4509.
212. Sharma, S.D., Hofflin, J.M., and Remington, J.S. (1985) In vivo recombinant interleukin 2 administration enhances survival against a lethal challenge with *Toxoplasma gondii*. *J. Immunol.* **135**, 4160–4163.
213. Geleziunas, R., Schipper, H.M., and Wainberg, M.A. (1992) Pathogenesis and therapy of HIV-1 infection of the central nervous system. *AIDS* **6**, 1411–1426.
214. Jacobson, M.A., Hardy, D., Connick, E., Watson, J., and DeBruin, M. (2000) Phase 1 trial of a single dose of recombinant human interleukin-12 in human immunodeficiency virus-infected patients with 100-500 CD4 cells/microL. *J. Infect. Dis.* **182**, 1070–1076.
215. Araujo, F.G., Hunter, C.A., and Remington, J.S. (1997) Treatment with interleukin 12 in combination with atovaquone or clindamycin significantly increases survival of mice with acute toxoplasmosis. *Antimicrob. Agents Chemother.* **41**, 188–190.
216. Hofflin, J.M. and Remington, J.S. (1987) In vivo synergism of roxithromycin (RU 965) and interferon against *Toxoplasma gondii*. *Antimicrob. Agents Chemother.* **31**, 346–348.

VIII
Cytokines in Viral Infections

19

Viroceptors

Virus-Encoded Receptors for Cytokines and Chemokines

Grant McFadden

1. INTRODUCTION

Viruses that propagate within vertebrate hosts have continuously coevolved with both the innate and acquired arms of the immune system for countless millennia *(1–3)*. Successful viruses generally exploit multiple strategies to survive in the hostile environment encountered within complex tissues of immunocompetent hosts. One of these strategies involves the synthesis of specific viral proteins that interact with critical immune molecules to either inhibit or modulate their antiviral activities *(4,5)*. Critical targets for viral subversion include ligands and receptors of the cytokine and chemokine networks *(6–9)*, a strategy that has been particularly effective for members of the poxvirus *(10–15)* and herpesvirus *(16–20)* families.

In order to systematize the growing family of virus-encoded gene products that modulate cytokines or their receptors, several terms have been proposed to indicate whether a given viral protein is more closely related to a host ligand or receptor. Thus, "virokines" are considered to be secreted viral proteins that mimic host cytokines, growth factors, or related extracellular immune regulators, whereas "viroceptors" are usually either cell associated or secreted but are thought to be derived from either host receptors or related immune ligand-binding molecules *(21,22)*. In this chapter, we focus only on examples of the viroceptor class of viral immunoregulatory proteins that are targeted toward cytokines and chemokines.

These viroceptors can be divided operationally into those that are secreted, usually as soluble glycoproteins, from virus-infected cells (Table 1 and 2) and those that localize to the infected cell surface (Table 3). In some cases, these viral proteins are thought to have been acquired from known cellular genes by ancestral cDNA capture events (and, thus, are true homologs of the cellular version), whereas in other cases, there is either low or no sequence similarity to host proteins. In the latter case, the viral proteins were sometimes identified by their operational ability to bind and inactivate known cytokines, rather than by any direct sequence relationship with the currently published database of known cellular cytokine receptors. With the rapid proliferation of current sequencing efforts, however, host homologs of some of these "orphan" viral cytokine-binding proteins may yet be discovered. In the following section, the various classes of viroceptors are considered according to either the cytokine receptors they mimic or the specific cytokines they bind and inhibit.

From: *Cytokines and Chemokines in Infectious Diseases Handbook*
Edited by: M. Kotb and T. Calandra © Humana Press Inc., Totowa, NJ

Table 1
Secreted Viroceptors That Mimic Cellular Receptors

Type	Example (virus)	Features
TNF-R	M-T2, S-T2 (MYX, SFV)	Inhibits rabbit TNF
TNF-R	CrmB (CPV, VaV)	Inhibits TNF, LT-α
TNF-R	CrmC (CPV, VV)	Inhibits TNF
TNF-R	CrmD (CPV, EV)	Inhibits TNF, LT-α
TNF-R	CrmE (CPV)	Inhibits human TNF
TNF-R	UL144 (HCMV)	TNF-R homolog
IL-1β-R	B15R (VV, CPV, EV)	Inhibits IL-1β and fever response
IFN-γ-R	M-T7 (MYX, SFV)	Inhibits rabbit IFN-γ and binds chemokines
	B8R (VV, CPV, EV, VaV)	Inhibits IFN-γ
IFN-α/β-R	B18R (VV, CPV, EV)	Inhibits type I IFN
	136R (YLDV)	Putative IFN-α/β-BP
CSF-1-R	BARF1 (EBV)	Inhibits CSF-1

Note: See Section 11 for explanation of abbreviations.

Table 2
Secreted Viroceptors That Bind Chemokines and Cytokines

Type	Example (virus)	Features
Chemokine-BP (CBP)	M-T7 (MYX, SFV)	Binds C, CC, CXC chemokines
	M-T1 (MYX, SFV)	Inhibits CC-chemokines
	C23L/B29R (VV-Lister, RPV)	Inhibits CC chemokines
	G3R (VaV)	Inhibits CC chemokines
	D1L/H5R (CPV)	Inhibits CC chemokines
	M3 (γ68HV)	Broad spectrum chemokine inhibitor
Cytokine-BP	gp38 (TPV)	Inhibits IL-2, IL-5, IFN-γ, TNF
GM-CSF/IL-2-BP	GIF (OV)	Inhibits GM-CSF, IL-2
IL-18-BP	MC53L, MC54L (MCV)	Inhibits IL-18
	D7L (EV, VV,CPV,VaV)	Inhibits IL-18
	14L (YLDV)	Putative IL-18 inhibitor

Note: See Section 11 for explanations of abbreviations.

2. SECRETED VIRAL TNF RECEPTORS

Tumor necrosis factor (TNF) is a potent proinflammatory cytokine produced by activated macrophages and T-cells (*see* refs. *23–29* for details). Three structurally and functionally related forms of TNF have been identified and are termed TNF (cachectin), lymphotoxin-α (LT-α), and lymphotoxin-β (LT-β). These TNF family ligands are active as trimers and induce pleiotropic effects on the immune system, as well as modulating the early host responses to virus infection. Two of the known cellular

Table 3
Cell Surface Viroceptors: Viral Chemokine Receptors

Type	Example (Virus)	Features
GPCR homologs	orf74 (HHV-8/KSHV)	Constitutive signaling CCR-CXCR
(Herpesviruses)	ECRF3/orf74 (HVS)	Functional CXCR
	orf74 (γ68HV)	Putative CXCR
	orf74 (EHV-2)	Putative CXCR
	E1 (EHV-2)	Functional CCR
	E6 (EHV-2)	Putative CCR
	US28 (HCMV)	Functional CCR-CX3CR
	US27 (HCMV)	Putative receptor
	UL78, UL33 (HCMV)	Putative CCR
	M78, M33 (MCMV)	Putative CCR
	R78, R33 (RaCMV)	Putative CCR
	U12, U51 (HHV-6, -7)	Functional CCR
GPCR homologs	K2R (SPV)	Putative CCR
(poxviruses)	Q2/3L (CaPV)	Putative CCR
	7L,145R (YLDV)	Putative CCR

Note: See Section 11 for explanation of abbreviations.

receptors for TNF are termed type 1 (p55) and type 2 (p75), both of which are members of a larger TNF-receptor superfamily. Members of this receptor superfamily transduce signals that can lead to apoptosis, inflammation, necrosis, or growth, depending on the cellular context. All possess multiple cysteine-rich domain (CRD) repeat motifs within their N-terminal extracellular ligand binding region. Each CRD consists of about 40 amino acids with 6 cysteine residues in a conserved spacing pattern. The TNF family members play pivotal roles in establishing the inflammatory and immune responses and TNF/LT-α and TNF/LT-β, in particular participate in a variety of antiviral activities.

The first documented example of a TNF-receptor-related protein encoded by a DNA virus was the S-T2 gene of Shope fibroma virus (SFV), a poxvirus that induces benign fibromas in rabbits *(30,31)*. Related genes have subsequently been identified in other poxviruses, including myxoma virus (M-T2) *(32,33)* cowpox virus (crmB, crmC, crmD, crmE) *(34–37)* variola virus (crmB) *(38,39)*, ectromelia virus (crmD), and vaccinia virus (crmC), although the vaccinia virus genes are disrupted and nonfunctional in some strains *(40,41)*. Like the cellular TNF receptors, the S-T2 and M-T2 proteins each contain four CRDs and a signal sequence *(31,33,42)*. None of the poxvirus family members has any obvious transmembrane domain, but several vaccinia strains exhibit cell surface TNF inhibitors, which remain to be characterized *(43)*. The role of M-T2 in virus virulence was confirmed by disrupting both copies of the M-T2 gene in the myxoma virus genome *(33)*.

Purified M-T2 protein effectively bound and inhibited rabbit TNF, but was unable to inhibit cellular lysis mediated by either murine or human TNF *(44)*. The binding affinity of M-T2 for TNF ligand is similar to that of secreted version of mammalian TNF receptors (K_d =170–195 pM), indicating that M-T2 can compete with cellular receptors to sequester TNF *(45)*. M-T2 is secreted from infected cells both as a 40-kDa monomer and as a disulfide-linked 80-kDa dimer, whereas the TNF-ligand itself is functional as a trimer. Both forms of M-T2 can bind TNF with comparable affinity but only the dimer inhibits TNF-mediated cell lysis efficiently *(45)*. Deletion studies on the M-T2 protein have indicated that only three of the four N-terminal CRDs, which are related to other TNF-receptor superfamily members, are essential for TNF inhibition *(46)*.

M-T2 has also been ascribed an intracellular role in blocking apoptosis in myxoma virus-infected lymphocytes. This antiapoptotic activity can be distinguished from TNF binding because C-terminal truncated versions of M-T2 that lack the third and fourth copies of the CRDs are unable to bind TNF but still inhibit apoptosis in virus infected T-cells *(47)*. Although many viral inhibitors of apoptosis have been documented *(48–51)*, M-T2 is the first viral protein discovered to have this unique dual function of extracellular cytokine inhibition and intracellular apoptosis inhibition *(47)*.

All of the characterized TNF viroceptors are from the poxviruses (reviewed in refs. *32, 52*, and *53*) except for one example in the herpesvirus family. The Toledo strain of human cytomegalovirus (HCMV) encodes a protein with CRDs characteristic of a TNF-receptor superfamily protein *(54)*. This putative HCMV viroceptor (UL144) is found only in the low-passage, virulent Toledo strain, and not in the genome of the AD169 standard laboratory strain, indicating that UL144 may have a role in survival within infected tissues *(55,56)*.

3. SECRETED VIRAL INTERLEUKIN-1β RECEPTORS

Interleukin (IL)-1-α and IL-β are pleiotropic proinflammatory cytokines that, along with TNF, play a critical role in mediating the early host responses to tissue injury and virus infection. The vaccinia virus genome encodes a protein designated B15R (strain WR) that possesses characteristic structural immunoglobulin domains and shares approx 30% amino acid similarity with the extracellular region of cellular type II IL-1 receptors. The vaccinia (and related cowpox) virus B15R gene product is a secreted glycoprotein that binds IL-1β, but not IL-1α or IL-1RA (the naturally occurring receptor antagonist of IL-1) with an affinity K_d=234 pM, comparable to the cellular receptor *(57,58)*. Expression of B15R from vaccinia virus was shown to inhibit the biological activity of IL-1β in vitro *(57,58)*.

The precise role of B15R in poxvirus virulence has been controversial. Vaccinia virus constructs with disruptions in the B15R gene caused a more pronounced disease phenotype (and increased morbidity) in mice but no alteration in host mortality when the virus is administered intranasally *(57)*. In contrast, infection of mice with the B15R-deficient virus by an intracranial route resulted in a marked decrease in lethality compared to infection with wild-type virus *(58)*. Later, it was shown that B15R plays a pivotal role during poxvirus infection in modulating the fever response during vaccinia virus infection *(59)*. Further clarification of this issue might come from studies with other poxviruses that express B15R-like genes, such as ectromelia virus in the mouse model *(60)*.

4. SECRETED VIRAL IFN-γ RECEPTORS

The interferons (IFNs) not only render cells resistant to viral infection, but they possess additional immunoregulatory properties also, such as the stimulation of the antigen-presentation pathways and the activation of critical effector cells such as macrophages, cytotoxic T-lymphocytes (CTLs), and natural killer (NK) cells *(61)*. Interferons can trigger the antiviral state in an autocrine or paracrine fashion by engaging interferon receptors on the surface of cells, generally in a species-specific fashion. Receptor signaling leads to activation of the JAK/STAT signal transduction pathway, which, in turn, is responsible for transcriptionally regulating the expression of a large number of genes that mediate the antiviral state *(62,63)*. Two classes of interferon have been identified, termed type I and type II. Type I interferons include IFN-α (leukocyte) and IFN-β (fibroblast), whereas the type II class is represented solely by IFN-γ, a product of activated T-lymphocytes and NK cells. The importance of both interferon pathways in immune defense against viruses has been validated in a variety of ways. For example, mice in which the interferon-receptor genes have been disrupted are severely impaired in their ability to handle virus infections *(64)*. Viruses have developed multiple strategies to counteract the adverse effects of type I and II interferons at both the intracellular and extracellular levels *(65)*.

The first indication that viruses can exploit an extracellular decoy strategy to target an interferon ligand directly was provided by the discovery that myxoma virus expresses a soluble, secreted IFN-γ receptor homolog *(66)*. This protein, M-T7, exhibits 30% amino acid sequence identity with the extracellular, ligand-binding domain of the human IFN-γ-receptor α chain, including all of the eight structurally important cysteine residues *(67)*. M-T7 directly binds and inhibits IFN-γ in a species-specific fashion *(66,68)*. M-T7 is secreted from myxoma virus-infected cells beginning at early times postinfection and rapidly accumulates (10^7 molecules/infected cell/h) as a stable, soluble glycoprotein in the extracellular environment *(68)*. M-T7 protein binds rabbit IFN-γ with an affinity comparable to the cellular receptor (K_d=1.2 n*M*) and is, therefore, a physiologically relevant IFN-γ inhibitor *(67,69)*. A T7 knockout mutant virus produced only nonlethal disease symptoms associated with a reduction in the ability of the virus to disseminate within the infected rabbit *(70)*. The loss of M-T7 expression in myxoma virus was also associated with a dramatic alteration of leukocyte flux into infected lesions, suggesting additional anti-immune properties for the M-T7 protein apart from the inhibition of IFN-γ *(70)*. Vaccinia vectors that are deleted for the IFN-γ receptor gene are also attenuated in vivo. *(71)*.

The genomes of a wide variety of orthopoxviruses, including vaccinia, cowpox, ectromelia, and variola viruses, also encode genes with homology to cellular IFN-γ receptors *(66,70,72)*. In contrast to M-T7, which binds and inhibits rabbit but not human or murine IFN-γ *(68)*, the homologs from other poxviruses display a broader species specificity *(72–74)*. The original species-specificity profile of each virus has implications for the evolutionary history of the orthopoxviruses *(72–75)*.

There have been several reports of poxvirus-secreted proteins that bind not only IFN-γ, but other ligands as well. As will be considered in a later section, the M-T7 protein of myxoma also binds promiscuously with a range of chemokines representing the three major chemokine subfamilies (CXC, CC, and C) via the conserved, heparin-binding motif at the C-terminus of many of these chemokines *(76)*. IFN-γ-binding activity has been documented by a 35-kDa secreted protein species expressed from tanapoxvirus-infected cells *(77)*. The usage of multifunctional domains may actually be a more common property of viroceptors than is currently appreciated in the literature. Such multifunctional viroceptors have been shown to possess generalized anti-inflammatory properties in animal models of inflammation outside the context of viral infections *(78)*.

5. SECRETED VIRAL IFN-α/β INHIBITORS

Experiments using transgenic mice have shown that type I interferons are pivotal for the control of infections resulting from many viruses *(64,79,80)*. The B18R gene of vaccinia (strain WR) encodes an IFN-α/β viroceptor *(81,82)*. This protein contains amino-acid-sequence motifs characteristic of the immunoglobulin superfamily, but has relatively low sequence similarity to the known interferon receptors. Nevertheless, the B18R protein has been shown to bind and functionally inhibit various type I interferons *(81–84)*. This inhibitory activity is characterized by broad species specificity, which is consistent with the wide host range exhibited by vaccinia *(82,84)*. Vaccinia B18R is important for virus virulence, because both a natural deletion variant (vaccinia strain Lister) and an engineered mutant of strain WR unable to express functional B18R protein each produce an attenuated disease phenotype in mice *(82)*. Related IFN-α/β-binding activities have also been observed for other orthopoxviruses, such as cowpox and ectromelia *(81,82)*.

Interferon-α binds type I interferon receptor via a single high-affinity site at the N-terminus of the ligand. In contrast, the interaction of B18R with IFN-α_1 and -α_2 is mediated by both the N- and C-terminal domains of the interferons, perhaps explaining the unusual broad species specificity of the vaccinia protein *(83)*. Another relevant feature of the B18R protein is that it is not only secreted from infected cells as soluble protein, but is also detected in a cell surface form *(85,86)*. Therefore, it is possible that B18R may act not only by sequestering IFN-α/β but also by interfering with signal transduction by type I interferon receptors *(86,87)*.

6. SECRETED VIROCEPTOR FOR COLONY-STIMULATING FACTOR-1

The *BARF1* gene product expressed by Epstein–Barr virus (EBV) is a secreted viral protein that is distantly related to the c-fms oncogene and that binds the pleiotropic cytokine, colony-stimulating factor-1 (CSF-1) *(88)*. CSF-1 is an important regulator for the differentiation of monocyte/macrophage and plays a critical role during reproductive gland development *(89,90)*. Thus, BARF1 has been suggested to represent a virus-specific strategy against the antiviral activities of activated macrophages *(88)*. In addition, the BARF1 gene has been implicated in the oncogenic potential of EBV *(91–95)*, although *BARF*1 gene knockout constructs remain competent for transformation of B-cells and latency *(96)*. Nevertheless, *BARF*1 was capable of blocking CSF-1-induced release of IFN-α from monocytes, consistent with an ability to bind and inhibit CSF-1 *(96)*. In fact, it is reasonable to propose that *BARF*1 compromises the potency of monocytes/macrophages as antiviral effector cells by specifically reducing their capacity to elaborate type I interferons *(96)*.

7. SECRETED VIRAL CHEMOKINE-BINDING PROTEINS

Chemokines comprise a growing superfamily of small proinflammatory proteins that function to activate and mobilize cells of the immune system to sites of trauma or infection *(97,98)*. Chemokines are currently classified based on conserved structural moieties and the receptors through which they impart their biological activity *(99,100)*. They exert proinflammatory and antiviral activities by signaling through specialized serpentine receptors belonging to the superfamily of G-protein-coupled receptors that span the cell surface membrane seven times.

A unique strategy used by certain poxviruses and herpesviruses for counteracting chemokine involve soluble chemokine-binding proteins (CBPs) *(6–8,14,101,102)*. These secreted 35- to 40-kDa viral glycoproteins function as extracellular chemokine scavengers but do not exhibit any sequence similarity to known chemokines or chemokine receptors. The related subject of virus-encoded chemokine mimics (which are technically classified as virokines) that can also antagonize chemokine functions is not covered in this chapter, but has been reviewed elsewhere *(6,7)*. Chemokine functions in vivo depend both on high-affinity interactions with target leukocyte G-protein-coupled receptors and lower-affinity interactions with glycosaminoglycans located on cell surfaces and throughout the extracellular matrix *(103,104)*. Thus, effective antagonism of chemokine functions can occur by disruption of either the low- or high-affinity chemokine-binding sites *(105)*. As previously mentioned, the M-T7 protein binds not only IFN-γ but also a wide spectrum of chemokines *(76,101)*. Binding studies using IL-8-deletion mutants revealed that purified M-T7 interacts with the low-affinity GAG-binding domain but not the high-affinity receptor-binding domain of IL-8 *(76)*. It has, therefore, been suggested that M-T7 may disrupt the presentation of chemokine gradients within infected tissues by competitively blocking chemokine–GAG interactions rather than occluding chemokine–receptor interactions *(101)*. Interestingly, the related T7-like protein of vaccinia does not bind chemokines, suggesting an evolutionary divergence between related proteins from different poxviruses *(106)*.

Another mechanistic class of poxvirus CBP was detected by physical binding studies and have been designated as T1/35K or vCCI (viral CC chemokine inhibitor) *(106–108)*. Related proteins have now been detected in many poxviruses, including variola (smallpox), cowpox, racoonpox, Shope fibroma, myxoma virus, camelpox, ectromelia (mousepox), rabbitpox, and some strains of vaccinia viruses *(see Table 2) (106–108)*. This class of viral CBP binds to a broad spectrum of CC chemokines with high affinity and at least one CXC chemokine IL-8, but with lower affinity. Binding of T1/35K/vCCI family members to CC chemokines effectively prevents the ability of these ligands to bind and trigger chemokine receptor signaling in responsive cells with inhibition constants (K_i) in the subnanomolar range *(106,108,109)*. However, none of these CBPs will neutralize CXC chemokines such as IL-8 in vitro, suggesting that CC chemokines are the preferential targets of inhibition in vivo *(106,108,109)*.

Members of the T1/35K/vCCI-CBP family were shown to potently inhibit CC chemokine-stimulated migration of monocytic cells, suggesting that these viral proteins function in vivo by blocking monocyte/macrophage trafficking into virus-infected tissues *(106,108,109)*. Purified CBP (VV-35 kDa) from vaccinia virus, for example, effectively blocks eotaxin-stimulated infiltration of eosinophils in a guinea pig skin model of inflammation *(106)*. Using knockout virus analysis, at least two of these family members have been demonstrated to dramatically block leukocyte chemotaxis during poxvirus infection. European rabbits infected with recombinant myxoma or rabbitpox virus variants deficient in T1/35K expression display a reduction in monocyte/macrophage and lymphocyte infiltrates into dermal lesions surrounding the primary infection site during the early stages of infection *(107,110)*, suggesting specific inhibition of CC-chemokine-mediated migration of inflammatory cells into virus-infected sites during the early acute phase of poxvirus infections. However, the gene knockout variants of both myxoma virus or rabbitpox virus had little effect in reducing mortality in the infected rabbit hosts despite these potent antichemokine properties *(110,111)*. Perhaps the most notable aspect of this family of CBPs is the apparent lack of sequence similarity to any known cellular proteins, including seven-transmembrane spanning chemokine receptors *(106–108)*. The structure of one member of this CBP family, namely the p35 chemokine inhibitor from cowpox, was determined and revealed a novel arrangement of twin β-sheets that suggests a novel mechanism of chemokine inhibition *(112)*. In fact, an Fc-fusion construct with the cowpox p35 protein has been shown to block allergen-induced hyperreactivity in a mouse model of asthma *(113)*.

More recently, a novel CBP from γ68-herpesvirus was identified and shown to have unique chemokine-binding spectrum *(114,115)*. It seems likely that other members of this growing CBP superfamily of viroceptors remain to be uncovered.

8. VIRAL BINDING PROTEINS THAT INHIBIT MULTIPLE CYTOKINES

In addition to the previously cited example of M-T7 protein, which binds IFN-γ as well as chemokines, several other secreted viral proteins interact with multiple classes of host cytokines. For example, the major secreted 38-kDa protein from cells infected with tanapoxvirus inhibits not only IFN-γ but also IL-2 and IL-5 *(77)*. Although the virus gene remains to be identified, the protein apparently also reduces TNF-induced upregulation of cellular adhesion genes *(116)*.

Another example of multiple cytokine inhibition by a single viral protein species is the GIF protein of orf virus, which binds and inhibits both granulocyte–macrophage colony stimulating factor (GM-CSF) and IL-2 *(117,118)*. This inhibition was shown to be species specific and exhibited picomolar binding affinities with the ovine cytokines *(118)*. The importance of IL-2 inhibition by GIF is likely mediated at the level of activated CTLs and NK cells. The observation that GM-CSF expressed by recombinant vaccinia virus causes increased antigen-presenting cells in regional lymph nodes *(119)* suggests that GM-CSF inhibition will favor virus escape from immune recognition.

9. VIRAL IL-18-BINDING PROTEINS

Interleukin-18 is a critical proinflammatory cytokine produced by activated macrophages and serves to promote IFN-γ secretion by reactive lymphocytes and NK cells *(120,121)*. Like IL-1 and TNF, IL-18 plays a major role in the early inflammatory responses to pathogens *(122)*, and it is clear that all three of these cytokines have been targeted for modulation by a variety of viruses. For example, when a cellular inhibitor of IL-18, termed IL-18 binding protein (IL-18BP), was first identified, it was noted that a related family of genes were encoded by a variety of poxviruses *(123,124)*. The suggestion that these viral IL-18BP homologs would be soluble inhibitors of IL-18 was subsequently demonstrated with the IL-18BPs from *Molluscum contagiosum* virus *(125,126)*, ectromelia virus *(127–129)*, vaccinia virus *(128)*, variola virus *(123)*, and cowpox virus *(128,129)*, of which all bind and inhibit IL-18 with nanomolar or subnanomolar affinities. The biological importance of IL-18 inhibition by poxviruses that express IL-18BPs likely includes protection against the activation of lymphocytes that elaborate IFN-γ upon IL-18 stimulation, such is Th1 cells, CTLs, and NK cells. More viruses continue to be discovered that encode putative IL-18BPs, such as Yaba-like disease virus of monkeys *(130)*. The role of these viral anti-IL18 proteins in viral pathogenesis and as anti-inflammatory reagents will probably be a focus of numerous future investigations.

10. VIRAL CHEMOKINE RECEPTORS

Nearly two dozen host chemokine receptors have been identified on migratory leukocytes such as monocytes, dendritic cells, neutrophils, T-lymphocytes, B-lymphocytes, NK cells, basophils, and eosinophils *(100)*. The unique receptor distribution profiles on each of these multiple cell types provides a wide diversity of antiviral responses and makes chemokine receptors common targets for pathogenic subversion. Some viruses, such as HIV, exploit cellular chemokine receptors as coreceptors for entry into target cells. In addition, many members of the herpesvirus and poxvirus family encode their own versions of viral chemokine receptors (vCRs) *(see* Table 3). Although these vCRs were initially thought to play a role only in immune evasion, there is growing indirect evidence pointing to more diverse roles, including viral replication, cellular tropism, and virus dissemination during infection. In this chapter, only a few representative vCRs are considered for illustrative purposes, but more comprehensive reviews of this topic have been recently published *(1,2,6,7,16,20)*.

Human cytomegalovirus (HCMV) encodes three open reading frames (ORFs), designated US27, US28 and UL33, with sequence similarity to the G-protein-coupled receptor superfamily *(131)*. Of these, the functional properties of US28 have been more extensively characterized. US28 is expressed as an early gene during lytic infection and is nonessential for viral replication in cultured cells *(132,133)*. US28 is 33% identical to human CCR1 and binds with high affinity to multiple CC chemokines, as well as the sole known CX_3C chemokine, fractalkine, but shows no detectable affinity for CXC chemokines *(134–136)*. CC chemokines induce transient Ca^{2+} mobilization in US28-expressing cells, suggesting that it is a functional signaling receptor *(134)*, but more recent data suggests that US28 can mediate constituitive activation of phospholipase C and necrosis factor (NF)-κB *(137)*. It has been claimed that US28 sequesters CC chemokines from the microenvironment in virus-infected lesions, but this model of chemokine depletion remains to be proven as a *bona fide* antihost strategy *(132,138)*. US28 has also been shown to substitute as a coreceptor for infection by certain strains of human immunodeficiency virus (HIV) *(139,140)*, which at least demonstrates the potential to synergystically bolster each virus during coinfections. Interestingly, US28 has been associated with exacerbated vascular smooth muscle cell migration in HCMV-infected cells in response to CC chemokine gradients, suggesting a potential role for HCMV infection in vascular disease *(141)*.

It remains feasible that US28 could promote trafficking of infected cells to secondary sites of infection and thus promote virus dissemination. Such a strategy has been proposed for other vCRs, such as UL33 of HCMV and its homologous genes in mouse murine cytomegalovirus (MCMV)(M33) and rat RaCMV(R33) *(142–144)*. The UL33 family of vCRs share notable amino acid conservation with the U12 ORF of human herpesvirus (HHV)-6 and HHV-7 *(142,143,145)*. M33 and UL33 are dispensable for viral propagation in vitro, but the expression of M33 does appear to be important for efficient MCMV propagation within the salivary gland *(142)*. The UL78 in mouse CMV is a constituent of the virion particle *(146)*, whereas the version from rat CMV (R78) is essential for maximal replication in vitro and for full virulence in infected rats *(147)*.

Herpesvirus saimiri (HVS) is a T-lymphotropic γ-herpesvirus that induces fatal lymphoproliferative diseases in New World primates. HVS encodes a vCR, designated ECRF3/orf 74, which is conserved and collinear with orthologous genes found in a variety of γ-herpesviruses *(148)*. ECRF3/orf 74 can be induced into intracellular Ca^{2+} signaling by a variety of CXC chemokines, but not CC chemokines *(149)*. HVS primarily infects and induces transformation in T-lymphocytes, but it is still unclear how ECRF3/orf 74 might provide an advantage for virus replication or survival.

The closely related orf 74 gene product of Kaposi sarcoma herpesvirus (KSHV, or HHV-8) can promiscuously bind a broad spectrum of CXC chemokines with high affinity and several CC chemokines with moderate to low affinity *(150–152)*. One notable feature of KSHV orf74 is that it possesses constitutive signaling activity even in the absence of ligand stimulation *(150,153)*. In KSHV orf74-expressing fibroblasts, this constitutive signaling resulted in cellular proliferation, transformation, and secretion of the potent angiogenic molecule vascular endothelial growth factor

(150,154,155). The constitutive activation of KSHV orf74 has been mimicked by a valine substitution (D138V) within the DRY sequence motif of the second extracellular loop of CXCR2 *(156)*. One interesting feature of KSHV orf74 is the ability to densitize heterologous serpentine receptors *(157)*, but the in vivo significance of this remains unclear.

Several CXC chemokines, such as IFN-γ-inducible protein-10 (IP-10) and stromal-cell-derived factor-1α (SDF-1α), act as inverse agonists, by blocking the constitutive signaling and transforming activity of KSHV orf74 *(158–160)*. In contrast, certain CXC chemokines, like IL-8 and growth-related gene protein GROα, augment the signaling levels of KSHV orf74 even further *(158,161)* as does HIV-1 tat *(162)*. Note, however, that KSHV orf74, like many other herpesvirus vCRs, is expressed primarily in the terminal lytic phase of the viral life cycle *(163)*, so it is unclear how the viral protein contributes to tumorogenesis, but transgenic mice that express KSHV orf74 in hematopoietic cells develop KS-like lesions *(164)*.

Other lymphotrophic herpesviruses, like equine herpesvirus-2 (EHV-2) and murine γ68-herpesvirus (γ68HV), also encode orf74 homologs, but their biological properties remain less characterized *(165–167)*. Mice chronically infected with γ68HV develop a lymphoproliferative disease that is amenable to experimental studies of viral pathogenesis and thus may serve as a useful animal model for studying the role of vCRs in vivo *(168,169)*.

Potential vCRs have also been identified within genomes of several poxviruses. Swinepox virus (SPV) encodes two examples, K2R and C3L, that share features typical of seven-transmembrane chemokine receptors, except that C3L lacks a significant portion of the N-terminus *(170)*. The Q2/3L ORF of capripox virus is another putative vCR *(171)*. Interestingly, Yaba-like disease virus (YLDV) encodes two closely related vCRs similar to primate CCR8, but their biological roles also remain to be studied *(130)*.

11. ABBREVIATIONS

BP	Binding protein	IFNα,β,γ	Interferon-α,β,γ
CaPV	Capripox virus	IFNα,β,γ-R	Interferon-α,β,γ-receptor
CBP	Chemokine binding protein	IL-1β-R	Interleukin-1β-receptor
CCR	CC chemokine receptor	KSHV	Kaposi sarcoma
CPV	Cowpox virus		herpesvirus (aka HHV-8)
CRD	Cysteine-rich domain	LT-α	Lymphotoxin-α
Crm	Cytokine response modifier	MCMV	Murine cytomegalovirus
CSF-1-R	Colony-stimulating	MCV	*Molluscum contagiosum* virus
	factor-1 receptor	MYX	Myxoma virus
CTL	Cytotoxic T lymphocyte	ORF	Open reading frame
CXCR	CXC chemokine receptor	OV	Orf virus
CX3CR	CXXXC-chemokine receptor	RaCMV	Rat cytomegalovirus
EBV	Epstein–Barr virus	RPV	Rabbitpox virus
EHV-2	Equine herpesvirus-2	SFV	Shope fibroma virus
EV	Ectromelia virus	SPV	Swinepox virus
γ68HV	γ68-Herpesvirus	TNF	Tumor necrosis factor
GM-CSF	Granulocyte/macrophage	TNF-R	TNF-receptor
	colony stimulating factor	TPV	Tanapox virus
GPCR	G-protein coupled receptor	VaV	Variola virus
HCMV	Human cytomegalovirus	vCR	Viral chemokine receptor
HHV-6,7,8	Human herpesvirus-6,7,8	VV	Vaccinia virus
HVS	Herpesvirus saimiri	YLDV	Yaba-like disease virus

REFERENCES

1. Tortorella, D., Gewurz, B.E., Furman, M.H., Schust, D.J., and Ploegh, H.L. (2000) Viral subversion of the immune system. *Ann. Rev. Immunol.* **18,** 861–926.
2. Alcamí, A. and Koszinowski, U.H. (2000) Viral mechanisms of immune evasion. *Immunol. Today* **21(9),** 447–455.
3. Kotwal, G.J. (1997) Microorganisms and their interaction with the immune system. *J. Leukocyte Biol.* **62(4),** 415–429.
4. Smith, G.L. (1994) Virus strategies for evasion of the host response to infection. *Trends Microbiol.* **2,** 81–88.
5. Spriggs, M.K. (1994) Poxvirus-encoded soluble cytokine receptors. *Virus Res.* **33(1),** 1–10.
6. Murphy, P.M. (2001) Viral exploitation and subversion of the immune system through chemokine mimicry. *Nature* **2(2),** 116–122.
7. Lalani, A.S., Barrett, J., and McFadden, G. (2000) Modulating chemokines: more lessons from viruses. *Immunol. Today* **21(2),** 100–106
8. Smith, G.L. (1996) Virus proteins that bind cytokines, chemokines or interferons. *Curr. Opin. Immunol.* **8,** 467–471.
9. Barry, M. and McFadden, G. (1997) Virus encoded cytokines and cytokine receptors. *Parasitology* **115,** S89–S100.
10. Smith, G.L. (1993) Vaccinia virus glycoproteins and immune evasion. *J. Gen. Virol.* **74(Pt. 9).** 1725–1740.
11. Nash, P., Barrett, J., Cao, J.-X., Hota-Mitchell, S., Lalani, A.S., Everett, H., et al. (1999) Immunomodulation by viruses: the myxoma virus story. *Immunol. Rev.* **168,** 103–120.
12. Alcamí, A., Symons, J.A., Khanna, A., and Smith, G.L. (1998) Poxviruses: capturing cytokines and chemokines. *Semin. Virol.* **8(5),** 419–427.
13. McFadden, G., Graham, K., Ellison, K., Barry, M., Macen, J., Schreiber, M., et al. (1995) Interruption of cytokine networks by poxviruses: lessons from myxoma virus. *J. Leukocyte Biol.* **57,** 731–738.
14. Kotwal, G.J. (2000) Poxviral mimicry of complement and chemokine system components: what's the end game? *Immunol. Today* **21(5),** 242–248.
15. Niemialtowski, M.G., Toka, F.N., Malicka, E., Spohr de Faundez, I., Gierynska, M., and Schollenberger, A. (1997) Orthopoxviruses and their immune escape. *Rev. Med. Virol.* **7,** 35–47.
16. Pease, J.E. and Murphy, P.M. (1998) Microbial corruption of the chemokine system: an expanding paradigm. *Semin. Immunol.* **10,** 169–178.
17. Davis-Poynter, N.J. and Farrell, H.E. (1996) Masters of deception: a review of herpesvirus immune evasion strategies. *Immunol. Cell Biol.* **74,** 513–522.
18. Ganem, D. (1997) KSHV and Kaposi's sarcoma: The end of the beginning? *Cell* **91,** 157–160.
19. Murphy, P.M. (1997) Pirated genes in Kaposi's sarcoma. *Nature* **385,** 296–299.
20. Dairaghi, D.J., Greaves, D.R., and Schall, T.J. (1998) Abduction of chemokine elements by herpesviruses. *Semin. Virol.* **8,** 377–385.
21. McFadden, G. (1995) Viroceptors, Virokines and Related Immune Modulators Encoded by DNA Viruses, R. G. Landes, Austin, TX.
22. Barry, M. and McFadden, G. (1997) In Cytokines in Health and Disease (Remick, D.G., and Friedland, J.S., eds.), Marcel Dekker, New York, pp. 251–261.
23. Sedgwick, J.D., Riminton, D.S., Cyster, J.G., and Korner, H. (2000) Tumor necrosis factor: a master-regulator of leukocyte movement. *Trends Immunol. Today* **21(3),** 110–113.
24. Gravestein, L.A. and Borst, J. (1998) Tumor necrosis factor receptor family members in the immune system. *Semin. Immunol.* **10(6),** 423–434.
25. Chan, F.K.-M., M.Siegel, R., and Lenardo, M.J. (2000) Signaling by the TNF receptor superfamily and T cell homeostasis. *Immunity* **13,** 419–422.
26. Locksley, R.M., Killeen, N., and Lenardo, M.J. (2001) The TNF and TNF receptor superfamilies: integrating mammalian biology. *Cell* **104(4),** 487–501.
27. Smith, C.A., Farrah, T., and Goodwin, R.G. (1994) The TNF receptor superfamily of cellular and viral proteins: activation, costimulation and death. *Cell* **76,** 959–962.
28. Ware, C.F., VanArsdale, S., and VanArsdale, T.L. (1996) Apoptosis mediated by the TNF-related cytokine and receptor families. *J. Cell. Biochem.* **60,** 47–55.
29. Baker, S.J. and Reddy, E.P. (1996) Transducers of life and death: TNF receptor superfamily and associated proteins. *Oncogene* **12,** 1–9.
30. Upton, C. and McFadden, G. (1986) Tumorigenic poxviruses: Analysis of viral DNA sequences implicated in the tumorigenicity of Shope fibroma virus and malignant rabbit virus. *Virology* **152(2),** 308–321.
31. Smith, C.A., Davis, T., Anderson, D., Solam, L., Beckman, M.P., Jerzy, R., et al. (1990) A receptor for tumor necrosis factor defines an unusual family of cellular and viral proteins. *Science* **248(4958),** 1019–1023.
32. McFadden, G., Schreiber, M., and Sedger, L. (1997) Myxoma T2 protein as a model for poxvirus encoded TNF receptor homologs. *J. Neuroimmunol.* **72,** 119–126.
33. Upton, C., Macen, J.L., Schreiber, M., and McFadden, G. (1991) Myxoma virus expresses a secreted protein with homology to the tumor necrosis factor receptor gene family that contributes to viral virulence. *Virology* **184(1),** 370–382.
34. Hu, F.-Q., Smith, C.A., and Pickup, D.J. (1994) Cowpox virus contains two copies of an early gene encoding a soluble secreted form of the Type II TNF receptor. *Virology* **204(1),** 343–356.
35. Loparev, V.N., Parsons, J.M., Knight, J.C., Panus, J.F., Ray, C.A., Buller, R.M.L., et al. (1998) A third distinct tumor necrosis factor receptor of orthopoxviruses. *Proc. Nat. Acad. Sci. USA* **95(7),** 3786–3791.

36. Saraiva, M. and Alcami, A. (2001) CrmE, a novel soluble tumor necrosis factor receptor encoded by poxviruses. *J. Virol.* **75(1)**, 226–233.

37. Smith, C.A., Hu, F.-Q., Smith, T.D., Richards, C.L., Smolak, P., Goodwin, R.G., et al. (1996) Cowpox virus genome encodes a second soluble homologue of cellular TNF receptors, distinct from CrmB, that binds TNF but not LTa. *Virology* **223(1)**, 132–147.

38. Massung, R.F., Esposito, J.J., Liu, L.I., Qi, J., Utterback, T.R., Knight, J.C., et al. (1993) Potential virulence determinants in terminal regions of variola smallpox virus genome. *Nature* **366(6457)**, 748–751.

39. Massung, R.F., Liu, L.I., Qi, J., Knight, J.C., Yuran, T.E., Kerlavage, A.R., et al. (1994) Analysis of the complete genome of smallpox variola major virus strain Bangladesh-1975. *Virology* **201(2)**, 215–240.

40. Goebel, S.J., Johnson, G.P., Perkus, M.E., Davis, S.W., Winslow, J.P., and Paoletti, E. (1990) The complete DNA sequence of vaccinia virus. *Virology* **179(1)**, 247–266.

41. Howard, S.T., Chan, Y.C., and Smith, G.L. (1991) Vaccinia virus homologues of the Shope fibroma virus inverted terminal repeat proteins and a discontinuous ORF related to the tumour necrosis factor receptor family. *Virology* **180(2)**, 633–647.

42. Smith, C.A., Davis, T., Wignall, J.M., Din, W.S., Farrah, T., Upton, C., et al. (1991) T2 open reading frame from Shope fibroma virus encodes a soluble form of the TNF receptor. *Biochem. Biophys. Res. Commun.* **176(1)**, 335–342

43. Alcamí, A., Khanna, A., Paul, N.L., and Smith, G.L. (1999) Vaccinia virus strains Lister, USSR and Evans express soluble and cell-surface tumour necrosis factor receptors. *J. Gen. Virol.* **80**, 949–959.

44. Schreiber, M. and McFadden, G. (1994) The myxoma virus TNF-receptor homologue inhibits TNFα in a species specific fashion. *Virology* **204**, 692–705.

45. Schreiber, M., Rajarathnam, K., and McFadden, G. (1996) Mxyoma virus T2 protein, a tumor necrosis factor (TNF) receptor homolog, is secreted as a monomer and dimer that each bind rabbit TNFα, but the dimer is a more potent TNF inhibitor. *J. Biol. Chem.* **271(23)**, 13,333–13,341.

46. Schreiber, M. and McFadden, G. (1996) Mutational analysis of the ligand binding domain of M-T2 protein, the tumor necrosis factor receptor homologue of myxoma virus. *J. Immunol.* **157(10)**, 4486–4495

47. Schreiber, M., Sedger, L., and McFadden, G. (1997) Distinct domains of M-T2, the myxoma virus TNF receptor homolog, mediate extracellular TNF binding and intracellular apoptosis inhibition. *J. Virol.* **71(3)**, 2171–2181.

48. Cuff, S. and Ruby, J. (1996) Evasion of apoptosis by DNA viruses. *Immunol. Cell Biol.* **74(6)**, 527–537.

49. Roulston, A., Marcellus, R.C., and Branton, P.E. (1999) Viruses and apoptosis. *Ann. Rev. Microbiol.* **53**, 577–628.

50. McFadden, G. and Barry, M. (1998) How poxviruses oppose apoptosis. *Semin. Virol.* **8**, 429–442

51. Turner, P.C. and Moyer, R.W. (1998) The control of apoptosis by poxviruses. *Semin. Virol.* **8(6)**, 453–469

52. Xu, X., Nash, P., and McFadden, G. (2000) Myxoma virus expresses a TNF receptor homolog with two distinct functions. *Virus Genes* **21(1–2)**, 97–109.

53. Cunnion, K.M. (1999) Tumor necrosis factor receptors encoded by poxviruses. *Mol. Genet. Metab.* **67(4)**, 278–282.

54. Cha, T.A., Tom, E., Kemble, G.W., Duke, G.M., Mocarski, E.S., and Spaete, R.R. (1996) Human cytomegalovirus clinical isolates carry at least 19 genes not found in laboratory strains. *J Virol.* **70**, 78–83.

55. Benedict, C.A., Butrovich, K.D., Lurain, N.S., Corbeil, J., Rooney, I., Schneider, P., et al. (1999) A novel viral TNF receptor superfamily member in virulent strains of human cytomegalovirus. *J. Immunol.* **162**, 6967–6970.

56. Lurain, N.S., Kapell, K.S., Huang, D.D., Short, J.A., Paintsil, J., Winkfield, E., et al. (1999) Human cytomegalovirus UL144 open reading frame: Sequence hypervariability in low-passage clinical isolates. *J. Virol.* **73(12)**, 10,040–10,050.

57. Alcamí, A. and Smith, G.L. (1992) A soluble receptor for interleukin-1β encoded by vaccinia virus: a novel mechanism of virus modulation of the host response to infection. *Cell* **71(1)**, 153–167.

58. Spriggs, M.K., Hruby, D.E., Maliszewski, C.R., Pickup, D.J., Sims, J.E., Buller, R.M., et al. (1992) Vaccinia and cowpox viruses encode a novel secreted interleukin-1 binding protein. *Cell* **71(1)**, 145–152.

59. Alcamí, A. and Smith, G.L. (1996) A mechanism for the inhibition of fever by a virus. *Proc. Nat. Acad. Sci. USA* **93(20)**, 11,029–11,034.

60. Smith, V.P. and Alcamí, A. (2000) Expression of secreted cytokine and chemokine inhibitors by ectromelia virus. *J. Virol.* **74(18)**, 8460–8471.

61. Gresser, I. (1997) Wherefore interferon? *J. Leukocyte Biol.* **61**, 567–574.

62. Pestka, S. (1997) The interferon receptors. *Semin. Oncol.* **24**, 918–940.

63. Bach, E.A., Aguet, M., and Schreiber, R.D. (1997) The interferon-receptor: a paradigm for receptor signaling. *Ann. Rev. Immunol.* **15**, 563–591.

64. van den Broek, M.F., Muller, U., Huang, S., Aguet, M., and Zinkernagel, R.M. (1995) Antiviral defense in mice lacking both α/β and γ interferon receptors. *J. Virol.* **69**, 4792–4796

65. Goodbourn, S., Didcock, L., and Randall, R.E. (2000) Interferons: cell signalling, immune modulation, antiviral response and virus countermeasures. *J. Gen. Virol.* **81**, 2341–2364.

66. Upton, C., Mossman, K., and McFadden, G. (1992) Encoding of a homolog of the interferon-γ receptor by myxoma virus. *Science* **258(5086)**, 1369–1372.

67. Mossman, K., Barry, M., and McFadden, G. (1994) Interferon-γ receptors encoded by poxviruses, in *Viroceptors, Virokines and Related Immune Modulators* (McFadden, G., ed.), R.G. Landes, Austin, TX.

68. Mossman, K., Upton, C., and McFadden, G. (1995) The myxoma virus soluble interferon-γ receptor homolog, M-T7, inhibits interferon-γ in a species specific manner. *J. Biol. Chem.* **270(7)**, 3031–3038

69. Mossman, K., Barry, M., and McFadden, G. (1997), in *Gamma Interferon: A Pleitropic Cytokine with Antiviral Activity* (Karupiah, G., ed.), R.G. Landes, Austin, TX, pp. 175–188.

70. Mossman, K., Nation, P., Macen, J., Garbutt, M., Lucas, A., and McFadden, G. (1996) Myxoma virus M-T7, a secreted homolog of the interferon-γ receptor, is a critical virulence factor for the development of myxomatosis in European rabbits. *Virology* **215(1),** 17–30.

71. Verardi, P.H., Jones, L.A., Aziz, F.H., Ahmad, S., and Yilma, T.D. (2001) Vaccinia virus vectors with an inactivated gamma interferon receptor homolog gene (B8R) are attenuated in vivo without a concomitant reduction in immunogenicity. *J. Virol.* **75(1),** 11–18.

72. Alcamí, A. and Smith, G.L. (1995) Vaccinia, cowpox and camelpox viruses encode soluble gamma interferon receptors with novel broad species specificity. *J. Virol.* **69(8),** 4633–4639.

73. Mossman, K., Upton, C., Buller, R.M., and McFadden, G. (1995) Species specificity of ectromelia virus and vaccinia virus interferon-γ binding proteins. *Virology* **208(2),** 762–769.

74. Alcamí, A. and Smith, G.L. (1996) Soluble interferon-γ receptors encoded by poxviruses. *Comp. Immunol. Microbiol. Infect. Dis.* **19,** 305–317.

75. Puehler, F., Weining, K.C., Symons, J.A., Smith, G.L., and Staeheli, P. (1998) Vaccinia virus-encoded cytokine receptor binds and neutralizes chicken interferon-gamma. *Virology* **248(2),** 231–240.

76. Lalani, A.S., Graham, K., Mossman, K., Rajarathnam, K., Clark-Lewis, I., Kelvin, D., et al. (1997) The purified myxoma virus gamma interferon receptor homolog, M-T7, interacts with the heparin binding domains of chemokines. *J. Virol.* **71(6),** 4356–4363.

77. Essani, K., Chalasani, S., Eversole, R., Beuving, L., and Birmingham, L. (1994) Multiple anti-cytokine activities secreted from tanapox virus-infected cells. *Microb. Pathogen.* **17(5),** 347–353.

78. Liu, L.Y., Lalani, A., Dai, E., Seet, B., Macauley, C., Singh, R., et al. (2000) The viral anti-inflammatory chemokine-binding protein M-T7 reduces intimal hyperplasia after vascular injury. *J. Clin. Invest.* **105(11),** 1613–1621.

79. van den Broek, M.F., Muller, U., Huang, S., Zinkernagel, R.M., and Aguet, M. (1995) Immune defence in mice lacking type I and/or type II interferon receptors. *Immunol. Rev.* **148,** 5–18.

80. Deonarain, R., Alcami, A., Alexiou, M., Dallman, M.J., Gewert, D.R., and Porter, A.C.G. (2000) Impaired antiviral response and alpha/beta interferon induction in mice lacking beta interferon. *J. Virol.* **74(7),** 3404–3409.

81. Colamonici, O.R., Domanski, P., Sweitzer, S.M., Larner, A., and Buller, R.M.L. (1995) Vaccinia virus B18R gene encodes a type I interferon-binding protein that blocks interferon α transmembrane signaling. *J. Biol. Chem.* **270(27),** 15,974–15,978

82. Symons, J.A., Alcamí, A., and Smith, G.L. (1995) Vaccinia virus encodes a soluble type I interferon receptor of novel structure and broad species specificity. *Cell* **81,** 551–560.

83. Liptáková, H., Kontsekova, E., Alcami, A., Smith, G.L., and Kontsek, P. (1997) Analysis of an interaction between the soluble vaccinia virus-coded Type I interferon (IFN)-receptor and human IFN-α1 and IFN-α2. *Virology* **232,** 86–90.

84. Vancova, I., La Bonnadiere, C., and Kontsek, P. (1998) Vaccinia virus protein B18R inhibits the activity and cellular binding of the novel type interferon-delta. *J. Gen. Virol.* **79,** 1647–1649.

85. Ueda, Y., Morikawa, S., and Matsuura, Y. (1990) Identification and nucleotide sequence of the gene encoding a surface antigen indiced by vaccinia virus. *Virology* **177,** 588–594.

86. Alcamí, A., Symons, J.A., and Smith, G.L. (2000) The vaccinia virus soluble α/β interferon (IFN) receptor binds to the cell surface and protects cells from the antiviral effects of IFN. *J. Virol.* **74(23),** 11,230–11,239

87. Karupiah, G., Fredrickson, T.N., Holmes, K.L., Khairallah, L.H., and Buller, R.M.L. (1993) Importance of interferons in recovery from mousepox. *J. Virol.* **67(7),** 4214–4226.

88. Strockbine, L.D., Cohen, J.I., Farrah, T., Lyman, S.D., Wagener, F., DuBose, R.F., et al. (1998) The Epstein–Barr virus BARF1 gene encodes a novel, soluble colony-stimulating factor-1 receptor. *J. Virol.* **75(5),** 4015–4021.

89. Sapi, E. and Kacinski, B.M. (1999) The role of CSF-1 in normal and neoplastic breast physiology. *Exp. Biol. Med.* **220(1),** 1–8.

90. Pollard, J.W. (1997) Role of colony-stimulating factor-1 in reproduction and development. *Mol. Reprod. Dev.* **46(1),** 54–60.

91. zur Hausen, A., Brink, A.A., Craanen, M.E., Middledorp, J.M., Meijer, C.J., and van den Brule, A.J. (2000) Unique transcription pattern of Epstein–Barr virus (EBV) in EBV-carrying gastic adenocarcinomas: expression of the transforming BARF1 gene. *Cancer Res.* **60(10),** 2745–2748.

92. Decaussin, G., Sbih-Lemmali, F., de Turenne-Tessier, M., Bouquermouh, A., and Ooka, T. (2000) Expression of BARF1 gene encoded by Epstein–Barr virus in nasopharyngeal carcinoma biopsies. *Cancer Res.* **60(19),** 5584–5588.

93. Wei, M. X., de Turenne-Tessier, M., Decaussin, G., Benet, G., and Ooka, T. (1997) Establishment of a monkey kidney epithelial cell line with the BARF1 open reading frame from Epstein–Barr virus. *Oncogene* **14(25),** 3073–3081.

94. Wei, M.X., Moulin, J.C., Decaussin, G., Berger, F., and Ooka, T. (1994) Expression and tumorigenicity of the Epstein–Barr virus BARF1 gene in human Louckes B–lymphocyte cell line. *Cancer Res.* **54(7),** 1843–1848.

95. Wei, M.X. and Ooka, T. (1989) A transforming function of the BARF1 gene encoded by Epstein–Barr virus. *EMBO J.* **8(10),** 2897–2903.

96. Cohen, J.I. and Lekstrom, K. (1999) Epstein–Barr virus BARF1 protein is dispensable for B-cell transformation and inhibits alpha interferon secretion from mononuclear cells. *J. Virol.* **73(9),** 7627–7632.

97. Mackay, C.R. (2001) Chemokines: immunology's high impact factor. *Nature* **2(2),** 95–101.

98. Gerard, C. and Rollins, B.J. (2001) Chemokines and disease. *Nature* **2(2),** 108–115.

99. Murdoch, C. and Finn, A. (2000) Chemokine receptors and their role in inflammation and infectious disease. *Blood* **95(10),** 3032–3043.

100. Murphy, P.M., Baggiolini, M., Charo, I.F., Hebert, C.A., Horuk, R., Matsushima, K., et al. (2000) International union of pharmacology XXII. Nomenclature for chemokine receptors. *Pharmacol. Rev.* **52(1),** 145–176.

101. Lalani, A.S. and McFadden, G. (1997) Secreted poxvirus chemokine binding proteins. *J. Leukocyte Biol.* **62,** 570–576.
102. Mahalingam, S. and Karupiah, G. (2000) Modulation of chemokines by poxvirus infections. *Curr. Opin. Immunol.* **12(4),** 409–412.
103. Witt, D.P. and Lander, A.D. (1994) Differential binding of chemokines to glycosaminoglycan subpopulations. *Curr. Biol.* **4(5),** 394–400.
104. Clark-Lewis, I., Kim, K.S., Rajarathnam, K., Gong, J.H., Dewald, B., Moser, B., et al. (1995) Structure–activity relationships of chemokines. *J. Leukocyte Biol.* **57,** 703–711.
105. McFadden, G. and Kelvin, D. (1997) New strategies for chemokine inhibition and modulation: you take the high road and I'll take the low road. *Biochem. Pharmacol.* **54,** 1271–1280.
106. Alcamí, A., Symons, J.A., Collins, P.D., Williams, T.J., and Smith, G.L. (1998) Blockade of chemokine activity by a soluble chemokine binding protein from vaccinia virus. *J. Immunol.* **160,** 624–633.
107. Graham, K.A., Lalani, A.S., Macen, J.L., Ness, T.L., Barry, M., Liu, L.-Y., et al. (1997) The T1/35kDa family of poxvirus secreted proteins bind chemokines and modulate leukocyte influx into virus infected tissues. *Virology* **229(1),** 12–24.
108. Smith, C.A., Smith, T.D., Smolak, P.J., Friend, D., Hagen, H., Gerhart, M., et al. (1997) Poxvirus genomes encode a secreted soluble protein that preferentially inhibits β chemokine activity yet lacks sequence homology to known chemokine receptors. *Virology* **236(2),** 316–327.
109. Lalani, A.S., Ness, T.L., Singh, R., Harrison, J.K., Seet, B.T., Kelvin, D.J., et al. (1998) Functional comparisons among members of the poxvirus T1/35kDa family of soluble CC-chemokine inhibitor glycoproteins. *Virology* **250,** 173–184.
110. Lalani, A.S., Masters, J., Graham, K., Liu, L., Lucas, A., and McFadden, G. (1999) Role of the myxoma virus soluble CC-chemokine inhibitor glycoprotein, M-T1, during myxoma virus pathogenesis. *Virology* **256(2),** 233–245.
111. Martinez-Pomares, L., Thompson, J.P., and Moyer, R.W. (1995) Mapping and investigation of the role in pathogenesis of the major unique secreted 35-kDa protein of rabbitpox virus. *Virology* **206,** 591–600.
112. Carfi, A., Smith, C.A., Smolak, P.J., McGrew, J., and Wiley, D.C. (1999) Structure of a soluble secreted chemokine inhibitor vCCI (p35) from cowpox virus. *Proc. Nat. Acad. Sci. USA* **96(22),** 12,379–12,383
113. Dabbagh, K., Xiao, Y., Smith, C., Stepick-Biek, P., Kim, S.G., Lamm, W.J., et al. (2000) Local blockade of allergic airway hyperreactivity and inflammation by the poxvirus-derived pan-CC-chemokine inhibitor vCCI. *J. Immunol.* **165(6),** 3418–3422.
114. Parry, B.C., Simas, J.P., Smith, V.P., Stewart, C.A., Minson, A.C., Efstathiou, S., et al. (2000) A broad spectrum secreted chemokine binding protein encoded by a herpesvirus. *J. Exp. Med.* **191(3),** 573–578.
115. van Berkel, V., Barrett, J., Tiffany, H.L., Fremont, D.H., Murphy, P.M., McFadden, G., et al. (2000) Identification of a gammaherpesvirus selective chemokine binding protein that inhibits chemokine action. *J. Virol.* **74(15),** 6741–6747.
116. Paulose, M., Bennet, B.L., Manning, A.M., and Essani, K. (1998) Selective inhibition of TNF-alpha induced cell adhesion molecular gene expression by tanapox virus. *Microb. Pathogen.* **25(1),** 33–41.
117. Haig, D.M. (1998) Poxvirus interference with the host cytokine response. *Vet. Immunol. Immunopathol.* **63,** 149–156.
118. Deane, D., McInnes, C.J., Percival, A., Wood, A., Thomson, J., Lear, A., et al. (2000) Orf virus encodes a novel secreted protein inhibitor of granulocyte-macrophage colony-stimulating factor and interleukin-2. *J. Virol.* **74(3),** 1313–1320.
119. Kass, E., Parker, J., Schlom, J., and Grenier, J.W. (2000) Comparative studies of the effects of recombinant GM-CSF and GM-CSF administered via a poxvirus to enhance the concentration of antigen-presenting cells in regional lymph nodes. *Cytokine* **12(7),** 960–971.
120. Lebel-Binay, S., Berger, A., Zinzindohoue, F., Cugnenc, P.H., Thiounn, N., Fridman, W.H., et al. (2000) Interleukin-18: biological properties and clinical implications. *Eur. Cytokine Netw.* **11(1),** 15–25.
121. Dinarello, C.A. (2000) Interleukin-18, a proinflammatory cytokine. *Eur. Cytokine Netw.* **11(3),** 483–486.
122. Sugawara, I. (2000) Interleukin-18 (IL-18) and infectious diseases, with special emphasis on diseases induced by intracellular pathogens. *Microbes Infect.* **2(10),** 1257–1263.
123. Novick, D., Kim, S.-H., Fantuzzi, G., Reznikov, L.L., Dinarello, C.A., and Rubinstein, M. (1999) Interleukin-18 binding proteins: a novel modulator of the Th1 cytokine response. *Immunity* **10,** 127–136.
124. Dinarello, C.A. (2000) Targeting interleukin 18 with interleukin 18 binding protein. *Ann. Rheum. Dis.* **59(Suppl. 1),** 17–20.
125. Xiang, Y. and Moss, B. (1999) Identification of human and mouse homologs of the MC51L-53L-54L family of secreted glycoproteins encoded by the Molluscum contagiosum poxvirus. *Virology* **257(2),** 297–302.
126. Xiang, Y. and Moss, B. (1999) IL-18 binding and inhibition of interferon g induction by human poxvirus-encoded proteins. *Proc. Nat. Acad. Sci. USA* **96(20),** 11,537–11,542.
127. Born, T., Morrison, L. A., Esteban, D. J., VandenBos, T., Thebeau, L. G., Chen, N., Spriggs, M. K., Sims, J. E., and Buller, R. M. L. (2000) A poxvirus protein that binds to and inactivates IL-18, and inhibits NK cell response, *J. Immunol.* **164(6),** 3246–3254
128. Smith, V.P., Bryant, N.A., and Alcamí, A. (2000) Ectromelia, vaccinia and cowpox viruses encode secreted interleukin-18-binding proteins. *J. Gen. Virol.* **81(Pt. 5),** 1223–1230.
129. Calderara, S., Xiang, Y., and Moss, B. (2001) Orthopoxvirus IL-18 binding proteins: affinities and antagonist activities. *Virology* **279(1),** 22–26.
130. Lee, H.-J., Essani, K., and Smith, G.L. (2001) The genome sequence of yaba-like disease virus, a yatapoxvirus. *Virology* **281(2),** 170–192.
131. Chee, M.S., Satchwell, S.C., Preddie, E., Weston, K.M., and Barrell, B.G. (1990) Human cytomegalovirus encodes three G protein-coupled receptor homologues. *Nature* **344,** 774–777.

132. Vieira, J., Schall, T.J., Corey, L., and Geballe, A.P. (1998) Functional analysis of the human cytomegalovirus US28 gene by insertion mutagenesis with the green fluorescent protein gene. *J. Virol.* 72(10), 8158–8165

133. Zipeto, D., Bodaghi, B., Laurent, L., Virelizier, J.-L., and Michelson, S. (1999) Kinetics of transcription of human cytomegalovirus chemokine receptor US28 in different cell types. *J. Gen. Virol.* **80**, 543–547.

134. Gao, J.L. and Murphy, P.M. (1994) Human cytomegalovirus open reading frame US28 encodes a functional β receptor. *J. Biol. Chem.* **269**, 28,539–28,542.

135. Neote, K., DiGregorio, D., Mak, J.Y., Horuk, R., and Schall, T.J. (1993) Molecular cloning, functional expression, and signaling characteristics of a C-C- chemokine receptor. *Cell* **72**, 415–425.

136. Kledal, T.N., Rosendike, M.M., and Schwartz, T.W. (1998) Selective recognition of the membrane-bound CX3C chemokine, fractalkine, by the human cytomegalovirus-encoded broad-spectrum receptor US28. *FEBS Lett.* **441**, 208–214.

137. Casarosa, P., Bakker, R.A., Verzijl, D., Navis, M., Timmerman, H., Leurs, R., et al. (2001) Constitutive signaling of the human cytomegalovirus-encoded chemokine receptor US28. *J. Biol. Chem.* **276(2)**, 1133–1137.

138. Bodaghi, B., Jones, T.R., Zipeto, D., Vita, C., Sun, L., Laurent, L., et al. (1998) Chemokine sequestration by viral chemoreceptors as a novel viral strategy: withdrawal of chemokines from the environment of cytomegalovirus-infected cells. *J. Exp. Med.* **188(5)**, 855–866.

139. Pleskoff, O., Treboute, C., Brelot, A., Heveker, N., Seman, M., and Alizon, M. (1997) Identification of a chemokine receptor encoded by human cytomegalovirus as a cofactor for HIV-1 entry. *Science* **276**, 1874–1878.

140. Ohagen, A., Li, L., Rosenweig, A., and Gabuzda, D. (2000) Cell-dependent mechanisms restrict the HIV type 1 coreceptor activity of US28, a chemokine receptor homolog encoded by human cytomegalovirus. *AIDS Res. Hum. Retroviruses* **16(1)**, 27–35.

141. Streblow, D.N., Soderberg-Naucler, C., Vieira, J., Smith, P., Wakabayashi, E., Ruchti, F., et al. (1999) The human cytomegalovirus chemokine receptor US28 mediates vascular smooth muscle cell migration. *Cell* **99**, 511–520.

142. Davis-Poynter, N.J., Lynch, D.M., Vally, H., Shellam, G.R., Rawlinson, W.D., Barrell, B.G., et al. (1997) Identification and characterization of a G protein-coupled receptor homolog encoded by murine cytomegalovirus. *J. Virol.* **71**, 1521–1529.

143. Margulies, B.J., Browne, H., and Gibson, W. (1997) Identification of the human cytomegalovirus G protein-coupled receptor homologue encoded by UL33 in infected cells and enveloped virus particles. *Virology* **225**, 111–125.

144. Beisser, P.S., Vink, C., Van Dam, J.G., Grauls, G., Vanherle, S.J.V., and Bruggeman, C.A. (1998) The R33 G protein-coupled receptor gene of rat cytomegalovirus plays an essential role in the pathogenesis of viral infection. *J. Virol.* **72(3)**, 2352–2363.

145. Isegawa, Y., Ping, Z., Nakano, K., Sugimoto, N., and Yamanishi, K. (1998) Human herpesvirus 6 open reading frame U12 encodes a functional β-chemokine receptor. *J. Virol.* **72(7)**, 6104–6112.

146. Oliveria, S.A. and Shenk, T.E. (2001) Murine cytomegalovirus M78 protein, a G protein-coupled receptor homologue, is a constituent of the virion and facilitates accumulation of immediate-early viral mRNA. *PNAS* **98(6)**, 3237–3242.

147. Beisser, P.S., Grauls, G., Bruggeman, C.A., and Vink, C. (1999) Deletion of the R78 G protein-coupled receptor gene from rat cytomegalovirus results in an attenuated, syncytium-inducing mutant strain. *J. Virol.* **73(9)**, 7218–7230.

148. Nicholas, J., Cameron, K.R., and Honess, R.W. (1992) Herpesvirus saimiri encodes homologues of G-protein coupled receptors and cyclins. *Nature* **355**, 362–365.

149. Ahuja, S.K. and Murphy, P.M. (1993) Molecular piracy of mammalian interleukin-8 receptor type B by herpesvirus saimiri. *J. Biol. Chem.* **268(28)**, 20,691–20,694.

150. Arvanitakis, L., Geras-Raaka, E., Varma, A., Gershengorn, M.C., and Cesarman, E. (1997) Human herpesvirus KSHV encodes a constitutively active G-protein-coupled receptor linked to cell proliferation. *Nature* **385**, 347–349.

151. Rosenkilde, M.M. and Schwartz, T.W. (2000) Potency of ligands correlates with affinity measured against agonist and inverse agonists but not against neutral ligand in constitutively active chemokine receptor. *Mol. Pharmacol.* **57(3)**, 602–609.

152. Cesarman, E., Mesri, E.A., and Gershengorn, M.C. (2000) Viral G-protein-coupled receptor and Kaposi's sarcoma: a model of paracrine neoplasia?, *J. Exp. Med.* **191(3)**, 417–421.

153. Munshi, N., Ganju, K.R., Avraham, S., Mesri, E.A., and Groopman, J.E. (1999) Kaposi's sarcoma-associated herpesvirus-encoded G protein-coupled receptor activation of c-Jun amino-terminal kinase/stress-activated protein kinase and lyn kinase is mediated by related adhesion focal tyrosine kinase/proline-rich tyrosine kinase 2. *J. Biol. Chem.* **274(45)**, 31,863–31,867.

154. Bais, C., Santomasso, B., Coso, O., Arvanitakis, L., Raaka, E.G., Gutkind, J.S., et al. (1998) G-protein coupled receptor of Kaposi's sarcoma-associated herpesvirus is a viral oncogene and angiogenesis activator. *Nature* **391(6662)**, 86–89.

155. Sodhi, A., Montaner, S., Patel, V., Zohar, M., Bais, C., Mesri, E.A., et al. (2000) The Kaposi's sarcoma-associated herpes virus G protein-coupled receptor up-regulates vascular endothelial mitogen-activated protein kinase and p38 pathways acting on hypoxia-inducible factor 1 alpha. *Cancer Res.* **60(17)**, 4873–4880.

156. Burger, M., Burger, J.A., Hoch, R.C., Oades, Z., Takamori, H., and Schraufstatter, I.U. (1999) Point mutation causing consitutive signaling of CXCR2 leads to transforming activity similar to Kaposi's sarcoma herpesvirus-G protein-coupled receptor. *Immunology* **163**, 2017–2022.

157. Lupu-Meiri, M., Silver, R.B., Simons, A.H., Gershengorn, M.C., and Oron, Y. (2000) Constitutive signaling by Kaposi's sarcoma-associated herpesvirus G-protein-coupled receptor desensitizes calcium mobilizaton by other receptors. *J. Biol. Chem.* **276(10)**, 7122–7128.

158. Rosenkilde, M.M., Kledal, T.N., Brauner-Osborne, E., and Schwartz, T.W. (1999) Agonists and inverse agonists for the herpesvirus 8-encoded constitutively active seven-transmembrane oncogene product, ORF-74. *J. Biol. Chem.* **274(2)**, 956–961.

159. Geras-Raaka, E., Varma, A., Ho, H., Clark-Lewis, I., and Gershengorn, M.C. (1998) Human interferon-gamma-inducible protein 10 (IP-10) inhibits constitutive signaling of Kaposi's sarcoma-associated herpesvirus G protein-coupled receptor. *J. Exp. Med.* **188(2)**, 405–408

160. Rosenkilde, M.M., Kledal, T.N., Holst, P.J., and Schwartz, T.W. (2000) Selective elimination of high constitutive activity or chemokine binding in the human herpesvirus 8 encoded seven transmembrane oncogene orf74. *J. Biol. Chem.* **275(34)**, 26,309–26,315.

161. Gershengorn, M.C., Geras-Raaka, E., Varma, E., and Clark-Lewis, I. (1998) Chemokines activate Kaposi's sarcoma-associated herpesvirus G protein-coupled receptor in mammalian cells in culture. *J. Clin. Invest.* **102**, 1469–1472.

162. Yen-Moore, A., Hudnall, S.D., Rady, P.L., Wagner, R.F., Jr., Moore, T.O., et al. (1999) Differential expression of the HHV-8 vGCR cellular homolog gene in AIDS-associated and classic Kaposi's sarcoma: potential role of HIV-1 tat. *Virology* **267**, 247–251.

163. Kirshner, J.R., Staskus, K., Haase, A., Lagunoff, M., and Ganem, D. (1999) Expression of the open reading frame 74 (G-protein-coupled receptor) gene of Kaposi's sarcoma (KS)-associated herpesvirus: implications for KS pathogenesis. *J. Virol.* **73**, 6006–6014.

164. Yang, B.T., Chen, S.C., Leach, M.W., Manfra, D., Homey, B., Wiekowski, M., et al. (2000) Transgenic expression of the chemokine receptor encoded by human herpesvirus 8 induces an angioproliferative disease resembling Kaposi's Sarcoma. *J. Exp. Med.* **191**, 445–454

165. Telford, E.A., Watson, M.S., Aird, H.C., Perry, J., and Davison, A.J. (1995) The DNA sequence of equine herpesvirus 2. *J. Mol. Biol.* **249**, 520–528.

166. Virgin, H.W., Latreille, P., Wamsley, P., Hallsworth, K., Weck, K.E., Dal Canto, A.J., and Speck, S.H. (1997) Complete sequence and genomic analysis of murine gammaherpesvirus 68. *J. Virol.* **71(8)**, 5894–5904

167. Camarda, G., Spinetti, G., Bernardini, G., Mair, C., Davis-Poynter, N., Capogrossi, M.C., et al. (1999) The equine herpesvirus 2 E1 open reading frame encodes a functional chemokine receptor. *J. Virol.* **73**, 9843–9848

168. Sunil-Chandra, N.P., Arno, J., Fazakerley, J., and Nash, A.A. (1994) Lymphoproliferative disease in mice infected with murine gammaherpesvirus 68. *Am. J. Pathol.* **145(4)**, 818–826.

169. Virgin, H.W. and Speck, S.H. (1999) Unraveling immunity to g-herpesviruses: a new model for understanding the role of immunity in chronic virus infection. *Curr. Opin. Immunol.* **11**, 371–379.

170. Massung, R.F., Jayarama, V., and Moyer, R.W. (1993) DNA sequence analysis of conserved and unique regions of swinepox virus: identification of genetic elements supporting phenotypic observations including a novel G protein-coupled receptor homologue. *Virology* **197(2)**, 511–528.

171. Cao, J.X., Gershon, P.D., and Black, D.N. (1995) Sequence analysis of HindIII Q2 fragment of capripoxvirus reveals a putative gene encoding a G-protein-coupled chemokine receptor homologue. *Virology* **209(1)**, 207–212.

20

Chemokines and Chemokine Receptors in HIV Infection

Paolo Lusso

1. INTRODUCTION

Human immunodeficiency virus (HIV), the causative agent of the acquired immunodeficiency syndrome (AIDS), is a member of the *Lentiviridae* subfamily of retroviruses *(1)*. HIV is a complex retrovirus that contains a diploid RNA genome, approx 9600 nucleotides in length. In addition to the typical retroviral genes (*gag, pol, env*), the HIV genome contains several nonstructural genes encoding small regulatory proteins that modulate viral expression and play an important role in the interaction with the infected host *(1)*. Three branches in the phylogenetic tree of HIV-1 have been defined: M (main), N (new), and O (outlier). Among them, group M is the most widespread, being responsible for more than 99% of the infections worldwide. At least nine distinct genotypes (or clades) have been identified within group M (labeled A through K), as well as a growing number of intermediate genotypes, chimeric viruses most likely resulting from mixed infections in endemic areas *(2)*.

Both in vitro and in vivo, HIV infects primarily T-lymphocytes of the CD4+ subtype, as well as cells of the mononuclear phagocytic system, although many other cell types are likely to play a role in the viral spread and pathogenic effects. For example, dendritic cells seem to be critical for mucosal transmission of HIV by binding viral particles via surface lectinlike molecules, such as DC-SIGN, and by transporting them to regional lymph nodes *(3)*. Infection with HIV invariably results in viral persistence lasting for the entire lifetime of the individual. However, the natural course of the infection is commonly slow, with a mean time of progression to symptomatic disease, in the absence of therapy, of more than 8 yr after primary infection. Thus, in most patients, there is a long asymptomatic phase during which an apparent equilibrium is reached between the pathogen and the host, even though viral replication is never fully suppressed and subtle immunological abnormalities can be consistently detected *(4)*.

It is generally believed that the level of HIV expression in vivo depends on a balance among conflicting forces, some of which favor viral replication, whereas others keep it under control. The cytokine network has been implicated as a major factor controlling the ability of HIV to spread productively throughout the body *(5)*. The interactions among HIV, cytokines, and immune system cells form a very intricate web that has only partially been unraveled and that may hold a key to understanding some of the basic mechanisms of HIV-induced pathogenesis, as well as to identifying novel pathways toward effective therapies and vaccines. Within the realm of cytokines, however, a unique place is occupied by chemokines (*chemo*tactic cyto*kines*) that entertain a very intimate and unprecedented relation with HIV *(6)*. Indeed, the evolutionary choice of HIV to exploit chemokine receptors as critical gateways for gaining access into cells *(7)* has turned chemokines, the physiologi-

From: *Cytokines and Chemokines in Infectious Diseases Handbook*
Edited by: M. Kotb and T. Calandra © Humana Press Inc., Totowa, NJ

cal ligands of such receptors, into natural antiviral agents that seem to play a fundamental role in modulating the course of HIV infection.

The chemokine superfamily encompasses a large number of small (approx 8 kDa) cytokines involved in the development and homeostasis of different organ systems, particularly the hematopoietic system, as well as in the generation of both innate and adaptive immune responses *(8)*. Furthermore, chemokines may play a role in angiogenesis and tissue repair mechanisms. Four families of chemokines have been recognized, each showing a distinctive cysteine motif: the CXC (or α family, characterized by two N-terminal cysteines separated by a single amino acid residue, the CC (or β) family, in which the two cysteines are contiguous, the C (or γ family, featuring a single-cysteine motif, and the CX_3C (or δ family, in which the two cysteines are separated by three intervening residues *(8)*. Functionally, two major groups of chemokines can be distinguished: the so-called "housekeeping" or homeostatic chemokines, which are generally expressed constitutively under physiological conditions and play an essential role in development and homeostasis, and the proinflammatory chemokines, which are typically inducible and play an essential role in inflammation and immune responsiveness. Chemokines recognize and activate cellular receptors belonging to the seven-transmembrane-domain, G-protein-coupled superfamily *(9)*. Intracellular signaling through chemokine receptors is generally mediated by heterotrimeric G-proteins that activate different cascades of signal conduction. A characteristic feature of the chemokine system is a remarkable degree of redundancy, with several chemokines recognizing a single receptor and several receptors recognized by a single chemokine. On the basis of ligand specificity, chemokine receptors can be classified into three major groups: specific (featuring a single high-affinity ligand), shared (with multiple ligands within a single chemokine family), and promiscuous (with multiple ligands within different families) *(9)*. In addition to cellular chemokines and receptors, virus-encoded homologs have been described *(10)*. Generally, these viral chemokines and chemokine receptors are genetically reprogrammed in order to function as either decoys or other molecular devices to fight the immune system and/or alter the life-span and activation state of infected cells *(10)*.

This chapter is focused on the extraordinary convergence between the fields of HIV and chemokines, which has led to a more precise understanding of the mechanism of HIV entry into cells and has opened new avenues for the development of effective strategies to fight AIDS, the most dreadful epidemics of the last century.

2. 1995–1996: CHEMOKINES ENCOUNTER HIV

The first connection between HIV and chemokines was established in December 1995, when Cocchi and colleagues identified three chemokines of the CC family, namely RANTES, macrophage inflammatory protein (MIP)-1α, and MIP-1β, as specific inhibitors of both human (HIV-1 and HIV-2) and simian (SIV) immunodeficiency viruses *(11)*, culminating a long quest for the identification of the CD8[+] T-cell-derived soluble HIV-suppressive factors that had been postulated almost a decade earlier by Walker and colleagues *(12)*. Shortly thereafter, in May 1996, Feng and colleagues, who were independently investigating the nature of cellular determinants of HIV susceptibility, identified a chemokine-receptorlike molecule, initially referred to as "fusin," as a critical cofactor (or "coreceptor") for HIV-1 entry into cells *(13)*. The extraordinary time coincidence of these two seminal discoveries triggered an authentic chain reaction of experimental observations that permitted one to lift the veil, within a period of only a few months, on several long-unsolved questions in HIV biology.

2.1. A Chain Reaction of "Breakthroughs"

In the original report on the HIV-suppressive activity of RANTES, MIP-1α, and MIP-1β *(11)*, the three chemokines were described as being selectively inhibitory for one of the two major biological subsets of HIV-1 isolates, variously defined as non-syncytia-inducer, slow/low, or macrophage-tropic, which are generally unable to grow in continuous T-cell lines *(14)*. Conversely, CXCR4/fusin was found to serve as an entry cofactor exclusively for T-cell-line-tropic (syncytia-inducer, rapid/ high or T-cell-tropic) HIV-1 strains *(13)*. Thus, it was obvious that two elements were missing to complete the picture. Again, with a striking time coincidence, a novel chemokine receptor with the ability to selectively bind RANTES, MIP-1α and MIP-1β, designated CCR5, was independently reported in the early spring of 1996 by two groups, one led by Parmentier in Belgium and one by Murphy in the United States *(15,16)*. Capitalizing on these reports, five independent research groups rushed to the identification of CCR5 as the major coreceptor used by non-T-cell-line-tropic HIV-1 isolates *(7)*. Prompted by this startling "domino effect," the CXC chemokine SDF-1 was swiftly identified as a specific ligand for fusin *(17,18)* that was thenceforth renamed CXCR4. Several other potential HIV coreceptors (i.e., CCR2b, CCR3, CCR8, CX_3CR1, GPR1, STRL33/Bonzo, GPR15/ BOB, APJ, and the LT_{B4} receptor) were identified both during 1996 and in the following years using in vitro assays of coreceptor function *(7)*, but their in vivo biological relevance is still under scrutiny.

Thus, before the end of 1996, the picture was virtually complete, showing two major HIV coreceptors, CCR5 and CXCR4, that can be specifically blocked by their physiological ligands. Finally, the last major fruit of this extraordinary season was the discovery of a genetic trait—a deletion within the coding sequence of the *CCR5* gene (CCR5-Δ32) that, in the homozygous form, confers near-complete protection from HIV infection *(19,20)*, providing the first conclusive evidence that resistance to HIV can be genetically determined.

2.2. A New Classification System for HIV-1

The observation that HIV-1 isolates differ in their ability to use two chemokine receptors (CCR5 and CXCR4) provided a key to elucidate the physiological basis of the biological variability of HIV-1, which was recognized for more than a decade *(14)*. A novel classification system was therefore proposed, based on the ability of individual isolates to use either CCR5 alone (CCR5-using or R5 variants), CXCR4 alone (CXCR4-using or X4 variants), or both CCR5 and CXCR4 simultaneously (dual-tropic or X4R5 variants) *(7)*. This function-based classification system has progressively replaced the old (and inaccurate) nomenclature that identified clear-cut functional groups of isolates based on their cellular tropism (T-cell-tropic vs macrophage-tropic) or the ability to induce giant multinucleated cell formation (syncytia-inducer vs non-syncytia-inducer), whereas it is now evident that these biological properties, with the exception of the ability to grow in continuous T-cell lines, are essentially shared by all the different subtypes of HIV-1 isolates.

2.3. New Insights into the Mechanism of HIV Entry

The recognition that chemokine receptors serve as critical coreceptors for both primate and feline immunodeficiency viruses has led to a better understanding of the process of viral entry into cells. According to the currently accepted model, HIV sequentially interacts with two cellular receptors, CD4 and a chemokine receptor—a strategy that allows the effective concealment and protection of conserved, antibody-vulnerable envelope elements. The virion surface exposes protein spikes formed by the oligomeric aggregation of the envelope glycoproteins, most likely in a trimeric form *(21)*. The initial interaction occurs with CD4 and involves the external envelope glycoprotein, gp120. The precise contact interface between CD4 and gp120 has been recently mapped with the solution of the X-ray crystal structure of a trimolecular complex formed by a truncated, variable loop-deleted HIV-1 gp120 core, a two-domain fragment of human CD4 and a single-chain neutralizing human antibody that recognizes a gp120 region widely overlapping with the putative coreceptor-binding site *(22)*. The CD4-binding site is located in a recessed cavity at the junction between the two major domains of gp120 (inner and outer, with respect to the structure of the trimer), which partly explains its poor immunogenicity in both naturally infected patients and vaccinated subjects. Binding to CD4 induces dramatic conformational changes in gp120 that result in the creation, stabilization, or exposure of previously cryptic structures, including a so-called "bridging sheet" that contains the primary site for coreceptor contact. Thus, the coreceptor-binding affinity of unbound gp120 is low, but it dramatically increases when gp120 is bound to CD4 *(22)*. In turn, binding to the chemokine receptor displaces gp120 from the central axis of the oligomer, allowing the transmembrane envelope glycoprotein, gp41, to undergo a series of conformational changes leading to the exposure of its amino-terminal "fusion domain," to the formation of a fusion-active "hairpin" structure, and, eventually, to the fusion between the viral and cellular membranes *(21)*. Each of these discrete steps represents a potential target for novel therapeutic agents capable of blocking the HIV entry/fusion process, as well as of novel strategies for the development of protective vaccines. Unfortunately, the production of antibodies against these conformation-dependent envelope structures, even during natural infection, is rather inefficient.

3. CHEMOKINE RECEPTORS IN HIV INFECTION: PIVOTAL ROLE OF CCR5

At all stages of the infection, the ability of HIV to replicate in the host is critically dependent upon the availability of specific coreceptors on the membrane of specific cellular subsets, as wells as upon their differential utilization by the viral strains circulating in the body. Thus, any genotypic or phenotypic host factors modulating the expression of chemokine receptors and their chemokine ligands can markedly affect the transmission, the tissue tropism and, ultimately, the pathogenic effects of HIV.

3.1. Genetic Polymorphisms of HIV Coreceptors: Effects on Viral Transmission and Pathogenesis

Soon after the connection between HIV and the chemokine world was established, genetic studies on individuals who remain uninfected despite frequent unprotected sexual contacts with HIV-infected partners led to the identification of a genetic trait—CCR5-Δ32/Δ32—that confers a high degree of protection from HIV infection *(19,20)*. The CCR5-Δ32 allele is characterized by a 32-base-pair deletion within the coding sequence of the *CCR5* gene. This deletion causes a reading frame shift that introduces a premature stop codon, resulting in a defective receptor that is not even expressed on the cellular surface. Only a handful of cases of CCR5-Δ32 homozygotes infected with HIV has been reported, and the infectious viral strains were consistently expressing an X4 phenotype *(23,24)*. By contrast, heterozygotes CCR5-Δ32/+, whose cells express reduced levels of CCR5, are not endowed with a reduced risk of infection, although their disease course is delayed *(19)*. These observations clearly attest to the central role of CCR5 in HIV infection. It is remarkable that the complete absence of CCR5 in CCR5-Δ32/Δ32 subjects is not associated with any disease or developmental problem, most likely as a result of the redundancy of the chemokine system *(8,9)*. This fascinating "experiment of nature" provides an important rationale for pursuing CCR5-targeted therapeutic strategies.

A second CCR5 polymorphism that introduces a premature stop codon, CCR5-m303, was described in exposed uninfected subjects, although no homozygotes have so far been identified and, thus, HIV resistance was only seen in double heterozygotes CCR5-Δ32/m303 *(25)*. Several other genetic polymorphisms, in both coding and noncoding regions of chemokine-receptor genes (CCR2, CCR5, CX_3CR1), have been linked to measurable effects on the pace (either slower or faster) of HIV disease progression in large cohort studies *(26)*. However, none was associated with resistance to HIV infection and, furthermore, some of these associations remain controversial. One of the most solid observations involves a variant allele of the CCR2 gene (*CCR2-64I*), which was linked to a slower progression to AIDS. Such mutation is not *per se* biologically relevant, because CCR2 is not an important HIV coreceptor, but it is in linkage dysequilibrium with a polymorphism in the CCR5 promoter region (59653-T), which is apparently associated with a reduced expression of CCR5 *(27)*.

Preliminary evidence indicates that chemokine-receptor alleles may also influence the response to antiretroviral therapy *(28)*, suggesting that chemokine-receptor genetic testing could be useful for identifying patients at risk of therapeutic failure.

3.2. In Vivo Utilization of Coreceptors by HIV-1

Despite the considerable number of chemokine receptors and related orphan molecules that, in vitro, can function as HIV or SIV coreceptors, a large body of evidence indicates that only two molecules, CCR5 and CXCR4, play a major role in vivo *(29)*. In particular, CCR5 is the most widely used coreceptor among wild HIV-1 isolates, whereas CXCR4 is used by a more restricted range of viral strains, with some variability among different viral clades. In contrast, there is still debate on the possible biological significance of some "minor" coreceptors in specific anatomical sites or during specific phases of the infection *(7)*. During the natural history of clade-B HIV-1 infection, the virus evolution follows a characteristic pattern, with the invariable predominance of R5 strains during the early clinical stages *(30)*. Subsequently, a "phenotypic switch" to CXCR4 usage may occur, often associated with increasing coreceptor promiscuity, generally at the time when the first immunological and clinical signs of disease progression appear *(30)*. The emergence of X4 strains has long been recognized as a negative prognostic factor *(14)*. However, even within clade B (which is dominant in North America and Europe) in which X4 strains are generally more prevalent than in other clades, a viral phenotypic switch is observed in only about 50% of the subjects *(14,31)*. This proportion is markedly lower in other clades, such as clade C (10–15%) *(32,33)*. Moreover, the acquisition of CXCR4 usage is rarely associated with a loss of CCR5 usage. Altogether, these observations demonstrate that, at variance with a diffused belief, the emergence of CXCR4-tropic variants is not a requirement for the development of AIDS. Thus, the traditional concept that X4 (syncytia-inducer) HIV-1 variants are inherently more aggressive and pathogenic than R5 ones is currently under revision. In this respect, an important argument is provided by the clinical observations in a few HIV-infected CCR5-Δ32 homozygotes. Although in subjects with wild-type CCR5, an early switch to CXCR4 usage is invariably associated with a high viral load and a rapid disease progression, infected CCR5-Δ32/Δ32 subjects, who harbor CXCR4-using strains since the onset of infection, show no increase in viral load nor rapid progression to AIDS *(24)*.

Despite the extraordinary advancements in this area, several questions regarding the in vivo evolution of HIV-1 remain unsolved. Why are the transmission and the early-stage replication of HIV-1 so obviously skewed in favor of CCR5 usage? Why do the CXCR4-using strains fail to emerge for several years or decades even though CXCR4 usage can be acquired by small amino acid changes within the variable loops of gp120, most notably the V3 loop, and in spite of the striking infidelity of the HIV replication machinery? The most reasonable explanation for this apparent paradox is the existence, in vivo, of a strong negative selective pressure against the utilization of CXCR4 by HIV. Such pressure would then progressively disappear when the immune system starts to lose its functional competence. However, the nature of the putative selective factor(s) is still largely unknown. Although the CXCR4 ligand, SDF-1, may hinder the mucosal transmission of X4 variants, it is unlikely to play a selective role after the establishment of persistent infection (*see* Section 4). Another possible mechanism is related to the documented preferential association between CD4 and CCR5 on the cell surface, even in cells coexpressing CXCR4 *(34)*. Because CCR5 is expressed by interleukin (IL)-2-stimulated, proliferating CD4$^+$ T-cells, which likely constitute the major source of virus reproduction in vivo, this skewed composition of the HIV-receptor complex would selectively favor the replication and spread of R5 strains.

4. ROLE OF CHEMOKINES IN HIV-INFECTED PATIENTS: A NATURAL MECHANISM OF PROTECTION?

The evolutionary choice of CCR5 as a primary entry coreceptor renders HIV vulnerable to the inhibitory action of its natural ligands, RANTES, MIP-1α, and MIP-1β, three highly diffused chemokines of the proinflammatory group, which are rapidly produced in response to a variety of inflammatory stimuli, including persistent HIV infection. Llikewise, the endogenous production of

Table 1
HIV-Inhibitory Chemokines

Chemokines	High-affinity receptors	HIV-variant specificity	Biological relevance
RANTES	CCR3, CCR5	R5	Major
MIP-1α, MIP-1β	CCR5	R5	Major
SDF-1	CXCR4	X4	Major
MCP-1, 2, 3, 4	CCR2b	X4,R5	Minor
Eotaxin	CCR3	X4,R5	Minor
I-309	CCR8	X4,R5	Minor
Fractalkine	CX$_3$CR1	X4	Minor
Apelin	APJ	X4	Minor
CXCR16	STRL33/Bonzo	X4	Minor
LARC	CCR6[a]	X4,R5	Minor
MDC	CCR4[a]	X4,R5	Minor

[a]CCR4 and CCR6 are not known to serve as HIV coreceptors; therefore, the inhibitory action of their ligand chemokines has been attributed to indirect mechanisms.

SDF-1, a "housekeeping" chemokine that is constitutively expressed in selected anatomical sites, may profoundly influence the transmission and spread of the less frequent biological variants of HIV, which use CXCR4. In addition to these major HIV-inhibitory chemokines, other members of the superfamily can modulate HIV infection (*see* Table 1), at least in some experimental systems, either by blocking minor HIV coreceptors (e.g., I309) (Malnati et al., unpublished results) or by indirect (still unknown) mechanisms (e.g., MDC) *(35)*. However, the biological relevance of these second-line HIV-inhibitory chemokines in the course of HIV infection remains, at present, uncertain.

4.1. Genetic Polymorphisms of Chemokine Genes: Effects on Disease Progression

Indirect evidence supporting an in vivo regulatory role of the chemokines RANTES and SDF-1 in the course of HIV infection came from genetic studies performed in large patient cohorts. As seen for chemokine receptors, genetic polymorphisms of the RANTES- and SDF-1-encoding genes have been implicated as constitutive factors that may influence the pace of HIV disease progression. In particular, genetic variants of the RANTES promoter that may increase the basal production of the chemokine have been associated with a slower progression to AIDS *(36,37)*. Strikingly, however, the same variants were suggested to favor the transmission of HIV *(37)*, an effect possibly related to the induction of a "proinflammatory" milieu at the mucosal level. In the case of SDF-1, homozygosity for the SDF-1 3' A allele, a polymorphism within the 3' untranslated region of the gene, has been linked to a slower progression of HIV disease *(26)*, although the results of a recent meta-analysis have challenged this conclusion *(38)*.

4.2. Chemokines as Natural HIV Antagonists: In Vivo Expression and Correlation with Disease Progression

Since the discovery of the HIV-suppressive activity of chemokines, it has immediately become evident that these natural substances could provide an important in vivo mechanism of protective immunity against HIV-1. Chemokine-mediated inhibition of HIV-1 appears to result from a combination of two different mechanisms: direct receptor interference and receptor downmodulation. Thus, the endogenous production of chemokines in lymphoid tissue, mucosae, and other tissues may represent a critical factor for the in vivo transmission and spread of the infection. An increased expression of RANTES, MIP-1α, and MIP-1β was documented in HIV-infected lymph nodes, with particularly elevated concentrations of RANTES in T-cell-dependent extrafollicular areas *(39)*. Similarly, overexpression of CCR5-binding chemokines was reported in HIV-1-infected subjects, both in vivo and ex vivo, with a general correlation between higher chemokine levels and early stages of infection or lack of disease progression *(40–44)*. It has to be emphasized that ex vivo studies, particularly when cells are stimulated with antigens or mitogens, primarily measure the functional reservoir of chemokine secretion, rather than the actual level of secretion occurring in vivo. Regardless, these chemokines may provide an effective control on the local spread of the most prevalent HIV-1 strains, those using CCR5, thereby potentially contributing to the typically slow pace of disease progression observed in most infected individuals. Although the exact mechanisms underlying the enhanced secretion of CCR5-binding chemokines in the course of HIV infection are still unknown at present, the current evidence supports the hypothesis of a complementary action of both cognate and innate immune responses. The former consist of antigen-specific CD4$^+$ and CD8$^+$ T-cell responses, which are known to be associated with the secretion of inflammatory chemokines *(43,44)*; the latter include less well-defined native responses to chronic inflammation, which involve a wider range of cell types and can be induced by HIV itself, as well as by other concurrent infections *(45)*.

As mentioned earlier, the CXCR4 ligand, SDF-1, may play a role in selectively hindering the transmission and spread of CXCR4-using HIV-1 strains. This chemokine is, indeed, highly expressed in the epithelium of the genital mucosa, as well as in the lamina propria of the small intestine, where HIV actively replicates during primary infection *(46)*. By contrast, the endogenous secretion of SDF-1 in blood cells and lymphoid tissues is generally low and, thus, this chemokine is unlikely to contribute to the selective suppression of X4 variants following the establishment of a persistent systemic infection.

4.3. Role of Chemokines in Vaccine-Elicited Protection from Primate Immunodeficiency Virus Infection

The search for an effective human AIDS vaccine has been so far quite frustrating, although some successes have been achieved in experimental nonhuman primate models *(47)*. However, no consistent and reliable correlates of vaccine-induced protection have been identified. Interestingly, evidence is accumulating to suggest that the level of chemokine secretion, measured either in vivo or ex vivo, may provide a reliable correlate of protection. This novel area of investigation was inaugurated by Lehner et al. in 1996, who measured high amounts of CD8$^+$ T cell-derived soluble SIV-suppressive factors, mainly consisting of CCR5-binding chemokines, in protected macaques that had received a targeted iliac-lymph-node SIV subunit vaccine *(48)*. Similar results were subsequently obtained in other animal studies using a variety of immunization protocols *(29)*. Of note, CCR5 and its ligands are preferentially associated with Th1-polarized responses, which are essential in the control of intracellular pathogens like retroviruses. Again, a cooperative effect of native and cognate immune mechanisms has been postulated in the generation of this chemokine response, with the participation of both antigen-specific and nonspecific secretive cells *(29)*. Remarkably, a similar phenotype has been linked with natural resistance to HIV, as suggested by the high prevalence of a high-RANTES, low-CCR5 phenotype in exposed, uninfected subjects, associated with Th1 polarization and decreased susceptibility of CD4$^+$ T-cells to HIV-1 infection *(49)*.

5. CHEMOKINES AS NEW THERAPEUTIC PRINCIPLES AGAINST HIV

The encounter between HIV and the chemokine system has opened new perspectives for the therapy of AIDS. The need for an improvement of the current drug-combination regimens, based on viral enzyme (i.e., reverse transcriptase and protease) inhibitors, is underscored by the important drawbacks and limitations that still characterize these therapies, including rapid rebound after withdrawal, increasing emergence and transmission of multidrug resistance, often severe side effects, difficulties in schedule compliance, and, most importantly, lack of virus eradication even after long-term effective treatment *(50)*. Although all of the currently licensed antiretroviral drugs block HIV after its penetration into the target cell, coreceptor inhibitors would target the early interactions between the virus and the cell membrane, thereby locking HIV outside its target cells. Thus, the introduction of CCR5-targeted agents as components of a multidrug cocktail could be extremely valuable, particularly during the early phase of the infection, when aggressive therapeutic regimens might have the greatest long-term impact on virus control and, ultimately, eradication. At present, no coreceptor-targeted drug is yet available for clinical use, but a few compounds have already shown promising results in preclinical studies.

One of the major hurdles on the way toward developing safe and effective coreceptor inhibitors is the risk of interfering with the physiology of the chemokine system, thereby causing potentially harmful side effects. This risk is of particular concern when targeting housekeeping chemokine receptors, such as CXCR4, that are involved in vital homeostatic functions. Conversely, the use of proinflammatory chemokine agonists may result in inflammatory side effects. In addition, one has to consider that the seven-transmembrane-domain, G-protein-coupled receptor superfamily, to which chemokine receptors belong, is widely distributed in higher organisms, with vital molecules in nearly every system. Thus, a critical issue is the selectivity of candidate drug inhibitors, which must bind to the target chemokine receptor but not to other related receptors in the body.

5.1. Inhibitors of CCR5

Because of the pivotal role it plays in the transmission and spread of HIV-1 in vivo, the CCR5 coreceptor represents the prime target for new therapeutic strategies *(29)*, also in consideration of the apparent lack of immunologic alterations associated with its congenital deficiency. Different approaches to target CCR5 have been proposed, with particular emphasis on the need to produce nonsignaling molecules in order to avoid inflammatory side effects, as well as putative enhancing effects on the replication of X4 HIV strains *(51)*. Another issue that has attracted considerable attention is the risk that, by blocking the CCR5-mediated viral entry pathway, one would exert a selective pressure on HIV, favoring the acquisition of CXCR4 usage and, thereby, accelerating the disease progression. A switch toward CXCR4 usage has indeed been observed in a few infected chimeric severe combined immunodeficiency (SCID) mice, repopulated with human peripheral blood mononuclear cells, upon treatment with modified RANTES analogs *(52)*. However, this concern may have been largely overemphasized because the strong selective forces that hinder the emergence of CXCR4-using viral strains in asymptomatic HIV-infected patients (*see* Subheading 3.2.) will most likely prevent a phenotypic switch even during administration of CCR5-targeted therapeutic agents.

A list of potential therapeutic agents targeting the CCR5 receptor is presented in Table 2. They include the natural chemokines, either in their native, soluble form *(11)* or with an endoplasmic reticulum-localization tag for intracellular trapping of CCR5 *(53)*, full-length *(54–57)*, or small-peptide *(58)* chemokine derivatives and chemokine-unrelated small molecules *(59,60)*. A strategy that has been widely pursued in order to improve the antiviral activity of native chemokines was the modification of the amino-terminal region, which contains the primary determinants for receptor activation. Chemically modified chemokines such as amino-oxypentane (AOP)-RANTES and *N*-nonanoyl (NNY)-RANTES are powerful R5 HIV inhibitors, with activity in the picomolar to low nanomolar range *(52,54)*, although they generally maintain agonistic functions, associated with a striking ability to downmodulate CCR5 expression. By contrast, RANTES analogs bearing natural amino acid substitutions are generally less potent, but have the advantage of being suitable for use in gene therapy delivery systems. Among the latter, a particularly promising molecule is C1.C5-RANTES, which possesses an increased anti-HIV potency, relative to the wild-type molecule, without agonistic functions on both CCR3 and CCR5 *(57)*.

A different approach is the derivation of small synthetic peptides mimicking the tridimensional structure of the functional regions of CCR5-binding chemokines. Recently, peptides derived from

Table 2
Potential Inhibitors of HIV Entry Targeting Chemokine Receptors

Molecules	Target receptors
RANTES, MIP 1-α, MIP 1-β, LD78β	CCR5
AOP-RANTES, NNY-RANTES	CCR5
C1.C5-RANTES, L-RANTES, RANTES$_{3-68}$, RANTES$_{9-68}$	CCR5
RANTES-derived synthetic peptides	CCR5
TAK-779 (quaternary ammonium derivative)	CCR5
SCH-C (piperazine derivative)	CCR5
E913 (spirodiketopiperazine derivative)	CCR5
SDF 1-α	CXCR4
Met-SDF-1	CXCR4
SDF-1-derived synthetic peptides	CXCR4
T22, T134, T-140, TC-14012 (polyphemusin derivatives)	CXCR4
ALX40-4C	CXCR4
AMD3100, AMD3329 (bicyclam analogs)	CXCR4
1-Deoxynojirimycin (saccharide decoy)	CXCR4
Intrakines (RANTES, SDF-1)	CCR5,CXCR4
Anticoreceptor antibodies (humanized)	CCR5,CXCR4
NSC 651016 (distamycin analogue)	CCR5, CXCR4
Baicalin (flavonoid derivative)	CCR5, CXCR4

the N-loop region of RANTES were shown to block HIV-1 infection and fusion, as well as to antagonize RANTES in a lymphocyte chemotaxis assay *(58)*, formally demonstrating that the antiviral and signaling functions of RANTES can be uncoupled. Interestingly, a retroinverted D-peptide mimetic, inherently resistant to digestion by proteases and, thus, potentially more stable in vivo, showed an HIV- and chemotaxis-inhibitory activity similar to that of its L-counterpart *(58)*. Although linear peptides based on the natural amino acid sequence generally possess a low specific activity, this information could be instrumental for the design of highly potent small-peptide inhibitors. Indeed, the lesson that we can learn from the tridimensional structure of a naturally selected ligand, such as RANTES, may teach us how to rationally design inhibitors with the best fitness for the target receptor.

Considerable attention, particular by large pharmaceutical industries, is currently focused on nonpeptidic small molecules with the selective ability to bind CCR5. The first nonpeptidic compound reported to display anti-HIV activity was a quaternary ammonium derivative, TAK-779 *(59)*. More recently, a specific oxime-piperidine CCR5 antagonist, SCH-C (SCH 351125), was identified by high-throughput screening *(60)*, which shows a broad and potent antiviral activity in vitro against primary R5 HIV-1 isolates (with specific activity in the low nanomolar range) while having no effect on CXCR4-using strains. Importantly, SCH-C displays a favorable pharmacokinetic profile in rodents and primates, with an oral bioavailability of 50–60% and a serum half-life of 5–6 h. The main potential drawback of this molecule is related to the observation of cardiac side effects (QT prolongation) that might reflect cross-recognition of a CCR5-related receptor molecule expressed in cardiomyocytes. Nevertheless, SCH-C is, at present, the most promising coreceptor-targeted drug for the treatment of HIV infection.

5.2. Inhibitors of CXCR4

Although the exact significance of CXCR4 as a therapeutic target is still debated, several molecules against this receptor are under investigation for potential use in preventing the emergence and spread of CXCR4-using variants in patients with advanced HIV disease *(see* Table 2). Even though SDF-1, the only known CXCR4 ligand, represents an obvious candidate, its specific activity against

HIV-1 is generally low, when compared to that of CCR5-binding chemokines *(30)*, a phenomenon that might be related to a rapid amino-terminal cleavage and functional inactivation by cathepsin G present on the surface of lymphocytes *(61)*. Several peptidic compounds, such as T22, T134, and ALX40-4C, as well as amino-glycoside conjugates of L-arginine, such as R4K and R3G, have been identified as CXCR4 antagonists and display anti-HIV activity in vitro. At present, however, the most potent and specific small-molecule HIV inhibitor targeting CXCR4 is the bicyclam derivative AMD3100 *(62)*. Strikingly, this drug was already recognized as an effective antiviral agent before the discovery of HIV coreceptors and is currently in phase II clinical experimentation.

The major concern in the development of CXCR4-targeted agents is the risk of causing severe side effects related to the crucial role of this housekeeping receptor in organ development and homeostasis. Indeed, both CXCR4 and SDF-1 knockout mice exhibit a lethal phenotype, with severe defects not only in the hematopoietic system, particularly in the B-lymphoid and myeloid compartments, but also in other tissues, such as the heart and the brain *(63,64)*. Moreover, it has to be underscored that a large number of CXCR4-using HIV-1 isolates are promiscuous in nature, as they can penetrate cells via alternative coreceptors, including CCR5 and/or CCR2b, CCR3, CCR8, APJ, or others. Thus, blockade of CXCR4 alone might prove insufficient to limit the in vivo spread of most X4 viral strains.

6. CONCLUSIONS

The extraordinary advances made during the past 5 yr in the field of HIV biology, primarily the elucidation of the complex and intimate interactions that occur between this virus and the chemokine system, have raised a cautious optimism on the possibility of developing increasingly effective strategies for the control of HIV infection. Specifically, with the availability of specific blockers of the two main HIV coreceptors, CCR5 and CXCR4, it will possible to design highly efficacious multidrug therapeutic protocols targeting at least three distinct steps in the viral life cycle: entry, reverse transcription, and maturation. The implementation of such protocols might eventually lead to the achievement of the ultimate goal of antiviral treatment, which is still beyond the reach of the current therapeutic weapons: HIV eradication.

REFERENCES

1. Luciw, P.A. (1996) Human immunodeficiency viruses and their replication, *in Fields Virology* (Fields, B.N., Knipe, D.M., and Howley, P.M. ed.). Lippincott–Raven, Philadelphia, pp. 1881–1952.
2. Essex, M. (1999) Human immunodeficiency viruses in the developing world. *Adv. Virus Res.* **53,** 71–88.
3. Geijtenbeek, T.B., van Vliet, S.J., van Duijnhoven, G.C., Figdor, C.G. and van Kooyk, Y. (2001) DC-SIGN, a dendritic cell-specific HIV-1 receptor present in placenta that infects T cells in trans-a review. *Placenta* **22,** S19–S23.
4. Miedema, F., Petit, A.J., Terpstra, F.G., Schattenkerk, J.K., de Wolf, F., Al, B.J., et al. (1988) Immunological abnormalities in human immunodeficiency virus (HIV)-infected asymptomatic homosexual men. HIV affects the immune system before CD4⁺ T helper cell depletion occurs. *J. Clin. Invest.* **82,** 1908–1914.
5. Poli G. (1999) Cytokines and the human immunodeficiency virus: from bench to bedside. *Eur. J. Clin. Invest.* **29,** 723–732.
6. Lusso, P. and Gallo, R.C. (1997) Chemokines and HIV infection. *Curr. Opin. Infect. Dis.* **10,** 12–17.
7. Berger, E.A., Murphy, P.M., and Farber, J.M. (1999) Chemokine receptors as HIV-1 coreceptors: roles in viral entry, tropism, and disease. *Annu. Rev. Immunol.* **17,** 657–700.
8. Loetscher, P., Moser B., and Baggiolini, M. (2000). Chemokines and their receptors in lymphocyte traffic and HIV infection. *Adv. Immunol.* **74,** 127–180.
9. Premack, B.A. and Schall, T.J. (1996). Chemokine receptors: gateways to inflammation and infection. *Nat. Med.* **2,** 1174–1178.
10. Murphy, P.M. (2001) Viral exploitation and subversion of the immune system through chemokine mimicry. *Nat. Immunol.* **2,** 116–122.
11. Cocchi, F., DeVico, A.L., Garzino-Demo, A., Arya, S.K., Gallo, R.C., and Lusso, P. (1995) Identification of RANTES, MIP-1α, MIP-1β as the major HIV-suppressive factors produced by CD8⁺ T cells. *Science* **270,** 1811–1815.
12. Walker, C.M., Moody, D.J., Stites, D.P., and Levy, J.A. (1986) CD8⁺ lymphocytes can control HIV infection in vitro by suppressing virus replication. *Science* **234,** 1563–1566.
13. Feng, Y., Broder, CC., Kennedy, P.E., and Berger, E.A. (1996) HIV-1 entry cofactor. Functional cDNA cloning of a seven-transmembrane, G protein-coupled receptor. *Science* **272,** 872–877.

14. Koot, M., Keet, I.P., Vos, A.H.V., de Goede, R.E.Y., Roos, M.T.L., Coutinho, R.A., et al. (1993). Prognostic value of HIV-1 syncytium-inducing phenotype for rate of CD4+ cell depletion and progression to AIDS. *Ann. Intern. Med.* **118,** 681–688.

15. Samson, M., Labbe, O., Mollereau, C., Vassart, G., and Parmentier, M. (1996) Molecular cloning and functional expression of a new human CC-chemokine receptor gene. *Biochemistry* **35,** 3362–3367.

16. Combadiere, C., Ahuja, S.K., Tiffany, H.L., and Murphy, P.M. (1996) Cloning and functional expression of CC CKR5, a human monocyte CC chemokine receptor selective for MIP-1α, MIP-1β, and RANTES. *J. Leukocyte Biol.* **60,** 147–152.

17. Oberlin, E., Amara, A., Bachelerie, F., Bessia, C., Virelizier, J.L., Arenzana-Seisdedos, F., et al. (1996) The CXC chemokine SDF-1 is the ligand for LESTR/fusin and prevents infection by T-cell-line-adapted HIV-1. *Nature* **382,** 833–835.

18. Bleul, C.C., Farzan, M., Choe, H., Parolin, C., Clark-Lewis, I., Sodroski, J., et al. (1996) The lymphocyte chemoattractant SDF-1 is a ligand for LESTR/fusin and blocks HIV-1 entry. *Nature* **382,** 829–833.

19. Liu, R., Paxton,W.A., Choe, S., Ceradini, D., Martin, S.R., Horuk, R., et al. (1996) Homozygous defect in HIV-1 coreceptor accounts for resistance of some multiply-exposed individuals to HIV-1 infection. *Cell* **86,** 367–377.

20. Samson, M., Libert, F., Doranz, B.J., Rucker, J., Liesnard, C., Farber, C-M., et al. (1996) Resistance to HIV-1 infection in caucasian individuals bearing mutant alleles of the CCR-5 chemokine receptor gene. *Nature* **382,** 722–725.

21. Chan, D.C. and Kim, P.S. (1998) HIV entry and its inhibition. *Cell* **93,** 681–684.

22. Kwong, P.D., Wyatt, R., Robinson, J., Sweet, R.W., Sodroski, J., and Hendrickson, W.A. (1998) Structure of an HIV gp120 envelope glycoprotein in complex with the CD4 receptor and a neutralizing human antibody. *Nature* **393,** 648–659.

23. Michael, N.L., Nelson, J.A., Kewal Ramani, V.N., Chang, G., O'Brien, S.J., Mascola, J.R., et al. (1998) Exclusive and persistent use of the entry coreceptor CXCR4 by human immunodeficiency virus type 1 from a subject homozygous for CCR5 delta32. *J. Virol.* **72,** 6040–6047.

24. Sheppard, H.W. Celum, C., Michael, N.L., O'Brien, S., Dean, M., Carrington, M., et al. (2002) HIV-1 infection in individuals with the CCR5-Delta32/Delta32 genotype: acquisition of syncytium-inducing virus at seroconversion. *J. Acquired Immune Defic. Syndrome* **29,** 307–313.

25. Quillent, C., Oberlin, E., Braun, J., Rousset, D., Gonzalez-Canali, G., Metais, P., et al. (1998) HIV-1-resistance pheno-type conferred by combination of two separate inherited mutations of CCR5 gene. *Lancet* **351,** 14–18.

26. Hogan, C.M. and Hammer, S.M. (2001) Host determinants in HIV infection and disease. Part 2: genetic factors and implications for antiretroviral therapeutics. *Ann. Intern. Med.* **134,** 978–996.

27. Kostrikis, L.G., Huang, Y., Moore, J.P., Wolinsky, S.M., Zhang, L., Guo, Y., et al. (1998) A chemokine receptor CCR2 allele delays HIV-1 disease progression and is associated with a CCR5 promoter mutation. *Nat. Med.* **4,** 350–353.

28. Lathey, J.L., Tierney, C., Chang, S.Y., D'Aquila, R.T., Bettendorf, D.M., Alexander, H.C., et al. (2001) Associations of CCR5, CCR2, and stromal cell-derived factor 1 genotypes with human immunodeficiency virus disease progression in patients receiving nucleoside therapy. *J. Infect. Dis.* **184,** 1402–1411.

29. Lusso, P. (2000) Chemokines and viruses: the dearest enemies. *Virology* **273,** 228–240.

30. Scarlatti, G., Tresoldi, E., Bjorndal, A., Fredriksson, R., Colognesi, C., Deng, H.K., et al. (1997) In vivo evolution of HIV-1 coreceptor usage and sensitivity to chemokine-mediated suppression. *Nat. Med.* **3,** 1259–1265.

31. deRoda Husman, A.M., van Rij, R.P., Blaak, H., Broersen, S., and Schuitemaker, H. (1999) Adaptation to promiscuous usage of chemokine receptors is not a prerequisite for human immunodeficiency virus type 1 disease progression. *J. Infect. Dis.* **180,** 1106–1115.

32. Peeters, M., Vincent, R., Perret, J.L., Lasky, M., Patrel, D., Liegeois, F., et al. (1999). Evidence of differences in MT2 cell tropism according to genetic subtypes of HIV-1: syncytium-inducing variants seem rare among subtype C HIV-1 viruses. *J. Acquir. Immune Defic. Syndr. Hum. Retrovirol.* **20,** 115–121.

33. Ping, L.H., Nelson, J.A., Hoffman, I.F., Schock, J., Lamers, S.L., Goodman, M., et al. (1999) Characterization of V3 sequence heterogeneity in subtype C human immunodeficiency virus type 1 isolates from Malawi: underrepresentation of X4 variants. *J. Virol.* **73,** 6271–6281.

34. Xiao, X., Wu, L., Stantchev, T.S., Feng, Y.R., Ugolini, S., Chen, H., et al. (1999). Constitutive cell surface association between CD4 and CCR5. *Proc. Natl. Acad. Sci. USA* **96,** 7496–7501.

35. Pal, R., Garzino-Demo, A., Markham, P. D., Burns, J., Brown, M., Gallo, R. C., et al. (1997) Inhibition of HIV-1 infection by the b-chemokine MDC. *Science* **278,** 695–698.

36. Liu, H., Chao, D., Nakayama, E.E., Taguchi, H., Goto, M., Xin, X., et al. (1999) Polymorphism in RANTES chemokine promoter affects HIV-1 disease progression. *Proc. Natl. Acad. Sci. USA* **96,** 4581–4585.

37. McDermott, D.H., Beecroft, M.J., Kleeberger, C.A., Al-Sharif, F.M., Ollier, W.E., Zimmerman, P.A., et al. (2000) Chemokine RANTES promoter polymorphism affects risk of both HIV infection and disease progression in the Multicenter AIDS Cohort Study. *AIDS* **14,** 2671–2678.

38. Ioannidis, J.P.A., Rosenberg, P.S., Goedert, J.J., Ashton, L.J., Benfield, T.L, Buchbinder, S.P., et al. (2001) Effects of CCR5-Δ32, CCR2-64I, and SDF-1 3' A alleles on HIV-1 disease progression: an international meta-analysis of indi-vidual-patient data. *Ann. Intern. Med.* **135,** 782–795.

39. Trumpfheller, C., Tenner-Racz, K., Racz, P., Fleischer, B., and Frosch, S. (1998) Expression of macrophage inflamma-tory protein (MIP)-1alpha, MIP-1beta, and RANTES genes in lymph nodes from HIV+ individuals: correlation with a Th1-type cytokine response. *Clin. Exp. Immunol.* **112,** 92–99.

40. Triozzi, P.L., Bresler, H.S., and Aldrich, W.A. (1998) HIV type 1-reactive chemokine-producing CD8+ and CD4+ cells expanded from infected lymph nodes. *AIDS Res. Hum. Retrovir.* **14,** 643–649.

41. Malnati, M., Tambussi, G., Clerici, E., Polo, S., Algeri, M., Nardese, V., et al. (1997) Increased plasma levels of the C-C chemokine RANTES in patients with primary HIV-1 infection. *J. Biol. Regul. Homeostasis Aging* **11,** 40–42.

42. Cocchi, F., DeVico, A.L., Yarchoan, R., Redfield, R., Cleghorn, F., Blattner, W.A., et al. (2000) Higher macrophage inflammatory protein (MIP)-1alpha and MIP-1beta levels from CD8+ T cells are associated with asymptomatic HIV-1 infection. *Proc. Natl. Acad. Sci. USA* **97,** 13,812–13,827.

43. Garzino-Demo, A., Moss, R.B., Margolick, J.B., Cleghorn, F., Sill, A., Blattner, W.A., et al. (1999) Spontaneous and antigen-induced production of HIV-inhibitory beta-chemokines are associated with AIDS-free status. *Proc. Natl. Acad. Sci. USA* **96,** 11,986–11,991.

44. Ferbas, J., Giorgi, J.V., Amini, S., Grovit-Ferbas, K., Wiley, D.J., Detels, R., and Plaeger, S. (2000) Antigen-specific production of RANTES, macrophage inflammatory protein (MIP)-1alpha, and MIP-1beta in vitro is a correlate of reduced human immunodeficiency virus burden in vivo. *J. Infect. Dis.* **182,** 1247–1250.

45. Grivel, J.C., Ito, Y., Fagà, G., Santoro, F., Shaheen, F., Malnati, M.S., et al. (2001) Suppression of CCR5- but not CXCR4-tropic HIV-1 in lymphoid tissue by human herpesvirus 6. *Nat. Med.* **7,** 1232–1235.

46. Agace, W.W., Amara, A., Roberts, A.I., Pablos, J.L., Thelen, S., Uguccioni, M.G., et al. (2000) Constitutive expression of stromal derived factor-1 by mucosal epithelia and its role in HIV transmission and propagation. *Curr. Biol.* **10,** 325–328.

47. Mascola, J.R. and Nabel, G.J. (2001) Vaccines for the prevention of HIV-1 disease. *Curr. Opin. Immunol.* **13,** 489–495.

48. Lehner, T., Wang,Y., Cranage, M., Bergmeier, L.A., Mitchell, E., Tao, L., et al. (1996) Protective mucosal immunity elicited by targeted iliac lymph node immunization with a subunit SIV envelope and core vaccine in macaques. *Nat. Med.* **2,** 767–775.

49. Paxton, W.A., Liu, R., Kang, S., Wu, L., Gingeras, T.R., Landau, N.R., et al. (1998) Reduced HIV-1 infectability of CD4+ lymphocytes from exposed-uninfected individuals: association with low expression of CCR5 and high production of beta-chemokines. *Virology* **244,** 66–73.

50. Richman, D.D. (2001) HIV chemotherapy. *Nature* **410,** 995–1001.

51. Kinter, A., Catanzaro, A., Monaco, J., Ruiz, M., Justement, J., Moir, S., et al. (1998) CC-chemok ines enhance the replication of T-tropic strains of HIV-1 in CD4+ T cells: role of signal transduction. *Proc. Natl. Acad. Sci. USA* **95,** 11,880–11,885.

52. Mosier, D.E., Picchio, G.R., Gulizia, R.J., Sabbe, R., Poignard, P., Picard, L., et al. (1999) Highly potent RANTES analogues either prevent CCR5-using human immunodeficiency virus type 1 infection in vivo or rapidly select for CXCR4-using variants. *J. Virol.* **73,** 3544–3350.

53. Yang, A.G., Bai, X., Huang, X.F., Yao, C., and Chen, S. (1997) Phenotypic knockout of HIV type 1 chemokine coreceptor CCR-5 by intrakines as potential therapeutic approach for HIV-1 infection. *Proc. Natl. Acad. Sci. USA* **94,** 11,567–1,1572.

54. Simmons, G., Clapham, P.R., Picard, L., Offord, R.E., Rosenkilde, M.M., Schwartz, T.W., et al. (1997) Potent inhibition of HIV-1 infectivity in macrophages and lymphocytes by a novel CCR5 antagonist. *Science* **276,** 276–279.

55. Proost, P., De Meester, I., Schols, D., Struyf, S., Lambeir, A.M., Wuyts, A., et al. (1998) Amino-terminal truncation of chemokines by CD26/dipeptidyl-peptidase IV. Conversion of RANTES into a potent inhibitor of monocyte chemotaxis and HIV-1 infection. *J. Biol. Chem.* **273,** 7222–7227.

56. Ylisastigui, L., Vizzavona, J., Drakopoulou, E., Paindavoine, P., Calvo, C.F., Parmentier, M., et al. (1998) Synthetic full-length and truncated RANTES inhibit HIV-1 infection of primary macrophages. *AIDS* **12,** 977–984.

57. Polo, S., Nardese, V., DeSantis, C., Arcelloni, C., Paroni, R., Sironi, F., et al. (2000) Enhancement of the HIV-1 inhibitory activity of RANTES by modification of the N-terminal region: dissociation from CCR5 activation. *Eur. J. Immunol.* **30,** 3190–3198.

58. Nardese, V., Longhi, R., Polo, S., Sironi, F., Arcelloni, C., Paroni, R., et al. (2001) Structural determinants of HIV-1 blockade and CCR5 recognition in RANTES. *Nat. Struct. Biol.* **8,** 611–615.

59. Baba, M., Nishimura, O., Kanzaki, N., Okamoto, M., Sawada, H., Iizawa, Y., et al. (1999) A small-molecule, nonpeptide CCR5 antagonist with highly potent and selective anti-HIV-1 activity. *Proc. Natl. Acad. Sci. USA* **96,** 5698–5703.

60. Strizki, J.M., Xu, S., Wagner, N.E., Wojcik, L., Liu, J., Hou, Y., et al. (2001) SCH-C (SCH 351125), an orally bioavailable, small molecule antagonist of the chemokine receptor CCR5, is a potent inhibitor of HIV-1 infection in vitro and in vivo. *Proc. Natl. Acad. Sci. USA* **98,** 12,718–12,723.

61. Delgado, M.B., Clark-Lewis, I., Loetscher, P., Langen, H., Thelen, M., Baggiolini, M., et al. (2001) Rapid inactivation of stromal cell-derived factor-1 by cathepsin G associated with lymphocytes. *Eur. J. Immunol.* **31,** 699–707.

62. Schols, D., Struyf, S., Van Damme, J., Este, J.A., Henson, G., and De Clercq, E. (1997) Inhibition of T-tropic HIV strains by selective antagonization of the chemokine receptor CXCR4. *J. Exp. Med.* **186,** 1383–1388.

63. Nagasawa, T., Hirota, S., Tachibana, K., Takakura, N., Nishikawa, S., Kitamura, Y., et al. (1996) Defects of B-cell lymphopoiesis and bone-marrow myelopoiesis in mice lacking the CXC chemokine PBSF/SDF-1. *Nature* **382,** 635–638.

64. Ma, Q., Jones, D., Borghesani, P.R., Segal, R.A., Nagasawa, T., Kishimoto, T., et al. (1998) Impaired B-lymphopoiesis, myelopoiesis, and derailed cerebellar neuron migration in CXCR4- and SDF-1-deficient mice. *Proc. Natl. Acad. Sci. USA* **95,** 9448–9453.

21

Cytokines in Viral Hepatitis

Mala K. Maini and Antonio Bertoletti

1. INTRODUCTION

Hepatitis B (HBV) virus and hepatitis C virus (HCV) are the two major causes of chronic liver inflammation worldwide, leading to cirrhosis and hepatocellular carcinoma. It has been estimated that 300 million people are HBV carriers, with cases particularly concentrated in Asia and Africa. HCV has infected around 100 million people and is the major causative agent of liver disease in the West, with an estimated prevalence of HCV infection in the general U.S. population of around 12% (1,2).

The two infections have very different virological characteristics. HBV, a member of the hepadnavirus family, is a DNA virus that uses a reverse transcriptase for replication from a pregenomic RNA template. The genome of HBV is a circular partially double-stranded DNA molecule and the complete DNA strand is approximately 3200 nucleotides long, containing 4 open reading frames encoding the viral envelope, nucleocapsid, polymerase, and X proteins (2).

Hepatitis C virus is a single-stranded RNA virus of positive polarity with a genome of 9500 nucleotides. It contains a large open reading frame encoding a precursor polyprotein of approximately 3000 amino acids, which is processed to produce structural proteins (core and envelopes 1 and 2) and at least 6 nonstructural proteins (NS2, NS3, NS4A, NS4B, NS5BA, NS5B). HCV shows a similar genetic organization to the flaviviridae and shares some sequence homology with members of this family (3,4).

Despite these differences in genetic organization and replication, both viruses are preferentially hepatotropic, not directly cytopathic, and elicit liver diseases that share a similar natural history. In both infections, disease severity varies greatly from person to person. In some subjects, the immune system is able to completely control infection and clear the virus from the bloodstream either without clinically evident liver disease or with an acute inflammation of the liver (acute hepatitis) that usually resolves without long-term clinical sequelae. Other patients fail to clear the virus and, instead, develop chronic infection. It has been calculated that around 15–25% of subjects infected with HCV will overcome the virus and the remaining 75–85% will develop a chronic infection (1). The rate of HBV chronicity has been estimated to be lower, with less than 10% of adult subjects unable to control the virus after acute infection (5). However, such estimates do not take into account the fact that most acute HBV and HCV infections are clinically inapparent and also that virus-specific antibody, used to calculate the number of infected people, could have different rates of disappearance in the two infections (6). Most patients with chronic HBV or HCV infection do not develop symptoms or life-threatening liver disease, but about 10–20% can develop liver cirrhosis and 1–5% develop a liver cancer called hepatocarcinoma.

From: *Cytokines and Chemokines in Infectious Diseases Handbook*
Edited by: M. Kotb and T. Calandra © Humana Press Inc., Totowa, NJ

In addition to their similar profiles of clinical manifestations, both infections are characterized by a central role for the immune system in the control of virus and in the pathogenesis of liver damage. In both infections, the ability to mount efficient helper and cytotoxic responses seems to be critical in the clearance of virus from the bloodstream (reviewed in refs. *5* and *7–9*). Furthermore, because neither virus is directly cytopathic, the immune system, specifically cytotoxic T-cells, have been implicated not only as the mediators of protection but also as the principal effectors of liver damage *(10)*.

Because most of the functions of the immune system are regulated and mediated by cytokines *(11)*, it is clear that these low-molecular-weight proteins will be involved in several aspects of the pathogenesis of HBV and HCV infection. Three different aspects of the interactions between cytokines and hepatitis viruses will be covered in this chapter:

First, direct cytokine-mediated inhibition of viral replication and the strategies that HCV and HBV have evolved to escape these antiviral effects will be reviewed. Cytokines will then be reviewed in the context of their regulation of the immune system and, therefore, in shaping the antiviral immune response against HBV and HCV. Finally, evidence for the role of different cytokines in mediating liver damage directly will be discussed.

1.1. Direct Antiviral Effect of Cytokines

The best characterized cytokines with known direct antiviral functions are interferon (IFN)-α and IFN-β (type I IFNs), tumor necrosis factor (TNF)-α, and IFN-γ *(12)*. Over 30 genes have been shown to be activated in a cell by IFN-α/β *(13,14)* and the recent advent of oligonucleotide arrays has enabled the identification of many new type I IFN-inducible genes *(15)*. The best characterized IFN-I-induced gene products able to produce a cellular antiviral state are the *(11)* (2'–5') oligoadenylate synthetase, Mx proteins, and double-stranded RNA-activated protein kinase (PKR) *(12,14,16)*. (2'–5') oligoadenylate synthetase seems to exert antiviral activity by the production of a cellular RNAase that degrades viral transcripts, whereas Mxa protein is able to inhibit viral replication by binding to viral ribonucleoprotein complexes *(17)*. Host cell protein synthesis is inhibited by PKR, consequently blocking viral replication.

The antiviral pathways elicited by TNF-α and IFN-γ overlap with those activated by IFN-α and IFN-β *(12)*. TNF-α is a weak antiviral cytokine alone, but is synergistic with IFNs. IFN-γ is also a strong inducer of nitric oxide synthase, which mediates an antiviral effect by modifying a number of molecules essential for replication *(18)*.

1.2. Early Production of Cytokines During Natural HBV and HCV Infection

One of the first defense mechanisms that an infected host is able to mount against viral infections is the production of IFN-α and IFN-β. These cytokines reach very high levels immediately after viral infection and were originally identified as antiviral proteins, even though they also have important immunomodulatory effects. The importance of the IFN-α/β pathway in the early stage of viral infection has been deduced primarily from cell culture systems or experimental infections in mice *(12)*. To date, there is no in vitro culture system able to sustain infection and replication of HBV or HCV *(5,19)*, and it is, therefore, impossible to test directly whether these viruses are strong or weak inducers of cytokines of the innate immune system (IFN-I and TNF-α). Furthermore, the only available animal model of HBV and HCV is the chimpanzee, where these early events of the immune response are difficult to study. Given these limitations, the picture of the early production of cytokines after infection, derived from human studies, is still controversial.

In one study, expression of type I interferon-induced MxA protein was studied as a marker of IFN-α and IFN-β production in subjects with acute hepatitis A, B, and C. Mx-A protein levels were found to be raised in hepatitis A but not in HBV- or HCV-infected subjects in this study, suggesting that HBV and HCV are poor interferon inducers *(20)*. However, in a different study, patients with acute HBV infection were found to harbor large quantities of IFN-α producing cells within the liver *(21)*. One limitation of these studies is that patients are usually studied after the onset of clinical symp-

Table 1
Cytokines Production and Activation of Cytokines Related Genes

	Chronic HBV infection		Chronic HCV infection	
	Cytokine level	Inducible genes	Cytokine level	Inducible genes
IFN-α	↓mRNA *(24)*	↓activation *(24–27)*	↓mRNA *(24)*	↑activation *(25)*
IFN-β	↓mRNA *(24)*	Weak activation *(25)*	↑mRNA *(24)*	↑activation *(25)*
TNF-α	↑production *(28)*	—	↑production *(29,30)*	—
IFN-γ	Preferential Th0 *(31,32)*	↓activation *(25)*	Preferential Th1 *(31,33)*	↑activation *(25,34,35)*

toms. Studies in chimpanzees *(22)* and humans *(23)* have shown that, at least in HBV infection, virus clearance is already almost complete at this stage. Therefore, it is very unlikely that investigations performed in symptomatic hepatitis patients have been able to detect the real early events of the innate immune response such as IFN-α and IFN-β production.

A large number of studies have analyzed activation of innate antiviral pathways in chronically infected patients (*see* Table 1). Enhanced expression of IFN-α and IFN-β-regulated genes has been shown in chronic HCV infection *(25)*. However, a direct analysis of type I interferon mRNA from liver and peripheral blood of chronic HCV patients showed an increase only in mRNA for IFN-β not IFN-α *(24)*. Despite the presence of IFN-α producing cells within the infected liver *(21,36)*, patients with chronic HBV seem to exhibit weaker hepatic activation of IFN-α and IFN-β-regulated genes *(26,27)* than that found in HCV infected subjects *(25)*. In fact, intrahepatic levels of IFN-α and IFN-β in chronic HBV infection have been reported to be identical to levels present within normal livers *(24)*.

These data are in agreement with initial reports showing low levels of interferon in the serum of patients with chronic HBV *(37,38)* and could be explained by the ability of HBV to inhibit IFN-β production *(39)* and block the activation of IFN-α mediated pathways. This inhibition has been explained by the ability of the carboxy-terminal portion of the HBV core antigen to bind to particular DNA sequences in the regulatory elements of IFN-α *(39)*. Furthermore, expression of the terminal part of HBV polymerase protein in transfected human cells has been shown to block IFN pathways *(40)* and could explain the lower activation of IFN-inducible genes in HBV-compared to HCV-infected patients *(25)*. Therefore, even though we are not yet able to depict precisely the dynamics and relative quantities of IFN-α and IFN-β production during HBV and HCV infection, the data generated in humans seem to support a quantitative difference, with a more pronounced activation of the type I IFN system in HCV-infected livers in comparison with HBV-infected livers.

Other cytokines with direct antiviral effects produced during natural infections are TNF-α and IFN-γ. TNF-α could be produced in the first stage of infection by activated monocytes and lymphocytes, whereas IFN-γ is the classical antiviral cytokine produced by the lymphocytes of the adaptive immune system, and its contribution to early events is restricted to production by NK cells *(12,16)*. Production of TNF-α has been observed during HBV *(28,41)* and HCV infection *(29,30)* but because of its weak direct antiviral effect and ability to cause direct cell damage, its has been associated more with the pathogenesis of liver damage. Therefore, this cytokine will be discussed more extensively in the section dedicated to liver injury.

Interferon-γ, in addition to mediating various immunomodulatory functions (discussed below), is the most important antiviral cytokine produced by the cells of the adaptive immune system: helper (CD4) and cytotoxic (CD8) T-lymphocytes *(42,43)*. Antigen-specific T-cells with direct antiviral activity are able to produce IFN-γ (and are defined as having a T-helper or cytotoxic profile type 1 or 0 of cytokine production), whereas cells that do not produce IFN-γ do not have direct antiviral effect (and are defined as having a type 2 cytokine profile) *(44)*. During infection with HBV or HCV, the ability to mount a helper *(45–49)* and cytotoxic T-cell response with a type 1 profile of cytokine production has been linked with successful containment of both infections (reviewed in refs. *7–9* and *50*).

T-Helper cells specific for HBV nucleocapsid antigen and able to produce IFN-γ have been observed in patients able to resolve acute HBV infection *(23,49,51)*. Cytotoxic T-cells present in these subjects are able to produce IFN-γ *(52,53)*, and control of HBV viremia in chronically infected patients is also associated with the ability to expand IFN-γ-producing CD8 cells after recognition of HBV antigens *(54)*. A similar profile of CD4 *(48,55)* and CD8 cells *(56,57)* producing IFN-γ after stimulation with peptides representing HCV epitopes has been observed in patients recovering from acute HCV infection. Conversely, activation of an HCV-specific CD4 response with a type 2 profile of cytokine production seems to play a role in the development of HCV chronicity *(58)*. Therefore, a large body of work indicates that high levels of IFN-γ are produced selectively by virus-specific T-cells in association with control of HBV and HCV. The quantity of these IFN-γ-producing cells, or their ability to expand promptly after antigen-specific encounter, seems to be reduced in chronic HBV and HCV infection (reviewed in refs. *7–9* and *50*). Whether this is the cause or effect of chronicity still needs to be determined.

1.3. Are Cytokines Able to Inhibit HBV and HCV Replication?

What are the relative sensitivities of HBV and HCV viruses to the antiviral effects of cytokines? Have these viruses developed specific mechanisms to counteract cytokine-mediated antiviral effects? A precise answer to these questions would need, as for the analysis of cytokine production, a reliable in vitro culture system or a well-characterized animal model, both of which are currently still lacking. However, the transgenic mouse model of HBV infection developed in the laboratory of Frank Chisari, has highlighted some peculiar features of the effect of cytokines on HBV and has suggested that these effects could be shared by other viruses that choose hepatocytes as their target cell. In this transgenic mouse model of HBV infection, it has been extensively demonstrated that the intrahepatic induction of IFN-α/β, TNF-α, and IFN-γ downregulates HBV replication *(59)*. Treatment of HBV transgenic mice with a potent inducer of the type I IFN system clears HBV replicative intermediates from the hepatocyte cytoplasm *(60)*. Furthermore, infection of transgenic mice with unrelated hepatotropic viruses is able to inhibit HBV replication by IFN-α/β-dependent mechanisms *(60–62)*. Inhibition of HBV replication could also be achieved by injection of HBV-specific cytotoxic T-lymphocytes, mediated by the secretion of IFN-γ and TNF-α *(63)*. In addition to inhibiting viral replication, this model has shown that cytokines are able to selectively degrade replicating HBV genomes, thereby clearing the virus without the absolute need for destruction of infected cells *(64)*.

Interestingly, clearance of a large proportion of HBV from the liver occurs before the peak of acute liver disease in chimpanzees, demonstrating that noncytopathic antiviral pathways contribute to viral control in an animal model closely related to the human disease *(22)*. A further hint that cytokine-mediated inhibition of HBV replication is operative during human HBV infection comes from results obtained in patients studied before the onset of acute hepatitis *(23)*. In these subjects, the fall in serum HBV-DNA is not proportional to the level of liver damage, suggesting that inhibition of HBV replication without destruction of infected cells is a central mechanism of control. This noncytopathic mechanism of viral clearance is not peculiar to HBV. Effective clearance of duck HBV *(65)* and woodchuck hepatitis virus *(66)*, both hepadnavirus viruses, have also been shown to occur without massive liver lysis. Furthermore, control of murine cytomegalovirus (CMV) infection *(67)* and *Listeria monocytogenes (68)* in the liver seem to be primarily mediated by IFN-γ production rather than perforin-dependent pathways. Lymphochoriomeningitis virus (LCMV) is also cleared from hepatocytes by noncytopathic mechanisms that are not operative in nonparenchymal cells or splenocytes *(69)*.

The possibility that divergent cytokine-mediated antiviral pathways are activated in different cell types has been recently studied by microarray analysis, showing that IFN-γ regulates distinct sets of genes in macrophages and fibroblasts *(70)*. Furthermore, the observation that the IFN-γ and TNF-α-induced downregulation of HBV expression is mediated by a novel RNA-binding protein called LA

(71,72) suggests that this may be a cytokine-mediated antiviral mechanism peculiar to hepatocytes. The potential cell-type specificity of cytokine-induced antiviral mechanisms is a field that remains to be fully evaluated, which could have implications for the strategies that HBV and HCV may have evolved to persist in the infected host. However, the work in the transgenic mouse model of HBV *(59)* and in chimpanzees *(22)* suggests that HBV may be particularly sensitive to antiviral effects activated by high levels of cytokines in hepatocytes. This idea is reinforced by the finding of high frequencies of HBV-specific CD8 cells in the liver of patients controlling HBV replication without signs of liver pathology *(54)*. These human data support the idea that antiviral cytotoxic T lymphocytes (CTLs) could inhibit HBV replication by noncytopathic cytokine-mediated mechanisms.

We do not know whether HCV has the same susceptibility as HBV to the antiviral pathways activated in hepatocytes by cytokines. Control of HCV infection has been associated with the presence of a multispecific CTLs response in chimpanzees and CTL have been found in the liver without any sign of liver disease *(73)*. However, it is not clear whether these virus-specific CTLs suppress HCV by cytokine-mediated mechanisms or by specific lysis of infected cells. Furthermore, the persistence of HCV in the face of strong activation of classical IFN-γ mediated pathways *(25)* and the poor response to IFN-α therapy *(74)* suggest that HCV, or some specific subtypes, may not be as sensitive as HBV to intracellular IFN-mediated antiviral pathways.

It has been observed that patients infected with different genotypes of HCV have variable response rates to IFN-α treatment *(74)*. In particular, the number of mutations in the carboxy-terminal region of the NS5A gene (between amino acids 2209 and 2248), termed the "interferon-sensitivity determining region" (ISDR), seems to correlate with response to treatment *(75,76)*. This observation has stimulated work to elucidate the function of this nonstructural region of HCV and has led to the recognition that NS5A can bind and inhibit one of the classical genes induced by IFNs, the double-stranded RNA-activated protein-kinase (PKR) *(77)*. However this property is not exclusive to the NS5A region (*see* Fig. 1), having also been seen with the envelope protein E2, particularly in HCV genotype 1 *(78)*. In HCV genotype 1, the virus strain most resistant to IFN-α therapy, the E2 protein contains a 12-amino-acid sequence similar to the phosphorylation site of PKR that is able to inhibit the kinase activity of PKR, thereby blocking its inhibitory effect on protein synthesis. This inhibition could account for the resistance of patients infected with genotypes 1 to IFN-α treatment, but not for those infected with genotypes 2 and 3. It is possible that the combined interaction of NS5A and E2 with PKR constitute one important strategy, in addition to others *(79)*, that allows HCV to circumvent the antiviral effect of interferons, thus perhaps partly accounting for its ability to persist in the infected host.

It is interesting to note, however, that all of these studies have been quite controversial *(80,81)*. The presence of mutations in the ISDR of NS5A that should increase their sensitivity to IFN-α-mediated inhibition have not been confirmed in non-Japanese patients responding to IFN treatment *(82)*. Similarly, a lack of correlation between resistance to IFN treatment and the presence of PKR-inhibitory activity in the HCV E2 sequence has also been found in other groups of patients *(81)*. This apparent controversy can be reconciled with the idea that HCV and HBV may have developed, during their coevolution with human populations, several different properties to increase their chances of resisting the antiviral effects of cytokines. However, because IFNs can stimulate multiple alternative antiviral pathways *(70)*, it is highly likely that the inhibition of specific IFN-activated antiviral pathways by HCV proteins will not be absolute, but will only increase the chance of persistence. The fact that antiviral cytokines can also stimulate different intracellular pathways according to cell type adds further complexity to this system. Because HCV seems capable of infecting extrahepatic sites, it might escape the activation of the IFN system simply by changing its host cell type to one in which different pathways of virus inhibition operate and blocking mechanisms may be more active. It is clear that this scenario is purely speculative at the moment, but it stresses the importance of developing a cell culture system or small-animal model where such possibilities can be tested.

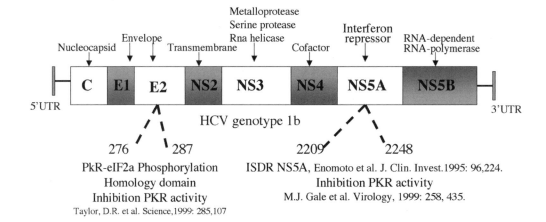

Fig. 1. Location of interferon-sensitivity determining regions (ISDR) within HCV genome.

2. CYTOKINES AND REGULATION OF HOST RESPONSE DURING VIRAL HEPATITIS

Cytokines are an essential component of the antiviral immune response not only because they possess direct antiviral effects but also because of their important immunoregulatory role in the adaptive immune response. During infection with HBV and HCV, several lines of evidence indicate that a key component of the adaptive immune response able to control these viruses is the profound expansion of IFN-γ-producing CD4 and CD8 cells (Th1 and Tc1 response). The cytokines that have the potential to promote the initial development of this adaptive immune response are interleukin (IL)-12, IFN-α, and IFN-β *(12)*. IL-12 has been proposed to be the dominant cytokine inducing Th1 responses *(83)*, but it is not induced by all viruses, and IL-12-independent T-cell IFN-γ responses have been observed *(84,85)*. Recent detailed analysis during LCMV infection has shown that IFN-α/ β production are also able to promote IFN-γ production by T-cells. In this mouse model of virus infection, two divergent patterns can be observed: One where IFN-γ production by CD8 cells is dependent on IFN-α and IFN-β production but completely IL-12 independent; a second where, in the absence of class I interferons, IL-12 is produced and the IFN-γ-producing T-cell response develops equally successfully *(86)*.

The data on HBV and HCV infections indirectly support the possibility that both pathways could be active. The higher production of IFN-α and IFN-β found in HCV chronic infection could explain the prominent T-helper-1 cytokine profile that characterizes the intrahepatic environment of HCV-infected livers. In livers infected with HCV, the majority of liver-infiltrating T-cells produce IFN- γ but not IL-4 or IL-5 *(31)*, and IFN-γ mRNA is upregulated, whereas IL-4 mRNA and IL-10 mRNA are found inconsistently *(33)*. Moreover, high levels of the chemokine IP-10, which is upregulated by IFN-γ production, have been found in the serum *(34)* and the liver of chronic hepatitis C patients *(25,34,35)*. All of these data show that an adaptive immune response preferentially producing IFN-γ is present during HCV infection, probably promoted by the high levels of type I interferons in these patients. Although we do not have direct data on the production and influence of IL-12 in HCV infection, it is likely that this cytokine does not play a major role in shaping the HCV-specific adaptive immune response. Indirect support for this speculation comes from the poor response of chronic hepatitis C patients to treatment with IL-12 *(87)*.

In contrast, IL-12-dependent induction of a Th1 response has been observed during HBV infection. Serum levels of IL-12 are higher in chronic asymptomatic HBV carriers than in uninfected subjects. Furthermore, increased levels of serum IL-12 are associated with control of high-level HBV replication, HBeAg seroconversion, and increases in serum Th1-cytokines *(88)*. Therefore, it is likely that IL-12 is active in the maturation of the HBV-specific adaptive immune response. Theoretically, this production could compensate for the defective influence exerted on the maturation of the adaptive immune response by the low levels of IFN-α and IFN-β usually present in chronic HBV patients. However, in patients with high levels of HBV replication, neither IL-12 nor IFN-α/β seem able to promote the complete maturation of a Th1-like-adaptive immune response, as observed in subjects with chronic HCV infection. Evidence for the presence of an adaptive immune response with elements of a Th2-type maturation derives from a number of studies. The isotype of the anti-HBV-specific antibody response present in patients with chronic HBV infection with high levels of virus replication is consistent with the presence of a Th2-type response *(32)*. Moreover, the cytokine environment in chronically HBV-infected liver has a Th2 bias, because a high proportion of non-HBV-specific liver infiltrating lymphocytes (CD4 as well CD8) produce low levels of IFN-γ but high levels of IL-4 and IL-5 *(31)*. Defects in the production of IFN-α and IFN-β or of IL-12 could cause these findings, but virological factors, secreted during HBV replication, have also been shown to have profound immunomodulatory functions.

During its replicative stage, HBV produces a secretory form of the nucleocapsid antigen called HBeAg that is not necessary for replication or infection *(89,90)*, but could modulate the development of the HBV-specific T-cell response. Experiments in transgenic mice have shown that HBeAg, in contrast to the nonsecretory HBcAg, stimulates a Th2-like response *(91)*. This ability to preferentially induce a Th2-like T-cell response could represent one important strategy that HBV has adopted to increase its chances of survival. For example, it has been demonstrated that HBeAg can cross the placenta and act as a "partial tolerogen" in newborn mice, resulting in the persistence of only HBeAg-specific cells of Th2 type *(92,93)*. Thus, the chronicity of HBV infection resulting from the vertical transmission of virus from mother to baby could be the consequence of a predominant HBeAg-specific Th2 response. By contrast, in the acute resolving hepatitis B of adults, the balance is toward the development of an HBcAg-specific Th1 response, acting to resolve the infection *(49,94)*.

The Th1-like cells are able to inhibit viral replication through the secretion of IFN-γ and TNF-α, but these cytokines could also exacerbate the level of liver injury. In contrast, Th2 cytokines are classical anti-inflammatory cytokines and have been shown to increase antiapoptotic proteins, promoting target cell survival *(95)*. Therefore, during natural HBV infection, the balance between the induction of Th1 and Th2 cytokines may influence not only the ability to control the virus but also the degree of liver injury. Loss of HBeAg antigen during chronic HBV infection is often associated with an exacerbation of liver injury *(96)*, and acute infection with HBeAg negative HBV mutants has been associated with fulminant hepatitis *(97–99)*. It is possible that these scenarios are the result of the lack of HBeAg-specific Th2-like cells that can potentially modulate and inhibit the HBcAg-specific Th1-like response. It is important to note that the influence of the secretory HBeAg in the maturation of a Th2-like T-cell response is not absolute, but can be modulated by the genetic background of the host or by IFN-α and IL-12. For example, treatment of HBeAg transgenic mice with IFN-α *(91)* or IL-12 *(100)* is capable of skewing the HBeAg-Th2 cells toward the Th1 subset.

Thus, the lack of an efficient IFN-γ-producing T-cell response during persistent HBV infection is multifactorial. It might depend not only on the relative balance of HBeAg/HBcAg production but also on the secretion of immunomodulatory cytokines. In conclusion, the data in the HBV system reinforce the importance of the secretion of early cytokines such as IFN-α/β and IL-12 in the promotion and maturation of an efficient antiviral adaptive immune response, despite the presence of viral factors with immunomodulatory features. Furthermore, the observation that the Th1–Th2 balance can be modified by IFN-α and IL-12 in mice may have important implications for treatment of patients with chronic HBV infection with new immunotherapeutic strategies. If the aim of the future therapy for chronic viral infection is to be the reconstitution of an immune response with features similar to that present in subjects controlling infection, it will be important to consider the cytokine milieu in which the initial priming of the adaptive immune response takes place.

3. CYTOKINES AND LIVER DAMAGE

In addition to their direct antiviral effect and ability to immunomodulate the adaptive immune response, cytokines are likely to play an essential role in the pathogenesis of liver damage during HBV and HCV infection. Because neither virus is directly cytopathic, cytotoxic T-cells have been implicated not only as the mediators of protection but also as the principal effectors of liver damage. It has always been hypothesized that recognition of HBV- and HCV-infected hepatocytes by antigen-specific human leukocyte antigen (HLA) class I-restricted CTL is the principal event determining the intensity of liver damage (*see* reviews in refs. *5,7,8,* and *50*).

Information about this process is scarce, because the study of intrahepatic antigen-specific T-cells has been hampered by the difficulty in obtaining adequate cell numbers from liver biopsies. A new technique for direct evaluation of the quantity of virus-specific CD8 cells *(101)* has provided the opportunity to investigate in more detail the relationship between HBV- and HCV-specific T-cells and liver damage in humans. These new data, in addition to the demonstration that CTLs can clear virus-infected hepatocytes using noncytopathic mechanisms, have challenged the idea that liver damage is proportional to the quantity of virus-specific CTLs *(10)*. For example, during HCV infection of chimpanzees, animals able to clear the infection possess intrahepatic cytotoxic T-cells specific for several different HCV epitopes, in contrast to weaker responses found in animals developing chronic infection *(73)*. However, cytotoxic assays performed with CD8+ cells directly isolated from the liver showed HCV-specific cytotoxic activity that did not correlate with the level of liver damage. High levels of cytotoxic activity were demonstrable in animals with normal levels of alanine transaminase (ALT, a marker of liver cell damage), whereas ALT levels indicative of extensive liver damage were found in chimpanzees with no detectable intrahepatic CTL activity. HCV-specific CTL activity was found in a histologically and biochemically normal liver more than 1 yr after resolution of infection *(73)*.

Similar results were found during infection in man, where the quantity of HBV-specific CTL did not seem to be proportional to the extent of liver damage. Chronic-HBV-infected patients lacking evidence of liver damage but controlling HBV replication had functionally active HBV-specific CD8 cells both in the circulation and in the liver *(54)*, and lower frequencies of virus-specific CTLs were usually found in patients with liver disease as a result of HBV *(54)* or HCV *(102)*. These results strongly suggest that the bulk of intrahepatic CD8 cells are non-antigen-specific during active liver damage. A low frequency of antigen-specific cells is also likely to be present in the CD4 T-cell compartment, although equivalent ex vivo data are not yet available. No HBV- or HCV-specific CD4 cells were found after antigen-specific analysis of a large panel of clones derived from intrahepatic T-cells *(31)*, and when HCV-specific CD4 cells have been identified, they have only been isolated from a minority of patients analyzed *(103)*. These data therefore indicate that the quantity of virus-specific cells does not appear to be the only variable directly determining the extent of virus-induced liver pathology (*see* Fig. 2). Others mechanisms must be implicated and it is likely that cytokines, secreted by the large infiltrate of antigen nonspecific mononuclear cells, contribute to the chronic hepatic damage.

The importance of non-antigen-specific recruitment and cytokines in the pathogenesis of acute liver damage has been shown in a transgenic mouse model of fulminant hepatitis *(104)* and in the concanavalin A-induced model of hepatitis *(105–107)*. In the HBsAg-transgenic mouse model, fulminant hepatitis is initiated by the injection of a large quantity of CTL clones specific for HBsAg.

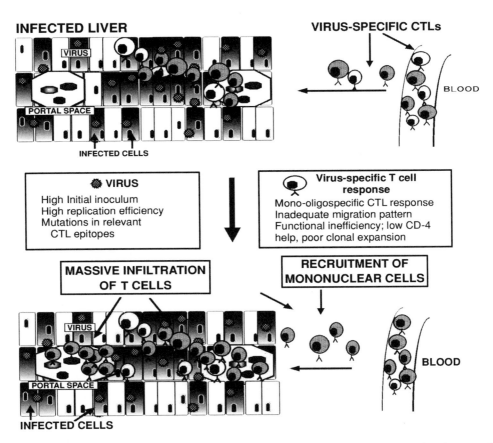

Fig. 2. Schematic model of liver inflammation following virus infection: recruitment of non-antigen-specific cells triggered by virus-specific CD8+ T cells.

Initially CTL clones trigger apoptosis of HbsAg-positive hepatocytes, but the destructive phenomenon that causes liver failure is the recruitment of large numbers of activated cells, mostly macrophages, that induce a delayed-type hypersensitivity reaction. This process is blocked by the injection of antibodies against IFN-γ *(104)*. In the concanavalin A-induced model of hepatitis, the development of hepatocyte injury seems to depend on TNF-α as well as IFN-γ, because neutralizing antibodies to either cytokine protect mice from liver failure *(105–108)*. Accordingly, high levels of TNF-α have been associated with the development of acute liver failure *(109)* and raised levels of TNF-α have been shown in chronic hepatitis C *(29,30)* and B infections *(110)*. However, analysis of mRNA transcripts in the liver of chronic hepatitis C patients did not find any relationship between TNF-α values and the activity of liver disease *(30)*.

Therefore, it is likely that hepatic damage is regulated and induced by more complex interactions between different cytokines. Other cytokines could also be involved: IL-18, secreted by activated macrophages, has, for example, a critical role in Fas-ligand-induced liver injury *(111)*. Soluble Fas ligand can be secreted by activated T-cells *(112)* and appears to stimulate IL-18 secretion from macrophages previously activated by IFN-γ *(111)*. IL-18 is a potent inducer of IFN-γ secretion *(113)* and augments the cytotoxic activities of NK and NK T-cells resident in the liver *(114)*. Therefore, liver damage during hepatitis could be triggered by virus-specific CD8 cells but caused by activated non-antigen specific cells *(see* Fig. 2). HBV and HCV-virus specific CD8 cells are capable of secreting IFN-γ and TNF-α and expressing Fas-L on their surface *(54,115–117)*. These cytokines and soluble molecules are not only able to control viral infections but could also trigger inflammatory phenomena, as observed in the different murine models of liver damage. It is possible that when virus-specific CTLs are faced by a quantity of virus that exceeds a certain threshold, they not only selectively lyse and/or inhibit viral replication in the infected cells but also potentially activate a cascade of events leading to liver damage.

This fine balance between infectious dose of virus and quantity of virus-specific CTLs has been explored in a mouse model of influenza virus infection *(118)*. In this experimental model, the same quantity of virus-specific CTLs could either promote virus clearance without any pathology or cause a lethal lung disease. The variable was the infectious dose of virus, and when the virus exceeded the clearance capacity of the virus-specific CTLs, lung pathology resulted. Interestingly, treatment with anti-IFN-γ antibody prevented the recruitment of large numbers of activated non-antigen-specific cells. IFN-γ seems to be central in most models of liver damage *(104,106)*. Therefore, it should not only be regarded as an anti-viral cytokine able to clear infection without causing liver damage *(62)*. It can also act as a typical proinflammatory cytokine, causing activation of macrophages *(119)*, increased susceptibility to TNF-mediated hepatic damage *(120)*, and initiating the recruitment of T-cells *(35,121,122)*, NK cells *(123)*, or NK T-cells *(124)* through the release of chemotactic cytokines. For example, IFN-γ induces secretion of the chemokine IP-10, that is upregulated in HBV and HCV chronic liver disease *(25,34,35)*. In line with these effects, transgenic mice that constitutively produce IFN-γ in the liver develop a form of chronic active hepatitis *(125)*. In addition, progressive liver injury in HCV infection correlates with high intrahepatic expression of Th1-type cytokines *(33)*, as does the organ damage in HLA-mismatched liver transplants *(126)*.

Recruitment of activated cells to the liver could also amplify the lysis of hepatocytes by Fas-mediated apoptosis. Activated cells express CD40L and engagement of the CD40 molecule constitutively expressed on hepatocytes would amplify Fas-dependent hepatocyte death *(127)*. Another mechanism whereby cytokines could regulate the amount of cell damage mediated by apoptosis has been described recently in autoimmune thyroid disease. Here, the destruction of thyrocytes during an inflammatory response is dependent on the cytokines produced by infiltrating lymphocytes. Thyrocytes express Fas-L in conditions of inflammation, but depending on whether Th1 or Th2 cytokines are produced, the consequences of Fas-L interaction are very different. IFN-γ induces thyrocytes to undergo Fas–Fas-L-mediated fratricide, whereas IL-4 produced by Th2 cells can cause upregulation of c-FLIP and Bcl-xl, which increase the resistance of cells to apoptosis *(128)*. It is therefore possible that the different cytokine profiles of non-antigen-specific cells present in HBV or HCV chronic hepatitis could also modulate the quantity of liver damage mediated by apoptosis. Apoptosis of liver cells has been shown to be an important phenomenon during both acute and chronic hepatitis *(129)*.

4. CONCLUSIONS

Cytokines are intimately involved in both the control and the pathogenesis of infection with the noncytopathic, hepatotropic viruses HBV and HCV. The role of non-lytic cytokine-mediated effects in the initial control of these viruses has been highlighted by recent studies of early events following infection. However, there is an urgent need for in vitro systems or small-animal models allowing better elucidation of the direct antiviral effects of cytokines in different cell types and of the escape mechanisms that these viruses have undoubtedly evolved.

There is accumulating evidence for the immunomodulatory effects of cytokines on these virus infections, where the balance between a Th1–Th2 response is critical in determining the degree of control versus liver pathology. In HCV infection, the type I interferons are likely to play a prominent part in promoting efficient IFN-γ production by cells of the adaptive immune response, whereas IL-12 and a viral secretory protein (HBeAg) appear to be more important in determining the nature of this response in HBV. In the future, it will be necessary to try to dissect the cytokine milieu associated with the initial priming of the adaptive immune response resulting in successful control of HBV and HCV infection.

The realization that antigen-specific CD8 cells can exert effective intrahepatic viral control without damage has underlined that these cells only constitute the first step in a cascade of events resulting in liver pathology. It is interesting to note that the only value that correlates with the amount of liver damage is the quantity of inflammatory infiltrate. T-cells may be activated by mechanisms independent of T-cell-receptor engagement and this could explain how non-antigen-specific cells might contribute through the secretion of cytokines. The relative significance of IFN-γ, TNF-α, IL-18 and other molecules yet to be described could be clarified by new techniques allowing thorough quantitative genomic and proteomic analysis of infected livers.

REFERENCES

1. Alter, M. (1997) Epidemiology of hepatitis. *C. Hepatology* **26**, 62S–65S.
2. Ganem, D. and Varmus, H. (1987) The molecular biology of the hepatitis B viruses. *Annu. Rev. Biochem.* **56**, 651–693.
3. Choo, Q., Kuo, G., Weiner, A., Overby, L., Bradley, D., and Houghton, M. (1989). Isolation of a cDNA clone derived from a blood-borne non-A, non-B viral hepatitis genome. *Science* **244**, 359–362.
4. Houghton, M., Weiner, A., Han, J., Kuo, G., and Choo, Q.-L. (1991) Molecular biology of the hepatitis C viruses: implications for diagnosis, development and control of diesease. *Hepatology* **14**, 381–388.
5. Chisari, F. and Ferrari, C. (1995) Hepatitis B virus immunopathogenesis. *Ann. Rev. Immunol.* **13**, 29–60.
6. Takaki, A., Wiese, M., Maertens, G., Depla, E., Seifert, U., Liebetrau, A., et al. (2000) Cellular immune responses persist and humoral responses decreases two decades after recovery from a single-source outbreak of hepatitis Cl. *Nat. Med.* **6**, 578–582.
7. Cerny, A. and Chisari, F. (1999) Pathogenesis of chronic hepatitis C: immunological features of hepatitis injury and viral persistence. *Hepatology* **30**, 595–601.
8. Koziel, M. (1997) The role of immune responses in the pathogenesis of hepatitis C virus infection. *J. Viral Hepatitis* **4**, 31–41.
9. Maini, M. and Bertoletti, A. (2000) How can the cellular immune response control hepatitis B virus replication? *J. Viral Hepatitis* **7**, 321–326.
10. Bertoletti, A. and Maini, M. (2000) Protection or damage: a dual role for the virus-specific cytotoxic T lymphocyte response in hepatitis B and C infection? *Curr. Opin. Immunol.* **12**, 403–408.
11. Paul, W. and Seder, R. (1994). Lymphocyte responses and cytokines. *Cell* **76**, 241–251.
12. Biron, C. (1999). Initial and innate responses to viral infections-pattern setting in immunity or disease. *Curr. Opin. Microbiol.* **2**, 374–381.
13. Kalvakolanu, D. and Borden, E. (1996). An overview of the interferon system: signal transduction and mecchanism of action. *Cancer Invest.* **14**, 25–53.
14. Stark, G., Kerr, I., Williams, B., Silvermann, R., and Schreiber, R. (1998) How cells respond to interferons. *Annu. Rev. Biochem.* **67**, 227–264.
15. Der, S., Zhou, A., Williams, B., and Silvermann, R. (1998). Identification of genes differentialy regulated by intreferon alpha, beta, or gamma using oligonucleotide arrays. *Proc. Natl. Acad. Sci USA* **95**, 15623–15628.
16. Biron, C. (1997) Activation and function of natural killer cell responses during viral infections. *Curr. Opin. Immunol.* **9**, 24–34.
17. Haller, O., Frese, M., and Kochs, G. (1998) Mx proteins: mediators of innate resistance to RNA viruses. *Rev. Sci. Technol.* **17**, 220–228.
18. Reiss, C. and Komatsu, T. (1998) Does nitric oxide play a critical role in viral infections? *J. Virol.* **72**, 4547–4551.
19. Cohen, J. (1999) The scientific challenge of hepatitis C virus. *Science* **285**, 26–30.
20. Jakschies, D., Zachoval, R., Muller, R., Manns, M., Nolte, K., Hochkeppel, H.K., et al. (1994) Strong transient expression of the type I interferon-induced MxA protein in hepatitis A but not in acute hepatitis B and C. *Hepatology* **19**, 857–865.
21. Nouri-Aria, K., Arnold, J., Davison, F., Portmann, B., Meager, A., Morris, A.G., et al. (1991) Hepatic interferon-alpha gene transcripts and products in liver specimens from acute and chronic hepatitis B virus infection. *Hepatology* **13**, 1029–1034.
22. Guidotti, L.G., Rochford, R., Chung, J., Shapiro, M., Purcell, R., and Chisari, F.V. (1999) Viral clearance without destruction of infected cells during acute HBV infection. *Science* **284**, 825–829.
23. Webster, G., Reignat, S., Maini, M., Whalley, S., Ogg, G., King, A., et al. (2000) Incubation phase of acute Hepatitis B in man: dynamic of cellular immune mechanism. *Hepatology* **32**, 1117–1124.
24. Castelruiz, Y., Larrea, E., Boya, P., Civeira, M., and Prieto, J. (1999) Interferon alpha subtypes and levels of type I interferons in the liver and peripheral mononuclear cells in patients with chronic hepatitis C and controls. *Hepatology* **29**, 1900–1904.
25. Patzwahl, R., Meier, V., Ramadori, G., and Mihm, S. (2001) Enhanced expression of interferon-regulated genes in the liver of patients with chronic hepatitis C infection: detection by suppression-subtractive hybridization. *J. Virol* **75**, 1332–1338.
26. Ikeda, T., Lever, A., and Thomas, H. (1986) Evidence for a deficiency of interferon production in patients with chronic hepatitis B virus infection acquired in adult life. *Hepatology* **6**, 962–965.
27. Poitrine, A., Chousterman, S., Chousterman, M., Naveau, S., Thang, M.-N., and Chaput, J.C. (1985) Lack of in vivo activation of the interferon system in HBsAg-positive chronic active hepatitis. *Hepatology* **5**, 171–174.

28. Sheron, N., Lau, J., Daniels, H., Goka, J., Eddlestone, A., Alexander, G.J., et al. (1991) Increased production of tumor necrosis factor alpha in chronic hepatitis B infection. *J. Hepatol.* **12**, 251–255.
29. Tilg, H., Wilmer, A., Vogel, W., Herold, M., Nolchen, B., Judmaier, G., et al. (1992) Serum levels of cytokines in chronic liver diseases. *Gastroenterology* **103**, 264–274.
30. Larrea, E., Garcia, N., Qiang, C., Civeira, M., and Prieto, J. (1996) Tumor necrosis factor α gene expression and the response to interferon in chronic hepatitis C. *Hepatology* **23**, 210–217.
31. Bertoletti, A., D'Elios, M.M., Boni, C., De Carli, M., Zignego, A.L., durazzo, M., et al. (1997) Different cytokine profiles of intraphepatic T cells in chronic hepatitis B and hepatitis C virus infections. *Gastroenterology* **112**, 193–199.
32. Maruyama, T., McLachlan, A., Iino, S., Koike, K., Kurokawa, K., and Milich, D.R. (1993). The serology of chronic hepatitis B infection revisited. *J. Clin. Invest.* **91**, 2586–2595.
33. Napoli, J., Bishop, G.A., McGuinness, P.H., Painter, D.M., and McCaughan, G.W. (1996) Progressive liver injury in chronic hepatitis C infection correlates with increased intrahepatic expression of Th1-associated cytokines. *Hepatology* **24**, 759–765.
34. Narumi, S., Tominaga, Y., Tamaru, S., Shimai, S., Okamura, H., Nishiojin, K., et al. (1997). Expression of IFN-inducible protein-10 in chronic hepatitis. *J. Immunol.* **158**, 5536–5544.
35. Shields, P., Morland, C., Salmon, M., Qin, S., Hubscher, S., and Adams, D.H. (1999). Chemokine and chemokine receptor interaction provide a mechanism for selective T cell recruitment to speific liver compartments within hepatitis C infected liver. *J. Immunol.* **163**, 6236–6243.
36. Dienes, H., Hess, G., Woorsdorfer, M., Rossol, S., Gallati, H., Ramadori, G., et al. (1991) Ultrastructural localization of intrferon-producing cells in the livers of patients with chronic hepatitis B. *Hepatology* **13**, 321–326.
37. Wheelock, E., Schenker, S., and Combes, B. (1968) Absence of circulating interferon in patients with infectious and serum hepatitis. *Proc. Soc. Exp. Biol. Med.* **128**, 251–253.
38. Tolentino, P., Dianzani, F., Zucca, M., and Giacchino, R. (1975) Decreased interferon response by lymphocytes from children with chronic hepatitis. *J. Infect. Dis.* **132**, 459–461.
39. Whitten, T., Quets, A., and Schloemer, R. (1991) Identification of the hepatitis B virus factor that inhibits expression of the beta interferon gene. *J. Virol.* **65**, 4699–4704.
40. Foster, G., Ackrill, A., Goldin, R., Kerr, I., Thomas, H., and Stark, G.R. (1991) Expression of the terminal protein region of hepatitis B virus inhibits cellular responses to interferons α and γ and double stranted RNA. *Proc. Natl. Acad. Sci. USA* **88**, 2888–2892.
41. Yoshioka, K., Kakumu, S., Arao, M., Tsutsumi, Y., and Inoe, M. (1989) Tumor necrosis factor alpha production by peripheral blood mononuclear cells of patients with chronic liver disease. *Hepatology* **10**, 769–773.
42. Biron, C. (1994). Cytokines in the generation of immune responses to, and resolution of, virus infection. *Curr. Opin. Immunol.* **6**, 530–538.
43. Muller, U., Steinhoff, U., Reis, L., Hemmi, S., Pavlovic, J., et al. (1994) Functional role of type I and type II interferons in antiviral defense. *Science* **264**, 1918–1921.
44. Mosmann, T.R. and Sad, S. (1996). The expanding universe of T-cell subsets: Th1, Th2 and more. *Immunol. Today* **17**, 138–146.
45. Ferrari, C., Penna, A., Bertoletti, A., Valli, A., Antoni, A., D., Giuberti, T., et al. (1990) Cellular immune response to hepatitis B virus encoded antigens in acute and chronic hepatitis B virus infection. *J. Immunol.* **145**, 3442–3449.
46. Jung, M., Spengler, U., Schraut, W., Hoffman, R., Zachoval, R., Eisenburg, J., et al. (1991) Hepatitis B virus antigen-specific T-cell activation in patients with acute and chronic hepatitis B. *J. Hepatol.* **13**, 310–317.
47. Lohr, H.F., Weber, W., Schlaak, J., Goergen, B., Meyer zum Buschenfelde, K.H., and Gerker, G. (1995) Proliferative response of CD4+ T cells and hepatitis B virus clearance in chronic hepatitis with or without hepatitis B e-minus hepatitis B virus mutants. *Hepatology* **22**, 61–68.
48. Missale, G., Bertoni, R., Lamonaca, V., Valli, A., Massari, M., Moric, C., et al. (1996) Different clinical behaviors of acute hepatitis C virus infection are associated with different vigor of the anti-viral cell-mediated immune response. *J. Clin. Invest.* **98**, 706–714.
49. Penna, A., Del Prete, G., Cavalli, A., Bertoletti, A., D'Elios, M.M., Sorrentino, R., et al. (1997). Predominant T-helper 1 cytokine profile of hepatitis B virus nucleocapsid-specific T cells in acute self-limited hepatitis B. *Hepatology* **25**, 1022–1027.
50. Chisari, F. (1997) Cytotoxic T cells and viral hepatitis. *J. Clin. Invest.* **99**, 1472–1477.
51. Penna, A., Artini, M., Cavalli, A., Levrero, M., Bertoletti, A., Pilli, M., et al. (1996) Long-lasting memory T cell responses following self-limited acute hepatitis B. *J. Clin. Invest.* **98**, 1185–1194.
52. Maini, M.K., Boni, C., Ogg, G.S., King, A.S., Reignat, S., Lee, C.K., et al. (1999) Direct ex vivo analysis of hepatitis B virus-specific CD8+ T cells associated with the control of infection. *Gastroenterology* **117**, 1386–1396.
53. Jung, M., Hartmann, B., Gerlach, J., Diepolder, H., Gruber, R., Schraut, W., et al. (1999) Virus-specific lymphokine production differs quantitatively but not qualitatively in acute and chronic hepatitis B infection. *Virology* **261**, 165–172.
54. Maini, M.K., Boni, C., Lee, C.K., Larrubia, J.R., Reignat, S., Ogg, G.S., et al. (2000) The role of virus-specific CD8+ cells in viral control and liver damage during persistent hepatitis B virus (HBV) infection. *J. Exp. Med.* **191**, 1269–1280.
55. Diepolder, H.M., Zachoval, R., Hoffmann, R.M., Wierenga, E., Santantonio, T., Jung, M.C., et al. (1995) Possible mechanism involving T-lymphocyte response to non-structural protein 3 in viral clearance in acute hepatitis C virus infection. *Lancet* **346**, 1006–1007.

56. Lechner, F., Wong, D., Dunbar, P., Chapman, R., Chung, R., Dohrenwend, P., et al. (2000) Analysis of succesful immune responses in person infected with hepatitis C virus. *J. Exp. Med.* **191,** 1499–1512.
57. Chang, K.-M., Thimme, R., Melpolder, J., Oldach, D., Pemberton, J., Moorhead-Loudis, J., et al. (2001) Differential CD4+ and CD8+ T-cell responsiveness in hepatitis C virus infection. *Hepatology* **33,** 267–276.
58. Tsai, S.L., Liaw, Y.F., Chen, M.H., Huang, C.Y., and Kuo, G.C. (1997). Detection of type 2-like T-helper cells in hepatitis C virus infection: implications for hepatitis C virus chronicity. *Hepatology* **25,** 449–458.
59. Guidotti, L., and Chisari, F. (1999) Cytokine-induced viral purging-role in viral pathogenesis. *Curr. Opin. Microbiol.* **2,** 388–391.
60. McClary, H., Koch, R., Chisari, F., and Guidotti, L. (2000) Relative sensitivity of hepatitis B virus and other cytokines to the antiviral effects of cytokines. *J. Virol.* **74,** 2255–2264.
61. Cavanaugh, V.J., Guidotti, L.G., and Chisari, F.V. (1998) Inhibition of hepatitis B virus replication during adenovirus and cytomegalovirus infections in transgenic mice. *J. Virol.* **72,** 2630–2637.
62. Guidotti, L.G., Borrow, P., Hobbs, M., Matzke, B., Gresser, I., Oldstone, M.B., et al. (1996) Viral cross-talk: intracellular inactivation of the hepatitis B virus during an unrelated viral infection of the liver. *Proc. Natl. Acad. Sci. USA* **94,** 4589–4594.
63. Guidotti, L.G., Ishikawa, T., Hobbs, M.V., Matzke, B., Schreiber, R., and Chisari, F.V. (1996) Intracellular inactivation of the hepatitis B virus by cytotoxic T lymphocytes. *Immunity* **4,** 25–36.
64. Guidotti, L. and Chisari, F. (1996). To kill or to cure: options in host defense against viral infection. *Curr. Opin. Immunol.* **8,** 478–483.
65. Jilbert, A., Wu, T., England, J., Hall, P., Carp, N., O'Connell, A.P., et al. (1992) Rapid resolution of duck hepatitis B virus infections occurs after massive hepatocellular involvment. *J. Virol.* **66,** 1377–1388.
66. Kajino, K., Jilbert, A.R., Saputelli, J., Aldrich, C.E., Cullen, J., and Mason, W.S. (1994) Woodchuck hepatitis virus infections: very rapid recovery after prolonged viremia and infection of virtually every hepatocyte. *J. Virol.* **68,** 5792–5803.
67. Tay, C. and Welsh, R. (1997) Distinct organ-dependent mechanisms for the control of murine cytomegalovirus infection by natural killer cells. *J. Virol.* **71,** 267–275.
68. Kagi, D., Ledermann, B., Burki, H., Hengartner, H., and Zinkernagel, R. (1994) CD8+ T-cell mediated protection against an intracellular bacterium by perforin-dependent cytotoxicity. *Eur. J. Immunol.* **24,** 3068–3072.
69. Guidotti, L.G., Borrow, P., Brown, A., McClary, H., Koch, R., and Chisari, F.V. (1999) Noncytopathic clearance of lymphocytic choriomeningitis virus from the hepatocyte. *J. Exp. Med.* **189,** 1555–1564.
70. Presti, R., Popkin, D., Connick, M., Paetzold, S., and Virgin H., IV. (2001) Novel cell type-specific antiviral mechanism of interferon γ action in macrhopages. *J. Exp. Med.* **193,** 483–496.
71. Heise, T., Guidotti, L., Cavanaugh, V., and Chisari, F. (1999) Hepatitis B virus RNA binding proteins associated with cytokine-induced clearance of viral RNA from the liver of transgenic mice. *J. Virol.* **73,** 474–481.
72. Heise, T., Guidotti, L., and Chisari, F. (1999) La autoantigen specifically recognizes a predicted stem-loop in hepatitis B virus RNA. *J. Virol.* **73,** 5767–5776.
73. Cooper, S., Erickson, A., Adams, E., Kansopon, J., Weiner, A., Chien, D.Y., et al. (1999) Analysis of a succesful immune response against Hepatitis C virus. *Immunity* **10,** 439–449.
74. Conjeevaram, H., Everhart, J., and Hoofnagle, J. (1995). Predictors of a sustained biochemical response to interferon alpha therapy in chronic hepatitis C. *Hepatology* **22,** 1326–1329.
75. Enomoto, N., Sakuma, I., Asahina, Y., Kurosaki, M., Murakami, T., Yamamoto, C., et al. (1996) Mutations in the nonstructural protein 5A gene and response to interferon in patients with chronic hepatitis C virus 1b infection. *N. Engl. J. Med.* **334,** 77–81.
76. Enomoto, N., Sakuma, I., Asahina, Y., Kurosaki, M., Murakami, T., Yamamoto, C., et al. (1995) Comparison of full-length sequences of interferon-sensitive and resistant hepatits C virus 1b. *J. Clin. Invest.* **96,** 224–230.
77. Gale, M., Jr., Korth, M.J., Tang, N-M., Tan, S.L., Hopkins, D.A., Dever, T.E., et al. Evidence that hepatitis C virus resistance to interferon is mediated through repression of the PKR protein Kinase by the nonstructural 5A protein. *Virology* **230,** 217–227.
78. Taylor, D., Shi, S., Romano, P., Barber, G., and Lai, M. (1999) Inhibition of the interferon-inducible protein-kinase PKR by HCV E2 protein. *Science* **285,** 107–109.
79. Heim, M., Moradpour, D., and Blum, H. (1999) Expression of hepatitis C virus proteins inhibits signal transduction through the Jak- STAT pathway. *J. Virol.* **73,** 8469–8475.
80. Herion, D. and Hoofnagle, J. (1997) The interferon sensitivity determining region: all hepatitis C virus isolates are not the same. *Hepatology* **25,** 769–771.
81. Abid, K., Quadri, R., and Negro, F. (2000) Hepatitis C virus, the E2 envelope protein, and α-interferon resistance. *Science* **287,** 1555a.
82. Zeuzem, S., Lee, J., and Roth, W. (1997) Mutations in the nonstructural 5A gene of european hepatitis C virus isolates and response to interferon alpha. *Hepatology* **25,** 740–744.
83. Trincheri, G. (1995) Interleukin 12: a pro-inflammatory cytokine with immune regulatory functions that bridge innate resistance and antigen-specific adaptive immunity. *Annu. Rev. Immunol.* **13,** 251–276.
84. Oxenius, A., Karrer, U., Zinkernagel, R., and Hengartner, H. (1999) IL-12 is not required for induction of type 1 cytokine responses in viral infection. *J. Immunol.* **162,** 965–973.
85. Schijins, V., Haagmans, B., Wierda, C., Kruithof, B., Heijnen, I., et al. (1998). Mice lacking IL-12 develop polarized Th1 cells during viral infection. *J. Immunol.* **160,** 3958–3964.
86. Cousens, L., Peterson, R., Hsu, S., Dorner, A., Altman, J., Ahmed, R., et al. (1999) Two roads diverged: interferon α/β and interleukin 12-mediated pathways in promoting T cell interferon γ responses during viral infection. *J. Exp. Med.* **189,** 1315–1327.

87. Lee, J., Teuber, G., von Wagner, M., Roth, W., and Zeuzem, S. (2000). Antiviral effect of human recombinant interleukin-12 in patients infected with hepatitis C virus. *J. Med. Virol.* **60**, 264–268.
88. Rossol, S., Marinos, G., Carucci, P., Singer, M.V., Williams, R., and Naoumov, N.V. (1997) Interleukin-12 induction of Th1 cytokines is important for viral clearance in chronic hepatitis B. *J. Clin. Invest.* **99**, 3025–3033.
89. Schlicht, H., Salfeld, J., and Schaller, H. (1987) The pre-C region of the duck hepatitis B virus encodes a signal sequence which is essential for the synthesis and secretion of processed core protein but not for virus formation. *J. Virol.* **61**, 3701–3709.
90. Chang, C., Enders, G., Sprengel, R., Peters, N., Varmus, H., and Ganem, D. (1987) Expression of the precore region of an avian hepatitis B virus is not required for viral replication. *J. Virol.* **61**, 3322–3325.
91. Milich, D.R., Schodel, F., Hughes, J.L., Jones, J.E., and Peterson, D.L. (1997) The hepatitis B virus core and e antigens elicit different Th cell subsets: antigen structure can affect Th cell phenotype. *J. Virol.* **71**, 2192–2201.
92. Milich, D.R., Peterson, D.L., Schodel, F., Jones, J.E., and Hughes, J.L. (1995) Characterization of self-reactive T cells that evade tolerance in hepatitis B e antigen transgenic mice. *Eur. J. Immunol.* **25**, 1663–1672.
93. Milich, D., Jones, J., Hughes, J., Price, J., Raney, A., and McLachlan, A. (1990). Is a function of the secreted hepatitis B e antigen to induce immunotolerance in vivo? *Proc. Natl. Acad. Sci. USA* **87**, 6599–6603.
94. Maruyama, T., Schodel, F., Iino, S., Koike, K., Yasuda, K., Peterson, D., et al. (1994) Distinguishing between acute and symptomatic chronic hepatitis B infection. *Gastroenterology* **106**, 1006–1015.
95. Stassi, G., Di Liberto, D., Todaro, M., Zeuner, A., Ricci-Vitiani, L., Stoppacciaro, A., et al. (2000) Control of target cell survival in tyroid autoimmunity by T helper cytokines via regulation of apoptotic proteins. *Nat. Immunol.* **1**, 483–487.
96. Brunetto, M., Giarin, M., Oliveri, F., Chiaberge, E., Baldi, M., Alfarano, A., et al. (1991) Wild-type and e antigen-minus hepatitis B viruses and course of chronic hepatitis. *Proc. Natl. Acad. Sci. USA* **88**, 4186–4190.
97. Liang, T., Hasegawa, K., Rimon, N., Wands, J., and Ben-Porath, E. (1991) A hepatitis B virus mutant associated with an epidemic of fulminant hepatitis. *N. Engl. J. Med.* **324**, 1705–1709.
98. Omata, M., Ehata, T., Yokosuka, O., Hosoda, K., and Ohto, M. (1991) Mutations in the precore region of hepatitis B virus DNA in patients with fulminant and severe hepatitis. *N. Engl. J. Med.* **324**, 1699–1704.
99. Carman, W., Fagan, E., Hadziyannis, S., Karayiannis, P., Tassolopoulos, N., Williams, R., et al. (1991) Association of a precore variant of hepatitis B virus with fulminant hepatitis. *Hepatology* **14**, 219–222.
100. Milich, D.R., Wolf, S.F., Hughes, J.L., and Jones, J.E. (1995) Interleukin 12 suppresses autoantibody production by reversing helper T-cell phenotype in hepatitis B e antigen transgenic mice. *Proc. Natl. Acad. Sci. USA* **92**, 6847–6851.
101. Altman, J.D., Moss, P.A.H., Goulder, P.J.R., Barouch, D.H., McHeyzer Williams, M.G., Bell, J.I., et al. (1996). Phenotypic analysis of antigen-specific T lymphocytes. *Science* **274**, 94–96.
102. He, X.-S., Rehermann, B., Lopez-Labrador, F.X., Boisvert, J., Cheung, R., Mumm, J., et al. (1999) Quantitative analysis of hepatitis C virus-specific CD8+ T cells in peripheral blood and liver using peptide-MHC tetramers. *Proc. Natl. Acad. Sci. USA* **96**, 5692–5697.
103. Minutello, M.A., Pileri, P., Unutmaz, D., Censini, S., Kuo, G., Houghton, M., et al. (1993) Compartmentalization of T lymphocytes to the site of disease: intrahepatic CD4+ T cells specific for the protein NS4 of hepatitis C virus in patients with chronic hepatitis C. *J. Exp. Med.* **178**, 17–25.
104. Ando, K., Moriyama, T., Guidotti, L.G., Wirth, S., Schreiber, R., Schlicht, H.J., et al. (1993) Mechanisms of class I restricted immunopathology. A transgenic mouse model of fulminant hepatitis. *J. Exp. Med.* **178**, 1541–1554.
105. Tiegs, G., Hentschel, J., and Wendel, A. (1992) A T-cell dependent experimental liver injury in mice inducible by concanavallin A. *J. Clin. Invest.* **90**, 196–203.
106. Kusters, S., Gantner, F., Kunstle, G., and Tiegs, G. (1996). Interferon gamma plays a critical role in T cell-dependent liver injury in mice initiated by concanavalin A. *Gastroenterology* **111**, 462–471.
107. Mizuhara, H., O'Neill, E., Seki, N., Ogawa, T., Kusonoki, C., Otsuka, K., et al. (1994). T Cell activation-associated hepatic injury: mediation by tumor necrosis factors and protection by interleukin 6. *J. Exp. Med.* **179**, 1529–1537.
108. Gantner, F., Leist, M., Lohse, A., Germann, P., and Tiegs, P. (1995). Concavallin-A induced T cell mediated hepatic injury in mice: role of tumor necrosis factor. *Hepatology* **21**, 190–198.
109. Muto, Y., Meager, A., Eddleston, A., Nouri-Aria, K., Alexander, G., et al. (1988) Enhanced tumor necrosis factor and interleukin-1 in fulminant hepatic failure. *Lancet* **9**, 72–74.
110. Sheron, N., Lau, J., Daniels, H., Goka, J., Eddleston, A., Alexander, G.J., et al. (1991) Increased production of tumor necrosis factor alpha in chronic hepatitis B infection. *J. Hepatol.* **12**, 251–255.
111. Tsutsui, H., Kayagaki, N., Kuida, K., Nakano, H., Hayashi, N., Takeda, K., et al. (1999) Caspase-1-independent, Fas/Fas Ligand-mediated IL-18 secretion from macrophages causes acute liver injury in mice. *Immunity* **11**, 359–367.
112. Kayagaki, N., Kawasaki, A., Ebata, T., Ohmoto, H., Ikeda, S., Inoue, S., et al. (1995) Metalloproteinase-mediated release of human Fas ligand. *J. Exp. Med.* **182**, 1777–1783.
113. Okamura, H., Tsutsui, H., Komatsu, T., Yutsudo, M., Hakura, A., Tanimoto, T., et al. (1995) Cloning of a new cytokine that induces IFN-γ production. *Nature* **378**, 88–91.
114. Dao, T., Mehal, W., and Crispe, I. (1998) IL-18 augments perforin-dependent cytotoxicity of liver NK-T cells. *J. Immunol.* **161**, 2217–2222.
115. Barnaba, V., Franco, A., Paroli, M., Benvenuto, R., De Petrillo, G., burgio, V-L., et al. (1994) Selective expansion of cytotoxic T lymphocytes with a CD4+CD56+ surface phenotype and a T helper type 1 profile of cytokine secretion in the liver of patients chronically infected with Hepatitis B virus. *J. Immunol.* **152**, 3074–3087.
116. Koziel, M., Dudley, D., Afdhal, N., Grakoui, A., Rice, C., Choo, O.L., et al. (1995) HLA class I-restricted cytotoxic T lymphocytes specific for hepatitis C virus. Identification of multiple epitopes and characterization of patterns of cytokine release. *J. Clin. Invest.* **96**, 2311–2321.

117. Ando, K., Hiroishi, K., Kaneko, T., Moriyama, T., Muto, Y., Kayagaki, N., et al. (1997) Perforin, Fas/Fas ligand, and TNF-alpha pathways as specific and bystander killing mechanisms of hepatitis C virus-specific human CTL. *J. Immunol.* **158,** 5283–5291.
118. Moskophidis, D. and Kioussis, D. (1998) Contribution of virus-specific CD8+ cytotoxic T cells to virus clearance or pathologic manifestations of influenza virus infection in a T cell receptor transgenic mouse model. *J. Exp. Med.* **188,** 223–232.
119. Young, H. and Hardy, K. (1995). Role of interferon-γ in immune cell regulation. *J. Leukocyte Biol.* **58,** 373–381.
120. Morita, M., Watanabe, Y., and Akaike, T. (1995) Protective effect of hepatocyte growth factor on interferon-gamma-induced cytotoxicity in mouse hepatocytes. *Hepatology* **21,** 1585–1593.
121. Taub, D., Conlon, K., Lloyd, A., Oppenheim, J., and Kelvin, D. (1993) Preferential migration of activated CD4+ and CD8+ T cells in response to MIP-1α and MIP-1β. *Science* **260,** 355–357.
122. Cook, D., Beck, M., Coffman, T., Kirby, S., Sheridan, J., Pragnell, I.B., et al. (1995) Requirement of MIP-1a for an inflammatory response to viral infection. *Science* **269,** 1583–1586.
123. Salazar-Mather, T., Orange, J., and Biron, C. (1998). Early murine cytomegalovirus (MCMV) infection induces liver natural killer (NK) cell inflammation and protection through macrophage inflammatory protein 1a (MIP-1a)-dependent pathways. *J. Exp. Med.* **187,** 1–14.
124. Kaneko, Y., Harada, M., Kawano, T., Yamashita, M., Shibata, Y., Gejyo, F., et al. (2000) Augmentation of Va14 NKT cell-mediated cytotoxicity by interleukin-4 in an autocrine mecchanism resulting in the development of Concanavalin A-induced hepatitis. *J. Exp. Med.* **191,** 105–114.
125. Toyonaga, T., Hino, O., Sugai, S., Wakasugi, S., Abe, K., Shichiri, M., et al. (1994) Chronic active hepatitis in transgenic mice expressing interferon-γ in the liver. *Proc. Natl. Acad. Sci USA* **91,** 614–618.
126. Marinos, G., Rossol, S., Carucci, P., Wong, P., Donaldson, P., Hussain, M.J., et al. (2000) Immunopathogenesis of hepatitis B virus recurrence after liver transplantation. *Transplantation* **69,** 1–10.
127. Afford, S., Randhawa, S., Eliopoulos, A., Hubscher, S., Young, L., and Adams, D.H. (1999) CD40 activation induces apoptosis in cultured human hepatocytes via induction of cell surface Fas ligand expression and amplifies Fas-mediated hepatocyte death during allograft rejection. *J. Exp. Med.* **189,** 441–446.
128. Stassi, G., Di Liberto, D., Todaro, M., Zeuner, A., Ricci-Vitiani, L., Stoppacciaro, A., et al. (2000) Control of target cell survival in thyroid autoimmunity by T helper cytokines via regulation of apoptotic proteins. *Nat. Immunol.* **1,** 483–488.
129. Guo, J., Zhou, H., Liu, C., Aldrich, C., Saputelli, J., Whitaker, T., et al. (2000) Apoptosis and regeneration of hepatocytes during recovery from transient hepadnavirus infections. *J. Virol.* **74,** 1495–1505.

IX
Cytokines as Therapeutic Agents in Infectious Diseases

22

Interferon-γ in the Treatment of Infectious Diseases

Steven M. Holland and John I. Gallin

1. INTRODUCTION

The interferons (IFNs) were identified and named for their interference with viral infections of eukaryotic cells *(1,2)*. They were divided into three categories, based on the predominant cells of origin: leukocytes (now known collectively as IFN-α), fibroblasts (now known as IFN-β), and T-cells (immune or IFN-γ). These interferons also had important differences in acid stability, molecular size, and activity. IFN-α and IFN-β, and the similar IFN-ω, share similar biochemical properties, gene proximity, induction, receptor, and signaling pathways and are collectively referred to as type I interferons. In contrast, IFN-γ is quite distinct in many of these features and is referred to as a type II interferon. However, all of the interferons have certain parts of the signaling pathways in common, and they all interfere with viral replication.

All interferons share the same basic signal transduction approach: The IFN molecule binds to a heterodimeric receptor on the cell surface, the polypeptide chains of which are constitutively associated with protein tyrosine kinase molecules of the Janus kinase family *(3,4)*. These signaling molecules transphosphorylate each other, leading to tyrosine phosphorylation of the respective ligand binding or α chains of the receptor. These phosphorylation steps lead to phosphorylation of the latent signal transduction and activator of transcription molecules (STATs) that then combine in various arrangements, and with other molecules translocate to the nucleus, and upregulate DNA transcription.

Among the most important molecules involved in the further refinement of intracellular signaling are the interferon regulatory factors (IRFs). These are a growing family of related transcriptional regulators that have DNA binding and protein–protein interacting domains and can act as activators or inhibitors of downstream signaling *(5)*.

2. IFN-γ

Although the discovery of the interferons was based on their role in viral infections, the overwhelming majority of subsequent work on IFN-γ has shown that it is critical for defense against intracellular infections, most notably those caused by mycobacteria, leishmania, and toxoplasmosis.

Interferon-γ is encoded by a single gene with three exons located on chromosome 12q14 in humans and chromosome 10 in mouse. It is produced by lymphocytes (CD4+, CD8+, natural killer [NK] cells) as well as macrophages and perhaps neutrophils *(6)* in response to interleukin (IL)-12 and IL-18, among others *(7,8)*. IFN-γ induces hundreds of genes, including its own inducers *(9,10)* as well as enzymes important in the killing of intracellular organisms, including the ATP receptor P2X7 *(11,12)*. IFN-γ activates neutrophils and macrophages to produce superoxide and nitric oxide, increase sur-

From: *Cytokines and Chemokines in Infectious Diseases Handbook*
Edited by: M. Kotb and T. Calandra © Humana Press Inc., Totowa, NJ

face display of major histocompatibility complex (MHC) antigens and Fc receptors, decrease lysosomal pH, and increase the intracellular concentration of certain antibiotics *(13,14)*. IFN-γ potently upregulates MHC class 2 expression and has been implicated in the etiology of aplastic anemia *(15)*. However, the effects of IFN-γ, and its inducer IL-12 on bone marrow transplantation and graft versus host disease (GVHD) are surprisingly salutary *(16,17)*. IFN-γ is not needed for acute GVHD in animal models *(18)*.

Aguet et al. *(19)* cloned the ligand-binding chain of the IFN-γ receptor, initially referred to as IFNγRα, but now as IFNγR1. Bohni et al. *(20)* showed that this receptor was not species-specific in its intracellular signaling (i.e., human receptors could use the intracellular signaling molecules of murine cells), whereas the ligand–receptor interaction was species-limited (i.e., human and mouse IFN-γ do not activate each other's receptors). Hemmi et al. *(21)* and Soh et al. *(22)* identified an accessory factor needed for IFN-γ signal transduction as IFN-γRβ, now IFN-γR2. These two chains were shown to be necessary and sufficient for IFN-γ activation of cells, although there has been some discussion of a possible third chain that more potently mediates antiviral activity *(22)*. Bach et al. *(23)* showed that IFN-γR2 is specifically downregulated in mature CD4 cells of either Th1 or Th2 phenotype, providing a means of desensitization of mature T-cells to IFN-γ through modulation of the signaling chain.

Dighe et al. *(24)* created an autosomal dominant form of the IFN-γR1 by truncation of the intracellular domain of the molecule leading to unusual expression characteristics in murine cells. The mutant molecule was overabundant on the cell surface and retained its IFN-γ binding activity although it had lost its signaling capacity and receptor recycling motif. This led to a dominant negative inhibition of IFN-γ signaling.

Interferon-γ signals through a membrane-bound receptor composed of two chains, IFN-γR1 and IFN-γR2 which are constitutively bound to their respective Janus kinases Jak1 and Jak2 *(see* Fig. 1). On binding of homodimeric IFN-γ the Jaks reciprocally transphosphorylate leading to phosphorylation of the intracellular domain of IFN-γR1 at tyrosine 440 (Y440). This serves as a binding site for the latent activator of signal transduction and transcription 1 (STAT1), which is, in turn, phosphorylated. Phosphorylated STAT1 (STAT1-P) homodimerizes, creating a complex that moves to the nucleus and binds nuclear DNA at sites that contain γ activation sequences (GAS) *(14,25,26)*.

3. ANIMAL MODELS

The creation of IFN-γ deficient *(27)*, IFN-γR1-deficient *(28)*, and IFN-γR2-deficient *(29)* mice allowed precise exploration of IFN-γ in mouse innate and acquired immunity. Enhanced susceptibility to *Mycobacterium (M). bovis* presaged the discovery of the critical roles of IFN-γ in protection against mycobacteria. IFN-γ was also shown to have important roles in the activity of NK cells and in the control of cellular proliferation. The remarkable similarities of IFN-γ deficient, IFN-γR1-deficient, and IFN-γR2-deficient mice suggested that the IFN-γR and its ligand are relatively mutually monogamous and control a large number of host innate and acquired immune responses. However, neither IFN-γ nor its receptor components are required for normal growth, development, generation of delayed-type hypersensitivity, or protection from normal flora under normal conditions. Therefore, IFN-γ (as well as IFN-α and IFN-β) is a cytokine whose function is most readily apparent in the setting of infection. In contrast, some of the signaling molecules that they activate, most notably Jak1, are absolutely required for normal development *(30)*. During acute viral infection in mice IFN-α inhibits IFN-γ production through a pathway that is dependent on the type 1 IFN receptor and is STAT1 mediated *(31)*. In addition, IFN-α inhibits IL-12-mediated IFN-γ production, at least in mice.

Dighe et al. *(32)* showed that IFN-γ responsiveness is necessary for tumor rejection. Expression of an autosomal dominant (AD) negative IFN-γR1 (ADIFN-γR1) mutant impaired immune rejection of a fibrosarcoma (Meth A) and overcame resistance in immune animals. Dighe et al. *(33)* also created mice transgenic for ADIFN-γR1 mutants under specific promoters that targeted IFN-γ unresponsiveness to specific compartments (mature macrophage or T-cell) by placing the construct under the control of the human lysozyme or *lck* promoters, respectively. In animals with macrophages rendered unresponsive to IFN-γ, susceptibility to listeriosis was enhanced, both in terms of mortality and microbial burden. This was not markedly augmented by wholesale neutralization of IFN-γ, suggesting that the macrophage is the critical compartment for listeriacidal activity. In animals with the ADIFN-γR1 construct under the *lck* promoter, the total numbers of T-cells and B-cells were normal, indicating that IFN-γ responsiveness is not needed for lymphoid development. However, functional expression of the transgene was limited to the CD3+ T-cell compartment. When animals with T-cells unresponsive to IFN-γ were challenged with *Listeria*, there was no difference between transgenics and normals in terms of mortality or body burden of organisms. There was no skewing of Th phenotype in animals transgenic for CD3+ ADIFN-γR1, suggesting that the Th1 phenotype development is not dependent on T-cell IFN-γ responsiveness. More relevant to Th1 development is IFN-γ enhancement of IL-12 production. Muller et al. *(34)* and Van den Broek et al. *(35)* used type 1 and type 2 IFNR knockout animals to demonstrate that for vaccinia and Theiler's viruses, both IFN systems are essential and are functionally nonredundant. Whereas IFN-α and IFN-β are essential for early response to viruses, IFN-γ is typically produced later in the course of the immune response and is active against intracellular bacteria and parasites. In contrast to mice with defects affecting type 1 IFN or STAT1, which died very early after viral infection, Weck et al. *(36)* used the γ-herpesvirus 68 to show that IFN-γR-deficient mice had longer survival, depending on the age at which they were inoculated. IFN-γR-deficient mice eventually cleared virus from their viscera, but they developed large-vessel arteritis several weeks after inoculation, involving the entire thickness of the vessel, whereas control animals had no mortality from virus and formed no arteritis.

Yap and Sher *(37)* showed important hematopoietic and parenchymal IFN-γR contributions to immune function by the creation of reciprocal bone marrow chimeric mice. Whereas resistance to *Listeria* required only hematopoietic IFN-γR expression, resistance to toxoplasmosis required expression of the IFN-γR on both hematopoietic and somatic cells. This result shows a critical role in host defense for nonhematopoietic cells. The anticipated curative effect of bone marrow transplantation for IFN-γR deficiency should be considered in the context of these findings, because even though successfully transplanted patients will have normal leukocytes, they may still be at risk for infections that require somatic contributions.

4. HUMAN POLYMORPHISMS

Tanaka et al. *(38)* studied a polymorphism in the signal peptide of IFN-γR1 (G88A, leading to the conversion of amino acid 14 from Met to Val). They found significant overrepresentation of this polymorphism in Japanese patients with systemic lupus erythematosus (SLE) compared to normals. The presence of the polymorphism led to reduced human leukocyte antigen-DR (HLA-DR) expression in response to IFN-γ stimulation. The amino acid change occurs at the end of the signal peptide and may therefore impede maturation of the receptor. However, subsequently, Nakashima et al. *(39)* followed up this work on the IFN-γR1 by looking at another polymorphism seen in the IFN-γR2, as reported in the initial article by Soh et al. *(22)*. The IFN-γR2 polymorphism is an arginine to glutamine change at amino acid 64 (Arg64Gln). This polymorphism carried no independent risk of SLE, but when combined with the previously described polymorphism Val14Met in IFN-γR1, it conferred an odds ratio for SLE of 9.6, compared to individuals bearing homozygous Val14 and homozygous Arg64. Retrospectively, Nakashima et al. *(39)* also recognized that the effects previously ascribed to the Val14Met polymorphism in IFN-γR1 were only seen when that was associated with the homozygous Gln64 polymorphism in IFN-γR2. Therefore, this is an example of a phenotype (increased risk of SLE) conferred only in the presence of a complex genotype (polymorphisms in both IFN-γR1 and IFN-γR2). Whether this genotype has an infection-related phenotype as well has not been determined.

Multiple defects have been identified in the IFN-γR1 and IFN-γR2 (reviewed in Chapter 11 in this volume and in ref. *26*). These have, in general, been identified because of severe infections with intracellular organisms such as nontuberculous mycobacteria and salmonella, but have also been associated with severe viral infections as well *(40)*.

5. IFN-γ THERAPY

In humans, IFN-γ has used for infectious and noninfectious diseases since the mid-1980s (see Table 1). Nathan et al. *(41)* first demonstrated the ability of IFN-γ to upregulate the production of superoxide by macrophages in vitro. IFN-γ produced the same upregulation of hydrogen peroxide formation in patients with advanced malignancy *(42)*. These seminal articles suggested that IFN-γ has a critical role in host defense that is dependent on the NADPH oxidase, the cellular mechanism that transfers an electron from NADPH to molecular oxygen, resulting in the superoxide anion and the downstream metabolites hydrogen peroxide and bleach *(43)*. The recognition that IFN-γ-induced macrophage and neutrophil superoxide production led to experiments in patients with chronic granulomatous disease (CGD), in whom the NADPH oxidase is genetically deficient. Certain CGD patients actually responded to IFN-γ in vitro with increased superoxide production and bacterial killing *(44–46)*. In addition, IFN-γ upregulated the expression of the X-linked gene involved in CGD, gp91[phox] *(47)*. Ezekowitz et al. *(48)* and Sechler et al. *(45)*, showed partial correction of the superoxide production defect in CGD by in vivo administration of IFN-γ.

Schiff et al. *(49)* administered IFN-γ to normal volunteers and examined markers of cellular adhesion, cellular activation, and opsonic potential. Neutrophil expression of the high-affinity Fc-γ-receptor (FcγR1) peaked 48 h after IFN-γ treatment. Monocyte expression of Fc-γR1, Fc-γRII, Fc-γRIII, CD11a, CD11b, CD18, and HLA-DR increased over the same time-course. Neutrophil phagocytosis of opsonized killed bacteria was also enhanced due to upregulation of Fc-γRI. Lipopolysaccharide-binding protein in serum also increased. These data proved that IFN-γ has broad effects on cellular activation, trafficking, and opsonic activity, and these effects may underlie some of its benefits in terms of innate immunity.

5.1. Route and Dose Considerations

Aulitzky et al. *(50)* studied longitudinal administration of IFN-γ to patients with renal cell carcinoma. They looked at the downstream markers of IFN-γ activation β2 microglobulin and neopterin. Using these two markers, they showed robust activation by IFNγ following the first dose, but there was tachyphylaxis at high doses (500 μg) and daily administration. In contrast, alternate-day administration and lower dose levels (100 μg) retained responsiveness. These data were used to determine the dosing regimens that were used in the CGD trial (50 μg/m^2 subcutaneously three times weekly). Subsequently, Ahlin et al. *(51)* examined the effects of 50 μg/m^2 and 100 μg/m^2 IFN-γ on neutrophil responses in two small randomized groups of patients with CGD of several different genotypes. Doses were given on two successive days and effects monitored over 18 d. There was modest induction of superoxide production in some patients in both groups, an increase in CD64 (Fc-γR1) expression that was somewhat dose dependent, and a modest increase in aspergillicidal activity that was slightly greater at the higher dose than the lower one. Long-term therapy was not addressed.

Jaffe et al. *(52)* administered IFN-γ by aerosol to normal volunteers over a range of doses up to 1000 μg for up to 2 wk. They showed good tolerance of the drug and good local induction of macrophage activation. Peripheral blood monocyte activation was not detected with aerosol administration, nor was there induction of interferon inducible protein 10 (IP-10), an IFN-γ responsive chemokine. In contrast, systemically administered IFN-γ led to no induction of pulmonary macrophage IP-10. However, it is unclear whether this compartmentalization of immune response can be extrapolated to patients with ongoing pulmonary inflammation or those receiving chronic therapy.

Table 1
Documented Uses of Interferon-γ in Infectious Diseases

Infection prophylaxis in chronic granulomatous disease*
Delay of disease progression in severe osteopetrosis*
Disseminated nontuberculous mycobacterial infection
Pulmonary nontuberculous mycobacterial infection (aerosol)
Pulmonary multidrug resistant tuberculosis (aerosol)
Visceral leishmaniasis
Diffuse cutaneous leishmaniasis
Lepromatous leprosy (high rate of ENL)

*Uses approved by the Food and Drug Administration of the United States. Doses are given in the relevant sections of the text.

Kuzmann et al. *(53)* found expansion of γδ T-cells in patients receiving the aminobisphosphonates alendronate, ibandronate, and pamidronate, which in turn, led to a significant increase in IFN-γ production in vitro. This may have unanticipated clinical implications for those being treated with these drugs.

6. CHRONIC GRANULOMATOUS DISEASE

The above observations in superoxide production led to an international, double-blinded, placebo controlled trial of IFN-γ therapy as infection prophylaxis in CGD. This trial showed that IFN-γ reduced the number and severity of infections in CGD by about 70%, regardless of antibiotic prophylaxis or genetic subtype of CGD *(54)*. However, this pivotal study did not show that the administration of IFN-γ led to upregulation of superoxide formation in the recipients; that is, IFN-γ was clearly effective in reducing infections in CGD, but the mechanism was not shown to be through the induction of superoxide or changes in the in vitro killing of bacteria. There was augmentation of in vitro killing of aspergillus hyphae by CGD cells from patients treated with IFN-γ *(55)*. Therefore, the salutary effects of IFN-γ on infection susceptibility in CGD are likely independent of regulation of the NADPH oxidase. Despite the absence of a cellular mechanism, IFN-γ was licensed in the United States in 1991 for the prophylactic treatment of CGD. Long-term follow-up of patients who have received over 10 yr of IFN-γ (50 µg/m^2 subcutaneously three times weekly) has shown no unexpected toxicity or impairment of growth or development *(56,57)*. These long-term IFN-γ safety data include pediatric populations and suggest that long-term therapy is safe and well tolerated.

Studies of IFN-γ prophylaxis in CGD mice have confirmed the benefits seen in the human study and the absence of superoxide production through NADPH oxidase, but have still not shed light on the specific mechanism *(58)*. Understanding this mechanism is still quite important, as it is the largest patient population studied so far, and the same effect can be shown in mice and humans.

7. OSTEOPETROSIS

Osteopetrosis is a genetic disease in which bone becomes sclerotic, compromising bone marrow space and cranial nerve foramina. Patients suffer from anemia, blindness, deafness, and recurrent pathologic fractures. In addition, patients with osteopetrosis have recurrent infections and their neutrophils are partially defective in superoxide production, as evidenced by granulocyte–monocyte colony-forming units (GM-CFUs) that are low producers of superoxide (as determined by nitroblue tetrazolium [NBT] reduction). Osteoclasts are also thought to be low producers of superoxide as well, which may be related to their failure to correctly remodel bone. Key et al. *(59)* showed that IFN-γ increased bone resorption and superoxide production in humans with osteopetrosis. Treatment of rat calvaria in vitro with parathyroid hormone (PTH) led to an increase in NBT staining and calcium release, an effect inhibited by desferal manganese, suggesting that superoxide is important in bone resorption. Presumably the superoxide produced in bone is not from the NADPH oxidase, because CGD patients who are NADPH oxidase deficient do not get osteopetrosis, pathologic fractures, or severe anemia. IFN-γ was used in the treatment of osteopetrosis at the same dose as that used in patients with CGD (50 μg/m^2 subcutaneously three times weekly) (60,61). The study of IFN-γ for osteopetrosis found that bone resorption was increased, the incidence of infections was markedly decreased, GM-CFU NBT reduction was increased, the transfusion requirement diminished, and growth increased. The drug was well tolerated. All patients experienced some fever, and two had fever > 40°C. The severe fevers disappeared with reduction of the dose by 50%, and all patients tolerated drug well after 6 mo of therapy. Osteopetrosis has been accepted as a licensed indication for the use of IFN-γ in the United States.

8. TRAUMA AND BURNS

Because IFN-γ activates phagocytes to increased production of superoxide and general activation, there has been interest in whether IFN-γ can reduce infection rates in the acutely ill. Hershmann et al. (62) found cell surface HLA-DR, a marker of monocyte activation, significantly reduced in patients with severe injury or trauma. This abnormality in HLA-DR display was corrected by incubation of blood from injured patients in vitro with IFN-γ.

Polk et al. (63) administered either placebo or 100 μg IFN-γ subcutaneously daily for 10 d to 213 trauma patients at high risk for infection. IFN-γ significantly increased monocyte HLA-DR antigen expression and outcome predictive score. Although there were fewer severe complications and fewer deaths in the IFN-γ arm, these differences were not statistically significant. This tantalizing result suggested that IFN-γ might be useful in patients with severe trauma, but required a larger and perhaps differently structured trial to be proven.

Dries et al. (64) conducted a large multicenter, double-blinded, randomized controlled trial in 416 patients using a 21-d treatment arm. They found a significant benefit to IFN-γ treatment in terms of the number of deaths resulting from infection, and deaths overall. However, this effect was dominated by the results of one center, leaving the overall utility of IFN-γ in this setting unproven.

Kox et al. (65) treated 10 patients with sepsis or the systemic immune response syndrome (SIRS) with 100 μg sc IFN-γ daily if they had <30% of monocytes expressing HLA-DR, and continued IFN-γ until expression was >50% for three consecutive days. Eight patients responded within the first 24 h, and the remainder took 2–3 d. IFN-γ was associated with early rises in plasma tumor necrosis factor (TNF)-α and IL-6 levels, but there was no clear effect on mortality or morbidity.

To explore the possible benefits of IFN-γ in prophylaxis in burns, Wasserman et al. (66) conducted a randomized, double blind, placebo-controlled, phase III multicenter trial at 23 European burn centers. They enrolled 216 patients with severe burns to receive either 100 μg IFN-γ subcutaneously daily for up to 90 d or placebo. They found no differences between the groups in terms of death, infection rate, duration of intensive care stay, or overall hospitalization, or scar formation.

9. LEISHMANIASIS

Carvalho et al. (67) showed that active infection with visceral leishmaniasis suppressed cytokine production. Whereas mitogen-stimulated IFN-γ production was normal in patients with active visceral leishmaniasis, IFN-γ production in response to *Leishmania donovani* antigen was absent during the active disease, but normalized after successful chemotherapy. This suggested that restoration of IFN-γ systemically during visceral leishmaniasis might be therapeutic. Murrray et al. (68) demonstrated synergy of IFN-γ and sodium stibogluconate (Pentostam) in *L. donovani*-infected human macrophages in vitro and in mice in vivo.

Badaro et al. (69) used IFN-γ plus pentostam in patients with visceral leishmaniasis who had been refractory to pentostam alone. Six of eight patients with refractory visceral leishmaniasis responded to treatment with IFN-γ at doses of 100–400 μg/m^2/d in addition to pentostam 20 mg/kg/d for 10–40 d. In addition, nine treatment-naïve patients with severe visceral leishmaniasis were treated, eight of whom responded to treatment with IFN-γ plus pentostam. Responders had marked improvement in anemia, leukopenia, weight gain, diminution in spleen size, and reduction in organisms in splenic aspirates. No relapse or recurrence was seen in up to 8 mo. The major toxicity was fever. Badaro and Johnson *(70)* later treated several South American patients successfully with diffuse cutaneous leishmaniasis.

Sundar et al. *(71)* treated 15 Indian patients refractory to conventional therapy with 30 d of pentostam and IFN-γ. In the remaining 13 patients, IFN-γ plus antimony treatment was associated with daily fever but no other adverse reactions. Thirteen of the patients were cured; two patients withdrew for intolerance and subsequently died.

Sundar et al. *(72)* went on to show that in previously untreated patients with visceral leishmaniasis, IFN-γ plus antimonials dramatically shortened the time to parasitologic cure compared to antimonials alone (63% vs 10%, respectively, at 10 d). Further, they had 100% response in the combined-therapy group, all of whom had durable cures. This was a higher level of response than in the conventional monotherapy arm.

Sundar and Murray *(73)* tested IFN-γ monotherapy in visceral leishmaniasis in nine patients. After 20 d of IFN-γ therapy, four patients did not have parasitologic change. In the other five patients, parasite loads in splenic aspirates declined about 75% but did not resolve completely. Therefore, although IFN-γ induced some degree of clearing, it was unable to cure leishmaniasis as monotherapy. Sundar et al. *(74)* showed equivalence of short-course (15-d) therapy with IFN-γ plus stibogluconate to long-course combined therapy (30 d) and long-course conventional monotherapy with stibogluconate (30 d).

In summary, active visceral leishmaniasis is associated with antigen-specific immune suppression, but the cells are still IFN-γ responsive. IFN-γ has a potent synergistic effect on therapy with conventional antimonials, but is of relatively modest effect without concurrently administered antiparasitics. The mechanisms involved in this activity are unclear, but increased intracellular concentration of antiparasitics may be important.

10. MYCOBACTERIAL INFECTIONS

Hypersusceptibility to nontuberculous mycobacterial infections in patients with mutations affecting IFN-γ/IL-12 synthesis or response serves as human proof of concept for the central role of IFN-γ and IL-12 in mycobacterial control. However, the mechanism(s) remain elusive *(26)*.

Appelberg and Orme *(75)* showed that IFN-γ was mycobacteriostatic in mouse cells in vitro and suggested that its main effect was to enhance acidification of mycobacteria-containing vesicles. Toxic oxygen radicals were unnecessary for control of *M. bovis* infection in mouse bone marrow cells in vitro *(76)*. In mice lacking the NADPH oxidase (i.e., CGD mice) and hence unable to produce phagocyte superoxide in response to infection, there was no increased susceptibility to *M. avium* infection compared to wild-type animals *(77)*. For *M. tuberculosis*, the NADPH oxidase appears to be more important for early but not late control of infection in the lung *(78,79)*. In contrast, nitric oxide (NO) is critically important for mycobacterial control in mice *(77,78)*. Human cells are inconsistent in vitro in terms of IFN-γ-activated mycobacterial killing: Some studies show IFN-γ mycobactericidal and mycobacteriostatic activities *(80)* but others do not *(81)*. In one study, IFN-γ enhanced the growth of *M. avium* complex (MAC) in macrophages *(82)*.

Interferon-γ knockout (KO) mice develop widespread tuberculosis with very poor granulomatous response and die rapidly *(83,84)*. Interestingly, parenterally administered IFN-γ failed to restore normal resistance to tuberculosis. It is still unclear whether this reflects a critical role for IFN-γ in immune development, that systemically administered IFN-γ does not activate critical local defenses as well as IFN-γ supplied by local T-cells or NK cells, or a dose effect in these kinds of animal experiments

(83). Similar tuberculosis susceptibilities were seen in IFN-γR-deficient mice *(85)* and in mice lacking the IFN-γ-induced interferon regulatory factor-1 (IRF-1) *(86)*. Hypersusceptibility to MAC infection was reported in IFN-γ-deficient mice *(77)*. In wild-type mice infected with MAC, elevated prostaglandin E_2 production (an inhibitor of macrophage function) was successfully down regulated by IFN-γ, leading to enhanced mycobacterial clearance *(87)*.

Hussain et al. *(88)* found that soon after MAC infection of mice, macrophage levels of IFN-γR1 and IFN-γR2 begin to decline, followed by inhibition of the ability to activate STAT1. This, in turn, led to the decrease of inducibility of many IFN-γ responsive genes (e.g., IRF-1) and a relative inability of the cell to be activated to the antimycobacterial state. Ting et al. *(89)* showed that *M. tuberculosis* infection of human macrophages blocks certain distal effects of IFN-γ, including killing of *Toxoplasma gondii* and induction of Fc-γRI. *M. tuberculosis* also inhibits the association of STAT1 with the transcriptional coactivators cAMP response element binding (CREB) protein and p300. Irradiated whole organisms, isolated cell walls, and, to a lesser degree, the cell wall component lipoarabinomannan (LAM) have similar effects on live organisms. Therefore, in contrast to the case using murine macrophages and MAC, in this human system, *M. tuberculosis* inhibits distal aspects of IFN-γ signaling while leaving proximal processes (Jak-STAT interaction) intact.

10.1 Treatment of Mycobacterial Infections

Interferon-γ has been used as an adjuvant in the treatment of the three major human mycobacterial infections: *M. leprae*, *M. avium* complex, and *M. tuberculosis*.

10.1.1. Mycobacterium leprae

Nathan et al. *(90)* first used short-course, low-dose, intradermal IFN-γ in the treatment of lepromatous leprosy (1–10 μg daily for 3 d) in conjunction with antimycobacterials. Monocyte hydrogen peroxide production was enhanced, granuloma formation increased, local activation markers upregulated, and the cutaneous bacterial burden decreased.

Sampaio et al. *(91)* used longer-term IFN-γ therapy (10 mo) in conjunction with antimycobacterials, but noted a rate of erythema nodosum leprosum (ENL; a toxic inflammatory reaction in leprosy that can lead to neuropathy or death) in IFN-γ recipients that was much higher than in those receiving antimycobacterials alone (60% vs 17%, respectively). ENL correlated with TNF-α message and protein in peripheral blood and mononuclear cells. Thalidomide, long used clinically in the treatment of ENL, decreased TNF-α levels in cells and blood through what was thought to be destabilization of TNF-α mRNA *(93)*. When IFN-γ was given simultaneous with thalidomide and antimycobacterial chemotherapy to patients with lepromatous leprosy, there was no increase in clearance of infection over that observed with antimycobacterials alone *(94)*. Therefore, thalidomide appears to modulate the factors that underlie IFN-γ's effect on mycobacterial clearance. On the other hand, thalidomide blocked the development of ENL.

The fundamental causes of ENL are still unknown. It is clear that ENL is a response to the presence of organisms and does not occur in leprosy patients treated to clearance of bacillary loads *(93)*. ENL has not been seen in the therapy of other mycobacterial diseases for which long-term IFN-γ has been used, suggesting that ENL is leprosy-specific. Haslett et al. *(94)* have now shown that thalidomide enhances CD8+ T-lymphocyte proliferation as well as IL-12 and IFN-γ production. Bekker et al. *(94a)* used thalidomide in patients with tuberculosis and HIV and showed enhancement of antigen-specific proliferative responses, preferentially through CD8+ T-lymphocytes. In contrast to the experience in leprosy, the clinical trials in tuberculosis showed little, if any, effect of thalidomide on TNF-α levels, leaving the mechanism by which thalidomide affects ENL unclear. However, there is no requirement that the effect that thalidomide or IFN-γ has on one mycobacterial infection be mirrored in another one. Just as the manifestations and clinical course of tuberculosis are quite different from leprosy, so the effects of immunomodulating drugs may be quite divergent in the different diseases.

In the treatment of leprosy, IFN-γ only reduced bacterial load when combined with antimycobacterials. When used alone (i.e., in the absence of associated antimycobacterials), it induced immunological changes (e.g., granulomata, hydrogen peroxide production) but did not significantly affect clearing of the infection. Similar effects were seen with IFN-γ monotherapy of leishmaniasis *(73)*. Both IFN-γ and TNF-α significantly increase the intracellular concentration of the macrolide antibiotic azithromycin, a mechanism that may be relevant for other antibiotics as well *(95)*.

10.1.2. Mycobacterium avium *Complex and Other Nontuberculous Mycobacteria*

Squires et al. *(96,97)* were the first to use IFN-γ in the treatment of MAC infection. They treated six MAC-bacteremic AIDS patients with IFN-γ with or without concurrent antimycobacterials for up to 6 wk. In those patients who received IFN-γ plus antimycobacterials, there was a clear decline in mycobacteremia, but when IFNγ was used without concurrent antimycobacterials there was no change in bacterial counts. After discontinuation of IFN-γ, bacterial counts rebounded. These results were independent of CD4+ T-lymphocyte counts, indicating that the IFN-γ therapeutic activity was not significantly mediated by CD4+ T lymphocytes.

Holland et al. *(98)* used subcutaneous IFN-γ in the treatment of seven patients with treatment refractory disseminated MAC infection who did not have HIV infection or known malignancies. They found dramatic improvement in clinical condition, culture recovery of organisms, as well as histopathologic and radiographic evidence of disease. This was correlated with low in vitro IFN-γ production in response to the mitogen phytohemagglutinin (PHA). Importantly, this effect of IFN-γ was independent of CD4+ T-lymphocyte counts, suggesting that exogenously administered IFN-γ is able to overcome at least some of the defects associated with lymphocytopenia. The drug was well tolerated, although some dose reductions were required. Subsequent experience of the same authors in the treatment of refractory disseminated MAC infections in patients with intact IFN-γ receptors has shown an overall cure rate of about 60% (unpublished data).

Patients with autosomal recessive, complete defects in the IFN-γR have been identified and reported and there have been suggestions of IFN-γ benefit in some of these cases *(99,100)*. However, these benefits have not been demonstrable in vitro. In contrast, the patients with ADIFN-γR1 mutations respond well to IFN-γ therapy *(101)*. Patients with mutations in the IL-12 p40 gene *(102)* or the IL-12Rβ1 chain *(103,104)* are also highly responsive to IFN-γ therapy, as would be expected. In these patients, the IFN-γR pathways are intact, but because of the lack of IL-12-driven IFN-γ production, the IFN-γ receptor is understimulated *(105)*. For patients with known or suspected mutations in the IFN-γ receptors, the advisability of IFN-γ therapy depends on whether the specific mutation is complete, partial, or dominant (*see* Fig. 1). Patients with complete ADIFN-γR1 or complete ADIFN-γR2 deficiency demonstrate absolute refractoriness to IFN-γ stimulation in vitro and in vivo. In contrast, patients with partial defects, whether in IFN-γR1 or IFN-γR2, show in vitro response to addition of IFNγ at levels 10- to 100-fold higher than normal (*see* Chapter 11). Patients with the dominant forms of IFN-γR1 deficiency show attenuated IFNγ responsiveness in vitro at higher doses. IFN-γ therapy in vivo is clearly effective in patients with ADIFN-γR1 deficiency, even at the standard 50-μg/m^2 dose (Holland et al, unpublished observations). Some cases of ADIFN-γR1 deficiency are slow to respond and higher doses may be needed (Kumararatne personal communication).

Chatte et al. *(106)* used aerosolized IFN-γ, 500 μg, by nebulizer 3 d/wk in a 38-yr-old man with silicosis and severe cavitary MAC disease who had failed medical therapy. Aerosolized IFN-γ converted his smears to negative, although his cultures persisted positive. With the cessation of aerosolized IFN-γ, his sputum smears reverted to their previous level and his disease progressed fatally. This was the first report of aerosolized IFN-γ in the treatment of mycobacterial disease. The finding of rapid conversion of sputum to smear negative was remarkable in such a long-term refractory patient.

10.1.3. Mycobacterium tuberculosis

The experience with IFN-γ and tuberculosis is limited. Raad et al. *(107)* reported a patient with acute lymphocytic leukemia in remission with biopsy proven multidrug-resistant tuberculosis (MDRTB) involving the brain and spinal cord was steroid dependent because of infection-related edema. Subcutaneous IFN-γ allowed rapid reduction in steroid dose and led to cure without any

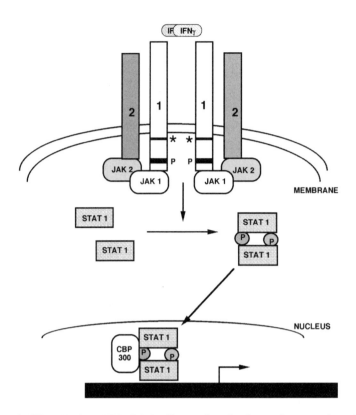

Fig. 1. Homodimeric IFN-γ binds to IFN-γR1, leading to dimerization and aggregation with IFN-γR2 molecules. The respective Janus kinases (JAKs) are brought together and transphosphorylate. This leads to the
phosphorylation of IFN-γR1 at Y440, shown by P. STAT1 binds to this site and becomes phosphorylated,
then homodimerizes and goes to the nucleus where it combines with CBP300 and upregulates IFN-γ responsive genes. * shows the site of 818del4 mutation in IFN-γR1.

exacerbation of central nervous system inflammation. The ability of IFN-γ to induce cure without an
exacerbation of local inflammation is encouraging in terms of its safety in the treatment of inflammatory diseases. This result was somewhat presaged by the experience in CGD, in which there was no
obvious exacerbation of inflammatory conditions in the randomized trial *(54)*. Condos et al. *(108)*
used IFN-γ aerosol (500 μg three times weekly for 4 wk) in five patients with long-standing MDRTB
refractory to medical therapy. All five showed clearing of the sputum smears within that month. With
this short course of therapy, no cultures converted and all patients returned to smear positive after
cessation of IFN-γ. Importantly, no patient worsened during therapy and there were no significant
systemic or local complaints. A placebo-controlled, randomized, multicenter prospective trial of aerosolized IFN-γ was conducted in pulmonary MDRTB but has not proven efficacy. A randomized trial
in severe or refractory pulmonary MAC infection is underway.

CONCLUSIONS

The mechanisms by which IFN-γ exerts its beneficial effects in the treatment of infectious diseases are easy to imagine but, so far, difficult to demonstrate. Even though we now have incontro-
vertible proof that IFN-γ is necessary for mycobacterial control, in particular, and the control of
intracellular infections in general, we still do not know why. This ignorance, in turn, leaves open
numerous hypotheses about mechanism of action in other disease states. However, the interferons are
critical components of normal host response and they can be therapeutically used in many diseases.

REFERENCES

1. Nagano, Y. and Kojima, Y.(1954) Pouvoir immunisant du virus vaccinal inactive par des rayons ultraviolets. *C. R. Soc. Biol. (Paris)* **148**, 1700–1702.
2. Isaacs, A. and Lindemann, J. (1957) Virus interferone. I: the interferons. *Proc. R. Soc. Biol. (Lond.)* **147**, 258–267.
3. David M. (1995) Transcription factors in interferon signaling. *Pharmacol. Ther.* **65(2)**, 149–161.
4. Frucht, D.M., Fan, S., Siegel, R.M., Visconti, R., and O'Shea, J.J. (2001) Cytokine signal transduction, in *Cytokine Therapeutics in Infectious Diseases* (Holland, S.M., ed.), Lippincott Williams & Wilkins, Philadelphia, pp. 295–322.
5. Nguyen, H., Hiscott, J., and Pitha, P.M. (1997) The growing family of interferon regulatory factors. *Cytokine Growth Factor Rev.* **8**, 293–312.
6. Wang, J., Wakeham, J., Harkness, R., and Xing, Z. (1999) Macrophages are a significant source of type 1 cytokines during mycobacterial infection. *J. Clin. Invest.* **103(7)**, 1023–1029.
7. Tomura, M., Maruo, S., Mu, J., Zhou, X.Y., Ahn, H.J., Hamaoka, T., et al. (1998) Differential capacities of CD4+, CD8+, and CD4-CD8– T cell subsets to express IL-18 receptor and produce IFN-gamma in response to IL-18. *J. Immunol.* **160**, 3759–3765.
8. Mountford, A.P., Coulson, P.S., Cheever, A.W., Sher, A., Wilson, R.A., and Wynn, T.A. (1999) Interleukin-12 can directly induce T-helper 1 responses in interferon-gamma (IFN-gamma) receptor-deficient mice, but requires IFN-gamma signalling to downregulate T-helper 2 responses. *Immunology* **97(4)**, 588–594.
9. Boehm, U., Klamp, T., Groot, M., and Howard, J.C. (1997) Cellular responses to interferon-g. *Annu. Rev. Immunol.* **15**, 749–795,
10. Pien, G.C., Satoskar, A.R., Takeda, K., Akira, S., and Biron, C.A. (2000) Cutting edge: selective IL-18 requirements for induction of compartmental IFN-gamma responses during viral infection. *J. Immunol.* **165(9)**, 4787–4791
11. Humphreys, B.D. and Dubyak, G.R. (1996) Induction of the P2z/P2X7 nucleotide receptor and associated phospholipase D activity by lipopolysaccharide and IFN-gamma in the human THP-1 monocytic cell line. *J. Immunol.* **157(12)**, 5627–5637.
12. Lammas, D.A., Stober, C., Harvey, C.J, Kendrick, N., Panchalingam, S., and Kumararatne, D.S. (1997) ATP-induced killing of mycobacteria by human macrophages is mediated by purinergic P2Z(P2X7) receptors. *Immunity* **7(3)**, 433–444.
13. Murray, H.W. (1996) Current and future clinical applications of interferon-gamma in host antimicrobial defense. *Intensive Care Med.* **22(Suppl. 4)**, S456–S461,
14. Darnell, J.E. Jr. (1998) Studies of IFN-induced transcriptional activation uncover the Jak–Stat pathway. *J. Interferon Cytokine Res.* **18**, 549–554.
15. Nistico, A. and Young, N.S. (1994) Gamma-interferon gene expression in the bone marrow of patients with aplastic anemia. *Ann. Intern. Med.* **120(6)**, 463–469.
16. Murphy, W.J., Welniak, L.A., Taub, D.D., Wiltrout, R.H., Taylor, P.A., Vallera, D.A., et al. (1998) Differential effects of the absence of interferon-gamma and IL-4 in acute graft-versus-host disease after allogeneic bone marrow transplantation in mice. *J. Clin. Invest.* **102(9)**, 1742–1748
17. Yang, Y.G., Dey, B.R., Sergio, J.J., Pearson, D.A., and Sykes, M. (1998) Donor-derived interferon gamma is required for inhibition of acute graft-versus-host disease by interleukin 12. *J. Clin. Invest.* **102(12)**, 2126–2135.
18. Saleem, S., Konieczny, B.T., Lowry, R.P., Baddoura, F.K., and Lakkis, F.G. (1996) Acute rejection of vascularized heart allografts in the absence of IFNgamma. *Transplantation* **62(12)**, 1908–1911.
19. Aguet, M., Dembic, Z., and Merlin, G. (1988) Molecular cloning and expression of the human interferon-gamma receptor. *Cell* **55(2)**, 273–280.
20. Bohni, R., Hemmi, S., and Aguet, M. (1994) Signaling steps involving the cytoplasmic domain of the interferon-gamma receptor alpha-subunit are not species-specific. *J. Biol.* **269(20)**, 14,541–14,545.
21. Hemmi, S., Bohni , R., Stark, G., Di Marco, F., and Aguet, M. (1994) A novel member of the interferon receptor family complements functionality of the murine interferon gamma receptor in human cells. *Cell* **76(5)**, 803–810.
22. Soh, J., Donnelly, R.J., Kotenko, S., Mariano, T. M., Cook, J. R., Wang, N., et al. (1994) Identification and sequence of an accessory factor required for activation of the human interferon gamma receptor. *Cell* **76(5)**, 793–802.
23. Bach, E.A., Szabo, S.J., Dighe, A.S., Ashkenazi, A., Aguet, M., Murphy, K. M., et al. (1995) Ligand-induced autoregulation of IFN-gamma receptor beta chain expression in T helper cell subsets. *Science* **270(5239)**, 1215–1218.
24. Dighe, A.S., Farrar, M.A., and Schreiber, R.D. (1993) Inhibition of cellular responsiveness to interferon-gamma (IFN gamma) induced by overexpression of inactive forms of the IFN gamma receptor. *J. Biol. Chem.* **268(14)**, 10,645–10,653.
25. Schindler, C. and Darnell, J.E., Jr. (1995)Transcriptional responses to polypeptide ligands: the JAK-STAT pathway. *Annu. Rev. Biochem.* **64**, 621–651,
26. Dorman, S.E. and Holland, S.M., (2000) Interferon-gamma and interleukin-12 pathway defects and human disease. *Cytokine Growth Factor Rev.* **11(4)**, 321–333.
27. Dalton, D.K., Pitts-Meek, S., Keshav, S., Figari, I.S., Bradley, A., and Stewart, T.A. (1993) Multiple defects of immune cell function in mice with disrupted interferon-gamma genes. *Science* **259(5102)**, 1739–1742.
28. Huang, S., Hendriks, W., Althage, A., Hemmi, S., Bluethmann, H., Kamijo. R., et al. (1993) Immune response in mice that lack the interferon-gamma receptor. *Science* **259(5102)**, 1742–1745

29. Lu, B., Ebensperger, C., Dembic, Z., Wang, Y., Kvatyuk, M., Lu, T., et al. (1998) Targeted disruption of the interferon-gamma receptor 2 gene results in severe immune defects in mice. *Proc. Natl. Acad. Sci. USA* **95**, 8233–8238.

30. Rodig, S.J., Meraz, M.A., White, J.M., Lampe, P.A., Riley, J.K., Arthur C.D., et al. (1998) Disruption of the Jak1 gene demonstrates obligatory and nonredundant roles of the Jaks in cytokine-induced biologic responses. *Cell* **93(3)**, 373–383.

31. Nguyen, K.B., Cousens, L.P., Doughty, L.A., Pien, G.C., Durbin, J.E., and Biron, C.A., (2000) Interferon a/b-mediated inhibition and promotion of interferon g: STAT1 resolves a paradox. *Nat. Immunol.* **1**, 70–76.

32. Dighe, A.S., Richards, E., Old, L.J., and Schreiber, R.D. (1994) Enhanced in vivo growth and resistance to rejection of tumor cells expressing dominant negative IFN gamma receptors. *Immunity* **1(6)**, 447–456.

33. Dighe, A.S., Campbell, D., Hsieh, C.S., Clarke, S., Greaves, D.R., Gordon, S., et al.(1995) Tissue-specific targeting of cytokine unresponsiveness in transgenic mice. *Immunity* **3(5)**, 657–666.

34. Muller, U., Steinhoff, U., Reis, L.F., Hemmi, S., Pavlovic, J., Zinkernagel, R.M., et al. (1994) Functional role of type I and type II interferons in antiviral defense. *Science* **264(5167)**, 1918–1921.

35. van den Broek, M.F., Muller, U., Huang, S., Zinkernagel, R.M., and Aguet., M. (1995) Immune defence in mice lacking type I and/or type II interferon receptors. *Immunol. Rev.* **148**, 5–18.

36. Weck, K,E., Dal Canto, A.J., Gould, J.D., O'Guin, A.K., Roth, K.A., Saffitz, J.E., et al.(1997) Murine gamma-herpesvirus 68 causes severe large-vessel arteritis in mice lacking interferon-gamma responsiveness: a new model for virus-induced vascular disease. *Nat. Med.* **3(12)**, 1346–1353.

37. Yap, G.S. and Sher, A. (1999) Effector cells of both nonhemopoietic and hemopoietic origin are required for interferon (IFN)-gamma- and tumor necrosis factor (TNF)-alpha-dependent host resistance to the intracellular pathogen, *Toxoplasma gondii*. *J. Exp. Med.* **189(7)**, 1083–1092.

38. Tanaka, Y., Nakashima, H., Hisano, C., Kohsaka, T., Nemoto, Y., Niiro, H., et al. (1999) Association of the interferon-gamma receptor variant (Val14Met) with systemic lupus erythematosus. *Immunogenetics* **49(4)**, 266–271.

39. Nakashima, H., Inoue, H., Akahoshi, M., Tanaka, Y., Yamaoka, K., Ogami, E., et al. (1999)The combination of polymorphisms within interferon-gamma receptor 1 and receptor 2 associated with the risk of systemic lupus erythematosus. *FEBS Lett.* **453(1–2)**, 187–190.

40. Dorman, S.E., Uzel, G., Roesler, J., Bradley, J.S., Bastian, J., Billman, G., et al.(1999) Viral infections in interferon-gamma receptor deficiency. *J. Pediatr.* **135(5)**, 640–643.

41. Nathan, C.F., Murray, H.W., Wiebe, M.E., and Rubin, B.Y. (1983) Identification of interferon-gamma as the lymphokine that activates human macrophage oxidative metabolism and antimicrobial activity. *J. Exp. Med.* **158(3)**, 670–689.

42. Nathan, C.F., Horowitz, C.R., de la Harpe, J., Vadhan-Raj, S., Sherwin, S.A., Oettgen, H.F., et al. (1985) Administration of recombinant interferon gamma to cancer patients enhances monocyte secretion of hydrogen peroxide. *Proc. Natl. Acad. Sci. USA* **82(24)**, 8686–8690.

43. Segal, B.H., Leto, T.L., Gallin, J.I., Malech, H.L., and Holland, S.M. (2000) Genetic, biochemical, and clinical features of chronic granulomatous disease. *Medicine (Balt.)* **79(3)**, 170–200.

44. Gallin, J.I., Sechler, J.M., and Malech, H.L. (1998) Reconstitution of defective phagocyte function in chronic granulomatous disease of childhood with recombinant human interferon-gamma. *Trans. Assoc. Am. Physicians* **101**, 12–17.

45. Sechler, J.M., Malech, H.L., White, C.J., and Gallin, J.I. (1988) Recombinant human interferon-gamma reconstitutes defective phagocyte function in patients with chronic granulomatous disease of childhood. *Proc. Natl. Acad. Sci. USA* **85(13)**, 4874–4878.

46. Ezekowitz, R.A, Orkin, S.H., and Newburger, P.E. (1987) Recombinant interferon gamma augments phagocyte superoxide production and X-chronic granulomatous disease gene expression in X-linked variant chronic granulomatous disease. *J. Clin. Invest.* **80(4)**, 1009–1016.

47. Newburger, P.E., Ezekowitz, R.A., Whitney, C., Wright, J., and Orkin, S.H.(1988) Induction of phagocyte cytochrome b heavy chain gene expression by interferon gamma. *Proc. Natl. Acad. Sci. USA* **85(14)**, 5215–5219.

48. Ezekowitz, R.A., Dinauer, M.C., Jaffe, H.S., Orkin, S.H., and Newburger, P.E. (1988) Partial correction of the phagocyte defect in patients with X-linked chronic granulomatous disease by subcutaneous interferon gamma. *N. Engl. J. Med.* **319(3)**, 146–151.

49. Schiff, D.E., Rae, J., Martin, T.R., Davis, B.H., and Curnutte, J.T. (1997) Increased phagocyte Fc gammaRI expression and improved Fc gamma-receptor-mediated phagocytosis after in vivo recombinant human interferon-gamma treatment of normal human subjects. *Blood* **90(8)**, 3187–3194.

50. Aulitzky, W., Gastl, G., Aulitzky, W.E., Nachbaur, K., Lanske, B., Kemmler, G., et al. (1987) Interferon-gamma for the treatment of metastatic renal cancer: dose-dependent stimulation and downregulation of beta-2 microglobulin and neopterinresponses. *Immunobiology* **176(1–2)**, 85–95.

51. Ahlin, A., Elinder, G., and Palmblad, J. (1997) Dose-dependent enhancements by interferon-gamma on functional responses of neutrophils from chronic granulomatous disease patients. *Blood* **89(9)**, 3396–3401.

52. Jaffee, H.A., Buhl, R., Mastrangeli, A., Holroyd, K.J., Saltini, C., Czerski, D., et al. (1991) Organ specific cytokine therapy: local activation of mononuclear phagocytes by delivery of an aerosol of recombinant interferon gamma to the human lung. *J. Clin. Invest.* **88**, 297–302.

53. Kunzmann, V., Bauer, E., Feurle, J., Weissinger, F., Tony, H.P., and Wilhelm, M., (2000) Stimulation of gammadelta T cells by aminobisphosphonates and induction of antiplasma cell activity in multiple myeloma. *Blood* **96(2)**, 384–392.

54. The International Chronic Granulomatous Disease Cooperative Study Group (1991) A controlled trial of interferon gamma to prevent infection in chronic granulomatous disease. *N. Engl. J. Med.* **324**, 509–516.

55. Rex, J.H., Bennett, J.E., Gallin, J.I., Malech, H.L., DeCarlo, E.S., and Melnick, D.A. (1991) In vivo interferon-gamma therapy augments the in vitro ability of chronic granulomatous disease neutrophils to damage *Aspergillus* hyphae. *J. Infect. Dis.* **163(4)**, 849–852.

56. Bemiller, L.S., Roberts, D.H., Starko, K.M., Curnutte, J.T. (1995) Safety and effectiveness of long-term interferon gamma therapy in patients with chronic granulomatous disease. *Blood Cells Mol. Dis.* **21**, 239–247.

57. Gallin, J.I., Farber, J.M., Holland, S.M., and Nutman, T.B. (1995) Interferon-gamma in the management of infectious diseases [clinical conference] [see comments]. *Ann. Intern. Med.* **123**, 216–224.

58. Jackson, S.H., Miller, G.F., Segal, B.H., Mardiney, M., III., Domachowske, J.B., Gallin, J.I., et al (2001) IFN-gamma is effective in reducing infections in the mouse model of chronic granulomatous disease (CGD). *J. Interferon Cytokine Res.* **21**, 567–573.

59. Key, L.L., Jr., Ries, W.L., Rodriguiz, R.M., and Hatcher, H.C., (1991) Recombinant human interferon gamma therapy for osteopetrosis. *J. Pediatr.* **121(1)**, 119–124.

60. Key, L.L, Jr., Rodriguiz, R.M., Willi, S.M., Wright, N.M., Hatcher, H.C., Eyre. D.R., et al. (1995)Long-term treatment of osteopetrosis with recombinant human interferon gamma. *N. Engl. J. Med.* **332(24)**, 1594–1599.

61. Madyastha, P.R., Yang, S., Ries, W.L., and Key, L.L., Jr. (2000) IFN-gamma enhances osteoclast generation in cultures of peripheral blood from osteopetrotic patients and normalizes superoxide production. *J. Interferon Cytokine Res.* **20(7)**, 645–652.

62. Hershman, M.J., Appel, S.H., Wellhausen, S.R., Sonnenfeld, G., and Polk, H.C., Jr. (1989) Interferon-gamma treatment increases HLA-DR expression on monocytes in severely injured patients. *Clin. Exp. Immunol.* **77(1)**, 67–70.

63. Polk, H.C., Jr., Cheadle, W.G., Livingston, D.H., Rodriguez, J.L., Starko, K.M., Izu, A.E., et al. (1992) A randomized prospective clinical trial to determine the efficacy of interferon-gamma in severely injured patients. *Am. J. Surg.* **163(2)**, 191–196.

64. Dries, D.J., Jurkovich, G.J., Maier, R.V., Clemmer, T.P., Struve, S.N., Weigelt, J.A., et al. (1994) Effect of interferon gamma on infection-related death in patients with severe injuries. A randomized, double-blind, placebo-controlled trial. *Arch. Surg.* **129**, 1031–1041.

65. Kox, W.J., Bone, R.C., Krausch, D., Docke, W.D., Kox S.N., Wauer, H., et al. (1997) Interferon gamma-1b in the treatment of compensatory anti-inflammatory response syndrome. A new approach: proof of principle. *Arch. Intern. Med.* **157(4)**, 389–393.

66. Wasserman, D., Ioannovich, J.D., Hinzmann, R.D., Deichsel, G., and Steinmann, G.G. (1998) Interferon-gamma in the prevention of severe burn-related infections: a European phase III multicenter trial. The Severe Burns Study Group. *Crit. Care Med.* **26(3)**, 434–439.

67. Carvalho, E.M., Badaro, R., Reed, S.G., Jones. T.C., and Johnson, W.D., Jr. (1985) Absence of gamma interferon and interleukin 2 production during active visceral leishmaniasis. *J. Clin. Invest.* **76(6)**, 2066–2069.

68. Murray, H.W., Berman, J.D., and Wright, S.D. (1988) Immunochemotherapy for intracellular Leishmania donovani infection: gamma interferon plus pentavalent antimony. *J. Infect. Dis.* **157(5)**, 973–978.

69. Badaro, R., Falcoff, E., Badaro, F.S., Carvalho, E.M., Pedral-Sampaio, D., Barral, A., et al. (1990) Treatment of visceral leishmaniasis with pentavalent antimony and interferon gamma. *N. Engl. J. Med.* **322(1)**, 16–21.

70. Badaro, R. and Johnson, W.D., Jr. (1993) The role of interferon-gamma in the treatment of visceral and diffuse cutaneous leishmaniasis. *J. Infect. Dis.* **167(Suppl 1)**, S13–S17.

71. Sundar, S., Rosenkaimer, F., and Murray, H.W. (1994) Successful treatment of refractory visceral leishmaniasis in India using antimony plus interferon-gamma. *J. Infect. Dis.* **170(3)**, 659–662.

72. Sundar, S., Rosenkaimer, F., Lesser, M.L., and Murray, H.W. (1995) Immunochemotherapy for a systemic intracellular infection: accelerated response using interferon-gamma in visceral leishmaniasis. *J. Infect. Dis.* **171(4)**, 992–996.

73. Sundar, S. and Murray, H.W. (1995) Effect of treatment with interferon-gamma alone in visceral leishmaniasis. *J. Infect. Dis.* **172(6)**, 1627–1629.

74. Sundar, S., Singh, V.P., Sharma, S., Makharia, M.K., and Murray, H.W. (1997) Response to interferon-gamma plus pentavalent antimony in Indian visceral leishmaniasis. *J. Infect. Dis.* **176(4)**, 1117–1119.

75. Appelberg, R. and Orme, I.M. (1993) Effector mechanisms involved in cytokine-mediated bacteriostasis of *Mycobacterium avium* infections in murine macrophages. *Immunology* **80**, 352–359

76. Flesch, I.E. and Kaufmann, S.H. (1998) Attempts to characterize the mechanisms involved in mycobacterial growth inhibition by gamma-interferon-activated bone marrow macrophages. *Infect. Immun.* **56**, 1464–1469.

77. Doherty, T.M. and Sher, A. (1997) Defects in cell-mediated immunity affect chronic, but not innate, resistance of mice to *Mycobacterium avium* infection. *J. Immunol.* **158**, 4822–4831.

78. Adams, L.B., Dinauer, M.C., Morgenstern, D.E., and Krahenbuhl, J.L. (1997) Comparison of the roles of reactive oxygen and nitrogen intermediates in the host response to *Mycobacterium tuberculosis* using transgenic mice. *Tuberc. Lung Dis.* **78**, 237–246.

79. Cooper, A.M., Segal, B.H., Frank, A.A., Holland, S.M., and Orme, I.M. (2000) Transient loss of resistance to pulmonary tuberculosis in p47(phox–/–) mice. *Infect. Immun.* **68**, 1231–1234.

80. Bermudez, L.E. snd Young, L.S. (1989) Oxidative and non-oxidative intracellular killing of Mycobacterium avium complex. *Microb. Pathol.* **7**, 289–298.

81. Denis, M., Gregg, E.O., and Ghandirian, E. (1990) Cytokine modulation of *Mycobacterium tuberculosis* growth in human macrophages. *Int. J. Immunopharmacol.* **12**, 721–727

82. Douvas, G.S., Looker, D.L., Vatter, A.E., and Crowle, A.J. (1985) Gamma interferon activates human macrophages to become tumoricidal and leishmanicidal but enhances replication of macrophage-associated mycobacteria. *Infect. Immun.* **50**, 1–8.

83. Flynn, J.L., Chan, J., Triebold, K.J., Dalton, D.K., Stewart, T.A., and Bloom, B.R. (1993) An essential role for inter-feron gamma in resistance to *Mycobacterium tuberculosis* infection. *J. Exp. Med.* **178,** 2249–2254.
84. Cooper, A.M., Dalton, D.K., Stewart, T.A., Griffin, J.P., Russell, D.G., and Orme, I.M. (1993) Disseminated tubercu-losis in interferon gamma gene-disrupted mice. *J. Exp. Med.* **178,** 2243–2247.
85. Kamijo, R., Le, J., Shapiro, D., Havell, E.A., Huang, S., Aguet, M., et al. (1993) Mice that lack the interferon-gamma receptor have profoundly altered responses to infection with Bacillus Calmette–Guerin and subsequent challenge with lipopolysaccharide. *J. Exp. Med.* **178,** 1435–1440.
86. Kamijo, R., Harada, H., Matsuyama, T., Bosland, M., Gerecitano, J., Shapiro, D., et al. (1994) Requirement for tran-scription factor IRF-1 in NO synthase induction in macrophages. *Science* **263,** 1612–1615.
87. Edwards, C.K., III., Hedegaard, H.B., Zlotnik, A., Gangadharam, P.R., Johnston, R.B., Jr., and Pabst, M.J. (1986) Chronic infection due to *Mycobacterium intracellulare* in mice: association with macrophage release of prostaglandin E2 and reversal by injection of indomethacin, muramyl dipeptide, or interferon-gamma. *J. Immunol.* **136,** 1820–1827.
88. Hussain, S., Zwilling, B.S., and Lafuse, W.P. (1999) *Mycobacterium avium* infection of mouse macrophages inhibits IFN-gamma Janus kinase-STAT signaling and gene induction by down-regulation of the IFN-gamma receptor. *J. Immunol.* **163(4),** 2041–2048.
89. Ting, L.M., Kim, A.C., Cattamanchi, A., and Ernst, J.D. (1999) *Mycobacterium tuberculosis* inhibits IFN-gamma tran-scriptional responses without inhibiting activation of STAT1.*J. Immunol.* **163(7),** 3898–3906.
90. Nathan, C.F., Kaplan, G., Levis, W.R., Nusrat, A., Witmer, M.D., Sherwin, S.A., et al. (1986) Local and systemic effects of intradermal recombinant interferon-gamma in patients with lepromatous leprosy. *N. Engl. J. Med.* **315,** 6–15.
91. Sampaio, E.P., Moreira, A.L., Sarno, E.N., Malta, A.M., and Kaplan, G. (1992) Prolonged treatment with recombinant interferon gamma induces erythema nodosum leprosum in lepromatous leprosy patients. *J. Exp. Med.* **175,** 1729–1737.
92. Sampaio, E.P., Kaplan, G., Miranda, A., Nery, J. A., Miguel, C.P., Viana, S.M., et al. The influence of thalidomide on the clinical and immunologic manifestation of erythema nodosum leprosum. *J. Infect. Dis.* **168,** 408–414.
93. Sampaio, E.P., Malta, A.M., Sarno, E.N., and Kaplan, G. (1996) Effect of rhuIFN-gamma treatment in multibacillary leprosy patients. *Int. J. Lepr. Other Mycobact. Dis.* **64,** 268–273.
94. Haslett, P.A., Klausner, J.D., Makonkawkeyoon, S., Moriera, A., Metatratip. P., Boyle, B., et al. (1999) Thalidomide stimulates T cell responses and interleukin 12 production in HIV-infected patients. *AIDS Res. Hum. Retroviruses* **15,** 1169–1179.
94a. Bekker, L.G., Haslett, P., Maartens, G., Steyn, L., and Kaplan, G. (2000) Thalidominde-induced antigen-specific immune stimulation in patients with human immunodeficiency virus type 1 and tuberculosis. *J. Infect. Dis.* **181,** 954–965.
95. Bermudez, L.E., Inderlied, C., and Young, L.S. (1991) Stimulation with cytokines enhances penetration of azithromycin into human macrophages. *Antimicrob. Agents Chemother.* **35,** 2625–2629.
96. Squires, K.E., Murphy, W.F., Madoff, L.C., and Murray, H.W. (1989) Interferon-gamma and *Mycobacterium avium–intracellulare* infection. *J. Infect. Dis.* **159,** 599–600.
97. Squires, K.E., Brown, S.T., Armstrong, D., Murphy, W.F., and Murray, H.W.(1992) Interferon-gamma treatment for *Mycobacterium avium–intracellular* complex bacillemia in patients with AIDS [letter]. *J. Infect. Dis.* **166,** 686–687.
98. Holland, S.M., Eisenstein, E.M., Kuhns, D.B., Turner, M.L., Fleisher, T.A., Strober, W., et al. (1994) Treatment of refractory disseminated nontuberculous mycobacterial infection with interferon gamma. A preliminary report. *N. Engl. J. Med.* **330,** 1348–1355.
99. Levin, M., Newport, M.J., D'Souza, S., Kalabalikis, P., Brown, I.N., Lenicker, H.M., et al. (1995) Familial dissemi-nated atypical mycobacterial infection in childhood: a human mycobacterial susceptibility gene? [see comments]. *Lan-cet* **345,** 79–83.
100. Vesterhus, P., Holland, S.M., Abrahamsen, T.G., and Bjerknes, R. (1998) Familial disseminated infection due to atypi-cal mycobacteria with childhood onset. *Clin. Infect. Dis.* **27,** 822–825.
101. Jouanguy, E., Lamhamedi-Cherradi, S., Lammas, D., Dorman, S.E., Fondaneche, M.C., Dupuis, S., et al. (1999) A human IFNGR1 small deletion hotspot associated with dominant susceptibility to mycobacterial infection; [see com-ments]. *Nat. Genet.* **21,** 370–378.
102. Altare, F., Lammas, D., Revy, P., Jouanguy, E., Doffinger, R., Lamhamedi, S., et al. (1998) Inherited interleukin 12 deficiency in a child with bacille Calmette–Guerin and *Salmonella enteritidis* disseminated infection. *J. Clin. Invest.* **102,** 2035–2040.
103. Altare, F., Durandy, A., Lammas, D., Emile, J.F., Lamhamedi, S., Le Deist, F., et al. (1998) Impairment of mycobacte-rial immunity in human interleukin-12 receptor deficiency. *Science* **280,** 1432–1435.
104. de Jong, R., Altare, F., Haagen, I.A., Elferink, D.G., Boer, T., van Breda Vriesman, P.J., et al. (1988) Severe mycobac-terial and *Salmonella* infections in interleukin-12 receptor-deficient patients. *Science* **280,** 1435–1438.
105. Holland, S.M. (2000) Treatment of infections in the patient with Mendelian susceptibility to mycobacterial infection. *Microbes Infect.* **13,** 1579–1590.
106. Chatte, G., Panteix, G., Perrin-Fayolle, M., and Pacheco, Y. (1995) Aerosolized interferon gamma for *Mycobacterium avium*-complex lung disease. *Am. J. Respir. Crit. Care Med.* **152,** 1094–1096.
107. Raad, I., Hachem, R., Leeds, N., Sawaya, R., Salem, Z., and Atweh, S. (1996) Use of adjunctive treatment with inter-feron-gamma in an immunocompromised patient who had refractory multidrug-resistant tuberculosis of the brain. *Clin. Infect. Dis.* **22,** 572–574.
108. Condos, R., Rom, W.N., and Schluger, N.W. (1997) Treatment of multidrug-resistant pulmonary tuberculosis with interferon- gamma via aerosol. [see comments]. *Lancet* **349,** 1513–1515.

23
Interleukin-2 for the Treatment of HIV Infection

Guido Poli, Claudio Fortis,
Adriano Lazzarin, and Giuseppe Tambussi

1. INTRODUCTION: HOMEOSTATIC ROLE OF INTERLEUKIN-2
IN THE HUMAN IMMUNE SYSTEM

Interleukin (IL)-2 was originally purified as a "T-cell growth factor" (TCGF) inducing the survival of human T-lymphocytes in vitro *(1)*. Shortly after this, a 19-kDa molecule was definitively named IL-2 *(2,3)* and was shown early to interact with a cell surface receptor identified by the anti-Tac monoclonal antibody (mAb) *(4,5)*. This mAb was later shown to recognize the α-chain (CD25) low-affinity receptor complex conferring high-affinity binding ($10^{-11} M$) to the β/γ-chain IL-2 receptor shared with other cytokines *(6,7)*. In 1983, the first DNA clone of IL-2 was obtained *(8)*.

Since its discovery, IL-2 was recognized as a potent regulator of survival, proliferation, and activation of several important immune effects in addition to T-lymphocytes (*see* Table 1). Recently, a number of unsuspected effects of IL-2 have emerged, mostly by animal studies, indicating an equally (if not superior role) of IL-2 in the elimination of T-cells crucial for the homeostasis of the immune system. Indeed, mice that had been genetically manipulated to avoid expression of IL-2 (i.e., IL-2 knockout, [KO], mice) showed an unpredicted phenotype characterized by a multiorgan lethal inflammatory disease with generalized lymphoadenopathy sustained by a profound activation of both T- and B-lymphocytes *(35)*. These mice frequently died of anemia or inflammatory bowel disease essentially caused by tissue infiltration of activated T-lymphocytes. Of interest for HIV pathogenesis, although both CD4+ and CD8+ T-cells were hyperactivated in IL-2 KO mice, CD4+ T-cells appeared to be the first subset involved, as reviewed in ref. *36*. A central defect in IL-2-deficient animals is likely related to the loss of a homeostatic control operated by the Fas (CD95)/Fas ligand (FasL) CD178 pathway, a major modulator of cell apoptosis. FasL interaction with a trimer of CD95 molecules expressed at the cell surface leads to the activation of caspase 8 (or FLICE) via the Fas adaptor death domain (FADD) present in the intracytoplasmic portion of the receptor; caspase activation leads to apoptosis of recently activated CD4+ T-cells, a process known as "activation-induced cell death" *(37)*. IL-2 directly operates in this process via upregulation of FasL expression concomitant with a downregulation of the intracellular FasL-inhibitory protein (FLIP) *(37)*. Therefore, animals lacking IL-2 are deficient in the Fas/FasL servomechanism crucial for avoiding the accumulation of activated T-cells that may become autoreactive upon chronic antigenic stimulation.

In addition to T- and B-cells, IL-2 can activate mononuclear phagocytes via the intermediate affinity ($10^{-9} M$) βγ receptor, resulting in the potentiation of tumoricidal and bactericidal capacity, also mediated by the release of proinflammatory molecules such as cytokines, prostaglandins, and thrombox-

From: *Cytokines and Chemokines in Infectious Diseases Handbook*
Edited by: M. Kotb and T. Calandra © Humana Press Inc., Totowa, NJ

Table 1
Effects of IL-2 Administration on Circulating PBMC Subsets

Cell subset	Effect	Ref.
CD4+ T-cells	↑ (absolute and %)	(9–17)
(CD4+ T-cells <200 µL)	=	(18,19)
CD8+ T-cells	↓ or = (absolute and %)	(11,18–23)
CD45Ra+ (naive) T-cells	↑ in % (late)	(20,21,24–27)
CD45Ro+ (memory) T-cells	↑ in % (early)	(20,21,24–27)
T-cell activation/proliferation		
(by Ki-67 expression)	↑ (CD4+, CD8+, CD16/CD56+ cells)	(28)
CD4/CD28+ or /CD26+ T-cells	↑ in %	(20–22,24)
CD4/CD25+ T-cells	↑ in %	(10,11,20,21,24,27,29,30)
CD8/HLA-DR+ T-cells	↑ in %	(10,11,28,30,31)
CD8/CD38+ T-cells	↑ in %	(21,22,28)
CD8/CD28+ T-cells	↑ in %	(21,24)
NK cells	↑ in %	(15,19)
CCR5/CXCR4 on CD4+ T-cells	↑	(32–34)

anes *(38)*. Natural killer (NK) cells are enhanced in their proliferative and cytotoxic activities and are induced to release cytokines and chemokines upon stimulation with IL-2 *(7,39,46)*. Expansion and activation of NK cells in the presence of IL-2 leads to the development of "lymphokine-activated killer" (LAK) cells showing an increased lytic potential against tumor cell targets and cells infected by a variety of viruses *(41,42)*. In this regard, however, recent studies have indicated that NK cells are more sensitive to IL-15 rather than IL-2 for their development *(43)*. The capacity of IL-2 of expanding and potentiating T-cell and NK cells in their lytic effector function has lead to its early experimental clinical use in patients affected by different forms of malignancies, resulting in a relative success at least against selected tumors, such as metastatic melanoma and renal cell carcinoma *(44,45)*. When T-cells were isolated from the areas surrounding the neoplastic masses (tumor infiltrating lymphocytes [TIL]), they were sensitive to the ex vivo expansion in the presence of IL-2 either alone or in synergy with other cytokines such as IL-4 or tumor necrosis factor-α (TNF-α), or by stimulation with anti-CD3 mAbs *(46,47)*. The experimental clinical protocols investigated in oncology have served as valuable models for the clinical use of IL-2 in human immunodeficiency virus (HIV)-infected individuals.

2. THE ROLE OF IL-2 IN HIV INFECTION IN VITRO AND EX-VIVO

The successful isolation of HIV, the etiological agent of AIDS, was firstly obtained with cord blood-derived or peripheral blood mononuclear cells (PBMCs) that had been previously activated with phytohemagglutinin and were then maintained in medium containing IL-2 *(48,49)*. Since then, T-cell activation (by IL-2 or other means) has been considered a *sine qua non* condition for productive HIV infection and replication, a general rule with some important exceptions. When antigen (Ag)-specific T-cell clones were transfected with a plasmid encoding the virus long terminal repeat (LTR; i.e., the region containing the regulatory sequence controlling HIV transcription) and the cells were subsequently activated by different stimuli, divergent effects were observed. Cell stimulation by phorbol esters resulted in strong T-cell proliferation and HIV-LTR activation, whereas IL-2 induced profound cell activation and proliferation but not HIV transcription *(50)*. This observation clearly demonstrated that T-cell activation and proliferation could be uncoupled from virus expression, a concept that has found recent validation in both macaques infected with simian immunodeficiency virus and in infected individuals *(51)*. Furthermore, the HIV-potentiating effect exerted by

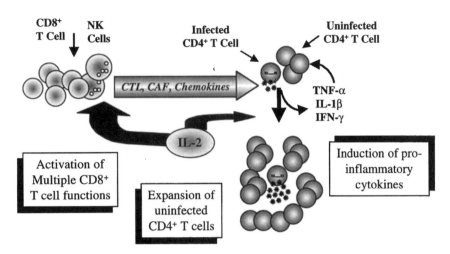

Fig. 1. Interleukin-2 activates immune effectors, mostly CD8[+] T-cells and NK cells, in both their specific (i.e., CTL), and nonlytic functions, including the release of HIV-inhibitory chemokines *(56)* and unidentified inhibitors described as "CD8 antiviral factor" (CAF) *(57)*. In addition, intermittent administration of IL-2 restores the quantitative defect of circulating and tissue CD4[+] T-cells caused by HIV infection. The proinflammatory effect of IL-2 is mostly accounted for by the release of cytokines such as TNF-α, IL-1, and others that are the principal cause of the clinical side effects (summarized in Table 2) and are also well-known activators of HIV replication *(58)*. This potentially deleterious effect is, however, overcome by a CD8-dependent antiviral effect *(55,57)*. IL-2-expanded CD4[+] T-cells are mostly uninfected, thus determining a dilution of those lymphocytes carrying integrated HIV proviruses (*see* Fig. 3).

IL-2 on infected PBMCs was mostly accounted for by the triggering of a proinflammatory cascade of cytokines, including TNF-α, TNF-β, IL-1β, and interferon-γ (IFN-γ) that were previously shown capable of activating HIV expression by acting at transcriptional and post-transcriptional steps in the virus life cycle *(52–54)*. Furthermore, when either PBMCs or lymph-node-derived mononuclear cells of HIV-infected individuals were stimulated ex vivo, IL-12, but not IL-2, activated HIV replication, whereas removal of CD8[+] cells (comprising both T-cells and a substantial fraction of NK cells) resulted in a strong upregulation of HIV replication by IL-2 that outscored IL-12 in terms of virus-inductive effects *(55)*. This observation indicated that IL-2 induced a CD8-related suppressor mechanism(s) that was dominant on cytokine-induced virus enhancement (*see* Fig. 1). It is conceivable that similar mechanisms may be operational in vivo and contribute to the significant expansion of circulating CD4[+] T-cells observed in most individuals receiving intermittent cycles of IL-2.

The recent demonstration that the seven-transmembrane domain receptors CCR5 and CXCR4 are crucial coreceptors required for HIV entry into CD4[+] cells *(56,59)*, raised the question of the potential role played by IL-2 on their cell surface expression and/or on the secretion of their related ligands, namely regulated upon activation normal T-cell-expressed and -secreted (RANTES), macrophage inflammatory protein-1α (MIP-1α) and MIP-1β for CCR5, and stromal cell-derived factor-1 (SDF-1) for CXCR4, exerting potent anti-HIV effects in vitro. Indeed, IL-2 stimulation induced the expression of several chemokine receptors, including CCR5, both on naive T-cells stimulated in vitro *(60)* as well as when administered in vivo to HIV-infected individuals *(32–34,61)* (*see* Fig. 1). However, the potent but transient upregulatory effect of IL-2 on CCR5 expression did not result in increased levels of plasma viremia. In contrast, prolonged incubation of monocyte-derived macrophages with IL-2 prior to infection resulted in decreased levels of expression of both CD4 and CCR5, with a consequent reduced HIV replication *(62)*. A number of additional studies have further substantiated the importance of IL-2 in the regulation of HIV chemokine coreceptors *(63–65)*.

3. IN VIVO EXPANSION OF CD4⁺ T-CELLS AND CONTROLLED VIREMIA BY INTERMITTENT CYCLES OF IL-2 AND ANTIRETROVIRAL THERAPY

Provision of IL-2 to infected individuals has been attempted since the early 1980s in order to correct the state of generalized immunodeficiency typical of this disease. In early clinical trials with IL-2, various routes of administration and doses were given with variable results. In 1985, Kern and colleagues administered increasing doses of intravenous (iv) IL-2 given as a bolus or by 4-h infusion to a small group of acquired immunodeficiency syndrome (AIDS) patients including individuals with lymphadenopathy syndrome *(66)*. A small phase I/II trial involving patients in advanced phases of infection was performed *(67)*. IL-2 improved delayed-type hypersensitivity (DTH) responses as well as the lymphocyte proliferative response to soluble Ags and allo-Ags and induced a transient lymphocytosis. In 1987, Volberding and colleagues *(68)* conducted the first relatively large phase I/II study on 87 AIDS patients, predominantly affected by Kaposi's sarcoma (KS). The individuals received variable doses (from 1×10^3 to 2 million international units (MIU/m^2) of IL-2 as a bolus every 48 h. No major alterations of immunological parameters were observed and the clinical results were quite discouraging: 3 patients had partial KS remissions, whereas the other 17 showed disease progression while on therapy *(68)*. In the early 1990s, Schwartz and colleagues *(9,69)* administered IL-2 at doses of up to 12 MIU/d for 5 d/wk for 30 d together with Zidovudine to 10 antiretroviral-naïve individuals with CD4⁺ T-cell counts >400 cells/mm^3. Six out of nine individuals studied 4–21 mo following the IL-2 administration period showed CD4⁺ T-cell counts higher than baseline, with a mean absolute increase of 135 cells/mm^3.

A major advancement in the clinical use of IL-2 occurred in 1995 when Kovacs and colleagues treated 23 patients with CD4⁺ T-cell counts >200 cells/mm^3 with 5-d or 21-d courses of continuos iv (civ) infusion of IL-2 at doses ranging from 1.8 to 24 MIU/d *(10)*. Dose-limiting side effects included capillary-leak syndrome, influenzalike symptoms, hepatic and renal dysfunction, thrombocytopenia, and neutropenia (*see* Table 2). No consistent changes in immunological variables or viral load (as measured by HIV-1 p24 Gag Ag or virus isolation from PBMCs) were observed. In the same study, 10 individuals with CD4⁺ T-cell counts >200 cells/mm^3 received repetitive cycles of IL-2 (civ IL-2 at the initial dose of 18 MIU/d for 5 d every 8 wk) together with current antiretroviral therapy (ART). Most individuals required dose reduction; however, 60% of the individuals showed an increase of CD4⁺ T-cell >50% of their individual baseline value. Viral load, measured by a branched DNA technique more sensitive than the standard HIV-1 p24 Gag Ag determination, increased transiently in some patients who received IL-2 *(10)*. The same authors provided more compelling evidence in a controlled trial involving 60 individuals with CD4⁺ T-cells >200 cells/mm^3 who were randomized to receive either ART alone or ART together with IL-2 (18 MIU/d, per civ for 5 d every 8 wk for a total of 6 mo) *(11)*. Patients were evaluated monthly up to 14 mo after randomization. Five out of 30 individuals withdrew from the study because of the IL-2-induced side effects, among which constitutional symptoms were the most common. Fifty-six percent of the individuals receiving IL-2 showed an increase of CD4⁺ T-cells >50% versus baseline at 48 wk, whereas this was not observed in the control group *(11)*. Again, no significant changes in viral load, measured by branched DNA, were observed.

Although intermittent civ IL-2 increased the CD4⁺ T-cell counts of infected individuals for prolonged periods, this route of administration is inconvenient for patients. Thus, several independent studies were aimed at the identification of a better modality of IL-2 administration preserving the full potency, in terms of increased CD4⁺ T-cell counts, observed with the highest doses but minimizing the side effects associated with the administration of the cytokine. In this regard, subcutaneous (sc) IL-2 administration either daily or twice a day (bid) has shown a similar range of biological and clinical effects than civ IL-2 in several independent studies, and it is better tolerated and convenient on an outpatient basis. In one study, 5-d cycles of sc IL-2 (3–18 MIU/d) were administered every 2 mo to 18 patients on ART *(71)*. The first three patients enrolled at 18 MIU/d manifested serious side

Table 2
IL-2-Related Side Effects

Grade 1	Grade 2	Grade 3	Grade 4
Weight gain	Fever	Fever	Neurological symptoms
Renal toxicity	Nausea	Nausea	
Diarrhea	Diarrhea		
Anorexia	Anorexia		
Asthenia	Asthenia		
Skin rash	Skin rash		
Myalgia	Myalgia		
Arthralgia	Hypotension		
Headache	Local inflammation		
Hypotension	Stomatitis		
Local inflammation	Hematological abnormalities		
Abdominal pain	Liver abnormalities		
Stomatitis			
Nasal congestion			
Neurological symptoms			
Coughing			
Insomnia			
Heart symptoms			
Hematological abnormalities			
Liver abnormalities			
Hypocalcemia			
hypomagnesiemia			

Source: ref. *70*.

effects including congestive heart failure and hypotension, and no additional individuals were included in this arm; the maximal tolerated dose was 15 MIU/d *(71)*. De Paoli and colleagues treated 10 ART-naïve individuals with CD4[+] T-cell counts ranging between 200 and 500 cells/mm^3; sc IL-2 (6 MIU/d) was administered at d 1–5 and 8–12 of a 28-d cycle for six cycles together with ART (Zidovudine plus dideoxyInosine), whereas six individuals received only ART. A superior increase of CD4[+] T-cell counts was observed in the IL-2-containing arm at 24 wk; IL-2 did not increase plasma viremia, confirming previous studies *(20)*. In a more recent controlled randomized trial, Levy and colleagues compared sc IL-2 (12 MIU/d) to an iv bolus of 2 MIU of IL-2 and to sc polyethileneglycol-conjugated IL-2 (PEG–IL-2; 3 MIU/m^2 bid) in 94 ART-naïve individuals with CD4[+] 250–550 cells/mm^3 who also received dual nucleoside analogs, whereas a control arm received ART alone *(21)*. Seven cycles of IL-2 were administered over 56 wk; a comparable increase in CD4[+] T-cell counts was observed in HIV-infected individuals receiving either the iv bolus or sc IL-2; the mean increases in CD4[+] T-cell counts versus baseline were 55, 564, and 676 cells/mm^3 in the control, sc, and iv bolus IL-2, respectively, whereas no significant changes in CD4[+] T-cell counts were noted in those receiving PEG–IL-2. Plasma viremia was comparably reduced in all arms, with approx 50% of individuals showing a reduction <500 copies of HIV RNA/mL, as determined by a polymerase chain-reaction (PCR)-based technique *(21)*. A similar trial was conducted on 60 antiviral-experience individuals by Tambussi and colleagues, who compared three IL-2-containing regimens and a control group receiving ART alone, in which Saquinavir hard-gel capsules was added to two nucleoside analogs *(70)*. Individuals in group A received civ IL-2 (12 MIU/d) for 5 d every 8 wk for two cycles, followed by sc IL-2 (7.5 MIU/bid) for 5 d every 8 wk for 4 cycles; in group B, sc IL-2 (7.5 MIU/bid) was administered for 6 cycles, whereas in group C sc IL-2 (3 MIU/bid) was given for 5 d every 4 wk for a total of 12 cycles. Therefore, all of the IL-2-containing regimens were administered equivalent cumulative doses of IL-2 over a 12-mo period. The mean CD4[+] T-cell counts absolute variation versus baseline were 698, 625, 726, and 103 cells for groups A, B, and C and control, respectively. No increase in either plasma viremia or in the number of genotypic mutations for inhibitors of both reverse transcriptase and viral protease were observed among patients treated with IL-2 *(70)*.

After the introduction of potent combinations of new antiretroviral cocktails in the clinical practice, several studies have demonstrated that IL-2 given in conjunction with HAART can increase the levels of circulating CD4[+] T-cells above the effect obtained by highly active antiretroviral therapy (HAART) alone. In one phase II randomized multicenter study *(30)*, individuals with CD4[+] T-cell counts between 200 and 500 cells/mm^3 were randomized to receive either HAART alone or HAART plus sc IL-2 (7.5 MIU/bid) for 5 d of an 8-wk cycle. The median percent change from baseline CD4[+] T-cell counts was 81% in the IL-2 plus HAART arm, but only 12% in those receiving HAART alone (*p*<0.001). Hengge and colleagues randomized 44 individuals with the same range of CD4[+] T-cell counts at baseline who were on stable HAART to receive sc IL-2 either 9 MIU/d for 5 d every 6 wk cycles (group A) or whenever their CD4[+] T-cell counts fell <1.25-fold their baseline values (group B); IL-2 was administered for 1 yr, whereas 20 matched controls formed the control group *(28)*. Fifty-eight out of 64 individuals completed the study (40/44 IL-2 recipients and 18/20 controls). A mean of 4.9 cycles were administered in group B; the median CD4[+] T-cell counts increased from 363 to 485 in group A and from 358 to 462 in group B, whereas no significant variations occurred in the control group *(28)*.

Limited information is currently available of the potential role of IL-2 plus HAART in individuals with more advanced HIV disease. Arnò and colleagues studied 25 individuals with CD4[+] T-cell counts ≤ 250 cells/mm^3 and with plasma viremia <500 copies of HIV RNA/mL. Thirteen of them, randomly chosen, received sc IL-2 (3 MIU/bid) for 5 d every 4 wk, for a total of 6 cycles together with HAART, whereas the 12 remainders continued to receive HAART alone *(24)*. After the first cycle, the dosage of IL-2 was reduced to 3 MIU/d for toxicity reasons. Eighteen individuals were then evaluated; the mean increases in CD4[+] T-cell counts were 105 and 30 cells in the IL-2 and control arms, respectively (the mean increase was statistically significant in the IL-2 group, but not in the control group) *(24)*.

Thus, the results of several independent randomized studies together convincingly demonstrate that intermittent administration of no less than 3 MIU/d IL-2 causes a sustained increases of the number of circulating CD4[+] T-lymphocytes in the majority of HIV-infected individuals receiving either ART or HAART. In this regard, an important aspect of IL-2 is its long-lasting effect once its administration is suspended. IL-2-boosted CD4[+] T-cells of infected individuals with >200 cells/mL at baseline frequently reach numbers of circulating cells superimposable to those of uninfected healthy individuals after 6–12 mo of therapy, whereas IL-2 suspension does not lead to a drop of CD4[+] T-cell counts for several months. These observations indicate that the effect of the cytokine is not a simple redistribution of CD4[+] T-cells from peripheral tissue to the blood compartment. Furthermore, readministration of IL-2 even after several months after its suspension induces, again, an increase of CD4[+] T-cells, indicating that there is no loss of responsiveness to the cytokine when administered on an intermittent 5-d-cycle basis *(72)*. Concerning the long-term effects of IL-2 administration, limited results have indicated an absence of alteration of the T-cell-receptor repertoire up to 18 mo after therapy *(10)*. By increasing the precursor frequency of certain Ag specificities, IL-2 may protect and expand residual immune function and prolong the time to onset of opportunistic infections (*see* Fig. 1). In this regard, a pooled intent-to-treat analysis *(73)* of 3 studies of intermittent civ IL-2 administration, involving 157 individuals, has indicated a decrease of approx 50% in viral load and in AIDS-defining events in those individuals who were originally randomized to receive IL-2 versus those who were not. Of interest, an unpredicted decreased viremia levels was observed in individuals who had received IL-2 during the trials, in spite of the fact that open-label IL-2 was received by up to 60% of individuals who did not receive the cytokine during the trial *(73)*. This observation suggests that IL-2 may indirectly exert an antiretroviral effect (likely via restoration of HIV-specific immunity) and that its potency may diminish over time. A formal demonstration of an antiviral effect of IL-2 therapy regardless of whether the individuals were receiving protease inhibitors as part of their ART was reported by Davey and colleagues *(74)*. Eighty-two individuals with 200–500 CD4+ T-cells and plasma viremia <10,000 copies of HIV RNA/mL were randomized to either ART or ART plus sc IL-2 (7.5 MIU/bid); on-treatment analysis was performed on 78 individuals, some of whom were receiving HAART. Sixty-seven percent of individuals receiving ART plus IL-2 showed a reduction of viremia <50 copies of HIV RNA/mL, whereas only 36% of patients treated with ART alone achieved this goal. The same trend was observed when the analysis was restricted to those individuals who received HAART together with or in the absence of IL-2 (with a 69% vs 44% reduction of viremia levels, respectively) *(74)*.

4. IMMUNOLOGICAL AND VIROLOGICAL CORRELATES OF INTERMIT-TENT IL-2 ADMINISTRATION

Administration of IL-2 is associated with a number of reversible dose-dependent symptoms (*see* Table 2). These undesired side effects are largely accounted for by the potent proinflammatory effect of IL-2 resulting in the upregulation of several cytokines *(75)* (*see* Table 3). A profound lymphopenia is typically observed 48–72 h after the beginning of IL-2 administration and is rapidly followed by lymphocytosis occurring between d 5 and d 8 at the end of a typical cycle of administration. A "step-by-step" increment of CD4+ T-cells is typically observed at the midpoints between two cycles of cytokine administration (*see* Fig. 2). The cumulative effect is a progressive reversal of the classical CD4+ T-cell lymphopenia observed in HIV-infected individuals, in terms of both absolute and relative numbers, achieving the restoration of a CD4/CD8 ratio >1 in most individuals that have begun to receive IL-2 when their CD4+ T-cell counts were >200 cells/μL *(72)*. It is interesting to note that this effect did not occur and, in contrast, both clinical deterioration and increased HIV replication were observed in individuals initiating IL-2 when in advanced stages of disease (<200 CD4+ T-cells/μL) *(10)*. This observation suggests that IL-2 may, indeed, exert multiple and contrasting effects in vivo as observed in vitro, and that such a balance may be tilted in favor or against HIV replication as a function of disease stage and concomitant ART. Introduction of HAART, in particular, has further changed this paradigm in that even individuals with very low CD4+ T-cell counts may respond to IL-2 therapy with stable increases of CD4+ T-cells in conditions of controlled virus replication *(24,25,81)*. HAART-treated individuals showing virological control but not an increment of peripheral CD4+ T-cells were shown to respond to IL-2 for this parameter, and this effect has been judged as an indication for the therapeutical use of IL-2 in advanced disease in France *(82)*.

The lack of rebounding virus replication at least in periphery in those individuals receiving IL-2 under conditions of incomplete virus suppression by the concomitant ART/HAART indicates that the viral dynamics in these individuals do not follow the "prey–predator" model that has been postulated to explain the paradoxical results of HAART-based clinical trials *(83)*. In some of these studies, rebound of viremia at therapy suspension or simplification was indeed quantitatively proportional to the extent of peripheral CD4+ T-cell expansion induced during HAART *(84)*. The underlying mechanisms evoked by IL-2 administration are unknown but likely effect several immunological functions resulting in the control of the multiple effects of HIV infection on the human immune system (*see* Table 4). In this regard, transient spikes of viremia were described as typically occurring at the end of the infusion/administration cycle and never resulting in an increased of steady-state viremia *(10)*. These bursts have been correlated to an increase of TNF-α levels *(73,74,85)* and/or to the downregulation of cellular transcription factors (Yin Yen-1, YY1, and LBP-1/LSF) *(86)* that have been described to play a negative role on HIV transcription *(87)*. In this latter study, the downregulatory effects were correlated to the induction of a proteolytic activity cleaving YY1 and, possibly, LBP-1/LSF, which did not abolish their DNA-binding capacity but removed the transactivating domain. In addition, we have described that IL-2 administration resulted in increased levels of a C-terminally truncated form of signal transducer and activator of transcription-5 (STAT-

Table 3
Expression of Cytokines and Other Soluble Factors
in Individuals Receiving IL-2

Cytokine/factor	IL-2 effect	Ref.
Serum Ig	↓	*(76)*
sCD25 (sIL-2Rα)	↑	*(9,15,29,34,77)*
sCD8	↑	*(34)*
sCD30	↑	*(20)*
IFN-α	↑	*(18)*
IFN-γ	↑	*(20,22,78)*
TNF-α	↑	*(79)*
TNF-α, IFN-γ, GM-CSF	Undetectable	*(13)*
IL-6	↑[a]	*(80)*
IL-4	↑	*(20,22)*
IL-13	↑	*(22)*
IL-16	↑	*(29)*
IL-10	=	*(20)*
RANTES, MIP-1α, MIP-1β	=	*(33,34)*
MCP-1 production by PBMCs	↓	*(22)*

[a]During IL-2 administration.

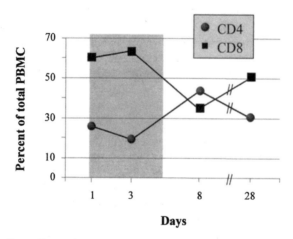

Days

Fig. 2. Differential effect of intermittent IL-2 administration on circulating CD4+ and CD8+ T-lymphocytes in a representative individual belonging to a larger cohort. Transient variations of these two PBMC subsets are typically observed during the administration of IL-2, with a relative decrease of circulating CD4+ T-cells 3 d after the beginning of the cycle. This effect is typically followed by a cellular rebound at the end of the cytokine administration (as indicated here at d 8). A re-equilibration of the two subsets is observed at the midpoint between two cycles (d 28), however with an absolute as well as relative gain of the CD4+ T-cell subset and a relative decrease of the number of CD8+ T-cells. (from ref. *70*).

5) that, together with STAT-1, was found constitutively expressed in most HIV-infected individuals *(88)*. As mentioned earlier, IL-2 has been reported to upregulate the apoptosis of activated murine CD4+ T-cells via upregulation of FasL and downregulation of the intracellular negative factor FLIP *(11)*. Because this latter effect appears controlled by STAT-5, it is possible that IL-2-mediated upregulation of C-terminally truncated STAT-5 may result in decreased levels of Fas-mediated apoptosis, as observed in individuals receiving low-dose IL-2 *(89)*.

Table 4
Potentially Beneficial and Detrimental Effects of IL-2 Therapy in HIV Infected Individuals

Beneficial	Detrimental
Expansion of uninfected memory and naive CD4+ T-cells	Substantial toxicity (reversible)
No increase of steady-state viremia	Viremia spikes during IL-2 administration
Decrease of PBMC-associated HIV DNA	Potential activation of underlying infections
Lack of interference with antiviral agents	Increased expression of proinflammatory cytokines
Potentiation of CD8+ lytic (CTL) and nonlytic antiviral activities	Upregulation of CCR5 expression on T-lymphocytes
Potentiation of NK/LAK activities	Emergence of latent autoimmune symptoms
Potentiation of CD4-dependent T-helper responses	

A reduction of latently infected cells by IL-2 administration in combination with either HAART or ART has been observed by independent investigators. Chun and colleagues have described a significant reduction in the ability of isolating replication-competent HIV from up to 360×10^6 resting memory CD4+ T-cells in individuals treated with HAART plus IL-2, but not in those receiving only HAART *(90)*. Unfortunately, this impressive finding did not translate into a significantly different outcome at therapy suspension in that a comparable viral rebound was observed in both HAART- and HAART plus IL-2-treated individuals *(85)*. A molecular analysis largely based on a heteroduplex tracking assay indicated that the rebounding virus was often diverse from the predominant circulating species present before therapy suspension *(91)*. This observation suggests that a different reservoir, perhaps less sensitive to the combined effect of HAART and IL-2, may have been the cellular source of the rebounding virus. However, additional studies indicated that IL-2 therapy did not expand different viral quasispecies versus that present before cytokine administration in six out of eight studied individuals *(92)*. In two individuals, a transient expansion of either a PBMC-associated HIV DNA species or of a uniquely clustered quasispecies unrelated to both plasma viremia and PBMCs was reported; the pre-IL-2 HIV variant nonetheless returned to be dominant after approx 30 d from IL-2 administration *(92)*. In the same study, evidence of a comparable decrease of HIV load in lymphoid tissue (mostly tonsils) was observed in both IL-2 recipient and control ART-treated individuals *(92)*. In addition, a profound decrease of lymph node-associated HIV RNA and DNA was reported in individuals receiving IL-2 and IFN-γ together with a five-drug HAART regimen *(81)*.

A progressive decrease of either HIV-infected CD4+ T-cell *(93)* or of PBMC-associated HIV DNA was observed in some individuals receiving ART plus IL-2, but not in those treated with antiretroviral agents only *(12,26,70,94)* (*see* Fig. 3). This effect likely reflected a dilution of infected CD4+ T-cells into an expanding pool of uninfected CD4+ T-cells, rather than an absolute elimination of HIV+ cells (*see* Fig 1). Nonetheless, this observation reinforces the hypothesis that IL-2 protects CD4+ T-cells from representing an expanded target population for the virus under conditions of incompletely controlled replication. Elucidation of these protective mechanisms would be of great value for IL-2 therapy as well as for monitoring the immunological profile of infected individuals receiving unrelated forms of therapy or vaccines.

In vivo, IL-2 administration induces both the redistribution and the activation of the main lymphocyte subsets, as reported in Table 1. In particular, an increased number of circulating CD4/CD25/CD28+ T-cells *(10,11,20–22,24,27,29,30)* with a concomitant reduction of CD8/HLA-DR/CD38+ T-cells *(10,11,21,22,28,30,31)* is the most common pattern described in individuals receiving intermittent cycles of IL-2 administration. Of note is the fact that an opposite pattern of these two PBMC subsets has been correlated to HIV disease progression in several studies *(95–97)*. In one study, a fourfold increase of CD4/CD25+ T-cells was observed after 12 mo of follow-up from the completion

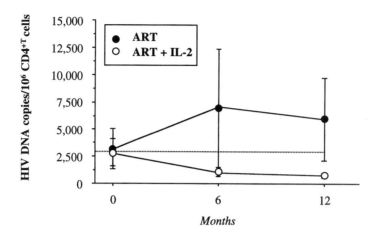

Fig. 3. Interleukin-2 induces a decrease of PBMC-associated HIV DNA. In a recent study from our group, as previously observed in others, a diminution of cell-associated HIV DNA (comprising both integrated and unintegrated forms) was observed in individuals receiving sc IL-2 plus ART, but not in those treated only with ART. Noteworthy, a substantial interpatient fluctuation of PBMC-associated HIV DNA was observed in the ART group, but not in those receiving the cytokine, in spite of the fact that the two groups of individuals had similar baseline features (from ref. *70*).

of a randomized study of sc IL-2 plus ART or HAART versus individuals who received only conventional therapy *(74)*. In contrast, no substantial differences were observed for other PBMC subsets, including CD8/CDC25[+], CD4/HLA-DR[+], and CD8/HLA-DR[+], between the two groups of patients *(74)*. Recently, CD4/CD25[+] T-cells have gained substantial attention in that they encompass cells with regulatory function involved both in auto-immunity and tolerance, as reviewed in ref. *98*. These cells depend on B7/CD28 interaction for their development *(99)* and express constitutively the CTLA-4 costimulatory molecule *(100,101)*. Therefore, it is conceivable that some effects mediated by IL-2 administration to HIV+ individuals is the result of the expansion and activation of these cells.

An increased number of PBMC expressing the three chains of the IL-2-receptor complex was found in HIV-infected individuals in comparison to both uninfected individuals and subjects with chronic hepatitis B virus infection *(102)*. In particular, α-, β-, and γ-chains were expressed mostly on CD8[+] T-cells, B-cells, monocytes, and, to a lesser extent, on approx 10% of CD4[+] T-lymphocytes *(102)*. Of interest, this pattern did not correspond to an increased responsiveness of these cells to IL-2, with the exception of B-lymphocytes, a feature that may be dependent on a relative defect of IL-2 during Ag-specific T-cell activation *(103)*. The recovery of T-cell functions induced by IL-2 is characterized in vivo by an increase of the skin test reactivity versus recall Ags *(13,28,31,76,104)* or HIV Ags *(28)*, and ex vivo by an increase of lymphoproliferative response to the same recall Ags and to mitogens *(14,21,104)* (*see* Table 5). However, some studies have reported a transient reduction of proliferative responses during the first week of treatment *(15,106,107)*.

As already mentioned, the cascade of soluble factors induced by IL-2 administration encompasses several proinflammatory cytokines as well as their soluble receptors, including the soluble α-chain of the IL-2R (sCD25) (*see* Table 3). In vivo, a positive correlation with peak levels of IL-2 and cytokine-induced side effects has been reported *(109)*, whereas no TNF-α, IFN-γ, or GM-CSF were detected in plasma/serum of individuals receiving ultralow doses of sc IL-2 (up to 1.2 MIU/m^2/d) *(13)*. However, in a recent study, we have observed a correlation between IL-2-related toxicity and the plasma levels of both IL-2 itself and TNF-α *(110)*.

Table 5
Effects of IL-2 Administration on Immune Function In Vivo or Ex Vivo

Cytokine/factor	IL-2 Effect	Ref.
Skin test	↑	*(13,28,31,76,104)*
Spontaneous PBMC proliferation	↑	*(17,105)*
LPA to PHA, anti-CD3 Ab, TT,	↑	*(14,21,104)*
STK, HIV°*	=/↓	*(15,106,107)*
Anti-HIV CTL	↑	*(12)*
	↓	*(107)*
Perforin, granzyme B in CD8+ T cells	↑	*(108)*
NK and/or LAK activity	↑	*(107)*
	=	*(10,21)*
Telomere restriction fragment length	↓ (transient)	*(92)*

° 11 HIV T helper epitopes derived from gag and env
* LPA: lymphoproliferative assay; PHA: phytohemagglutinin; TT: tetanus toxoid; STK: streptokinase

5. CONCLUSIONS AND PERSPECTIVES

The vanished goal of eradicating HIV infection by combining several antiretroviral agents has refocused most of the attention on the long-term management of HIV disease. In this context, the possibility of combining antiviral and immune-based approaches has a solid basis in the consolidated experience of IL-2 administration. Multiple trials on different cohorts of infected individuals have shown that intermittent administration of 3–12 MIU/d of IL-2 can restore normal levels of circulating CD4+ T-lymphocytes, a crucial parameter of immune function. Retrospective analysis of individuals who have received IL-2 in previous years is encouraging in the hypothesis that the observed increases of CD4+ T-cell counts are not a simple "cosmetic" change in the composition of PBMCs of these individuals. Hopefully, ongoing phase III clinical trials will address this fundamental question. An added value of IL-2 experimental therapy is its broader implication: Administration of a cytokine, a messenger protein that allows the intercellular communication among immune cells, as a drug to immunodeficient individuals may lead to the reconstitution of their immune responses, thus increasing their capacity to fight opportunistic infections and tumors.

ACKNOWLEDGMENTS

This study was possible because of the commitment of several physicians, nurses, and investigators of the San Raffaele Scientific Institute in Milano, but it would have not been possible without the collaboration of seropositive individuals willing to accept the side effects of IL-2. This study was supported by grants of the III National Program of Research Against AIDS of the Istituto Superiore di Sanità, Rome, Italy.

REFERENCES

1. Morgan, D.A., Ruscetti, F.W., and Gallo, R. (1976) Selective in vitro growth of T lymphocytes from normal human bone marrows. *Science* **193,** 1007–1008.
2. Smith, K.A. (1980) T-cell growth factor. *Immunol. Rev.* **51,** 337–357.
3. Watson, J. and Mochizuki, D. (1980) Interleukin 2: a class of T cell growth factors. *Immunol. Rev.* **51,** 257–278.
4. Robb, R.J., Munck, A., and Smith, K.A. (1981) T Cell growth factor receptors. Quantitation, specificity, and biological relevance. *J. Exp. Med.* **154,** 1455–1474.

5. Depper, J.M., Leonard, W.J., Robb, R.J., Waldmann, T.A., and Greene W.C. (1983) Blockade of the interleukin-2 receptor by anti-Tac antibody: inhibition of human lymphocyte activation. *J. Immunol.* **131,** 690–696.
6. Leonard, W.J. and O'Shea, J.J. (1998) Jaks and STATs: biological implications. *Annu. Rev. Immunol.* **16,** 293–322.
7. Waldmann, T.A. and Tagaya, Y. (1999) The multifaceted regulation of interleukin-15 expression and the role of this cytokine in NK cell differentiation and host response to intracellular pathogens. *Annu. Rev. Immunol.* **17,** 19–49.
8. Taniguchi, T., Matsui, H., Fujita, T., Takaoka, C., Kashima, N., Yoshimoto, R., et al. (1983) Structure and expression of a cloned cDNA for human interleukin-2. *Nature* **302,** 305–310.
9. Schwartz, D.H., Skowron, G., and Merigan, T.C. (1991) Safety and effects of interleukin-2 plus zidovudine in asymptomatic individuals infected with human immunodeficiency virus. *J. Acquired Immune Defic. Syndrome* **4,** 11–23.
10. Kovacs, J.A., Baseler, M., Dewar, R.J., Vogel, S., Davey, R.T., Jr., Falloon, J., et al. (1995) Increases in CD4 T lymphocytes with intermittent courses of interleukin- 2 in patients with human immunodeficiency virus infection. A preliminary study. *N. Engl. J. Med.* **332,** 567–575.
11. Kovacs, J.A., Vogel, S., Albert, J.M., Falloon, J., Davey, R.T., Jr., Walker, R.E., et al. (1996) Controlled trial of interleukin-2 infusions in patients infected with the human immunodeficiency virus. *N. Engl. J. Med.* **335,** 1350–1356.
12. Wood, R., Montoya, J.G., Kundu, S.K., Schwartz, D.H., and Merigan, T.C. (1993) Safety and efficacy of polyethylene glycol-modified interleukin-2 and zidovudine in human immunodeficiency virus type 1 infection: a phase I/II study. *J. Infect. Dis.* **167,** 519–525.
13. Jacobson, E.L., Pilaro, F., and Smith, K.A. (1996) Rational interleukin 2 therapy for HIV positive individuals: daily low doses enhance immune function without toxicity. *Proc. Natl. Acad. Sci. USA* **93,** 10,405–10,410.
14. Teppler, H., Kaplan, G., Smith, K.A., Montana, A.L., Meyn, P., and Cohn, Z.A. (1993) Prolonged immunostimulatory effect of low-dose polyethylene glycol interleukin 2 in patients with human immunodeficiency virus type 1 infection. *J. Exp. Med.* **177,** 483–492.
15. McMahon, D.K., Armstrong, J.A., Huang, X.L., Rinaldo, C.R., Jr., Gupta, P., Whiteside, T.L., et al. (1994) A phase I study of subcutaneous recombinant interleukin-2 in patients with advanced HIV disease while on zidovudine. *AIDS* **8,** 59–66.
16. Mazza, P., Bocchia, M., Tumietto, F., Costigliola, P., Coronado, O., Bandini, G., et al. (1992) Recombinant interleukin-2 (rIL-2) in acquired immune deficiency syndrome (AIDS): preliminary report in patients with lymphoma associated with HIV infection. *Eur. J. Haematol.* **49,** 1–6.
17. Schnittman, S.M., Vogel, S., Baseler, M., Lane, H.C., and Davey, R.T., Jr. (1994) A phase I study of interferon-alpha 2b in combination with interleukin- 2 in patients with human immunodeficiency virus infection. *J. Infect. Dis.* **169,** 981–989.
18. Klimas, N., Patarca, R., Walling, J., Garcia, R., Mayer, V., Moody, D., et al. (1994) Clinical and immunological changes in AIDS patients following adoptive therapy with activated autologous CD8 T cells and interleukin-2 infusion. *AIDS* **8,** 1073–1081.
19. Bernstein, Z.P., Porter, M.M., Gould, M., Lipman, B., Bluman, E.M., Stewart, C.C., et al. (1995) Prolonged administration of low-dose interleukin-2 in human immunodeficiency virus-associated malignancy results in selective expansion of innate immune effectors without significant clinical toxicity. *Blood* **86,** 3287–3294.
20. De Paoli, P., Zanussi, S., Simonelli, C., Bortolin, M.T., D'Andrea, M., Crepaldi, C., et al. (1997) Effects of subcutaneous interleukin-2 therapy on CD4 subsets and in vitro cytokine production in HIV+ subjects. *J. Clin. Invest.* **100,** 2737–2743.
21. Levy, Y., Capitant, C., Houhou, S., Carriere, I., Viard, J.P., Goujard, C., et al. (1999) Comparison of subcutaneous and intravenous interleukin-2 in asymptomatic HIV-1 infection: a randomised controlled trial. ANRS 048 study group. *Lancet* **353,** 1923–1929.
22. Zanussi, S., Simonelli C., Bortolin M.T., D'Andrea M., Crepaldi C., Vaccher E., et al. (1999) Immunological changes in peripheral blood and in lymphoid tissue after treatment of HIV-infected subjects with highly active anti-retroviral therapy (HAART) or HAART + IL-2. *Clin. Exp. Immunol.* **116,** 486–492.
23. Losso, M.H., Belloso, W.H., Emery, S., Benetucci, J.A., Cahn, P.E., Lasala, M.C., et al. (2000) A randomized, controlled, phase II trial comparing escalating doses of subcutaneous interleukin-2 plus antiretrovirals versus antiretrovirals alone in human immunodeficiency virus-infected patients with CD4+ cell counts >/=350/mm³. *J. Infect. Dis.* **181,** 1614–1621.
24. Arnò, A., Ruiz, L., Juan, M., Jou, A., Balague, M., Zayat, M.K., et al. (1999) Efficacy of low-dose subcutaneous interleukin-2 to treat advanced human immunodeficiency virus type 1 in persons with <250/µL CD4 T cells and undetectable plasma viral load. *J. Infect. Dis.* **180,** 56–60.
25. David, D., Nait-Ighil, L., Dupont, B., Maral, J., Gachot, B., and Theze, J. (2001) Rapid effect of interleukin-2 therapy in human immunodeficiency virus- infected patients whose CD4 cell counts increase only slightly in response to combined antiretroviral treatment. *J. Infect. Dis.* **183,** 730–735.
26. Zanussi, S., Simonelli, C., Bortolin, M.T., D'Andrea, M., Comar, M., Tirelli, U., et al. (1999) Dynamics of provirus load and lymphocyte subsets after interleukin 2 treatment in HIV-infected patients. *AIDS Res. Hum. Retroviruses* **15,** 97–103.
27. Simonelli, C., Zanussi, S., Sandri, S., Comar, M., Lucenti, A., Talamini, R., et al. (1999) Concomitant therapy with subcutaneous interleukin-2 and zidovudine plus didanosine in patients with early stage HIV infection. *J. Acquired Immune Defic. Syndrome Hum. Retrovir.* **20,** 20–27.
28. Hengge, U.R., Goos, M., Esser, S., Exner, V., Dotterer, H., Wiehler, H., et al. (1998) Randomized, controlled phase II trial of subcutaneous interleukin-2 in combination with highly active antiretroviral therapy (HAART) in HIV patients. *AIDS* **12,** F225–F234.
29. De Paoli, P., Zanussi, S., Caggiari, L., Bortolin M.T., D'Andrea M., Simonelli C. et al. (1999) Kinetics of lymphokine production in HIV+ patients treated with highly active antiretroviral therapy and interleukin 2. *J. Clin. Immunol.* **19,** 317–325.

30. Davey, R.T., Jr., Chaitt, D.G., Albert, J.M., Piscitelli, S.C., Kovacs, J.A., Walker, R.E., et al. (1999) A randomized trial of high- versus low-dose subcutaneous interleukin-2 outpatient therapy for early human immunodeficiency virus type 1 infection. *J. Infect. Dis.* **179**, 849–858.

31. Carr, A., Emery S., Lloyd A., Hoy J., Garsia R., French M., et al. (1998) Outpatient continuous intravenous interleukin-2 or subcutaneous, polyethylene glycol-modified interleukin-2 in human immunodeficiency virus-infected patients: a randomized, controlled, multicenter study. Australian IL-2 Study Group. *J. Infect. Dis.* **178**, 992–999.

32. Weissman, D., Dybul, M., Daucher, M.B., Davey, R.T., Jr., Walker, R.E., and Kovacs J.A. (2000) Interleukin-2 upregulates expression of the human immunodeficiency virus fusion coreceptor CCR5 by CD4+ lymphocytes in vivo. *J. Infect. Dis.* **181**, 933–938.

33. Blanco, J., Cabrera, C., Jou, A., Ruiz, L., Clotet, B. and Este, J.A. (1999) Chemokine and chemokine receptor expression after combined anti-HIV-1 interleukin-2 therapy. *AIDS* **13**, 547–555.

34. Zou, W., Foussat, A., Houhou, S., Durand-Gasselin, I., Dulioust, A., Bouchet, L., et al. (1999) Acute upregulation of CCR-5 expression by CD4+ T lymphocytes in HIV- infected patients treated with interleukin-2. ANRS 048 IL-2 Study Group. *AIDS* **13**, 455–463.

35. Horak, I., Lohler, J., Ma, A., and Smith, K.A. (1995) Interleukin-2 deficient mice: a new model to study autoimmunity and self-tolerance. *Immunol. Rev.* **148**, 35–44.

36. Hunig, T. and Schimpl, A. (1998) The IL-2 deficiency syndrome. A lethal disease caused by abnormal lymphocyte survival, in *Cytokine Knockouts* (Durum, S.K. and Muegge, K., eds.), Humana, Totowa, NJ, pp. 1–19.

37. Refaeli, Y., Van Parijs, L., London, C.A., Tschopp, J., and Abbas, A.K. (1998) Biochemical mechanisms of IL-2-regulated Fas-mediated T cell apoptosis. *Immunity* **8**, 615–623.

38. Espinoza-Delgado, I., Bosco, M.C., Musso, T., Gusella, G.L., Longo, D.L., and Varesio, L. (1995) Interleukin-2 and human monocyte activation. *J. Leukocyte Biol.* **57**, 13–19.

39. Ben Aribia, M.H., Leroy, E., Lantz, O., Metivier, D., Autran, B., Charpentier, B., et al. (1987) rIL 2-induced proliferation of human circulating NK cells and T lymphocytes: synergistic effects of IL 1 and IL 2. *J. Immunol.* **139**, 443–451.

40. Oliva, A., Kinter, A.L., Vaccarezza, M., Rubbert, A., Catanzaro, A., Moir, S., et al. (1998) Natural killer cells from human immunodeficiency virus (HIV)-infected individuals are an important source of CC-chemokines and suppress HIV-1 entry and replication in vitro. *J. Clin. Invest.* **102**, 223–231.

41. Mule, J.J., Shu, S., Schwarz, S.L., and Rosenberg, S.A. (1984) Adoptive immunotherapy of established pulmonary metastases with LAK cells and recombinant interleukin-2. *Science* **225**, 1487–1489.

42. Yu, T.K., Caudell, E.G., Smid, C., and Grimm, E.A. (2000) IL-2 activation of NK cells: involvement of MKK1/2/ERK but not p38 kinase pathway. *J. Immunol.* **164**, 6244–6251.

43. Liu, C.C., Perussia, B., and Young, J.D. (2000) The emerging role of IL-15 in NK-cell development. *Immunol. Today* **21**, 113–116.

44. Lanier, L.L. and Bakker, A.B. (2000) The ITAM-bearing transmembrane adaptor DAP12 in lymphoid and myeloid cell function. *Immunol. Today* **21**, 611–614.

45. Mingari, M.C., Ponte, M., Vitale, C., Bellomo, R. and Moretta, L. (2000) Expression of HLA class I-specific inhibitory receptors in human cytolytic T lymphocytes: a regulated mechanism that controls T-cell activation and function. *Hum. Immunol.* **61**, 44–50.

46. Rosenberg, S.A. (1984) Immunotherapy of cancer by systemic administration of lymphoid cells plus interleukin-2. *J. Biol. Response Modifiers* **3**, 501–511.

47. Rosenberg, S.A. (2000) Interleukin-2 and the development of immunotherapy for the treatment of patients with cancer. *Cancer J. Sci. Am.* **6(Suppl 1)**, S2–7.

48. Barre-Sinoussi, F., Chermann, J.C., Rey, F., Nugeyre, M.T., Chamaret, S., Gruest, J., et al. (1983) Isolation of a T-lymphotropic retrovirus from a patient at risk for acquired immune deficiency syndrome (AIDS). *Science* **220**, 868–871.

49. Gallo, R.C., Sarin, P.S., Gelmann, E.P., Robert-Guroff, M., Richardson, E., Kalyanaraman, V.S., et al. (1983) Isolation of human T-cell leukemia virus in acquired immune deficiency syndrome (AIDS). *Science* **220**, 865–867.

50. Hazan, U., Thomas, D., Alcami, J., Bachelerie, F., Israel, N., Yssel, H., et al. (1990) Stimulation of a human T-cell clone with anti-CD3 or tumor necrosis factor induces NF-kappa B translocation but not human immunodeficiency virus 1 enhancer-dependent transcription. *Proc. Natl. Acad. Sci. USA* **87**, 7861–7865.

51. Zhang, Z., Schuler, T., Zupancic, M., Wietgrefe, S., Staskus, K.A., Reimann, K.A., et al. (1999) Sexual transmission and propagation of SIV and HIV in resting and activated CD4+ T cells. *Science* **286**, 1353–1357.

52. Vyakarnam, A., McKeating, J., Meager, A., and Beverley, P.C. (1990) Tumour necrosis factors (α,β) induced by HIV-1 in peripheral blood mononuclear cells potentiate virus replication. *AIDS,* **4**, 21–27.

53. Ramilo, O., Bell, K.D., Uhr, J.W., and Vitetta, E.S. (1993) Role of CD25+ and CD25-T cells in acute HIV infection in vitro. *J. Immunol.* **150**, 5202–5208.

54. Kinter, A.L., Poli, G., Fox, L., Hardy, E., and Fauci, A.S. (1995) HIV replication in IL-2-stimulated peripheral blood mononuclear cells is driven in an autocrine/paracrine manner by endogenous cytokines. *J. Immunol.* **154**, 2448–2459.

55. Kinter, A.L., Bende, S.M., Hardy, E.C., Jackson, R., and Fauci, A.S. (1995) Interleukin 2 induces CD8+ T cell-mediated suppression of human immunodeficiency virus replication in CD4+ T cells and this effect overrides its ability to stimulate virus expression. *Proc. Natl. Acad. Sci. USA* **92**, 10,985–10,989.

56. Lusso, P. (2000) Chemokines and viruses: the dearest enemies. *Virology* **273**, 228–240.

57. Walker, C.M., Moody, D.J., Stites, D.P., and Levy, J.A. (1986) CD8+ lymphocytes can control HIV infection in vitro by suppressing virus replication. *Science* **234**, 1563–1566.

58. Poli, G. (1999) Laureate ESCI award for excellence in clinical science 1999. Cytokines and the human immunodeficiency virus: from bench to bedside. European Society for Clinical Investigation. *Eur. J. Clin. Invest.* **29**, 723–732.

59. Simmons, G., Reeves, J.D., Hibbitts, S., Stine, J.T., Gray, P.W., Proudfoot, A.E., and Clapham, P.R. (2000) Co-receptor use by HIV and inhibition of HIV infection by chemokine receptor ligands. *Immunol. Rev.* **177,** 112–126.
60. Loetscher, P., Seitz M., Baggiolini, M., and Moser, B. (1996) Interleukin-2 regulates CC chemokine receptor expression and chemotactic responsiveness in T lymphocytes. *J. Exp. Med.* **184,** 569–577.
61. Plana, M., Garcia, F., Gallart, T., Tortajada, C., Soriano, A., Palou, E., et al. (2000) Immunological benefits of antiretroviral therapy in very early stages of asymptomatic chronic HIV-1 infection. *AIDS* **14,** 1921–1933.
62. Kutza, J., Hayes, M.P., and Clouse, K.A. (1998) Interleukin-2 inhibits HIV-1 replication in human macrophages by modulating expression of CD4 and CC-chemokine receptor-5. *AIDS* **12,** F59–F64.
63. Bleul, C.C., Wu, L., Hoxie, J.A., Springer, T.A., and Mackay, C.R. (1997) The HIV coreceptors CXCR4 and CCR5 are differentially expressed and regulated on human T lymphocytes. *Proc. Natl. Acad. Sci. USA* **94,** 1925–1930.
64. Unutmaz, D., Xiang, W., Sunshine, M.J., Campbell, J., Butcher, E., and Littman D.R. (2000) The primate lentiviral receptor Bonzo/STRL33 is coordinately regulated with CCR5 and its expression pattern is conserved between human and mouse. *J. Immunol.* **165,** 3284–3292.
65. Inngjerdingen, M., Damaj, B., and Maghazachi, A.A. (2001) Expression and regulation of chemokine receptors in human natural killer cells. *Blood* **97,** 367–375.
66. Kern, P., Toy, J., and Dietrich, M. (1985) Preliminary clinical observations with recombinant interleukin-2 in patients with AIDS or LAS. *Blut* **50,** 1–6.
67. Ernst, M., Kern, P., Flad, H.D., and Ulmer, A.J. (1986) Effects of systemic in vivo interleukin-2 (IL-2) reconstitution in patients with acquired immune deficiency syndrome (AIDS) and AIDS- related complex (ARC) on phenotypes and functions of peripheral blood mononuclear cells (PBMC). *J. Clin. Immunol.* **6,** 170–181.
68. Volberding, P., Moody, D.J., Beardslee, D., Bradley, E.C., and Wofsy, C.B. (1987) Therapy of acquired immune deficiency syndrome with recombinant interleukin-2. *AIDS Res. Hum. Retroviruses* **3,** 115–124.
69. Schwartz, D.H. and Merigan, T.C. (1990) Interleukin-2 in the treatment of HIV disease. *Biotherapy* **2,** 119–136.
70. Tambussi, G., Ghezzi, S., Nozza, S., Vallanti, G., Magenta, L., Guffanti, M., et al. (2001) Efficacy of low-dose intermittent subcutaneous interleukin (IL)-2 in antiviral drug-experienced human immunodeficiency virus-infected persons with detectable virus load: a controlled study of 3 IL-2 regimens with antiviral drug therapy. *J. Infect. Dis.* **183,** 1476–1484.
71. Davey, R.T., Jr., Chaitt, D.G., Piscitelli, S.C., Wells, M., Kovacs, J.A., Walker, R.E., et al. (1997) Subcutaneous administration of interleukin-2 in human immunodeficiency virus type 1-infected persons. *J. Infect. Dis.* **175,** 781–789.
72. Miller, K.D., Spooner, K., Herpin, B.R., Rock-Kress, D., Metcalf, J.A., Davey, R.T., Jr., et al. (2001) Immunotherapy of HIV-infected patients with intermittent interleukin-2: effects of cycle frequency and cycle duration on degree of CD4(+) T-lymphocyte expansion. *Clin. Immunol.* **99,** 30–42.
73. Emery, S., Capra W.B., Cooper D.A., Mitsuyasu R.T., Kovacs J.A., Vig P., et al. (2000) Pooled analysis of 3 randomized, controlled trials of interleukin-2 therapy in adult human immunodeficiency virus type 1 disease. *J. Infect. Dis.* **182,** 428–434.
74. Davey, R.T., Jr., Murphy R.L., Graziano F.M., Boswell S.L., Pavia A.T., Cancio M., et al. (2000) Immunologic and virologic effects of subcutaneous interleukin 2 in combination with antiretroviral therapy: A randomized controlled trial. *JAMA* **284,** 183–189.
75. Lentsch, A.B., Miller, F.N., and Edwards, M.J. (1999) Mechanisms of leukocyte-mediated tissue injury induced by interleukin-2. *Cancer Immunol. Immunother.* **47,** 243–248.
76. Lane, H.C., Siegel, J.P., Rook, A.H., Masur, H., Gelmann, E.P., Quinnan, G.V., and Fauci, A.S. (1984) Use of interleukin-2 in patients with acquired immunodeficiency syndrome. *J. Biol. Response Modifiers* **3,** 512–516.
77. Piscitelli, S.C., Forrest A., Vogel S., Chaitt D., Metcalf J., Stevens R., et al. (1998) Pharmacokinetic modeling of recombinant interleukin-2 in patients with human immunodeficiency virus infection. *Clin. Pharmacol. Ther.* **64,** 492–498.
78. Khatri, V.P., Fehniger T.A., Baiocchi R.A., Yu F., Shah M.H., Schiller D.S., et al. (1998) Ultra low dose interleukin-2 therapy promotes a type 1 cytokine profile in vivo in patients with AIDS and AIDS-associated malignancies. *J. Clin. Invest.* **101,** 1373–1378.
79. Piscitelli, S.C., Wells, M.J., Metcalf, J.A., Baseler, M., Stevens, R. and Davey, R.T., Jr. (1996) Pharmacokinetics and pharmacodynamics of subcutaneous interleukin-2 in HIV-infected patients. *Pharmacotherapy* **16,** 754–759.
80. Piscitelli, S.C., Vogel, S., Figg, W.D., Raje, S., Forrest, A., Metcalf, J.A., et al. (1998) Alteration in indinavir clearance during interleukin-2 infusions in patients infected with the human immunodeficiency virus. *Pharmacotherapy* **18,** 1212–1216.
81. Lafeuillade, A., Poggi, C., Chadapaud, S., Hittinger, G., Chouraqui, M., Pisapia, M., et al. (2001) Pilot study of a combination of highly active antiretroviral therapy and cytokines to induce HIV-1 remission. *J. Acquired Immune Defic. Syndrome* **26,** 44–55.
82. Katlama, C., Duvivier, C., Chouquet, C., Autran, B., Carcelain, G., De Sa, M., et al. (2000) ILSTIM (ANRS 082)—a randomized comparative open-label study of interleukin-2 (IL2) in patients with CD4 <200 despite effective HAART. 7th Conference on Retroviruses and Opportunistic Infections, p. 177 (abstract).
83. De Boer, R.J. and Perelson, A.S. (1998) Target cell limited and immune control models of HIV infection: a comparison. *J. Theor. Biol.* **190,** 201–214.
84. de Jong, M.D., de Boer, R.J., de Wolf, F., Foudraine, N.A., Boucher, C.A., Goudsmit, J., et al. (1997) Overshoot of HIV-1 viraemia after early discontinuation of antiretroviral treatment. *AIDS* **11,** F79–F84.
85. Davey, R.T., Jr., Bhat N., Yoder C., Chun T.W., Metcalf J.A., Dewar R., et al. (1999) HIV-1 and T cell dynamics after interruption of highly active antiretroviral therapy (HAART) in patients with a history of sustained viral suppression. *Proc. Natl. Acad. Sci. USA* **96,** 15,109–15,114.
86. Bovolenta, C., Camorali, L., Lorini, A.L., Vallanti, G., Ghezzi, S., Tambussi, G., et al. (1999) In vivo administration of recombinant IL-2 to individuals infected by HIV down-modulates the binding and expression of the transcription factors ying-yang-1 and leader binding protein-1/Late simian virus 40 factor. *J. Immunol.* **163,** 6892–6897.

87. Margolis, D.M., Somasundaran, M., and Green, M.R. (1994) Human transcription factor YY1 represses human immunodeficiency virus type 1 transcription and virion production. *J. Virol.* **68**, 905–910.
88. Bovolenta, C., Camorali, L., Lorini, A.L., Ghezzi, S., Vicenzi, E., Lazzarin, A. and Poli, G. (1999) Constitutive activation of STATs upon In vivo human immunodeficiency virus infection. *Blood* **94**, 4202–4209.
89. Pandolfi, F., Pierdominici, M., Marziali, M., Livia, Bernardi, M., Antonelli, G., Galati, V., et al. (2000) Low-dose IL-2 reduces lymphocyte apoptosis and increases naive CD4 cells in HIV-1 patients treated with HAART. *Clin. Immunol.* **94**, 153–159.
90. Chun, T.W., Engel D., Mizell S.B., Hallahan C.W., Fischette M., Park S., et al. (1999) Effect of interleukin-2 on the pool of latently infected, resting CD4+ T cells in HIV-1-infected patients receiving highly active anti-retroviral therapy. *Nat. Med.* **5**, 651–655.
91. Chun, T.W., Davey, R.T., Jr., Ostrowski, M., Shawn Justement, J., Engel, D., Mullins, J.I., et al. (2000) Relationship between pre-existing viral reservoirs and the re-emergence of plasma viremia after discontinuation of highly active anti- retroviral therapy. *Nat. Med.* **6**, 757–761.
92. Kovacs, J.A., Imamichi H., Vogel S., Metcalf J.A., Dewar R.L., Baseler M., et al. (2000) Effects of intermittent interleukin-2 therapy on plasma and tissue human immunodeficiency virus levels and quasi-species expression. *J. Infect. Dis.* **182**, 1063–1069.
93. Dianzani, F., Antonelli, G., Aiuti, F., Turriziani, O., Riva, E., Capobianchi, M.R., et al. (2000) The number of HIV DNA-infected mononuclear cells is reduced under HAART plus recombinant IL-2. IRHAN Study Group. *Antiviral Res.* **45**, 95–99.
94. Clark, A.G., Holodniy, M., Schwartz, D.H., Katzenstein, D.A., and Merigan, T.C. (1992) Decrease in HIV provirus in peripheral blood mononuclear cells during zidovudine and human rIL-2 administration. *J. Acquired Immune Defic. Syndrome* **5**, 52–59.
95. Pantaleo, G., Koenig, S., Baseler, M., Lane, H.C., and Fauci, A.S. (1990) Defective clonogenic potential of CD8+ T lymphocytes in patients with AIDS. Expansion in vivo of a nonclonogenic CD3+CD8+DR+CD25- T cell population. *J. Immunol.* **144**, 1696–1704.
96. Liu, Z., Cumberland, W.G., Hultin, L.E., Prince, H.E., Detels, R., and Giorgi, J.V. (1997) Elevated CD38 antigen expression on CD8+ T cells is a stronger marker for the risk of chronic HIV disease progression to AIDS and death in the Multicenter AIDS Cohort Study than CD4+ cell count, soluble immune activation markers, or combinations of HLA-DR and CD38 expression. *J. Acquired Immune Defic. Syndrome Hum. Retrovir.* **16**, 83–92.
97. Shearer, G.M. (1998) HIV-induced immunopathogenesis. *Immunity* **9**, 587–593.
98. Shevach, E.M. (2000) Regulatory T cells in autoimmmunity. *Annu. Rev. Immunol.* **18**, 423–449.
99. Salomon, B., Lenschow, D.J., Rhee, L., Ashourian, N., Singh, B., Sharpe, A., et al. (2000) B7/CD28 costimulation is essential for the homeostasis of the CD4+CD25+ immunoregulatory T cells that control autoimmune diabetes. *Immunity* **12**, 431–440.
100. Read, S., Malmstrom, V., and Powrie F. (2000) Cytotoxic T lymphocyte-associated antigen 4 plays an essential role in the function of CD25(+)CD4(+) regulatory cells that control intestinal inflammation. *J. Exp. Med.* **192**, 295–302.
101. Takahashi, T., Tagami, T., Yamazaki, S., Uede, T., Shimizu, J., Sakaguchi, N., et al. (2000) Immunologic self-tolerance maintained by CD25(+)CD4(+) regulatory T cells constitutively expressing cytotoxic T lymphocyte-associated antigen 4. *J. Exp. Med.* **192**, 303–310.
102. David, D., Bani, L., Moreau, J.L., Treilhou, M.P., Nakarai, T., Joussemet, M., et al. (1998) Regulatory dysfunction of the interleukin-2 receptor during HIV infection and the impact of triple combination therapy. *Proc. Natl. Acad. Sci. USA* **95**, 11,348–11,353.
103. Moreau, J.L., Chastagner, P., Tanaka, T., Miyasaka, M., Kondo, M., Sugamura, K., et al. (1995) Control of the IL-2 responsiveness of B lymphocytes by IL-2 and IL-4. *J. Immunol.* **155**, 3401–3408.
104. Teppler, H., Kaplan, G., Smith, K., Cameron, P., Montana, A., Meyn, P., et al. (1993) Efficacy of low doses of the polyethylene glycol derivative of interleukin-2 in modulating the immune response of patients with human immunodeficiency virus type 1 infection. *J. Infect. Dis.* **167**, 291–298.
105. Vaith, P., Maas D., Feigl, D., Hauke, G., Lang, B., Oepke, G., et al. (1985) In vitro and in vivo studies with interleukin 2 (IL-2) and various immunostimulants in a patient with AIDS. *Immun. Infekt.* **13**, 51–63.
106. Kelleher, A.D., Roggensack, M., Emery, S., Carr, A., French, M.A., and Cooper, D.A. (1998) Effects of IL-2 therapy in asymptomatic HIV-infected individuals on proliferative responses to mitogens, recall antigens and HIV-related antigens. *Clin. Exp. Immunol.* **113**, 85–91.
107. Aladdin, H., Larsen, C.S., Moller, B.K., Ullum, H., Buhl, M.R., Gerstoft, J., et al. (2000) Effects of subcutaneous interleukin-2 therapy on phenotype and function of peripheral blood mononuclear cells in human immunodeficiency virus infected patients. *Scand. J. Immunol.* **51**, 168–175.
108. Zou, W., Foussat, A., Capitant, C., Durand-Gasselin, I., Bouchet, L., Galanaud, P., et al. (1999) Acute activation of CD8+ T lymphocytes in interleukin-2-treated HIV-infected patients. ANRS-048 IL-2 Study Group. Agence Nationale de Recherches sur le SIDA. *J. Acquired Immune Defic Syndrome* **22**, 31–38.
109. Piscitelli, S.C., Amatea, M.A., Vogel, S., Bechtel, C., Metcalf, J.A., and Kovacs, J.A. (1996) Effects of cytokines on antiviral pharmacokinetics: an alternative approach to assessment of drug interactions using bioequivalence guidelines. *Antimicrob. Agents Chemother.* **40**, 161–165.
110. Fortis, C., Soldini, L., Ghezzi, S., Colombo, S., Tambussi, G., Vicenzi, E., et al. (2002) Tumor necrosis factor-α, interleukin-2 (IL-2), and soluble IL-2 receptor levels in human immunodeficiency virus-1 infected individuals receiving intermittent cycles of IL-2. *AIDS Res. Hum. Retrovir.* **18**, 491–499.

24

Clinical Applications of G-CSF and GM-CSF in the Treatment of Infectious Diseases

Kai Hübel, David C. Dale, Richard K. Root, and W. Conrad Liles

1. INTRODUCTION

Infectious diseases remain a major cause of morbidity and mortality throughout the world, including the United States. The immune system represents the primary host defense against pathogenic bacteria, fungi, and parasites. The first line of defense is comprised primarily of polymorphnuclear granulocytes (PMNs), macrophages, natural killer (NK) cells, and cytotoxic lymphocytes. Upon activation, these cells can destroy and eliminate pathogenic microorganisms. The possibility of augmenting host defense has increased dramatically during the past two decades with the discovery and development of cytokines. The immunomodulatory effects of colony-stimulating factors (CSFs) on selected leukocyte populations have received increasing attention recently.

This chapter will focus on the properties of two cytokines, namely granulocyte colony-stimulating factor (G-CSF) and granulocyte–macrophage colony-stimulating factor (GM-CSF). Both have been subjects of significant investigation as therapeutic immunomodulatory agents to upregulate phagocyte function during infection. Despite overlapping biologic activities, the two factors do not appear to be derivatives of a common evolutionary ancestral regulatory molecule based on their respective amino acid sequence structures (1). Both cytokines are now available commercially in recombinant forms for clinical use worldwide.

2. G-CSF

2.1. Overview

Granulocyte-CSF is produced primarily by monocytes/macrophages, fibroblasts, and endothelial cells (2). Two different genes encoding the amino acid sequence of G-CSF were initially isolated independently from different tissue sources. Nagata et al. isolated cDNA for G-CSF, which encoded a predicted amino acid sequence of 177 amino acids from a squamous cell line (3). Because of alternative mRNA splicing sites, Souza et al. isolated a different cDNA for G-CSF that coded for a polypeptide of 174 amino acids from a bladder carcinoma cell line (4). The G-CSF gene is located on chromosome 17 q21–22 near other genes involved in the development of neutrophilic granulocytes, whereas the G-CSF receptor is encoded by a single gene on chromosome 1 p35–p34.3 (5). In its native form, the G-CSF protein is O-glycosylated with a molecular mass of approximately 20 kDa. Structurally, it is composed of four helices connected by amino acid loops, which contribute importantly to the molecule's three-dimensional structure (6). Approved pharmaceutical forms of G-CSF

From: *Cytokines and Chemokines in Infectious Diseases Handbook*
Edited by: M. Kotb and T. Calandra © Humana Press Inc., Totowa, NJ

for human use include a recombinant nonglycosylated protein expressed in *Escherichia coli* (Filgrastim; Amgen, Thousand Oaks, CA) and a glycosylated form expressed in Chinese hamster ovary cells (Lenograstim; Chugai Pharmaceuticals, Tokyo, Japan). Glycosylation stabilizes the molecule in vitro by suppressing polymerization and conformational changes *(7)*. Furthermore, it confers resistance to degradation by proteases in human serum *(8)*. Both forms have similar biological activities and bioavailability following subcutaneous or intravenous administration.

In healthy persons, serum levels of G-CSF are 25 ± 19.7 pg/mL. During the acute stage of an infection, serum levels of G-CSF increase by an average 30-fold; in endotoxin-induced shock, levels rise to approx 200 ng/mL *(9)*. This rise is mediated by bacterial products and inflammatory mediators, such as tumor necrosis factor-α (TNF-α) *(10)*. G-CSF may also be a negative feedback signal for the release of TNF-α; in rats, G-CSF suppresses sepsis-induced production of TNF-α *(11)*.

The major target cells of G-CSF are neutrophil precursors and mature neutrophils *(2)*. The essential role of G-CSF in the normal regulation of neutrophil development was demonstrated in the G-CSF "knockout" mouse. Mice rendered G-CSF deficient by targeted disruption of the G-CSF gene in embryonic stem cells developed chronic neutropenia, associated with a 50% reduction of granulocyte precursor cells in the bone marrow. G-CSF knockout mice exhibited a markedly impaired ability to control infection by *Listeria monocytogenes* and failed to developed sepsis-related neutrophilia *(12)*.

In addition to the critical role of G-CSF in the regulation of granulopoiesis, interest has focused on qualitative improvements in the host immune response, including specific neutrophil functional responses and cytokine production, mediated by G-CSF in vitro and in vivo. Administration of G-CSF has been shown to enhance chemotaxis, respiratory (oxidative) burst, phagocytosis, and bactericidal activity of neutrophils, as well as to stimulate surface expression of CD11b/CD18, FcγRII (CD32) and FcγRIII (CD64) on neutrophils *(13–15)*. These effects are apparent at a G-CSF dose of 0.5–1 µg/kg *(16)*. To evaluate the effects of G-CSF on neutrophil function, Allen et al. treated healthy human volunteers with G-CSF daily for 2 wk and employed a chemiluminescence system for differential measurement of oxidase and myeloperoxidase (MPO) dioxygenation activities in whole blood *(17)*. Opsonin-receptor-mediated phagocyte functions were also measured with this system. G-CSF induced a dose-dependent neutrophil leukocytosis and a proportional increase in oxidase activity per volume of blood. The specific oxidase activity per neutrophil was only mildly increased in response to G-CSF treatment and remained relatively constant throughout the treatment period. In contrast, G-CSF treatment caused large, time-dependent increases in phagocyte-mediated MPO-dependent responses *(17)*.

2.2. Effects of G-CSF in Animal Models of Infection

In an experimental animal model, pretreatment with G-CSF has been shown to prevent sepsis-related mortality in mice *(18)*. In various other neutropenic and non-neutropenic animal studies involving severe burns, intramuscular abscesses, streptococcal infections, pneumonias, viral infections, peritonitis, and sepsis, administration of G-CSF has been associated with reduced mortality (overview in refs. *19* and *20*). Rabbits with pneumonia induced 24 hours after transtracheal inoculation of *Pasteurella multocida* were treated with penicillin and either G-CSF (5–8 µg/kg) or placebo for 5 d *(21)*. Although overall survival was only slightly improved (G-CSF: 77%; placebo: 67%), G-CSF treatment was associated with significantly increased survival in a subgroup of animals with sepsis-induced neutropenia (G-CSF: 57%; placebo: 39%). Because the survival benefit occurred mostly within the first 24 h of treatment before significant differences in the mean white blood cell (WBC) count between the two groups existed, leukocytosis was an unlikely explanation for improved survival in the G-CSF-treated animals .

More pronounced survival benefits were observed in other studies in which G-CSF was administered earlier in the course of infection and at higher dosages (50–100 µg/kg equivalent to 5–10 µg/kg in humans). In a hemorrhage mouse model designed to examine the high risk of pneumonia in patients with severe hemorrhage, mortality induced by *Pseudomonas aeruginosa* pneumonia was reduced from 92% to 62% by prophylactic treatment with G-CSF *(22)*. A similar treatment scheme also

Table 1
Animal Models Reporting Efficacy of G-CSF for Treatment of Infection

Authors	Animal	Infection and treatment	Outcome in G-CSF animals
Smith et al. *(22)*	Rabbit	Pneumonia, penicillin/G-CSF vs penicillin/placebo in neutropenic animals	Significant increase in survival
Abraham et al. *(23)*	Mouse	Prophylactic G-CSF in pneumonia after hemorrhage	Mortality reduced from 92% to 62%
Dunne et al. *(25)*	Rat	Prophylactic G-CSF in *E. coli* peritonitis	Increased survival from 38% to 78%
Cairo et al. *(26)*	Rat, neonatal	G-CSF 72 h after inducing group B streptococcal sepsis	Significant increase in survival with G-CSF plus antibiotics
Lundblad et al. *(11)*	Rat	G-CSF 4 h after inducing intra-abdominal sepsis	Reduced mortality rate from 96% to 42%; no neutrophil-mediated tissue damage

reduced the mortality of pneumonia caused by *Klebsiella pneumonia* in rats suffering from acute ethanol intoxication from 90% to 10% *(23)*. In this study, G-CSF enhanced granulocyte recruitment to the lungs, which was inhibited by alcohol intake. Similar G-CSF-mediated effects were observed following experimental *Streptococcus pneumoniae* pneumonia in splenectomized mice with impaired bacterial clearance, where G-CSF improved bacterial clearance and decreased the number of viable pneumococci in tracheobronchial lymph nodes compared with saline-treated controls *(24)*.

Prophylactic administration of G-CSF also increased survival from 38% to 78% in non-neutropenic rodents with *E. coli* peritonitis *(25)*. Bactericidal activity was significantly increased in neutrophils recovered from the peritoneal cavities of G-CSF-treated animals compared to neutrophils recovered from control animals. These observations suggested that enhancement of the cellular arm of the immune response by G-CSF improved survival *(25)*.

In a model of neonatal sepsis, newborn rats were inoculated with group B streptococcus and simultaneously treated with G-CSF or placebo *(26)*. Treatment with appropriate antibiotics was initiated in some animals 24 h following inoculation with bacteria. Seventy-two hours after inoculation, animals that received neither antibiotics nor G-CSF had a survival rate of 4%. Animals treated with antibiotics alone had a 28% survival rate, whereas 91% of the rats treated with antibiotics and G-CSF survived.

Significant synergistic effects on survival by treatment with G-CSF plus antibiotics were confirmed by other studies in septic animals *(27)*. Although granulocyte-mediated lung injury was enhanced by G-CSF in animals administered HCl intratracheally or cyclophosphamide systemically *(28)*, treatment with G-CSF was not associated with increased neutrophil-related tissue damage in animal models of sepsis *(17)*.

Table 1 summarizes studies reporting efficacy of G-CSF in animal models of infection. On the basis of the above physiologic and animal studies, many clinical trials have analyzed the effects of G-CSF as an adjuvant to antibiotics in the treatment of human infections in both neutropenic and non-neutropenic patients.

2.3. Clinical Studies of G-CSF for the Prevention or Treatment of Infection

2.3.1. Therapeutic Use of G-CSF in Neutropenic Patients

Currently, G-CSF is widely employed therapeutically for the treatment of clinical neutropenia, including neutropenia secondary to chemotherapy, radiotherapy, or myelosuppressive drugs, as well as idiopathic neutropenia, leukemia associated with neutropenia, and aplastic anemia *(29–31)*. Based on randomized trials conducted in patients with chemotherapy-induced neutropenia, G-CSF has been approved to accelerate marrow recovery after standard-dose therapy for solid tumors and hematological malignancies *(32,33)*. Accelerated reversal of neutropenia leads to a decrease in the incidence of infection after standard regimens and fewer days with infectious and febrile neutropenic episodes during recovery from bone marrow transplantation. The decrease in morbidity is associated with shorter hospitalization times and reduced administration of parenteral agents *(34)*. Many ongoing studies are now focused on the use of G-CSF to accelerate myeloid recovery following dose-intensive chemotherapy, with the goal of improving overall survival for patients with various malignancies. Furthermore, many studies have investigated the mobilization of CD34+ hematopoietic stem cells from the marrow to the peripheral blood (PBSCs) for use in hematopoietic transplantation, in lieu of bone marrow cells (reviewed in ref. *35*). The results of these investigations have led to major changes in clinical practice, including an overall reduction in the duration of hospitalization as a result of the more rapid repopulation of marrow and recovery of blood counts in most patients receiving PBSC transplantation compared to patients receiving conventional bone marrow transplantation. However, it has yet to be established whether dose intensification of chemotherapy facilitated by the use of G-CSF or stem cell support affects remission rates or survival *(34)*.

Patients with congenital, idiopathic, or cyclic neutropenia have frequent and severe infections as a result of diminished neutrophil production and chronic neutropenia *(36)*. Prior to the availability of human growth factors, no predictably effective therapy was available for these disorders (review in ref. *37*). It is now known that more than 95% of these patients will respond promptly to G-CSF treatment *(37)*. In general, toxic and adverse events are not clinically troublesome and seldom necessitate discontinuing therapy *(38)*. However, data from the Severe Chronic Neutropenia International Registry have identified 23 of 249 patients with congenital neutropenia treated with G-CSF who have developed myelodysplasia or acute myelogenous leukemia within an average follow-up period of 4.5 yr *(38)*. In contrast, no malignant transformation has been observed in patients with cyclic or idiopathic neutropenia who were treated with G-CSF. However, the possibility of malignant transformation and other bone marrow alterations requires continued careful monitoring.

2.3.2. Use of G-CSF in Granulocyte Transfusion Therapy

Because neutropenia remains the major risk factor for the development of severe bacterial and fungal infections in patients undergoing hematopoietic stem cell transplantation and intensive chemotherapy of malignant diseases, the transfusion of normal neutrophils has long been considered as a logical approach to the treatment of such infections *(39)*. The infusion of granulocytes to restore host defense has been studied for more than 60 yr. Beginning early in this decade, several research groups began using hematopoietic growth factors to study their effects on neutrophil formation and function in normal subjects. It was quickly learned that G-CSF will rapidly and dramatically elevate the circulating neutrophil count in normal individuals. Administration of G-CSF to normal subjects allows for collection of $(40-80) \times 10^9$ neutrophils, a sufficient quantity of cells to increase the peripheral blood neutrophil counts to normal levels when transfused in severely neutropenic patients *(40)*. Moreover, neutrophil levels are maintained at or near normal levels for many hours after transfusion of cells from G-CSF-stimulated donors, possibly because G-CSF promotes cell survival by exerting an antiapoptotic effect on neutrophils *(41)*.

Recently, the feasibility of a community blood bank granulocyte transfusion program utilizing community donors stimulated with a single-dose regimen of subcutaneous G-CSF plus oral dexamethasone was examined *(42)*. The recipients of these transfusions were neutropenic hematopoietic stem cell transplantation patients with severe bacterial or fungal infections. Nineteen patients received 165 transfusions (mean: 8.6 transfusions/patients; range: 1–25). Ninety-four percent of the 175 donors providing transfusions were community donors, whereas only 6% of donors were relatives of the transfusion recipients. Sixty percent of the community donors initially contacted agreed to participate, and 98% of these individuals indicated a willingness to participate again. Adverse donor side effects, such as bone pain and headache, likely attributable to G-CSF and/or dexamethasone, were relatively common but usually no more than mild to moderate in degree. Bone pain, headache, and insomnia, most likely an effect of dexamethasone, occurred in 41%, 30%, and 30% of the donors, respectively. Transfusion of (81.9 ± 2.3 × 10^9 neutrophils (mean ± SD) resulted in a mean 1-h posttransfusion neutrophil increment of (2.6 ± 2.6) × 109/μL and restored the peripheral neutrophil count to the normal range in 17 of the 19 patients. The buccal neutrophil response, a measure of the capacity of neutrophils to migrate to tissue sites in vivo, was restored to normal in most patients following transfusion. Chills, fever, and arterial oxygen desaturation of ≥ 3% occurred in 7% of the transfusions, but these changes were not sufficient to limit therapy. Infection resolved in 8 of 11 patients with invasive bacterial infections or candidemia, indicating that transfusion of neutrophils can restore a severely neutropenic patient's blood neutrophil supply and neutrophil inflammation response, thereby reducing the risk of lethal infections.

2.3.3. Therapeutic Use of G-CSF in Neonatal Sepsis

Because of the immaturity of the immune system, neonates, especially those who are premature or have low birth weight, are predisposed to severe infections with bacterial pathogens—in particular, group B streptococci *(43)*. Neutropenia resulting from an exhaustion of the neutrophil reserves is believed to be a major pathogenic mechanism predisposing to such infection *(44)*. A randomized trial was performed in 42 newborns (26–40 wk of age) with presumed bacterial sepsis within the first 3 d of life *(45)*. The patients were randomized to receive either placebo (9 patients) or varying doses of G-CSF (1, 5, or 10 μg/kg every 24 h (27 patients), or 5 or 10 μg/kg every 12 h (6 patients) on d 1, 2, and 3). Intravenous G-CSF was well tolerated, with no acute toxicity recognized. A significant increase in the peripheral blood neutrophil count was observed within 24 h in patients receiving 5 or 10 μg doses every 12 and 24 h. This response was sustained through 96 h. An increase in the neutrophil storage pool was observed at these dosages, as well as an increase in expression of CD11b/CD18, a neutrophil phagocytic and adhesion receptor, at 24 h in patients receiving 10 μg/kg of G-CSF every 24 h. These studies demonstrate that administration of G-CSF to neonates is safe, and larger controlled clinical trials are underway to examine the effects of G-CSF on infectious morbidity and mortality in the newborn.

2.3.4. Use of G-CSF in Fungal Infections

The rates of opportunistic fungal infections have increased substantially in both Europe and North America *(46)*. Because neutrophils constitute the main mechanism of host defense against fungi, including *Candida* and *Aspergillus* species, these infections occur predominately in patients with neutropenia or impaired neutrophil function *(47)*. Because G-CSF not only increases neutrophil number but also modulates various physiological properties of the neutrophils, interest has been directed toward the potential use of G-CSF in the therapeutic approach to fungal infections. The administration of G-CSF (300 μg/d subcutaneously) to five healthy volunteers for 6 d significantly enhanced neutrophil-mediated damage of *Candida albicans* pseudohyphae by 33% ($p = 0.007$) on d 2 and by 44% ($p = 0.04$) on d 6 *(48)*. However, fungicidal activity against hyphae from either *Fusarium solani* or *Aspergillus fumigatus* did not significantly change during the study period. In a mouse model of subacute or chronic disseminated *Candida* infection, G-CSF was less effective, indicating that neutrophil recruitment and activation are crucial in acute candidiasis, whereas other host defense mechanisms control the outcome of less overwhelming *Candida* infection *(49)*. Controlled clinical trials would be necessary to establish a role for G-CSF as an adjunctive immunomodulatory agent in fungal infections.

2.3.5. Therapeutic Use of G-CSF in Non-Neutropenic Patients with Infections

The safety and survival data from animal models of infection, combined with the favorable toxicity profile in humans, have led to several clinical trials of G-CSF as adjunctive therapy in the treatment of infections in non-neutropenic patients. The rationale for these studies has been to enhance the number and functional activities of preformed neutrophils in order to promote recovery from or prevention of local or systemic infections. Sepsis prophylaxis is a promising indication for the use of G-CSF in non-neutropenic patients where the time-point for risk of infection is known or can be anticipated (surgery, trauma, burn, local infection). To date, information is available from several studies in patients with pneumonia and patients with insulin-dependent diabetes mellitus and foot infections, as well as small trials in a variety of other conditions (reviewed in ref. *50*).

2.3.5.1. PNEUMONIA

Pneumonia continues to be a leading cause of death in the United States, and resolution of infection is dependent on neutrophil function *(51)*. In a double-blind, controlled, multi-center trial with community-acquired bacterial pneumonia, 756 patients were enrolled to receive intravenous antibiotics plus either G-CSF (300 µg/d for up to 10 d; $n = 380$) or placebo ($n = 376$) *(52)*. Outcome measures included time to resolution of morbidity (TRM), 28-d mortality, length of stay, and adverse events. A microbial cause for pneumonia was identified in 56% of patients, and antimicrobial use was judged to be appropriate in 98% of the patients by an independent review group. Administration of G-CSF increased the peripheral blood neutrophil count threefold, but TRM, mortality, and length of hospitalization were not affected. However, the time to resolution of infiltrates was significantly more rapid in the G-CSF-treated group, and only one patient developed empyema as compared to six patients in the placebo group ($p = 0.068$). Not only was the administration of G-CSF safe and well tolerated, but also the development of sepsis-related organ failure acute respiratory distress syndrome (ARDS) and disseminated intravascular coagulopathy (DIC) was significantly ($p < 0.017$ and $p < 0.007$, respectively) reduced in the G-CSF recipients. The clinical benefits of G-CSF therapy appeared to be more pronounced in the subgroup of patients with multilobar pneumonia. In two recent studies, administration of G-CSF to patients with severe community-acquired pneumonia or nosocomial pneumonia did not alter morbidity or mortality *(53,54)*.

2.3.5.2. DIABETIC FOOT INFECTION

Foot infections are an important problem in diabetic patients. Extensive surgery and antibiotic therapy are often necessary to achieve resolution of infection. However, because of a lack of neutrophilia in diabetes and impaired superoxide generation in neutrophils from diabetic patients, G-CSF would appear to be a reasonable candidate for adjuvant therapy in the treatment of severe foot infections. Gough et al. conducted a randomized double-blind, placebo-controlled trial with G-CSF in 40 insulin-dependent diabetic patients with foot infections *(55)*. On admission, patients were randomly assigned to receive G-CSF ($n = 20$) or placebo ($n = 20$) for 7 d. Both groups were treated with similar antibiotic and insulin regimens. G-CSF treatment was associated with significantly earlier eradication of pathogens (median: 4 vs 8 d), quicker resolution of cellulitis (median: 7 vs 12 d), a shorter hospital stay (median: 10 vs 17.5 d), and a shorter duration of antibiotic treatment (median: 8.5 vs 14.4 d). No G-CSF-treated patient required surgery, whereas two placebo recipients underwent amputations and two required extensive debridement under anesthesia. G-CSF therapy was generally well tolerated. Neutrophil superoxide production was also measured and found to be low in the diabetic patients compared with normal controls at the start of therapy. After 7 d of G-CSF treatment, neutrophil superoxide production was significantly greater in the G-CSF group than in the placebo group. These encouraging results provide support for further studies of G-CSF in diabetic patients with severe infections.

2.3.5.3. HIV INFECTION

Neutropenia has been identified as an important independent risk factor for the development of infectious complications in human immunodeficiency virus (HIV)-infected individuals *(56)*. The administration of G-CSF has reversed or prevented neutropenia even during periods of full-dose myelotoxic therapy in HIV patients *(57)*. Furthermore, G-CSF has improved defective neutrophil function in vitro and in vivo in the setting of HIV infection *(57)*. In a study of 258 moderately neutropenic HIV-infected patients, G-CSF treatment significantly reduced the incidence of severe neutro-penia and bacterial infections *(58)*. G-CSF-treated patients also had 54% fewer severe bacterial infections, and 45% fewer days of hospitalization were required for the management of any bacterial infection. In another clinical study, 30 acquired immunodeficiency syndrome (AIDS) patients were randomized to receive 5 d of treatment with rifabutin, G-CSF, or both *(59)*. The capacity to kill *Mycobacterium avium* was assessed in neutrophils harvested from each patient before intervention, during therapy (d 4), and after therapy (d 7). A 90% reduction in *M. avium* growth was observed after therapy for patients treated with G-CSF alone ($p = 0.01$), whereas a reduction in growth of 59% and 11% were observed for patients treated with both agents ($p = 0.06$) and with rifabutin alone ($p = 0.84$), respectively.

Interleukin-2 (IL-2) production in HIV-infected patients is depressed and may contribute to de-creased lymphocyte proliferation and reduced generation of cytotoxic T-lymphocytes *(60)*. Adminis-tration of G-CSF to patients with advanced HIV infection has been shown to improve the production of IL-2 in whole blood ex vivo *(60)*.

2.3.5.4. TRAUMA AND SURGICAL PROPHYLAXIS

Various other smaller studies have shown beneficial effects of G-CSF therapy in non-neutropenic infectious conditions. In a pilot study with 20 polytraumatized patients and patients undergoing ma-jor surgery with a high risk of developing sepsis, prophylactic administration of G-CSF improved the neutrophil oxidative burst and reduced the number of episodes of sepsis (G-CSF: 0; placebo: 3) *(61)*. Thirty-seven patients who received G-CSF beginning the first day after liver transplantation had significantly reduced rejection, sepsis, and sepsis-related mortality compared with grafted patients who did not receive G-CSF *(62)*. Endo et al. treated 24 patients with sepsis-induced granulocytopenia who had failed to respond to antibiotics with low-dose G-CSF (75 µg/d) for 5 d *(63)*. Leukocyte counts increased ninefold in 19 survivors, whereas 5 nonresponders died. Thus, G-CSF may favor-ably modulate the host immune response during the "immune paralysis" of late sepsis.

Because esophagectomy for patients with esophageal carcinoma is associated with substantial infectious complications, the use of G-CSF to reduce the number of postoperative infections in this patient population was investigated *(64)*. Nineteen patients were treated perioperatively by daily administration of G-CSF for 10 d beginning 2 d before surgery. Their outcome was compared histori-cally with 77 patients with esophageal cancer who did not receive G-CSF. Within the first 10 d after surgery, 23 untreated patients but none of the G-CSF-treated patients developed infections (29.9% vs 0%; $p = 0.005$). Following cessation of G-CSF therapy, two cases of infection developed in the G-CSF-treated group compared to six additional cases of infection in the untreated group (10.5% vs 37.7%; $p < 0.05$). The rate of fatal hospital infections was reduced in the G-CSF group, but not significantly (G-CSF patients: 0%; historical controls: 9%). During G-CSF treatment, the investiga-tors found an increase in neutrophil phagocytosis, neutrophil oxidative burst, and protective serum cytokines, respectively, which might explain the reduced infection rate.

Table 2 provides an overview of studies examining the use of G-CSF for the treatment of clinical infections. To date, clinical studies indicate a potential use of G-CSF to reduce neutropenic and non-neutropenic infectious complications. However, only large controlled clinical trials will define the impact of G-CSF on the prevention and treatment of specific infections, particular in patients with compromised granulocyte reserves or function.

3. GM-CSF

3.1. Overview

The principal cellular sources of GM-CSF are monocytes/macrophages, fibroblasts and endothe-lial cells *(2)*. GM-CSF promotes growth and differentiation of multipotential hematopoietic progeni-tor cells and stimulates physiologic activity of neutrophils, eosinophils, and monocytes/macrophages

Table 2
Clinical Studies of G-CSF for the Prevention or Treatment of Infection.

Authors	Study population	Treatment	Outcome in G-CSF patients
Trillet-Lenoir et al. *(33)*	130 patients with small-cell lung CDE[a] chemotherapy	G-CSF vs placebo on d 4–17 cancer receiving	Significant decrease in neutropenic fever, parenteral antibiotics, infection-related hospitalization and delay of next cycle
Gillan et al. *(45)*	42 newborns with presumed bacterial sepsis	Prophylactic G-CSF versus placebo	Significant increase in blood neutrophils and functional activation of neutrophils in a subgroup of patients; no acute toxicity
Nelson et al. *(52)*	756 patients with community-acquired bacterial pneumonia	Antibiotics plus G-CSF or placebo	Significant acceleration of radiologic improvement; significant reduction of sepsis-related organ failures; no differences in TRM and mortality
Mitsuyasu *(58)*	258 HIV-infected patients	Prophylactic G-CSF	Significant decrease in severe neutropenia and bacterial infections
Gough et al. *(55)*	40 insulin-dependent diabetic patients with foot infections	Antibiotics plus G-CSF versus placebo	Significant improvement in eradication of pathogens, resolution of cellulitis, hospital stay and intravenous antibiotic treatment

[a]CDE: cyclophosphamide, doxorubicin, etoposide.

(2). However, GM-CSF appears not to play an essential role in normal neutrophil development, as shown by studies in the GM-CSF "knockout" mouse *(65)*. Mice lacking GM-CSF have impaired pulmonary homeostasis, manifested as alveolar proteinosis, and increased splenic hematopoietic progenitors. However, steady-state hematopoiesis is not impaired *(65)*. Murine GM-CSF was cloned in 1984, followed by the cloning of human GM-CSF in 1985 *(66)*. The single copy of the gene-encoding human GM-CSF is located on chromosome 5, region 5q21–5q32 *(67)*. Other genes in this area include those for M-CSF, interleukin (IL)-3, IL-4, and IL-5. In knockout mice lacking functional IL-3, GM-CSF, and IL-5, no hematological defect other than a reduced number of eosinophils was found, indicating a functional overlap with other cytokine systems for hematopoiesis *(68)*. Deletions in this region have been reported in therapy-related myelodysplastic syndromes, acute leukemias, and refractory anemia with morphologic abnormalities of the megakaryocytes *(69)*.

The initial GM-CSF polypeptide consists of 144 amino acids that undergoes cleavage of a 17-amino-acid segment from the amino terminus, resulting in a mature protein of 127 amino acids with 4 α-helices and two β-sheets in a bilobed configuration *(70)*. Because of glycosylation of two serine residues near the amino terminus and the variable N-linked addition of complex carbohydrate at two sides, the molecular weight varies between 14.5 and 35 kDa *(71)*. Commercial, nonglycosylated GM-CSF is expressed in *E. coli* (Molgramostim; Sandoz Ltd, Basel, Switzerland), and the commercial glycosylated form is a yeast-derived GM-CSF (Sargramostim; Immunex Corp., Seattle, WA). The lack or presence of glycosylation does not appear to affect the primary actions of the molecule but may alter its pharmacokinetics. In a study conducted in healthy volunteers, the serum concentration of the nonglycosylated form reached a higher level more rapidly, which also decreased more quickly than the glycosylated form *(72)*. Therefore, the profile of the side effects of both molecules are different. The glycosylated form has a lower incidence of side effects in humans than does the form derived from bacteria *(73)*.

To clarify the effects of glycosylated GM-CSF on neutrophil and monocyte function and the mechanisms of neutrophilia caused by this cytokine, recombinant human GM-CSF was administered to seven normal volunteers for periods of up to 14 d (74). Each subject received GM-CSF at a dose of $250 \mu g/m^2/d$ subcutaneously. This schedule of daily injection caused symptoms in all subjects. Itching and redness at the injection side, bone pain, and headache were the most common symptoms. In addition, all individuals developed eosinophilia. During treatment, blood neutrophil counts rose gradually to peak at a level 3.5-fold greater than baseline by d 14. Marrow aspirates on d 5 of GM-CSF treatment showed a statistically significant increase in the proportion of promyelocytes and myelocytes, accompanied by a significant decrease in band and segmented neutrophils. The transit time through the postmitotic marrow pool accelerated (normal = 6.4 d, GM-CSF = 3.9 d; $p < 0.01$). Treatment caused minimal effects on either the blood neutrophil half-life or the neutrophil turnover rate. The migration of neutrophils to skin chambers was significantly decreased by GM-CSF. The buccal neutrophil response was reduced during GM-CSF treatment in four of five subjects, but the responses were quite variable and the differences were not significant. Treatment increased expression of CD11b/CD18 but not Fcγ receptors. Treatment also stimulated the in vitro neutrophil respiratory burst in response to a variety of agonists, and this enhancement persisted for the duration of treatment.

3.2. Effects of GM-CSF in Animal Models of Infection

The protein sequence homology between human and murine GM-CSF is only 60% (66). Even monkeys have developed antibodies against GM-CSF following administration of human GM-CSF. Thus, animal models to study recombinant GM-CSF have been relatively limited (1,66).

Neutrophil production and function are compromised in neonatal rats during infection. The prophylactic intraperitoneal administration of murine GM-CSF to neonatal rats 6 h prior to a 90% lethal dose challenge of Staphylococcus aureus significantly improved survival (75). In another study in which human GM-CSF was given after infection to neonatal rats, GM-CSF-treated animals had a higher survival rate than control animals (76). In group B streptococcal infection, the administration of penicillin plus GM-CSF decreased the mortality rate substantially as compared to antibiotics alone (77). However, in a rat model of intraperitoneal infection by cecal ligation and puncture, GM-CSF failed to enhance survival above that of control animals (78). Moreover, the mortality rate was higher and animals died earlier after receiving GM-CSF. Inhibition of leukosequestration in the peritoneal cavity was also observed. The liver of GM-CSF-treated rats showed centrilobular degeneration and necrotic changes. These conflicting data raise questions concerning the immunomodulatory role of GM-CSF. In infection, no systemic GM-CSF levels can be detected, so it is likely that endogenous GM-CSF plays its major physiological role in the immediate vicinity of the cells by which it is secreted (79). Exposure of macrophages to GM-CSF primes them for enhanced release of inflammatory cytokines when triggered by lipopolysaccharides (LPS), including IL-1, TNF, and IL-6 (80). After intravenous challenge with endotoxin, mice pretreated with GM-CSF at a dose that did not induce neutrophilia exhibited a significant increase in TNF-α, and a nonlethal dose of endotoxin became lethal (81). In contrast, pretreatment with G-CSF in the same study raised the neutrophil count by 78% but did not enhance TNF-α expression.

A critical role for GM-CSF in pulmonary host defense was recently demonstrated in mice rendered deficient in GM-CSF by targeted gene disruption (82). In these mice, susceptibility to group B streptococcal pneumonia was increased. Additionally, administration of GM-CSF was therapeutically beneficial in a mouse model of disseminated M. avium complex (MAC) infection (83). MAC synthesizes superoxide dismutase, which can inactivate macrophage-derived superoxide anions as well as enzymes which can hinder superoxide production. However, stimulation of MAC-infected macrophages by GM-CSF was shown to increase production of reactive oxygen species and enhance mycobacteriostatic/mycobactericidal activity in vitro and in vivo. In this study, a significant reduction in the number of viable bacteria was observed in the blood, liver, and spleen of mice treated with a combination of GM-CSF and antimicrobial agents compared with control mice and those treated with GM-CSF or antimicrobials alone.

Table 3
Animal Studies Reporting Efficacy of GM-CSF for Treatment of Infection

Authors	Animal	Infection and treatment	Outcome in GM-CSF animals
Frenck et al. *(75)*	Rat, neonatal	Prophylactic GM-CSF prior to a 90% lethal dose of *S. aureus*	Significant increase in survival
Givner et al. *(77)*	Rat, neonatal	Penicillin alone versus penicillin + G-CSF	Significant decrease in mortality rate
Toda et al. *(75)*	Rat	GM-CSF in peritonitis	No enhanced survival; higher mortality rate compared to controls
Bermudez et al. *(83)*	Mouse	Antibiotics alone versus antibiotics + GM-CSF in disseminated *M. avium* complex infection	Significant reduction of bacteria in the blood, liver, and spleen
Liehl et al. *(84)*	Mouse	GM-CSF in *C. albicans* infection	Significant increase in survival and clearance of pathogen from the liver and spleen, but not from the kidney
Mayer et al. (85)	Mouse	Prophylactic GM-CSF in neutropenic mice with *C. albicans*, *P. aeruginosa*, or *S. aureus* infection	Protection against lethal infection

Considerable research efforts have been devoted toward the potential use of GM-CSF as an adjunctive treatment for fungal infection. In one study in mice, the use of GM-CSF led to significantly enhanced survival during 15 d associated with clearing of *C. albicans* from the liver and spleen, but not from the kidney *(84)*. In a neutropenic mouse model, GM-CSF was administered prophylactically prior to experimental *C. albicans*, *P. aeruginosa*, or *S. aureus* infection *(85)*. Prophylactic GM-CSF protected against lethal infection, resulting in increased numbers of survivors. In another study, GM-CSF was given to mice for 7 or 14 d beginning 4 wk after CD4+ T-lymphocyte depletion and infection with *P. carinii (86)*. As compared to a control group that did not receive GM-CSF treatment, the investigators found a significant decrease in the intensity of infection by histological examination of lung tissue and a reduced inflammation score (which did not reach statistical significance). Alveolar macrophages from mice treated with GM-CSF released significantly more TNF-α than cells from control mice after in vitro stimulation with LPS alone or with LPS plus murine recombinant interferon-γ (IFN-γ).

Table 3 provides an overview of animal studies examining the use of GM-CSF for treatment of infections. Overall, data from animal models of acute infection support a protective role for GM-CSF when administered prophylactically. However, the protective actions of GM-CSF may be accompanied and counterbalanced by an exaggerated systemic inflammatory cytokine response. In certain circumstances, especially when severe infection is already present, GM-CSF may have detrimental effects if administered alone, although it may be useful as an adjuvant to antibiotic therapy.

3.3. Studies of GM-CSF for the Prevention and Treatment of Infection

3.3.1. Therapeutic Use of GM-CSF in Neutropenic Patients

Similar to G-CSF, the predominant clinical use of GM-CSF is in the treatment of neutropenia. Its efficacy was evaluated in patients with cancer chemotherapy-induced myelosuppression *(87)*, patients who had been accidentally exposed to cesium-137 *(70)*, and patients undergoing bone marrow or peripheral hematopoietic stem cell transplantation (reviewed in ref. *88*). Moreover, considerable interest has focused recently on the use of GM-CSF for ex vivo expansion of hematopoietic stem and progenitor cells for a variety of applications, including in vitro tumor cell purging and the reduction in the volume of blood required for processing leukapheresis *(88)*.

In a retrospective study, the incidence of infection in patients receiving GM-CSF following autologous bone marrow transplantation was compared to a group of patients who did not receive GM-CSF treatment *(89)*. From the day of transplantation to 28 d posttransplantation, when both groups had severe neutropenia, 40% (38 of 95) of control patients developed infection compared to only 13% (6 of 46) of GM-CSF-treated patients (*p* = 0.001). In GM-CSF-treated patients, there was a trend toward fewer fungal infections, Gram-negative bacterial infections, and pulmonary infections. Patients who did not receive GM-CSF experienced more days of treatment with amphotericin B (*p* = 0.0305) and intravenous antibiotics (not significant). Two control patients, but no GM-CSF-treated patients, died because of infection before d 28. Along with other findings, these results demonstrate that prophylactic GM-CSF can reduce infectious complications in specific clinical settings.

Similar to G-CSF, GM-CSF has the ability to support engraftment following bone marrow or hematopoietic stem cell transplantation and to induce the mobilization of hematopoietic progenitor cells into the peripheral blood for collection and use in subsequent autotransplantation *(84)*. The latter procedure has facilitated further intensification of standard chemotherapy protocols in order to enhance tumor response to cytotoxic agents. Patients receiving hematopoietic stem cells collected following GM-CSF-induced mobilization experience faster recoveries of neutrophil counts and platelet counts, thereby reducing the costs for antibiotic therapy and platelet transfusions *(90)*. In leukemic patients receiving T-cell-depleted allogeneic bone marrow transplantation, GM-CSF may induce antileukemic mechanisms in monocytes, such as the secretion of pro-inflammatory mediators or the stimulation of antibody-dependent cellular cytotoxicity *(91)*. The use of GM-CSF in such patients may minimize the incidence of tumor relapse and accelerate engraftment.

As mentioned previously, GM-CSF exerts effects on a large population of target cells. Therefore, it is not surprising that investigators have tried administration of this growth factor to patients with aplastic anemia. Although GM-CSF treatment may be beneficial in the early stages of aplastic anemia, clinical results have been disappointing in later stages of disease associated with progressive hypocellularity of the bone marrow *(92)*. A greater benefit was evident when administration of GM-CSF was combined with other cytokines, such as IL-1 or IL-3, which act at earlier stages of hematopoietic development *(93)*.

Yoshida et al. examined the effects of long-term treatment with GM-CSF in 61 patients with myelodysplastic syndrome (MDS) who were randomized to receive GM-CSF on a daily schedule at a dose of 60 μg/m^2, 125 μg/m^2, or 250 μg/m^2 for 8 wk *(94)*. In all three groups, neutrophil counts and eosinophil counts increased within 1 wk after the start of treatment. There were no consistent changes in other cell lineages, including monocytes, lymphocytes, reticulocytes, or platelets, but peak levels of these cells were significantly higher as compared with the baseline levels. Infectious complications were reduced in the groups of patients receiving higher doses. In this trial, GM-CSF therapy was generally well tolerated, and no serious side effects were observed. However, as reported by Lieschke and Burgess, patients with MDS who have ≥ 14% marrow blasts before GM-CSF therapy are at risk of developing acute myeloid leukemia (AML) during GM-CSF treatment *(95)*.

3.3.2. Use of GM-CSF in Fungal Infections

Candida and *Aspergillus* species have been consistently noted as the most important opportunistic fungal pathogens in cancer patients *(96)*. GM-CSF has been shown to inhibit fungal growth in a number of systems. Specifically, GM-CSF increased the cytotoxicity of human monocytes and macrophages isolated from the lamina propria of the intestine against *C. albicans* *(97)*. Furthermore, the use of GM-CSF and pentoxifylline, a xanthine derivative that may preserve neutrophil migration during GM-CSF administration, was reported to be effective for treatment of a patient with invasive candidiasis resulting from *C. albicans* *(98)*.

The ability of proinflammatory cytokines to enhance the host immune response during fungal infection was evaluated in isolated neutrophils and buffy coat cells from healthy donors *(99)*. The study compared the differential effects of IFN-γ, G-CSF, and GM-CSF in vitro on hyphal damage of *A. fumigatus*, *F. solani*, and *C. albicans*. IFN-γ significantly enhanced neutrophil-mediated damage to the hyphal and pseudophyphal forms of the three opportunistic fungi studied. Additionally, IFN-γ also significantly enhanced the antifungal activity of buffy coat cells against all three fungi. The colony-stimulating factors G-CSF and GM-CSF were less effective. G-CSF increased hyphal damage mediated by both neutrophils and buffy coat cells against *F. solani*, and GM-CSF augmented the antifungal activity of buffy coat cells against hyphal forms of both *F. solani* and *C. albicans*. The observations provide further experimental support for the use of cytokines as an adjunct to conventional antifungal therapy in the treatment of infections because of opportunistic fungal pathogens.

3.3.3. Overview of Clinical Studies Investigating Administration of GM-CSF for Various Conditions

In vitro, GM-CSF potentiated the recruitment of blast cells into active phases of the cell cycle, thereby increasing their sensitivity to cell-dependent cytotoxic drugs like cytarabine *(90)*. This property has been part of the rationale for the use of GM-CSF in patients with AML *(100)*. Leukemic progenitor cells, which express GM-CSF receptors on their cell surface, can be triggered into S-phase by GM-CSF stimulation. However, based on current knowledge, GM-CSF should be used only in a subset of AML patients at high risk of infection and in those patients who relapse or are resistant to induction therapy (reviewed in ref. *101*). The risk of stimulating the leukemic clone with GM-CSF should be kept in mind, although the balance of evidence indicates that GM-CSF therapy does not affect relapse rates, frequency of remissions, or patient life expectancy *(101)*.

The possible induction of tumor cell cytotoxicity in leukocytes by GM-CSF may also help to destroy cytokeratin-positive cells, such as in micrometastases. In a pilot study of patients with gastric cancer, administration of GM-CSF activated monocytes, leading to a decrease in the number of cytokeratin-positive cells in the bone marrow *(102)*. GM-CSF treatment was also associated with a reduction in the risk of relapse *(102)*.

Oral mucositis in patients treated with intensive cancer chemotherapy or radiotherapy is a major cause of dose reduction or treatment delay. Mucosal damage can be caused directly by cytotoxic effects and indirectly by sustained neutropenia after cytostatic therapy. An impaired mucosal barrier predisposes to life-threatening infectious complications and sepsis. Therefore, there is a great need for effective prophylaxis and treatment of oral mucositis. Several studies have demonstrated the efficacy of GM-CSF therapy in the treatment of oral mucositis after chemotherapy or radiotherapy. Chi et al. evaluated the effects of GM-CSF on chemotherapy-induced oral mucositis in 20 patients with stage IV squamous cell carcinoma of the head and neck *(103)*. Patients were randomized to receive either 4 μg/kg/d GM-CSF subcutaneously from d 5 to 14 or no therapy. Administration of GM-CSF during the first cycle of chemotherapy significantly reduced the incidence, mean duration, and mean area under the curve of severe oral gross mucositis. These beneficial clinical effects continued when patients were crossed over to not receive GM-CSF in the second cycle of chemotherapy. Furthermore, GM-CSF administered in the second cycle to patients who did not receive GM-CSF during the first cycle reduced the incidence of severe mucositis. In a small phase II study, 14 patients undergoing surgery for oropharyngeal tumors received adjuvant radiotherapy at a dose of 2 Gy/d/wk to a total dose of 64 Gy *(104)*. All patients received GM-CSF treatment at the appearance of the mucositis at 30 Gy. Five patients who had already presented mucositis at 30 Gy improved their symptoms significantly during treatment with GM-CSF (from stage III to I or 0). Six patients had an improvement from stage III to II or I, whereas three patients had no measurable benefit by the treatment. A randomized phase III multicenter study of this treatment modality is in progress.

Beneficial modulation of host defense by GM-CSF has been demonstrated in a variety of clinical studies of infectious diseases. It has been well documented that GM-CSF can inhibit the intracellular replication of bacteria or protozoa. Macrophages, which provide a protected environment for microorganisms against extracellular concentrations of antibiotics because of limitations of endocytosis and membrane permeability, are activated by GM-CSF to allow higher intracellular concentrations of certain antimicrobial agents *(105)*. Quantitative and qualitative defects in leukocytes of HIV-infected

Table 4
Clinical Studies of GM-CSF for the Prevention or Treatment of Infection.

Authors	Study population	Treatment	Outcome in GM-CSF patients
Nemunaitis et al. (89)	141 neutropenic patients following autologous bone marrow transplantation	Prophylactic GM-CSF versus placebo	Significant decrease in infection and use of amphotericin B
Yoshida et al. (94)	61 patients with MDS[a]	Daily GM-CSF at doses of 60, 125, or 250 μg/m^2 for 8 wk	Significant increase in neutrophils and eosinophils; reduced infections in higher dose groups
Chi et al. (103)	20 patients with chemotherapy-induced mucositis	Prophylactic GM-CSF versus no therapy	Significant decrease in incidence and mean duration of severe mucositis
Skowron et al. (106)	20 HIV-infected patients with antiretroviral therapy	GM-CSF three times/week for 8 wk versus placebo	Increase of CD4+ count; trend toward decreased HIV RNA
Badaro et al. (107)	20 neutropenic patients with leishmaniasis	Supportive treatment with GM-CSF versus placebo for 10 d	Significant increase in neutrophils, eosinophils, monocytes, and platelets; significant decrease in secondary infections

[a]MDS myelodysplastic syndrome

patients, which may be exacerbated by antiviral therapy, contribute to the high incidence of opportunistic infections and neoplasms (90). Therapy with GM-CSF has been shown to increase both the number and the function of neutrophils, monocytes, and eosinophils in HIV-infected individuals, as well as to enhance the activity of certain antiretroviral drugs. In a randomized, double-blind study of 20 patients with AIDS receiving antiretroviral regimens, either GM-CSF or placebo was administered three times a week for 8 wk (106). GM-CSF was well tolerated and increased the CD4+ lymphocyte count. Furthermore, a trend toward decreased HIV RNA (i.e., "viral load") was noted in patients receiving GM-CSF. Inflammatory cytokines and surrogate markers of disease progression, such as IL-10 and soluble TNF receptors, remained stable during the course of GM-CSF treatment.

In acute visceral leishmaniasis, patients experience suppression of the immune system, associated with abnormal production of cytokines, such as IL-2, IL-3, IFN-γ, and GM-CSF. This altered regulation of cytokine production has been hypothesized to contribute to downregulation of the host antileishmanial response (107). Administration of exogenous GM-CSF might increase inhibition of leishmania proliferation in macrophages by altering the immune balance.

Table 4 provides an overview of reported clinical studies examining the use of GM-CSF for treatment of infectious diseases.

4. COMPARISON OF G-CSF AND GM-CSF TOXICITIES

The clinical use of the hematopoietic growth factors G-CSF and GM-CSF may be summarized as follows: (1) to increase the proliferation the normal hematopoiesis in marrow disorders, such as aplastic anemia, cyclic neutropenia, and myelodysplastic syndromes; (2) to reduce infectious complications by increasing the absolute neutrophil count and the neutrophil function in cancer patients after radiotherapy, conventional chemotherapy, or bone marrow or stem cell transplantation; (3) to enhance the number of circulating stem cells and neutrophils to allow stem cell transplantation and granulocyte transfusion; and (4) to recruit tumor cells into the S-phase of the cell cycle to increase their susceptibility to cytotoxic agents.

The clinical indications for the use of G-CSF and GM-CSF are very similar, and both growth factors have been shown to play a valuable therapeutic role. However, the reason that G-CSF is currently more widely employed clinically than GM-CSF is not only a result of marketing strategies but also the spectrum of potential side effects. Extensive experience has been gained worldwide with G-CSF therapy, and the most commonly reported side effect is mild to moderate bone and/or muskulosceletal pain, seen in 20–30% of recipients *(16,50)*. Aside from this effect, the safety profile of G-CSF appears to be fairly innocuous, even after years of administration in patients with severe chronic neutropenia. Aside from bone pain, the most common adverse effects have been anemia, splenomegaly, thrombocytopenia, and injection-side reactions *(108)*. Allergic reactions have been rarely reported. In clinical trials, up to 2% of the patients developed skin reactions consistent with a clinical diagnosis of cutaneous vasculitis (Sweet's syndrome) *(108)*. G-CSF has not produced dose-limiting side effects, and adverse events decrease following discontinuation of treatment.

In contrast to the anti-inflammatory characteristics of G-CSF, GM-CSF treatment has been associated with a greater number of more severe side effects because of its proinflammatory nature. The most frequently reported side effect is fever, which occurs in >20% of patients and can serve as a confounding factor in the evaluation of responses to the treatment of infection *(109)*. Fever is often accompanied by myalgias and a flulike syndrome. First-dose reactions, consisting of flushing, tachycardia, hypotension, musculoskeletal pain, dyspnea, nausea, vomiting, and arterial oxygen desaturation, have been reported in 5% of recipients *(110)*. High doses (>15 µg/kg) have been reported to cause a generalized capillary leak syndrome *(111)*.

Although there is no convincing evidence to date that either G-CSF or GM-CSF has caused malignant transformation or worsened the course of malignant diseases, careful evaluation of the clinical application of either agent is recommended. In a human skin carcinoma model, tumor progression to high-grade malignancy has been associated with constitutive expression and secretion of G-CSF and GM-CSF, both in vitro and in vivo *(112)*. The carcinoma cells expressed both G-CSF and GM-CSF receptors, and both G-CSF and GM-CSF stimulated cell proliferation and migration in vitro. Additionally, both proliferation and migration were inhibited by neutralizing antibodies to G-CSF and GM-CSF, respectively.

5. SUMMARY

In summary, both G-CSF and GM-CSF have the ability to upregulate phagocyte function. These cytokines play critical roles in the host defense response during infection. As demonstrated in experimental animal models of infection, G-CSF and GM-CSF can potentially be administered therapeutically to enhance pathogen eradication and decrease morbidity and/or mortality. However, this therapeutic potential must be substantiated in controlled clinical trials, which are required to define the proper role of G-CSF and GM-CSF therapy in the clinical management of specific infections.

ACKNOWLEDGMENT

This work was supported in part by a grant from Deutsche Krebshilfe, Germany.

REFERENCES

1. Metcalf, D. (1986) The molecular biology and functions of the granulocyte–macrophage colony-stimulating factors. *Blood* **67**, 257–267.
2. Liles, W.C. and Van Voorhis, W.C. (1995) Nomenclature and biologic significance of cytokines involved in inflammation and the host immune response. *J. Infect. Dis.* **172**, 1573–1580.
3. Nagata, S., Tsuchiya, M., Asano, S., Kaziro, Y., Yamazaki, T., Yamamoto, O., et al. (1986) Molecular cloning and expression of cDNA for human granulocyte colony-stimulating factor. *Nature* **319**, 415–418.
4. Souza, L.M., Boone, T.C., Gabrilove, J., Lai, P.H., Zsebo, K.M., Murdock, D.C., et al. (1986) Recombinant human granulocyte colony-stimulating factor: effects on normal and leukemic myeloid cells. *Science* **232**, 61–65.
5. Gabrilove, J.L. and Jakubowski, A. (1990) Hematopoietic growth factors: biology and clinical application. *J. Natl. Cancer Inst. Monogr.* **10**, 73–77.

6. Hill, C.P., Osslund, T.D., and Eisenberg, D.S. (1993) The structure of granulocyte colony-stimulating factor (r-hu-G-CSF) and its relationship to other growth factors. *Proc. Natl. Acad. Sci. USA* **90,** 5167–5171.

7. Oh-eda, M., Hasegawa, M., Hattori, K., Kuboniwa, H., Kojima, T., Orita, T., et al. (1990) O-linked sugar chain of human granulocyte colony-stimulating factor protects it against polymerization and denaturation allowing it to retain its biological activity. *J. Biol. Chem.* **265,** 11,432–11,435.

8. Nissen, C., Carbonare, V.D., and Moser, Y. (1994) In vitro comparison of the biological potency of glycosylated versus nonglycosylated rG-CSF. *Drug. Invest.* **7,** 346–352.

9. Kawakami, M., Tsursumi, H., Kumakawa, T., Abe, H., Hirai, M., Kurossawa, S., et al. (1990) Levels of serum granulocyte colony-stimulating factor in patients with infections. *Blood* **76,** 1962–1964.

10. Koeffler, H.P., Gasson, J., Ranyard, J., Souza, L., Shepard, M., and Munker, R. (1987) Recombinant human TNF-(stimulates production of granulocyte colony-stimulating factor. *Blood* **70,** 55–59.

11. Lundblad, R., Nesland, J.M., and Giercksky, K.E. (1996) Granulocyte colony-stimulating factor improves survival rate and reduces concentrations of bacteria, endotoxin, tumor necrosis factor, and endothelin-1 in fulminant intra-abdominal sepsis in rats. *Crit. Care Med.* **24,** 820–826.

12. Lieschke, G.J., Grail, D., Hodgson, G., Metcalf, D., Stanley, E., Cheers, C., et al. (1994) Mice lacking granulocyte colony-stimulating factor have chronic neutropenia, granulocyte and macrophage progenitor cell deficiency, and impaired neutrophil mobilization. *Blood* **84,** 1737–1746.

13. Carulli, G., Minnucci, S., Azzara, A., Angiolini, C., Sbrana, S., Caracciolo, F., et al. (1995) Granulocyte colony-stimulating factor (G-CSF) administration increases PMN CD32 (FcRII) expression and FcR-related functions. *Haematologica* **80,** 150–154.

14. Nathan, C.F. (1989) Respiratory burst in adherent human neutrophils: triggering by colony-stimulating factors CSF-GM and CSF-G. *Blood* **73,** 301–306.

15. Roilides, E., Walsh, T.J., Pizzo, P.A., and Rubin, M. (1991) Granulocyte colony-stimulating factor enhances the phagocytic and bactericidal activity of normal and defective human neutrophils. *J. Infect. Dis.* **163,** 579–583.

16. Itoh, Y., Kuratsuji, T., Tsunawaki, S., Aizawa, S., and Toyama, K. (1991) In vivo effects of recombinant human granulocyte colony-stimulating factor on normal neutrophil function and membrane effector molecule expression. *Int. J. Hematol.* **54,** 463–469.

17. Allen, R.C., Stevens, P.R., Price, T.H., Chatta, G.S., and Dale, D.C. (1997) In vivo effects of recombinant human granulocyte colony-stimulating factor on neutrophil oxidative functions in normal human volunteers. *J. Infect. Dis.* **175,** 1184–1192.

18. Gorgen, I., Hartung, T., Leist, M., Niehorster, M., Tiegs, G., Uhlig, S., et al. (1992) Granulocyte colony-stimulating factor treatment protects rodents against lipopolysaccharide-induced toxicity via suppression of systemic tumor necrosis factor-α. *J. Immunol.* **149,** 918–924.

19. Dale, D.C., Liles, W.C., Summer, W.R., and Nelson, S. (1995) Granulocyte colony-stimulating factor—role and relationships in infectious diseases. *J. Infect. Dis.* **172,** 1061–1075.

20. Nelson, S. (1995) Role of granulocyte colony-stimulating factor in the immune response to acute bacterial infection in the nonneutropenic host: an overview. *Clin. Infect. Dis.* **18,** 197–204.

21. Smith, W.S., Sumnicht, G.E., Sharpe, R.W., Samuelson, D., and Millard, F.E. (1995) Granulocyte colony-stimulating factor versus placebo in addition to penicillin G in a randomized blinded study of gram-negative pneumonia sepsis: analysis of survival and multisystem organ failure. *Blood* **86,** 1301–1309.

22. Abraham, E. and Stevens, P. (1992) Effects of granulocyte colony-stimulating factor in modifying mortality from *Pseudomonas aeruginosa* pneumonia after hemorrhage. *Crit. Care Med.* **20,** 1127–1133.

23. Nelson, S., Summer, W., Bagby, G., Nakamura, C., Steward, L., Lipscornb, G., et al. (1991) Granulocyte colony-stimulating factor enhances pulmonary host defences in normal and ethanol-treated rats. *J. Infect. Dis.* **164,** 901–906.

24. Hebert, J.C., O'Reilly, M., and Gamelli, R.L. (1990) Protective effect of recombinant human granulocyte colony-stimulating factor against pneumococcal infections in splenectomized mice. *Arch. Surg.* **125,** 1075–1078.

25. Dunne, J.R., Dunkin, B.J., Nelson, S., and White, J.C. (1996) Effects of granulocyte colony-stimulating factor in a nonneutropenic rodent model of *Escherichia coli* peritonitis. *J. Surg. Res.* **61,** 348–354.

26. Cairo, M.S., Mauss, D., Kommareddy, S., Norris, K., van de Ven, C., and Modanlou, H. (1990) Prophylactic or simultaneous administration of recombinant human granulocyte colony stimulating factor in the treatment of group B streptococcal sepsis in neonatal rats. *Pediatr. Res.* **27,** 612–616.

27. Nelson, S., Daifuku, R., and Andresen, J. (1994) Use of Filgrastim (r-metHuG-CSF) in infectious diseases, in *Filgrastim (r-metHuG-CSF) in Clinical Practice* (Morstyn, G. and Dexter, T.M., eds.), Marcel Dekker, New York, pp. 253–266.

28. King, J., Deboisblanc, B.P., Mason, C.M., Onofrio, J.M., Lipscomb, G., Mercante, D.E., et al. (1995) Effect of granulocyte colony-stimulating factor on acute lung injury in the rat. *Am. J. Respir. Crit. Care Med.* **151,** 302–309.

29. Hollingshead, L.M. and Goa, K.L. (1991) Recombinant granulocyte colony-stimulating factor (rG-CSF). A review of its pharmacological properties and prospective role in neutropenic conditions. *Drugs* **42,** 300–330.

30. Steward, W.P. (1993) Granulocyte and granulocyte–macrophage colony-stimulating factors. *Lancet* **342,** 153–157.

31. Dale, D.C. (1994) Potential role of colony-stimulating factors in the prevention and treatment of infectious diseases. *Clin. Infect. Dis.* **18(Suppl 2),** S180–S188.

32. Crawfort, J., Ozer, H., Stoller, R., Johnson, D., Lyman, G., Tabbara, I., et al. (1991) Reduction by granulocyte colony-stimulating factor of fever and neutropenia induced by chemotherapy in patients with small cell lung cancer. *N. Engl. J. Med.* **325,** 164–170.

33. Trillet-Lenoir, V., Green, J., Manegold, C., Von Pawel, J., Gatzemeier, U., Lebebau, B., et al. (1993) Recombinant granulocyte colony-stimulating factor reduces the infectious complications of cytotoxic chemotherapy. *Eur. J. Cancer.* **29A,** 319–324.

34. Frampton, J.E., Yarker, Y.E., and Goa, K.L. (1995) Lenograstim. A review of its pharmacological properties and therapeutic efficacy in neutropenia and related clinical settings. *Drugs* **49**, 767–793.
35. Welte, K., Gabrilove, J., Bronchud, M.H., Platzer, E., and Morstyn, G. (1996) Filgrastim (r-metHuG-CSF): the first 10 years. *Blood* **88**, 1907–1929.
36. Dale, D.C. (1998) The discovery, development and clinical applications of granulocyte colony-stimulating factor. *Trans. Am. Clin. Climatol. Assoc.* **109**, 27–36.
37. Welte, K. and Boxer, L.A. (1997) Severe chronic neutropenia: pathophysiology and therapy. *Semin. Hematol.* **34**, 267–278.
38. Freedman, M.H. (1997) Safety of long-term administration of granulocyte colony-stimulating factor for severe chronic neutropenia. *Curr. Opin. Hematol.* **4**, 217–224.
39. Pizzo, P.A. (1993) Management of fever in patients with cancer and treatment-induced neutropenia. *N. Engl. J. Med.* **328**, 1323–1332.
40. Dale, D.C., Liles, W.C., Llewellyn, C., Rodger, E., Bowden, R., and Price, T.H. (1998) Neutrophil transfusion therapy: characteristics and kinetics of cells from donors treated with a combination of G-CSF and dexamethasone. *Transfusion* **38**, 713–721.
41. Price, T.H., Bowden, R.A., Boeckh, M., Liles, W.C., Llewellyn, C., Fuller, F., et al. (1997) Neutrophil collection from community apheresis donors after granulocyte colony-stimulating factor and dexamethasone stimulation: feasibility and efficacy. *Blood* **90**, 137b (abstract).
42. Price, T.H., Bowden, R.A., Boeckh, M., Bux, J., Nelson, K., Liles, W.C., et al. (2000) Phase I/II trial of neutrophil transfusion from donors stimulated with G-CSF and dexamethasone for treatment of infections in hematopoietic stem cell transplantation patients. *Blood* **95**, 3302–3304.
43. Ferrieri, P. (1990) Neonatal susceptibility and immunity to major bacterial pathogens. *Rev. Infect. Dis.* **12(Suppl.),** S394–400.
44. Berger, M. (1990) Complement deficiency and neutrophil dysfunction as risk factors for bacterial infection in newborns and the role of granulocyte transfusion in therapy. *Rev. Infect. Dis.* **12 (Suppl),** S401–409.
45. Gillan, E.R., Christensen, R.D., Suen, Y., Ellis, R., van de Ven, C., and Cairo, M.S. (1994) A randomized, placebo-controlled trial of recombinant human granulocyte colony-stimulating factor administration in newborn infants with presumed sepsis: significant induction of peripheral and bone marrow neutrophilia. *Blood* **84**, 1427–1233.
46. Bohme, A. and Karthaus, M. (1999) Systemic fungal infections in patients with hematologic malignancies: indications and limitations of the antifungal armamentarium. *Chemotherapy* **45**, 315–324.
47. Diamond, R.D. (1993) Interactions of phagocytic cells with Candida and other opportunistic fungi. *Arch. Med. Res.* **24**, 361–369.
48. Gaviria, J.M., van Burk, J.-A.H., Dale, D.C., Root, R.K., and Liles, W.C. (1999) Modulation of neutrophil-mediated activity against the pseudohyphal form of *Candida albicans* by granulocyte colony-stimulating factor (G-CSF) administered in vivo. *J. Infect. Dis.* **179**, 1301–1304.
49. Kullberg, B.J., Netea, M.G., Vonk, A.G., and van der Meer, J.W. (1999) Modulation of neutrophil function in host defense against disseminated *Candida albicans* infection in mice. *FEMS Immunol. Med. Microbiol.* **26**, 299–307.
50. Root, R.K. and Dale, D.C. (1999) Granulocyte colony-stimualting factor and granulocyte–macrophage colony stimulating factor: comparisons and potential for use in the treatment of infections in nonneutropenic patients. *J. Infect. Dis.* **179 (Suppl 2),** S342–S352.
51. Smith, J.A. (1994) Neutrophils, host defense, and inflammation: a double-edged sword. *J. Leukocyte Biol.* **56,** 672–686.
52. Nelson, S., Belknap, S.M., Carlson, R.W., Dale, D., DeBoisblanc, B., Farkas, S., et al. (1998) A randomized controlled trial of filgrastim as an adjunct to antibiotics for treatment of hospitalized patients with community-acquired pneumonia. CAP study group. *J. Infect. Dis.* **178**, 1075–1080.
53. Nelson, S., Heyder, A.M., Stone, J., Bergeron, M.G., Daugherty, S., Peterson, G., et al. (2000) A randomized controlled trial of Filgrastim for the treatment of hospitalized patients with multilabor pneumonia. *J. Infect. Dis.* **182**, 970–973.
54. Root, R., Nelson, S., Dale, D., Martin, T., and Welch, W. (2000) A multicenter, double-blind, placebo-controlled study of Filgrastim (r-methuG-CSF) in the treatment of patients with multilobar community-acquired pneumonia (MLCAP). *Am. J. Respir. Crit. Care Med.* **161**, A91 (abstract).
55. Gough, A., Clapperton, M., Rolando, N., Foster, A.V., Philpott-Howard, J., and Edmonds, M.E. (1997) Randomized placebo-controlled trial of granulocyte-colony stimulating factor in diabetic foot infection. *Lancet* **350**, 855–859.
56. Hermans, P. (1999) HIV disease-related neutropenia: an independent risk factor for severe infections. *AIDS* **13 (Suppl 2),** S11–S17.
57. Frumkin, L.R. (1997) Role of granulocyte colony-stimulating factor and granulocyte–macrophage colony-stimulating factor in the treatment of patients with HIV infection. *Curr. Opin. Hematol.* **4**, 200–206.
58. Mitsuyasu, R. (1999) Prevention of bacterial infections in patients with advanced HIV infection. *AIDS* **13(Suppl. 2),** S19–S23.
59. George, S., Coffey, M., Cinti, S., Collins, J., Brown, M., and Kazanjian, P. (1998) Neutrophils from AIDS patients treated with granulocyte colony-stimulating factor demonstrate enhanced killing of *Mycobacterium avium. J. Infect. Dis.* **178**, 1530–1533.
60. Hartung, T., Pitrak, D.L., Foote, M., Shatzen, E.M., Verral, S.C., and Wendel, A. (1998) Filgrastim restores interleukin-2 production in blood from patients with advanced human immunodeficiency virus infection. *J. Infect. Dis.* **178**, 686–692.
61. Weiss, M., Gross-Weege, W., Schneider, M., Neidhardt, H., Liebert, S., Mirow, N., et al. (1995) Enhancement of neutrophil function by in vivo filgrastim treatment for prophylaxis of sepsis in surgical intensive care patients. *J. Crit. Care* **10**, 21–26.

62. Foster, P.F., Mital, D., Sankary, H.N., McChesney, L.P., Marcon, J., Koukoulis, G., et al. (1995) The use of granulocyte colony-stimulating factor after liver transplantation. *Transplantation* **59**, 1557–1563.

63. Endo, S., Inada, K., Inoue, Y., Yamada, Y., Takakuwa, T., Kasai, T., et al. (1994) Evaluation of recombinant human granulocyte colony-stimulating factor (rhG-CSF) therapy in granulopoietic patients complicated with sepsis. *Curr. Med. Res. Opin.* **13**, 233–241.

64. Schafer, H., Hubel, K., Bohlen, H., Mansmann, G., Hegener, K., Richarz, B., et al. (2000) Perioperative treatment with granulocyte colony-stimulating factor (G-CSF) in patients with esophageal cancer stimulates granulocyte function and reduces infectious complications after esophagectomy. *Ann. Hematol.* **79**, 143–151.

65. Seymour, J.F., Lieschke, G.J., Grail, D., Quilici, C., Hodgson, G., and Dunn, A.R. (1997) Mice lacking both granulocyte colony-stimulating factor (CSF) and granulocyte–macrophage CSF have impaired reproductive capacity, pertubed neonatal granulopoiesis, lung disease, amyloidosis, and reduced long-term survival. *Blood* **90**, 3037–3049.

66. Wong, G.G., Witek, J.S., Temple, P.A., Wilkens, K.M., Leary, A.C., Luxenberg, D.P., et al. (1985) Human GM-CSF: molecular cloning of the complementary DNA and purification of the natural and recombinant proteins. *Science* **228**, 810–815.

67. Huebner, K., Isobe, M., Croce, C.M., Golde, D.W., Kaufmann, S.E., and Gasson, J.C. (1985) The human gene encoding GM-CSF is at 5q21–q32, the chromosome region deleted in the 5q- anomaly. *Science* **230**, 1282–1285.

68. Hara, T. and Miyajima, A. (1996) Function and signal transduction mediated by the interleukin 3 receptor system in hematopoiesis. *Stem Cells* **14**, 605–618.

69. Gasson, J.C. (1991) Molecular physiology of granulocyte–macrophage colony-stimulating factor. *Blood* **77**, 1131–1145.

70. Ruef, C. and Coleman, D.L. (1990) Granulocyte–macrophage colony-stimulating factor: pleiotropic cytokine with potential clinical usefulness. *Rev. Infect. Dis.* **12**, 41–62.

71. Clark, S.C. (1988) Biological activities of human granulocyte–macrophage colony-stimulating factor. *Int. J. Cell. Cloning* **6**, 365–377.

72. Denzlinger, C., Tetzloff, W., Gerhartz, H.H., Pokorny, R., Sagebiel, S., Haberl, C., et al. (1993) Differential activation of the endogenous leukotriene biosynthesis by two different preparations of granulocyte–macrophage colony-stimulating factor in healthy volunteers. *Blood* **81**, 2007–2013.

73. Dorr, R.T. (1993) Clinical properties of yeast-derived granulocyte–macrophage colony stimulating factor. *Clin. Ther.* **15**, 19–29.

74. Dale, D.C., Liles, W.C., Llewellyn, C., and Price, T.H. (1998) Effects of granulocyte–macrophage colony-stimulating factor (GM-CSF) on neutrophil kinetics and function in normal human volunteers. *Am. J. Hematol.* **57**, 7–15.

75. Frenck, R.W., Sarman, G., Harper, T.E., and Buescher, E.S. (1990) The ability of recombinant murine granulocyte–macrophage colony-stimulating factor to protect neonatal rats from septic death due to *Staphylococcus aureus. J. Infect. Dis.* **162**, 109–114.

76. Wheeler, J.G. and Givner, L.B. (1992) Therapeutic use of recombinant human granulocyte–macrophage colony-stimulating factor in neonatal rats with type III group B streptococcal sepsis. *J. Infect. Dis.* **165**, 938–941.

77. Givner, L.B. and Nagaraj, S.K. (1993) Hyperimmune human IgG or recombinant human granulocyte–macrophage colony-stimulating factor as adjunctive therapy for group B streptococcal sepsis in newborn rats. *J. Pediatr.* **122**, 774–779.

78. Toda, H., Murata, A., Oka, Y., Uda, K., Tanaka, N., Ohashi, I., et al. (1994) Effect of granulocyte–macrophage colony-stimulating factor on sepsis-induced organ injury in rats. *Blood* **83**, 2893–2898.

79. Freund, M. and Kleine, H.D. (1992) The role of GM-CSF in infection. *Infection* **20(Suppl 2)**, S84–S92.

80. Heidenreich, S., Gong, J.H., Schmidt, A., Nain, M., and Gemsa, D. (1989) Macrophage activation by granulocyte/macrophage colony-stimulating factor. *J. Immunol.* **143**, 1198–1205.

81. Tiegs, G., Barsig, J., Matiba, B., Uhlig, S., and Wendel, A. (1994) Potentiation by granulocyte–macrophage colony-stimulating factor of lipopolysaccharide toxicity in mice. *J. Clin. Invest.* **93**, 2616–2622.

82. LeVine, A.M., Reed, J.A., Kurak, K.E., Cianciolo, E., and Whitsett, J.A. (1999) GM-CSF-deficient mice are susceptible to pulmonary group B streptococcal infection. *J. Clin. Invest.* **103**, 563–569.

83. Bermudez, L.E., Martinelli, J., Petrofsky, M., Kolonoski, P., and Young, L.S. (1994) Recombinant granulocyte–macrophage colony-stimulating factor enhances the effects of antibiotics against *Mycobacterium avium* complex infection in the beige mouse model. *J. Infect. Dis.* **169**, 575–580.

84. Liehl, E., Hildebrandt, J., Lam, C., and Mayer, P. (1994) Prediction of the role of granulocyte–macrophage colony-stimulating factor in animals and man from in vitro results. *Eur. J. Clin. Microbiol. Infect. Dis.* **13(Suppl 2)**, S9–S17.

85. Mayer, P., Schutze, E., Lam, C., Kricek, F., and Liehl, E. (1991) Recombinant murine granulocyte–macrophage colony-stimulating factor augments neutrophil recovery and enhances resistance to infections in myelosuppressed mice. *J. Infect. Dis.* **163**, 584–590.

86. Mandujano, J.F., D'Souza, N.B., Nelson, S., Summer, W.R., Beckerman, R.C., and Shellito, J.E. (1995) Granulocyte–macrophage colony stimulating factor and Pneumocystis carinii pneumonia in mice. *Am. J. Respir. Crit. Care Med.* **151**, 1233–1238.

87. Antman, K.S., Griffin, J.D., Elias, A., Socinski, M.A., Ryan, L., Cannistra, S.A., et al. (1988) Effect of recombinant human granulocyte–macrophage colony-stimulating factor on chemotherapy-induced myelosuppression. *N. Engl. J. Med.* **319**, 593–598.

88. Avanzi, G.C., Gallicchio, M., and Saglio, G. (1998) Hematopoietic growth factors in autologous transplantation. *Biotherapy* **10**, 299–308.

89. Nemunaitis, J., Buckner, C.D., Dorsey, K.S., Willis, D., Meyer, W., and Appelbaum, F. (1998) Retrospective analysis of infectious disease in patients who received recombinant human granulocyte–macrophage colony-stimulating factor versus patients not receiving a cytokine who underwent autologous bone marrow transplantation for treatment of lymphoid cancer. *Am. J. Clin. Oncol.* **21**, 341–346.

90. Scarffe, J.H. (1991) Emerging clinical use for GM-CSF. *Eur. J. Cancer* **27,** 1493–1504.
91. De Witte, T., Vreugdenhil, A., and Schattenberg, A. (1995) The role of recombinant granulocyte–macrophage colony-stimulating factor (GM-CSF) after T-cell deplete allogenic bone marrow transplantation, in *Granulocyte–Macrophage Colony-Stimulating Factor (GM-CSF). Current Use and Future Applications* (Nissen, N.I. and Dexter, T.M., eds.), Pennine, Cheshire, pp. 30–34.
92. Ruef, C. and Colemann, D.L. (1991) GM-CSF and G-CSF: cytokines in clinical applications. *Schweiz. Med. Wochenschr.* **121,** 397–412.
93. Moore, M.A. (1991) The clinical use of colony stimulating factors. *Annu. Rev. Immunol.* **9,** 159–191.
94. Yoshida, Y., Nakahata, T., Shibata, A., Takahashi, M., Moriyama, Y., Kaku, K., et al. (1995) Effects of long-term treatment with recombinant human granuolocyte-macrophage colony-stimulating factor in patients with myelodysplastic syndrome. *Leukocyte Lymphoma* **18,** 457–463.
95. Lieschke, G.J. and Burgess, A.W. (1992) Granulocyte colony-stimulating factor and granulocyte–macrophage colony-stimulating factor. *N. Engl. J. Med.* **327,** 99–106.
96. Bodey, G., Bueltmann, B., Duguid, W., Gibbs, D., Hanak, H., Hotchi, M., et al. (1992) Fungal infections in cancer patients: an internatonal autopsy survey. *Eur. J. Clin. Microbiol. Infect. Dis.* **11,** 99–109.
97. Smith, P.D., Janoff, E.N. and Wahl, S.M. (1993) Granulocyte–macrophage colony-stimulating factor augmentation of human monocyte effector and accessory cell function, in *Hemopoietic Growth Factors and Mononuclear Phagocytes* (Van Furth, R., ed.), Karger, Basel, pp. 79–89.
98. Montgomery, B., Bianco, J.A., Jacobsen, A., and Singer, J.W. (1991) Localization of transfused neutrophils to site of infection during treatment with recombinant human granulocyte–macrophage colony-stimulating factor and pentoxyfylline. *Blood* **78,** 533–534.
99. Gaviria, J.M., van Burik, J.-A.H., Dale, D.C., Root, R.K., and Liles, W.C. (1999) Comparison of interferon-gamma, granulocyte colony-stimulating factor, and granulocyte–macrophage colony-stimulating factor for priming leukocyte-mediated hyphal damage of opportunistic fungal pathogens. *J. Infect. Dis.* **179,** 1038–1041.
100. Hast, R., Bernell, P., Kimby, E., and Petrescu, A. (1995) rhGM-CSF in combination with standard induction chemotherapy for the treatment of acute myeloid leukemia—an overview, in *Granulocyte–Macrophage Colony-Stimulating Factor (GM-CSF). Current Use and Future Applications* (Nissen, N.I. and Dexter, T.M., eds.), Pennine, Cheshire, pp. 24–26.
101. Lanza, F., Rigolin, G.M., Castagnari, B., Moretti, S., and Castoldi, G. (1997) Potential clinical applications of rhGM-CSF in acute myeloid leukemia based on its biologic activity and receptor interaction. *Haematologica* **82,** 239–245.
102. Schlimok, G., Fackler-Schwalbe, I., Lindemann, F., Gruber, R., Flieger, D., Heiss, M., et al. (1995) GM-CSF in gastric cancer: monitoring of micrometastatic tumour cells in bone marrow, in *Granulocyte–Macrophage Colony-Stimulating Factor (GM-CSF). Current Use and Future Applications* (Nissen, N.I. and Dexter, T.M., eds.), Pennine Cheshire, pp. 20–24.
103. Chi, K.H., Chen, C.H., Chan, W.K., Chow, K.C., Cher, S., Yen, S.H., et al. (1995) Effect of granulocyte–macrophage colony-stimulating factor on oral mucositis in head and neck cancer patients after cisplatin, fluorouracil and leucovorin chemotherapy. *J. Clin. Oncol.* **13,** 2620–2628.
104. Masucci, G. (1996) New clinical applications of granulocyte–macrophage colony-stimulating factor. *Med. Oncol.* **13,** 149–154.
105. Silverstein, S.C., Cao, C., Rudin, D., Gao, P., and Neu, H. (1993) Organic anion transporters promote the secretion of anionic antibiotics from cells of the J774 macrophage-like cell line, in *Hemopoietic Growth Factors and Mononuclear Phagocytes* (Van Furth, R., ed.), Karger, Basel, pp. 134–139.
106. Skowron, G., Stein, D., Drusano, G., Melbourne, K., Bilello, J., Mikolich, D., et al. (1999) The safety and efficacy of granulocyte–macrophage colony-stimulating factor (Sargramostin) added to indinavir- or ritonavir-based antiretroviral therapy: a randomized double-blind, placebo-controlled trial. *J. Infect. Dis.* **180,** 1064–1071.
107. Badaro, R., Nascimento, C., Carvalho, J.S., Badaro, F., Russo, D., Ho, J.L., et al. (1994) Granulocyte–macrophage colony-stimulating factor in combination with pentavalent antimony for the treatment of visceral leishmaniasis. *Eur. J. Clin. Microbiol. Infect. Dis.* **13 (Suppl. 2),** S23–S28.
108. Decoster, G., Rich, W., and Brown, S.L. (1994) Safety profile of Filgrastim (r-metHuG-CSF), in Filgrastim (r-metHuG-CSF) in *Clinical Practice* (Morstyn, G. and Dexter, T.M., eds.), Marcel Dekker, New York, pp. 267–290.
109. Peters, W.P., Shogan, J.S., Shpall, E.J., Jones, R.B., and Kim, C.S. (1988) Recombinant human granulocyte–macrophage colony-stimulating factor produces fever. [letter]. *Lancet* **1,** 950.
110. Lieschke, G.J., Cebon, J., and Morstyn, G. (1989) Characterization of the clinical effects after the first dose of bacterially synthesized recombinant granulocyte–macrophage colony-stimulating factor. *Blood* **74,** 2634–2643.
111. Arnig, M., Kliche, K.O., and Schneider, W. (1991) GM-CSF therapy and capillary-leak syndrome. [letter]. *Ann. Hematol.* **62,** 83.
112. Mueller, M.M. and Fusenig, N.E. (1999) Constitutive expression of G-CSF and GM-CSF in human skin carcinoma cells with functional consequence for tumor progression. *Int. J. Cancer* **83,** 780–789.

X
Anticytokine-Based Therapy in Treatment of Infectious Diseases

25

Anticytokine Therapies in Patients with Severe Sepsis and Septic Shock

Pierre-Yves Bochud, Michel P. Glauser, and Thierry Calandra

1. INTRODUCTION

Considerable progress has been made in the understanding of the pathogenesis of inflammation and sepsis over the last 20 yr (1). One of the most significant achievement in this area has been the recognition of the central role played by the innate immune system in the host defenses against invasive pathogens. Innate immune responses are activated when a pathogen crosses the host natural defense barriers. Soluble factors (acute-phase proteins and components of the complement and coagulation systems) and pattern recognition receptors (CD14 and the Toll-like receptors [TLR]) expressed on cells of the myelo-monocytic lineage (monocytes, macrophages, neutrophils, dendritic cells) are essential components of the host defense system. When bound to pattern recognition receptors of innate immune cells, microbial products stimulate the production and release of a multitude of effector molecules, including cytokines, that serve to activate the inflammatory and immune responses whose aim is to eliminate the invasive micro-organism. The innate immune response must be tightly regulated. Failure to mount an appropriate defense response might have dramatic consequences for the host. On the one hand, quantitative or qualitative defects of the innate immune system may result in overwhelming infections, whereas disproportionate inflammatory reactions may lead to vascular collapse, tissue injury and multi-organ dysfunction, as is seen in patients with severe sepsis and septic shock. Numerous studies have shown that high levels of proinflammatory cytokines are associated with poor outcome in patients with septic shock. This has led investigators to postulate that treatment strategies aimed at modulating the production of proinflammatory cytokines or at inhibiting their activity, once they are released in tissues or in the systemic circulation, may improve the outcome of patients with severe sepsis or septic shock. In this chapter, we will review the results obtained in experimental animal models and in humans with anticytokine therapy.

2. PROINFLAMMATORY CYTOKINES

It is beyond the scope of this chapter to discuss the implication of every single proinflammatory cytokine in the pathogenesis of sepsis. Detailed information about the biological activities of many proinflammatory cytokines are available in several chapters of this book. Therefore, we will focus our attention on interventions aimed at inhibiting classical proinflammatory cytokines and some recently identified mediators of sepsis.

From: *Cytokines and Chemokines in Infectious Diseases Handbook*
Edited by: M. Kotb and T. Calandra © Humana Press Inc., Totowa, NJ

2.1. Anti-Tumor Necrosis Factor-α Monoclonal Antibodies

Administration of anti-tumor necrosis factor (TNF)-α antibodies was found to be protective in different animal models of endotoxemia (*see* Table 1). Blocking TNF-α protected mice injected either with low doses of lipopolysaccharide (LPS) given together with D-galactosamine *(2)* or with high doses of LPS (2–20 mg/kg) given alone *(6,8)*. Yet, it failed to prevent death when the LPS dose was greater than 50 mg/kg *(10)*. Of note, animals were protected only when anti-TNF-α antibodies were given either before or at the same time as LPS. Protection was lost when treatment was administered after the LPS. Anti-TNF-α antibodies also protected against death induced by the injection of *Escherichia coli, Staphylococcus aureus,* or Gram-positive cell walls or exotoxins *(11,18)* (*see* Table 1). However, it did not protect against an intravenous challenge with *Klebsiella pneumoniae (16)* or *Streptococcus pyogenes (20)*. Immunoneutralization of TNF-α also failed to prevent death in most experimental models of local infections such as peritonitis or pneumonia *(24,50)* (*see* Table 1). Yet, favorable results have been observed in a rat model of *Neisseiria meningitidis* peritonitis *(21)* and in a rat model of *Pseudomonas aeruginosa* sepsis *(21)*.

During the last decade, several clinical trials have evaluated the efficacy of anti-TNF-α antibodies in the treatment of severe sepsis and septic shock *(93–100)* (*see* Table 2). Anti-TNF-α therapy did not increase survival in two initial phase II studies that included 80 and 42 patients with severe sepsis and/or septic shock *(93–94)*. The efficacy and safety of another murine monoclonal antibody (BAYx1351) was then tested in three large multicenter studies. The North American Sepsis Trial (NORASEPT I) evaluated the role of BAYx1351 in 971 patients with severe sepsis or septic shock *(95)*. Patients were stratified in two groups based on the presence or absence of septic shock and randomized to receive a single infusion of 7.5 or of 15 mg/kg of anti-TNF-α monoclonal antibodies or placebo. Septic shock occurred in 49% of the subjects included in the study. Overall, mortality rates were similar in patients treated with anti-TNF-α antibodies or with placebo. However, within the prospectively defined subgroup of patients with septic shock, anti-TNF-α therapy was associated with a statistically significant reduction of mortality on d 3, 7, and 14, but not on d 28 (45.6% in the placebo group, 37.7% in patients who received 7.5 mg/kg of anti-TNF-α antibody [*p*=0.20], and 37.8% in patients who received 15 mg/kg anti-TNF-α antibody [*p*=0.15]). The International Sepsis Trial (INTERSEPT) evaluated the efficacy of BAYx1351 in patients with severe sepsis and septic shock enrolled in 40 European centers *(96)*. When the results of the NORASEPT I trial became available, the enrolment of patients without shock was discontinued. Patients were treated with a single infusion of 3 or 15 mg/kg of anti-TNF-α antibody or placebo. Of the 533 patients enrolled in the study, 420 were in septic shock. Mortality at d 28 was 39.5% in the placebo group, 31.5% in the 3-mg/kg anti-TNF-α group, and 42.4% in the 15 mg/kg anti-TNF-α group. In contrast to the NORASEPT I trial, anti-TNF-α did not reduce mortality at any time within the first 14 d of study. The second North American Sepsis Trial (NORASEPT II) included 1879 patients with septic shock who were randomized to receive either a single infusion of 7.5 mg/kg of anti-TNF-α monoclonal antibodies (BAYx1351) or placebo *(98)*. Once again, no significant beneficial effect of the anti-TNF-α antibodies was observed. Day 28 mortality was 40.3% in patients who received the anti-TNF-α antibody and 42.8% in patients who received placebo.

The failure of these three large trials of anti-TNF-α antibodies to decrease mortality of patients with severe sepsis and septic shock led some investigators to focus on more specific groups of patients. In fact, in one of the first anti-TNF-α trials, treatment improved survival in a subgroup of patients with elevated TNF-α levels *(100)*. Similarly, in the afelimomab phase II study, in which a F(ab')$_2$ murine monoclonal antibody with high affinity for TNF-α was given to 142 patients, mortality was reduced in a subgroup of patients with elevated circulating concentration of interleukin (IL)-6 (>1000 pg/mL), but not in the entire study population *(97)*. Based on these results, a phase III trial was conducted to evaluate the efficacy of afelimomab in septic patients with high IL-6 concentrations. Of 994 patients enrolled, 446 had circulating IL-6 levels above 1000 pg/mL at baseline and were randomized to receive afelimomab, administered as three infusions of 1 mg/kg/d for three consecutive days *(99)*. The study was terminated prematurely, when an interim analysis estimated that the primary efficacy end point (i.e., a reduction in the 28-d all-cause mortality in treated patients) would not be met. The mortality rate was 54.0% in patients who received afelimomab and 57.7% in control patients, a difference that was not statistically significant. More recently, the results of a large North American afelimomab phase III trial in 2634 septic patients have been reported in an abstract form *(93)*. At d 28, mortality was 32.3% in 1305 patients who received afelimomab and 35.9% in 1329 control patients (p=0.04).

A total of 6726 patients have been included in eight clinical trials of anti-TNF-α antibodies for the treatment of severe sepsis and septic shock. Only one of these studies showed a reduction of mortality *(100)*. Thus, monoclonal antibodies against TNF-α may exert beneficial effects in some patients with severe sepsis or septic shock. However, the impact of treatment is smaller than initially anticipated. Indeed, if the results of the eight studies are pooled, anti-TNF-α antibodies was associated with a 2.9% absolute reduction of lethality (36.7% vs 39.6%; p=0.01). However, such crude results should be considered with great caution, as patient characteristics and prognostic factors may differ between the two treatment groups in the pooled patient population.

2.2. Soluble TNF-α Receptors

Tumor necrosis factor-α exerts its biological effect via an interaction with two receptors coexpressed on most target cells: the TNF type I receptor (TNFR type I or TNFR p55) and the TNF type II receptor (TNFR type II or TNFR p75). These TNF receptors are shed from the membrane after cell activation and can be detected as soluble molecules in the circulation. Soluble TNF receptors are naturally occurring inhibitors of TNF-α. Fusion proteins have been produced that combined the extracellular portion of the TNF receptor and the Fc fragment of human IgG. These molecules act as decoy receptors, competing with membrane-bound TNF receptors for binding of TNF-α and thus preventing overstimulation of target cells. Soluble TNF receptor fusion protein p55 (sTNFR p55) was found to reduce mortality in various animal models of endotoxemia *(42)* and bacterial sepsis *(46)* *(see* Table 1). In contrast, no protective effect was observed when a sTNFR p75 was used in these experimental animal models *(44)*.

Three clinical studies have examined the safety and efficacy of soluble TNFR fusion proteins for the treatment of 1927 patients with severe sepsis or septic shock *(see* Table 2). The first study included 141 septic shock patients randomized to receive placebo or a single infusion of 0.15, 0.45, or 1.5 mg/kg of sTNFR p75 *(101)*. An unexpected significant dose-dependent increase in mortality was observed in patients who received sTNFR p75. Mortality was 30% in patients who received placebo or low-dose sTNFR p75, 48% in patients who received the middle dose of sTNFR p75, and 53% in those who received the highest of dose sTNFR p75. As the sTNFR appears to be more that 50 times as effective as monoclonal antibodies in inactivating TNF-α *(102)*, increased mortality may be related to an excessive and prolonged neutralization of TNF-α. Indeed, blocking TNF activity has been shown to be deleterious in experimental models of focal bacterial sepsis *(48,49)* *(see* Table 1). Alternatively, sTNFR p75–IgG construct might have acted as a TNF-α carrier resulting in the prolongation of the presence of TNF-α in the circulation *(107)*.

Four hundred ninety-eight patients, stratified into a severe sepsis and a refractory shock group, were randomized to receive a single dose of either 0.083, 0.043, or 0.008-mg/kg of sTNFR p55 *(102)*. The 0.008-mg/kg treatment arm was discontinued after an interim analysis showed that it was associated with a trend toward higher mortality. In the entire study population, sTNFR p55 did not improve survival. However, in the prospectively defined subgroup of patients with severe sepsis, there was 36% reduction in the 28-d all-cause mortality in patients treated with 0.083 mg/kg of sTNFR p55 (mortality 23%) when compared to the placebo recipients (mortality 36%; p=0.07). Yet, a large phase III trial of 1340 patients with severe sepsis did not confirm the favorable trend observed in the phase II study *(103)*.

Table 1
Effect of Blocking TNF, IL-1, MIF, IFN-γ, IL-12 or IL-18 in Different Animal Models of Sepsis

Cytokine	Therapy or type of mice	Microbial products or toxins	Experimental model and effect of therapy or gene deletion Systemic infections	Focal infections	Intracellular and fungal infections
TNF	Anti-TNF antibodies or TNF-deficient mice	Low-dose LPS/galactosamine and high-dose LPS: **beneficial** (2–9); Very high dose LPS: **no effect** (10); Peptidoglycan, SEB and TSST-1: **beneficial** (11,12)	E. coli: **beneficial** (13–17); S. aureus: **beneficial** (18) or harmful (19); K. pneumoniae and S. pyogenes: **no effect** (16,20)	Oral P. aeruginosa and N. meningitidis peritonitis: **beneficial** (21,22); E. coli and group B streptococcal peritonitis: **no effect** (2,7,23); CLP peritonitis: **harmful** (24) or no effect (10,25); S. pneumoniae and P. aeruginosa pneumonia: **harmful** (26–28)	L. monocytogenes, C. trachomatis, S. typhimurium, C. albicans, C. neoformans: **harmful** (4,29–39)
	sTNFR p55-IgG or TNFR p55-deficient mice	Low-dose LPS/galactosamine: **beneficial** (40–45); High-dose LPS: **beneficial** (8) or no effect (44,45)	E. coli: **beneficial** (46,47)	E. coli and S. pneumoniae peritonitis: **harmful** (41,43,49) or no effect (48,49); K. pneumoniae pneumonia: **harmful** (50)	L. monocytogenes: **harmful** (44,45)
	sTNFR p75 IgG or TNFR p75-deficient mice	Low-dose LPS/galactosamine and high-dose LPS: **no effect** (41,44,51)	E. coli: no effect (46)	S. pneumoniae pneumonia: **no effect** (48)	L. monocytogenes: **no effect** (44)
IL-1	IL-1 receptor antagonis	High-dose LPS: **beneficial** (52,53) or no effect (54)	E. coli and S. epidermidis: **beneficial** (54–56)	Subcutaneous K. pneumoniae: **harmful** (57)	
MIF	Anti-MIF antibodies or MIF-deficient mice	High-dose LPS: **beneficial** (58) SEB and TSST-1: **beneficial** (59,60)	E. coli peritonitis: **beneficial** (61)	CLP: **beneficial** (61)	
IFN-γ	Anti-IFN-γ antibodies, or IFN-γ or IFNγ-R-deficient mice	Low-dose LPS/galactosamine and high-dose LPS: **beneficial** (62–65) or no effect (66)	E.coli: **beneficial** (67)	E. coli peritonitis: **beneficial** (68); Colon ascendant stent peritonitis: **harmful** (69)	L. monocytogenes, S. typhimurium, Y. enterocolitica, M. tuberculosis, M. bovis: **harmful** (34,70–76)
IL-12	Anti-IL12 antibodies or IL-12-deficient mice	Low-dose LPS/BCG sensitization and high-dose LPS: **beneficial** (77,78)	Group B streptococcus: harmful (79)	CLP and E. coli peritonitis, K. pneumoniae pneumonia: **harmful** (78,80,81)	Y. enterocolitica, M. tuberculosis, C. neoformans: **harmful** (82–84)
IL-18	Anti-IL18 antibodies or IL-18-deficient mice	Low-dose LPS/P. acnes sensitization and high-dose LPS: **beneficial** (85–87)	S. aureus: **beneficial** (88)		S. typhimurium, Y. enterocolitica, M. tuberculosis, M. bovis: **harmful** (90,91)

Note: sTNFR: soluble tumor necrosis factor receptor fusion protein, LPS: lipopolysaccharide; CLP: cecal ligation and puncture; SEB: staphylococcal enterotoxin B; TSST-1: toxic shock syndrome toxin 1. Numbers in parenthesis are reference numbers.

Source: Adapted from refs. *1* and *92*.

Table 2
Clinical Trials of aAnticytokine Therapies

Authors (ref.)	Therapy	Type of study	Days of therapy	Inclusion criteria	No. of patients	Mortality Control group	Mortality Therapy group	Odd ratio (95% confidence interval)
Anti-TNF-a monoclonal antibodies								
Fisher et al., 1993 (93)	CB006	Open label, phase II	1	Severe sepsis or septic shock	80	32%	44%	0.58 (0.17–1.94)
Dhainaut et al., 1995 (94)	CDP571	Open label, phase II	1	Septic shock	42	60%	63%	0.90 (0.17–5.28)
Abraham et al., 1995 (95)	BAYx1351	Double blind, phase III	1	Severe sepsis or septic shock	971	33%	30%	1.13 (0.84–1.52)
Cohen, et al., 1996 (96)	BAYx1351	Double blind, phase III	1	Severe sepsis or septic shock	553	40%	37%	1.10 (0.74–1.62)
Reinhart et al., 1996 (97)	BAYx1351	Double blind, phase III	1	Septic shock	1878	43%	40%	1.11 (0.92–1.34)
Abraham et al., 1998 (98)	MAK195F	Open label, phase II	3	Severe sepsis or septic shock	122	41%	47%	0.79 (0.31–1.98)
Reinhart et al., 2001 (99)	MAK195F	Double blind, phase III	3	Severe sepsis or septic shock and IL-6 >1000 pg/mL	446	58%	54%	1.16 (0.78–1.71)
Panacek et al., 2000 (100)	MAK195F	Double blind, phase III	3	Sepsis or septic shock	2634	36%	32%	1.17 (0.99–1.38)
All studies					6726	40%	37%	1.13 (1.02–1.25)
Soluble TNF receptors								
Fisher et al., 1996 (101)	sTNFR p75	Double blind, phase II	1	Septic shock	141	30%	45%	0.52 (0.21–1.29)
Abraham et al., 1997 (102)	sTNFR p55	Double blind, phase II	1	Severe sepsis or septic shock	444	39%	35%	1.19 (0.77–1.84)
Abraham et al., 2001 (103)	sTNFR p55	Double blind, phase II	1	Severe sepsis or "early" septic shock	1342	28%	27%	1.08 (0.84–1.38)
All studies					1927	30%	31%	0.96 (0.79–1.18)
Interleukin-1 receptor antagonist								
Fisher et al., 1994 (104)	Antril	Open label, phase II	3	Severe sepsis or septic shock	99	44%	24%	2.44 (0.85–7.04)
Fisher et al., 1994 (105)	Antril	Double blind, phase III	3	Severe sepsis or septic shock	893	34%	30%	1.19 (0.88–1.62)
Opal et al., 1997 (106)	Antril	Double blind, phase III	3	Severe sepsis or septic shock	696	36%	33%	1.16 (0.84–1.60)
All studies					1688	36%	31%	1.25 (1.01–1.54)

Note: sTNFR: soluble tumor necrosis factor fusion protein, n.a.: not available.

385

2.3. Interleukin-1 Receptor Antagonist

Interleukin-1 receptor antagonist (IL-1ra) is a naturally occurring antagonist of IL-1. IL-1ra competes with IL-1 for binding to the IL-1 type I receptor and thus inhibits IL-1 biological activity. Administration of IL-1ra has been shown to improve survival in models of endotoxemia *(52,53)* and bacterial infections *(54)* (*see* Table 1). Three clinical studies have examined what was the effect of recombinant human IL-1ra in patients with severe sepsis or septic shock (*see* Table 2). In the phase II study, 96 patients with severe sepsis or septic shock were randomized to receive placebo or a 100-mg dose of IL-1ra followed by a 72-h perfusion with escalading doses of IL-1ra (17, 67, or 133 mg/h) *(104)*. IL-1ra reduced the mortality at d 28 in a dose-dependent fashion (44% in the placebo group vs 32%, 25%, and 16% in patients treated with a low, medium, or high dose of IL-1ra, respectively). Unfortunately, the beneficial effects of the phase II study were not confirmed in two large phase III studies. The first phase III trial included 893 patients with the sepsis syndrome randomized to receive placebo or IL-1ra (single injection of 100 mg followed by a 72-h infusion of 1 or 2 mg/kg/h) *(105)*. The mortality at d 28 was 34% in the placebo group and 31% and 29% in the 1 and 2 mg/h IL1-ra groups, respectively. A post hoc analysis revealed a trend toward favorable outcome in a subset of patients with certain organ dysfunctions and/or a predicted risk mortality of 24% or greater. A second phase III study was undertaken to confirm these findings. Six hundred ninety-six patients with severe sepsis or septic shock were randomized to receive either placebo or IL-1ra (single injection of 100 mg followed by a 72-h continuous infusion of 2 mg/h of IL-1ra) *(106)*. The study was discontinued for futility at an interim analysis. The 28-d mortality was reduced from 36.4% in the placebo group to 33.1% in patients treated with IL-1ra, but the difference was not statistically significant. Altogether, 1688 patients were enrolled in the three IL1-ra trials. A rough analysis of the crude mortality rates in the pooled data revealed that treatment with IL-1ra improved survival (30.6% compared to 35.5% in control patients; *p*=0.04). However, the comment that was made for the meta-analysis of the anti-TNF-α studies also applies for the pooled IL-1ra data.

2.4. Interferon-γ, Interleukin-12, and Interleukin-18

Functionally, the cytokines interferon-γ (IFN)-γ, IL-12, and IL-18 are closely related and have been shown to be critical for the host defenses against intracellular pathogens. IFN-γ exerts very potent priming effects on cells of the monocyte/macrophage lineage and upregulates the expression of numerous cell surface molecules and effector molecules. IL-12 plays an important role in the initiation of inflammatory responses. IL-12 and IL-18 share the capacity to stimulate natural killer (NK) cells and T-lymphocytes to produce IFN-γ. Infections with intracellular pathogens stimulate NK cells and T-cells to release IL-12, IL-18, and IFN-γ. IFN-γ, IL-12, and IL-18 have been shown to be integral components of the host response to LPS (*see* Table 1). Injection of recombinant IFN-γ increases TNF-α levels and mortality in mice after LPS challenge *(64)*. In contrast, mice treated with neutralizing antibodies to IFN-γ, IL-12, or IL-18 were protected from lethal endotoxemia, which was associated with reduction of TNF-α levels in most instances *(62,63,85)*. However, anti-IFN-γ antibodies did not protect against endotoxemia in a D-galactosamine-sensitized mouse model *(66)*. Inhibition of IFN-γ, IL-12, and IL-18 activity yielded diverse results in bacterial sepsis models. Neutralization of IFN-γ was protective in a model of systemic *E. coli* infection *(67)* as well as in an *E. coli* peritonitis model *(68)*. Mice with deletion of the IL-18 gene were protected from lethal *Streptococcus aureus* bacteremia *(88)*. In contrast, blocking IL-12 had deleterious effects in a model of group B streptococcal bacteremia *(79)* and in several models of pneumonia and intra-abdominal infections *(78)*. Mice deficient in the IFN-γ receptor were more sensitive than wilde-type mice to colonic stent peritonitis *(69)*. All studies of intracellular bacterial or fungal infections clearly showed that inhibiting IFN-γ, IL-12, and IL-18 had deleterious consequences, confirming the essential part of this family of cytokines in the host defenses against these pathogens *(70,82,91)*.

In agreement with the results obtained in animal models of infection, there has been many reports of severe infections due to intracellular pathogens (especially *Salmonella* species and *Mycobacte-*

rium species) in humans with mutations of the IFN-γ or IL-12 cytokine or cytokine receptor genes. Few clinical studies have examined the impact of modulating the expression of IFN-γ, IL-12, and IL-18 in patients with infectious diseases. The immunostimulatory properties of IFN-γ have been exploited to prevent infections in immunocompromised patients. Treatment with recombinant IFN-γ significantly reduced the number of serious infections in patients with chronic granulomatous disease *(108)*. In a multicenter study of 416 patients with severe injuries, recombinant IFN-γ was shown to reduce death caused by infections, but the effect was limited to a subset of patients randomized in one center *(109)*. In another study of 213 trauma patients, however, recombinant IFN-γ failed to decrease the rate of infection and did not reduce mortality *(110)*. Similar results were obtained in 216 patients with severe burns *(111)*.

2.5. Macrophage Migration Inhibitory Factor

The cytokine macrophage migration inhibitory factor (MIF) was identified in the early 1960s as a factor released by activated lymphocytes *(112,113)*. However, up until recently, its biological activities have remained mysterious. During the last 10 yr, it has become apparent that MIF is an important cytokine of the innate immune system (for a review, refer to Chapter 5). MIF was rediscovered as a constitutively expressed protein released by the anterior pituitary gland, macrophages, and T-cells after stimulation with microbial toxins, cytokines, and mitogens *(58,114–116)*. In addition to immune cells, MIF mRNA and protein as been detected in many organs, including the brain, kidney, lung, liver, ovary, testis, skin, and endocrine organs. MIF promotes inflammatory and immune responses of macrophages and T- and B-cells *(114,116)* and was found to act as an antagonist of glucocorticoids *(116,117)*. In fact, MIF and glucocorticoid hormones appear to function as integral component of a counterregulatory system that regulates inflammatory and immune responses.

Studies performed over the last 5 yr have established that MIF is an important effector molecule of experimental endotoxemia, toxic shock syndromes induced by Gram-positive exotoxins, and bacterial sepsis. When coinjected with LPS, recombinant MIF augmented lethality, whereas animals treated with anti-MIF antibodies before the LPS challenge were fully protected from death *(58)*. Improved survival was associated with reduction of the serum concentrations of TNF-α. Nearly identical results were acquired in mice with deletion of the *Mif* gene *(59)*. Mice treated with anti-MIF antibody or mice deficient in MIF after deletion of the *Mif* gene were observed to be resistant toxic shock syndromes induced by the toxic shock syndrome toxin 1 or by staphylococcal enterotoxin B *(59)*. Likewise, anti-MIF antibodies protected mice from lethal bacterial peritonitis induced by an intraperitoneal injection of *E. coli* or by cecal ligation and puncture *(61)*. Of note, anti-MIF antibody protected mice even when treatment was delayed by 8 h.

High levels of MIF have been detected in the circulation of patients with severe sepsis or septic shock caused by Gram-negative or by Gram-positive bacteria. Plasma concentrations of MIF were higher in patients with septic shock than in patients with severe sepsis or healthy controls *(61)*. In another study, serum levels were higher in patients with septic shock than in trauma patients and controls ($p<0.01$) and higher in nonsurvivors than in survivors ($p = 0.001$) *(118)*. There was a correlation between concentrations of MIF and cortisol and MIF and IL-6 in septic patients. Multivariate analysis showed that MIF concentrations were a better predictor of patients' outcome than acute respiratory distress syndrome (ARDS). Altogether, these results indicate that MIF plays a critical role in innate immune responses against Gram-negative and Gram-positive pathogens and may, therefore, be a candidate for therapeutic interventions in patients with severe sepsis and septic shock.

2.6. High Mobility Group 1

High-mobility group protein-1 (HMG-1) was initially described as a nonhistone nuclear protein-stabilizing nucleosome formation and regulating gene transcription and replication *(119)*. HMG-1 is also a membrane-bound protein shown to be implicated in neurite outgrowth *(120)*. More recently, HMG-1 was found to be secreted by cells and to act as a mediator of inflammation. HMG-1 does not circulate in healthy mice or humans. However, HMG-1 is secreted in a cytokinelike fashion by macrophages, monocytes, and pituitary cells after exposure to LPS, TNF-α, IL-1, and IFN-γ *(121)*. Kinetic studies has revealed that HMG-1 acts as a "late" mediator of inflammation. HMG-1 was released from culture macrophages more than 8 h after stimulation by endotoxin. In mice, serum levels of HMG-1 have been observed to increase 8–32 h after the injection of LPS *(121)*. Once released, HMG-1 enhances inflammatory response by stimulating the expression of proinflammatory cytokines *(122)*. When administered at low doses, HMG-1 potentiates LPS toxicity. However, injection of high doses of HMG-1 is lethal. Administered intratracheally in mice, HMG-1 produce acute lung injury with accumulation of neutrophils, lung edema, and local production of proinflammatory cytokines *(123)*. In septic patients, higher levels of HMG-1 were associated with increased mortality *(121)*. Blocking HMG-1 activity with neutralizing antibodies protected mice from lethal endotoxemia, even when the first injection of the antibodies was given 2 h after LPS challenge *(121)*. The administration of anti-HMG-1 antibodies either before or after endotoxin-reduced lung injuries, but did not decrease the production of proinflammatory cytokines *(123)*. The neutralization of HMG-1 has not been evaluated in experimental models of infections or in septic patients. However, the delayed production of HMG-1 after exposure to LPS makes it an interesting target for therapeutic interventions in humans..

3. CYTOKINES WITH ANTI-INFLAMMATORY PROPERTIES

Cytokines have been classified into two main classes based on whether they exert predominantly proinflammatory or anti-inflammatory activities. This classification is an oversimplification because cytokines often exhibit both proinflammatory and anti-inflammatory activities. In addition to the soluble TNF receptors and IL-1ra that are naturally occurring cytokines antagonists, IL-10, IL-4, IL-13, IL-6, transforming growth factor-β (TGF-β), and granulocyte colony-stimulating factor (G-CSF) are classical anti-inflammatory cytokines *(92)* (*see* Table 3). Of note, these cytokines also display proinflammatory and immunostimulatory activities.

3.1. IL-10, IL-4, IL-13, IL-6, TGF-β

Interleukin-10 has been shown to suppress cell-mediated immune responses and to inhibit T-cell proliferation and cytokine production by activated neutrophils, monocytes, macrophages, NK cells, and Th1 lymphocytes (reviewed in refs. *124* and *125*). The mechanisms by which IL-10 exerts its anti-inflammatory activities include the inhibition of nuclear factor (NF)-κB activity *(125)*, the promotion of TNF-α and IL-1 mRNA turnover *(126)*, the downregulation of the expression of TNFR *(127)* and an increased shedding of soluble p55 and p75 TNR receptors *(128)*. Like IL-10, IL-4 and IL-13 have been shown to suppress the production of several proinflammatory molecules including TNF-α and IL-1 *(129)*. The anti-inflammatory activity of IL-1 and IL-13 is not mediated by IL-10 *(130)*. IL-6 is produced in large amounts together with TNF-α and IL-1 during endotoxemia or acute infections and was, therefore, at first considered to be an exclusively proinflammatory cytokine. However, recent studies have shown that IL-6 inhibits the synthesis of TNF-α and IL-1 *(131)*. TGF-β was one of the first cytokines known to suppress monocyte and macrophage proinflammatory activities. On the other hand, TGF-β also stimulates the chemotaxis of inflammatory cells and promotes the production of proinflammatory mediators in response to tissue injury or inflammation.

The effects of recombinant IL-10, IL-13, and IL-4 have been tested in experimental models of sepsis (*see* Table 3). IL-10, IL-13 and IL-4 were found to improve survival in several mouse models of endotoxemia *(135,148)*. IL-6 and IL-10 have shown protective effects in models of toxic shock syndrome induced by the injection of staphylococcal enterotoxin B *(138,156)*. The role of the anti-inflammatory cytokines in the resolution of sepsis in models of focal infections is less clear. In a model of peritonitis, treatment with IL-10 had no effect, whereas inhibition of IL-10 with anti-IL-10 antibodies was deleterious, revealing the protective role of IL-10 *(141)*. Treatment with IL-10 had beneficial effects in a model of *P. aeruginosa* pneumonia *(140)*, whereas it exerted detrimental effects

Table 3
Effect of IL-10, IL-4, IL-13, IL-6, or G-CSF in Different Animal Models of Sepsis

Cytokine	Therapy or type of mice	Experimental model and effect of therapy or gene deletion		
		Microbial products or toxins	Focal or systemic infections	Intracellular and fungal infections
IL-10	Recombinant IL-10, anti-IL-10 antibodies, or IL-10-deficient mice	High-dose LPS: **beneficial** (*132–135*) SEB: **beneficial** (*136–138*)	Subcutaneous group B streptococcus and *P. aeruginosa* peritonitis: **beneficial** (*139,140*) CLP: **beneficial** (*141*) **or no effect** (*142*) *E. coli* and *B. fragilis* peritonitis: **no effect** (*143*) *S. pneumoniae* and *K. pneumoniae* pneumonia: **harmful** (*144*)	*L. monocytogenes*: harmful (*145,146*) **or no effect** (*146*) *C. albicans*: **harmful** (*147*)
IL-4	Recombinant IL-4, anti-IL-4 antibodies, or IL-4-deficient mice	Low-dose LPS/galactosamine: **beneficial** (*148*)	*P. aeruginosa* pneumonia and subcutaneous *B. burgdorferi*: **beneficial** (*149,150*) *S. aureus* arthritis: **harmful** (*151*)	*L. monocytogenes*: harmful (*152*) **or no effect** (*153*)
IL-6	Recombinant IL-6 or anti-IL-6 antibodies SEB: beneficial (*156*)	High-dose LPS: **beneficial** (*154*) **or no effect** (*155*) B streptococci: **beneficial** (*156–160*)	*E. coli* peritonitis, *S. pneumoniae* pneumonia, and subcutaneous group	*L. monocytogenes, M. tuberculosis*: **beneficial** (*161–164*) *S. typhimurium*: **harmful** (*165*) *C. albicans*: **harmful** (*169*) **or no effect** (*166*)
IL-13	Recombinant IL-13 or anti-IL-13 antibodies	Low-dose LPS/galactosamine or high dose LPS: **beneficial** (*148,167,168*)	CLP: **beneficial** (*169*)	*L. monocytogenes*: **beneficial** (*170*)
G-CSF	Recombinant G-CSF	Low-dose LPS/galactosamine or high-dose LPS: **beneficial** (*171*)	CLP and *E. coli* peritonitis: **beneficial** (*172–178*) *S. aureus* and *P. multocida* pneumonia: **beneficial** (*179–180*) *S. pneumoniae* pneumonia: **beneficial** (*181,182*) **or no effect** (*182,183*) *E. coli* pneumonia: **beneficial** (*184*) **or harmful** (*179*) *K. pneumoniae* pneumonia: **harmful** (*185*) Systemic *P. aeruginosa*: **no effect** (*186,187*)	

Note: LPS: lipopolysaccharide; CLP: cecal ligation and puncture; SEB: staphylococcal enterotoxin B; TSST-1: toxic shock syndrome toxin 1. Numbers in parenthesis are reference numbers.

Source: Adapted from refs. *1* and *92*.

389

when pneumonia was caused by *K. pneumoniae* and *S. pneumoniae (144,188)*. Experiments performed in IL-6-deficient mice or in mice treated with anti-IL-6 antibodies or with recombinant IL-6 have shown that IL-6 is required to cure bacterial infections *(157,158,162,164,189)* and to reduce mortality of staphylococcal enterotoxin B shock *(156)*. In contrast, IL-6 does not seem to play a critical role in shock induced by LPS or TNF-α *(157,190)*. None of these treatment modalities have yet been investigated in patients with severe sepsis or septic shock.

3.2. Granulocyte Colony-Stimulating Factor

Granulocyte colony-stimulating factor (G-CSF) stimulates the recruitment of myeloid progenitors from stem cells and thus regulates the development of neutrophils in the bone marrow and their release in the circulation. Moreover, G-CSF stimulates the expression of adhesion receptors, induces neutrophil chemotaxis, and enhances phagocytosis *(191)*. G-CSF has been shown to shorten the duration of neutropenia and reduce the incidence of infections after myelosuppressive chemotherapy *(192)*. Recent in vitro and in vivo data suggest that G-CSF also displays anti-inflammatory properties *(193,194)* (*see* Table 3). Pretreatment with recombinant human G-CSF protected mice from lethal endotoxemia *(171)*. G-CSF reduced mortality in a pig model of *P. aeruginosa* bacteremia, but the effect was not statistically significant because of the small number of animals enrolled in that study *(186,187)*. Favorable results have also been observed in experimental peritonitis models. Pretreatment with recombinant G-CSF reduced the concentrations of proinflammatory cytokines and improved survival in various models of *E. coli (177)* or polymicrobial peritonitis *(172,174,178)*. This favorable effect was sustained even when G-CSF was administered after the infection in rats models of peritonitis induced by cecal perforation *(173,175)*. G-CSF improved survival in some but not all pneumonia models. Favorable results have been observed in a dog *E. coli* pneumonia model *(184)*. In rabbits with *Pasteurella multocida* pneumonia, combined G-CSF and penicillin therapy administered after the onset of infection was associated with a trend toward improved survival *(169)*. Prophylactic administration of G-CSF was protective in a rat *S. aureus* pneumonia model, but was deleterious when pneumonia was the result of *E. coli (179)*. In two studies of pneumococcal pneumonia, recombinant G-CSF improved survival of splenectomized mice, but not consistently in sham-operated mice *(181,183)*. In another study, pretreatment with G-CSF protected mice from *S. pneumoniae* pneumonia, but only when infection was induced by a low inoculum of *S. pneumoniae (182)*. In contrast, pretreatment with G-CSF increased mortality in a mouse *K. pneumoniae* pneumonia model *(175)*, possibly because G-CSF increased *K. pneumoniae* polysaccharide production. In contrast to G-CSF, treatment with granulocyte–macrophage stimulating factor (GM-CSF) was shown to be deleterious in several experimental sepsis models *(173)*.

The anti-inflammatory and neutrophil-activating properties of G-CSF and encouraging results obtained in animal models of infections suggested the possibility that G-CSF might be a good candidate for treatment of non-neutropenic patients with severe sepsis or septic shock. Recombinant G-CSF has been evaluated to prevent severe infections in patients at risk of sepsis *(194)*. G-CSF prophylaxis was shown to reduce infections in patients with severe neurological trauma or hemorrhage *(195)* and in patients who had major neck or esophageal surgery *(196,197)*. In contrast, administration of G-CSF before and after liver transplantation was associated with an increased incidence of biopsy-proven rejection and nosocomial pneumonia, but it did not change survival *(198)*. In a randomized double-blind study that compared G-CSF and placebo in 40 patients with diabetic foot infections, therapy with G-CSF increased the clearance of the pathogens from the infected ulcer and the resolution of cellulitis and shortened the duration of intravenous antibiotherapy and hospital stay *(199)*. Large multicenter studies have been conducted in patients with community-acquired pneumonia. Seven hundred fifty-six patients with severe community-acquired pneumonia were randomized to receive G-CSF or placebo. Treatment with recombinant G-CSF fastened the resolution of pneumonia as assessed by chest X-rays, but did not to reduce the mortality and the length of hospital stay

(200). In a recent study including another 480 patients with multilobar pneumonia, treatment with recombinant G-CSF reduced mortality from 11.6% to 8.0% ($p = 0.18$) *(201)*. In a small study of patients with severe head injuries treated with high-dose barbiturate and hypothermia who presented with life-threatening infections, treatment with G-CSF reduced mortality when compared to historical controls *(202)*. The efficacy of human recombinant G-CSF has been evaluated in 18 patients with community-acquired or nosocomial pneumonia and sepsis or septic shock. G-CSF therapy or placebo was started more than 72 h after the diagnosis of pneumonia and was given for 5 d. Mortality was lower in G-CSF treated patients (3 of 12, 25%) than in placebo patients (4 of 6, 67%) *(203)*. However, the favorable results observed in these small studies have to be confirmed in large comparative double-blind trials. For more detailed information about G-CSF, readers should refer to Chapter 24.

4. GLUCOCORTICOIDS

Glucocorticoids are very powerful anti-inflammatory and immunosuppressive molecules. One of the mechanisms by which glucocorticoids exert their anti-inflammatory effects is the inhibition of cytokine gene transcription, including TNF-α, IL-1, IL-2, IL-3, IL-5, IL-6, IL-8, IL-12, IFN-γ, and GM-CSF, to cite only a few. This effect is mediated in part by a direct interaction between the ligand-activated glucocorticoid receptors and the transcription factors nuclear factor κB (NF-κB), activator protein 1 (AP-1), or cyclic AMP-responsive element-binding protein (CREB). Glucocorticoids was also reported to induce the transcription of the IκBα gene *(204,205)*, thereby augmenting the levels of the IκBα protein in the cytoplasm and decreasing the amount of NF-κB translocating to the nucleus and, thus, NF-κB-dependent cytokine gene activation. The effect of glucocorticoids on chromatin structure also may mediate some of the anti-inflammatory effects of steroids. Moreover, glucocorticoids may bind to several transcription corepressor molecules implicated in the regulation of the activity of histone deacetylase. This results in a compact coiling of DNA that impair the access of transcription factors to their specific binding sites and suppresses gene expression. Finally, glucocorticoids have been shown to decrease the stability of cytokine mRNA by binding to AU-rich sequences in the 3' untranslated region of cytokine genes.

The anti-inflammatory and immunosuppressive properties of glucocorticoids have been used successfully for the treatment of many autoimmune or inflammatory diseases. As inflammation is a central feature of severe sepsis and septic shock, it was logical to investigate the impact that steroids would have in the management of septic patients *(206)*. High doses of glucocorticoids were found to improve survival in several experimental sepsis models *(207–209)*. Promising results had been obtained in an initial study of 172 patients with septic shock randomized to receive high doses of methylprednisolone, dexamethasone, or placebo. Glucocorticoids were reported to reduce mortality from 38% to 10% *(210)*. However, as shown in Table 4, these favorable results were not confirmed in seven subsequent trials *(211–216)*. Three recent meta-analyses have indicated that high doses glucocorticoids did not improve *(223,224)* and sometimes even aggravated *(225)*, the outcome of patients with severe sepsis or septic shock. A major difference between experimental and clinical sepsis is the timing of glucocorticoid administration. In most animal models, glucocorticoids have been administered before or shortly after the onset of sepsis. When given before sepsis, glucocorticoids inhibit cytokine production and thus decrease inflammation *(226)*. However, recent data have indicated that glucocorticoids also may exert proinflammatory effects. For example, glucocorticoids can upregulate the expression of different proinflammatory cytokine receptors and, thus, have the capacity to act synergistically with proinflammatory cytokines *(226,227)*. Moreover, a potent proinflammatory cytokine, MIF, was recently shown to be induced rather than suppressed by glucocorticoids *(117)*. Finally, the effects of glucocorticoids may be dose dependent and thus may vary dependent on whether they are administered in physiological or pharmacological doses.

Despite absolute elevated plasma concentrations of cortisol, many septic patients suffer from a relative adrenocortical insufficiency. Relative cortisol insufficiency cannot be diagnosed based on

Table 4
Clinical Trials of Glucocorticoid Therapies

Authors (ref.)	Therapy	Type of study	Days of therapy	Inclusion criteria	No. of patients	Mortality Control group	Mortality Therapy group	Odd ratio (95% confidence interval)
Corticosteroids (high doses)								
Schummer et al., 1976 (210)	Methylprednisolone or dexamethasone	Double blind	1	Severe sepsis or septic shock[a]	172	38%	10%	5.53 (2.22–3.91)
Thompson et al., 1976 (211)	Methylprednisolone	Double blind	1	N.A.	60	78%	79%	0.97 (0.24–3.91)
Sprung et al., 1984 (212)	Methylprednisolone or dexamethasone	Double blind	1	Septic shock[a]	59	69%	77%	0.67 (0.16–3.07)
Lucas et al., 1984 (213)	Dexamethasone	Open label	2	Septic shock[a]	48	20%	22%	0.90 (0.18–4.64)
VA study, 1987 (214)	Methylprednisolone	Double blind	1	Sepsis or severe sepsis[a]	223	22%	21%	1.07 (0.53–2.13)
Bone et al., 1987 (215)	Methylprednisolone	Double blind	1	Severe sepsis or septic shock[a]	381	25%	34%	0.66 (0.41–1.05)
Luce et al., 1988 (216)	Methylprednisolone	Double blind	1	Severe sepsis or septic shock[a]	75	54%	58%	0.86 (0.31–2.35)
All studies					1018	33%	34%	0.96 (0.73–1.25)
Corticosteroids (low doses)								
Cooperative group 1963 (217)	Hydrocortisone	Double blind	6	Severe sepsis or septic shock[a]	194	33%	56%	0.38 (0.20–0.70)
Klastersky et al., 1971 (218)	Bethamethasone	Double blind	3	Disseminated cancer and life-threatening infection[a]	85	56%	52%	1.19 (0.46–3.06)
Bollaert et al., 1998 (219)	Hydrocortisone	Double blind	5	Septic shock	41	63%	32%	3.67 (0.85–16.74)
Briegel et al., 1999 (220)	Hydrocortisone	Double blind	6	Septic shock	40	30%	20%	1.71 (0.32–9.94)
Annane, 2000 (221)	Hydrocortisone and fludrocortisone	Double blind	7	Septic shock	299	N.A.	N.A.	N.A.
All studies (except 221)					360	41%	48%	0.74 (0.48–1.15)

Note: N.A.: not available.
[a]studies performed before the consensus conference definitions of sepsis, severe sepsis and septic shock (222)

the sole measurement of cortisol levels. A rapid corticotropin test has been proposed to evaluate the adrenocortical function in septic patients *(228)*. Several authors have found that a subnormal response to corticotropin stimulation was associated with a poor prognosis *(229–231)*. It was thus proposed that "stress" doses of glucocorticoids may improve the survival of patients with septic shock (*see* Table 4). However, studies of stress doses of glucocorticoids conducted in the 1960s and 1970s did not demonstrate a beneficial effect on the survival of patients with severe infections *(217,218)*. More recently, uncontrolled studies have shown that low doses of glucocorticoids improved hemodynamic parameter in septic patients *(232,233)*. Two comparative trials have examined the role of hydrocortisone (300–400 mg/d given for 5–6 d) in patients with septic shock. In a study of 40 septic shock patients, hydrocortisone reduced the median duration of vasopressor support from 7 d to 2 d ($p = 0.005$) but did not result in a statistically significant reduction of mortality (20% in the treatment group versus 30% in the control group) *(220)*. In the other study, stress doses of hydrocortisone were associated with a reduction of mortality (32% in 22 steroid-treated patients compared to 63% in 19 placebo patients; $p = 0.09$) *(219)*. A recent multicenter study compared the efficacy and safety of a 7-d combined hydrocortisone (50 mg intravenously every 6 h) and fludrocortisone (50 µg oral once a day) therapy or placebo in 299 patients with septic shock *(221)*. A short corticotropin test was performed in all patients at study entry. Mortality was reduced by 30% in patients treated with glucocorticoids in comparison to those who received placebo ($p = 0.03$). A subgroup analysis revealed that the reduction of mortality was significant in patients who did not respond to adrenocorticotropic hormone (ACTH) testing ($p = 0.02$), but not in those who responded ($p = 0.3$). Large randomized trials are necessary to confirm the possible beneficial effects of physiological doses of corticosteroids for the treatment of patients with septic shock.

5. NONSTEROIDAL ANTI-CYTOKINE THERAPIES

Pharmacological agents such as pentoxifylline, thalidomide, and chlorpromazine have been shown to have the capacity to decrease cytokine production, especially TNF-α, and have thus been tested as antisepsis therapies. In addition, other medications, including antibiotics, catecholamines, and anesthetics, were found to exhibit cytokine modulating properties.

5.1. Pentoxifylline

Pentoxifylline, a phosphodiesterase inhibitor, has been shown to exert multiple beneficial effects in sepsis *(232)*. In various animal models of endotoxemia in mice *(235–238)*, rats *(239)*, dogs *(240)*, and sheep *(241)*, pentoxifylline or its analogs reduced the circulating levels of TNF-α and improved survival. Favorable effects have been observed even when pentoxifylline was given up to 4 h after LPS *(235)*. Pentoxifylline also reduced mortality in mice injected with staphylococcal enterotoxin B and toxic shock syndrome toxin (TSST)-1 *(242)*. It decreased IL-1 and TNF levels and improved survival in rats with cecal perforation *(243,244)*. Pentoxifylline was observed to improve hemodynamics in a pig model of *E. coli* peritonitis *(245,246)*. However, less favorable results were obtained in other studies. Pentoxifylline failed to improve survival in rats with *E. coli* bacteremia *(247)* and in mice with endotoxemia, *K. pneumoniae*, or *C. albicans* sepsis *(246)*. The doses and route of administration of pentoxifylline can dramatically influence its effect on mortality. In a rat model of endotoxemia, pentoxifylline exerted beneficial effects when given in low doses, but was harmful at higher doses *(239)*. In a dog model of *E. coli* peritonitis, continuous infusion of pentoxifylline increased, in a dose-dependent fashion, the relative risk of death *(248)*. In contrast, low doses of pentoxifylline improved survival in rodent models of polymicrobial peritonitis *(249,250)*.

In humans, pentoxifylline has been used in patients with severe *Plasmodium falciparum* malaria. It was found to reduce blood levels of TNF-α, but had no impact on patients' outcome *(251)*. A limited number of studies with few patients enrolled have evaluated the impact of pentoxifylline in patients with severe sepsis and septic shock. Improvements of clinical parameters and reduction of proinflammatory cytokines were observed in the initial studies conducted with pentoxifylline *(252–*

257). More recent trials have yielded interesting results. Fifty-one surgical patients with severe sepsis were randomized to receive a continuous infusion of pentoxifylline or placebo *(258)*. Pentoxifylline improved hemodynamic and respiratory parameters, but did not affect mortality (pentoxifylline group: 30%; placebo group: 33%). In a study of 78 bacteremic premature infants who received a 6-d course of pentoxifylline or placebo, pentoxifylline-treated patients had lower TNF-α levels and mortality rates (1 of 40; 2.5%) than placebo patients (6 of 38; 16%; $p = 0.05$) *(259)*. Larger studies are needed to evaluate the role of pentoxifylline in septic patients.

5.2. Thalidomide and Chlorpromazine

First used as a sedative agent, thalidomide was withdrawn from the market more than 30 yr ago because of its dramatic teratogenic effects. More recently, clinicians regained interest in thalidomide because of its anti-inflammatory properties *(260)*. Thalidomide reduced TNF-α levels and mortality in rodents with endotoxemia *(238,261,262)*. Thalidomide has been used successfully for the treatment of dermatological disorders, including aphtous stomatitis, Behçet's syndrome, and chronic cutaneous systemic lupus erythematosus *(263)*. It was recently approved by the Food and Drug Administration (FDA) for the treatment of erythema nodosum leprosum *(264)*. In the last decade, many thalidomide studies have been performed in patients with the acquired immunodeficiency syndrome *(265)*. Thalidomide was shown to be efficacious for the treatment of wasting syndrome, oral and esophageal aphtous ulcers, chronic diarrhea, and Kaposi's sarcoma. No study have been conducted in patients with sepsis.

The immunomodulatory effects of antipsychotic drugs have been known since the 1950s. Chlorpromazine inhibition of TNF-α and IL-1 has been well documented *(266)*. Moreover, some reports suggested that chlorpromazine can also inhibit phospholipase A2 and reduce the proinflammatory effects of platelet-activating factor (PAF), thromboxane, and leukotrienes *(267,268)*. Chlorpromazine improved survival of mice *(246,269)*, guinea pigs *(269)*, rabbits *(267)*, and calves *(270)* injected with LPS. It has not been evaluated for the treatment of severe sepsis in humans.

6. OTHER THERAPIES FOR SEPSIS

In addition to the production of proinflammatory cytokines, microbial products can induce hypotension and tissue injuries as a result of the release of nitric oxide (NO), arachidonic acid metabolites (thromboxane A2, prostaglandins, leukotrienes), and the direct activation of the coagulation and complement cascades *(1)*. Thus, treatment strategies for the management of patients with severe sepsis is not limited to those modulating cytokine production. Numerous studies have investigated treatment modalities aimed at inhibiting diverse targets, including endotoxin *(271–277)*, NO *(278–280)*, bradykinin *(224,281)*, cyclo-oxygenase *(282–285)*, thromboxane *(286–289)*, prostaglandins *(290–294)* or platelet-activating factor *(295,296)*. None of these studies were shown to improve survival. Because of space limitations, these experimental therapies will not be discussed in this chapter, but have been reviewed elsewhere *(297,298)*.

Several studies have evaluated on whether treatment modalities aimed at correcting sepsis-induced coagulation abnormalities might influence patients' outcome. Several large-multicenter studies have been performed with antithrombin III, tissue factor pathway inhibitor, and activated protein C (APC). APC (also referred to as drotrecogin alfa) have so far yielded the most promising results. APC, a naturally occurring protein that promotes fibrinolysis and inhibits thrombosis, is an important modulator of coagulation and inflammation in sepsis *(299)*. Decreased levels of protein C have been reported to be associated with poor prognosis in patients with sepsis *(300)*. A prospective, double-blind, placebo-controlled, phase III trial of activated protein C (24 µg/kg body wt/h for a total duration of 96 h) or placebo has been conducted in 1690 patients with severe sepsis. The study was stopped at the second interim analysis because the differences in the mortality rates between the two groups exceeded the predetermined guideline for stopping the trial. Day-28 all-cause mortality rates was 24.7% in patients who received activated protein C and 30.8% in patients who received placebo ($p = 0.005$) *(301)*. However, the incidence of serious bleeding was higher in the activated protein C group than in the placebo group (3.5% vs 2.0%; $p = 0.06$).

7. CONCLUSIONS

Despite encouraging results in preclinical investigations, all recent experimental anticytokine therapies have had a modest impact on the outcome of patients with severe sepsis and septic shock. Several factors may account for the limited efficacy of anti-TNF and anti-IL-1 therapies in sepsis (reviewed in refs. *302–304*). First, it is perhaps not so surprising, because of the complexity of the cytokine network cascade induced by sepsis, that immunomodulatory therapies targeting one single mediator did not markedly improve patients' survival. Although TNF-α and IL-1 are important cytokines of the host defense system, many other effector molecules are likely to be contribute to the pathogenesis of the sepsis syndrome. Second, beyond obvious factors associated with species disparity, patients enrolled in clinical trials also differ quite significantly from experimental animals with sepsis. Preclinical studies have always been carried out in healthy animals with identical genetic backgrounds. By contrast, patients randomized in clinical trials differ with respect to their genetic makeup, age, underlying diseases, presence of comorbidities, and other key characteristics, including the microbial species causing the infection as well as the site, type and severity of infection. Moreover, in animal models, anticytokine therapy was most often administered before or together with the microbial extracts or the microbes themselves. In many models, the protective effect was frequently lost when treatment was started after the injurious stimuli. The timing of therapeutic intervention was very different in clinical trials. The immunomodulating agent was almost always infused at least hours, and sometimes days, after the onset of infection. Therefore, experimental therapy was probably administered after the peak of cytokine release. Cytokines measurements were performed in a limited number of trials. When available, these retrospective analyses have revealed that a minority of patients had detectable levels of cytokines in the blood when anti-TNF-α or anti-IL-1 therapy was administered. Time-course studies of cytokine release in septic patients have indicated that sepsis also induces a powerful anti-inflammatory response *(305)*. Thus, anti-inflammatory therapies administered during the compensatory, anti-inflammatory response could impair the host defenses. Indeed, blockade of proinflammatory cytokines was efficacious in models of hyperacute inflammation or fulminant sepsis. However, when given to animals with focal rather than systemic infections, such as peritonitis or pneumonia, for example, the same agents often exerted detrimental effects and increased lethality. Phase III clinical trials have included patients with both focal and systemic infections associated with different death rates. In theory, it is possible that the sickest patients benefited from anticytokine therapy, whereas those with less severe infections might have been harmed by it. The net overall results might have been an absence of protective effects as a result of opposite effects occurring in these highly heterogeneous groups of patients. The currently used definitions of sepsis, severe sepsis, and septic shock may, thus, not be very useful to identify patients likely to respond to novel therapeutic interventions. Classification of patients based primarily on biological factors of interest rather than on the sole clinical parameters may be an approach worth pursuing to detect those individuals most likely to respond to defined therapy *(302)*. However, despite the lack of encouraging results obtained with anti-TNF-α and anti-IL-1 therapies in sepsis, the concept of blocking cytokine has yielded impressive results for the treatment of patients with rheumatoid arthritis and Crohn's disease. Identification of new therapeutic targets for the treatment of septic shock remain essential. Recent investigations have shown that MIF, HMG-1 and, perhaps, the recently recognized TREM-1 receptor *(306)* might be targets for future therapeutic interventions. Furthermore, whole microbes or microbial products can also induce inflammation by a direct activation of the coagulation and the complement cascades. The exciting results obtained recently in humans with severe sepsis treated with activated protein C *(301)*, a naturally occurring inhibitor of coagulation, suggest the possibility of developing therapeutic interventions acting on various systems activated by microbial pathogens.

ACKNOWLEDGMENTS

This work was supported by grants from the Swiss National Science Foundation to T.C. (32-49129.96, 32-48916.96, 32-055829.98) and to P-Y.B. (81LA-65462). M.P.G. is recipient of a career award from the Bristol-Myers Squibb Foundation. T.C. is recipient of a career award from the Leenards Foundation.

REFERENCES

1. Heumann, D., Glauser M.P., and Calandra, T. (2001) The generation of inflammatory response, in *Molecular Medical Biology* (Sussmann, M., ed.), Academic, London, pp. 687–728.
2. Zanetti, G., Heumann, D., Gérain, J., Kohler, J., Abbet, P., Barras, C., et al. (1992) Cytokine production after intravenous or peritoneal Gram negative bacterial challenge in mice. Comparative protective efficacy of antibodies to TNFα and to LPS. *J. Immunol.* **148,** 1890–1897.
3. Fiedler, V. B., Loof, I., Sander, E., Voehringer, V., Galanos, C., and Fournel, M. A. (1991) Monoclonal antibody to tumor necrosis factor-α prevents lethal endotoxin sepsis in adult rhesus monkeys. *J. Lab. Clin. Med.* **120,** 574–588.
4. Marino, W. M., Dunn, A., Grail, D., Inglese, M., Noguchi, Y., Richards, E., et al. (1997) Characterization of tumor necrosis factor-deficient mice. *Proc. Natl. Acad. Sci. USA* **94,** 8093–8098.
5. Beutler, B., Milsark, I. W., and Cerami, A. (1985) Passive immunization against cachectin/tumor necrosis factor protects mice from lethal effect of endotoxin. *Science* **229,** 869–871.
6. Mathison, J.C., Wolfson, E., and Ulevitch, R.J. (1988) Participation of tumor necrosis factor in the mediation of bacterial lipopolysaccharide-induced injury in rabbits. *J. Clin. Invest.* **81,** 1925–1937.
7. Bagby, G. J., Plessala, K. J., Wilson, L. A., Thompson, K. J., and Nelson, S. (1991) Divergent efficacy of antibody to tumor necrosis factor-α in intravascular and peritonitis models of sepsis. *J. Infect. Dis.* 163, 83–88.
8. Jin, H., Yang, R., Marsters, S.A., Bunting, S.A., Wurm, F.M., Chamow, S. M., and Ashkenazi, A. (1994) Protection against rat endotoxic shock by p55 tumor necrosis factor (TNF) receptor immunoadhesin: comparison with anti-TNF monoclonal antibody. *J. Infect. Dis.* **170,** 1323–1326.
9. Emerson, T. E., Lindsey, D. C., Jesmok, G. J., Duerr, M. L., and Fournel, M. A. (1992) Efficacy of monoclonal antibody against tumor necrosis factor alpha in an endotoxemic baboon model. *Circ. Shock* **38,** 75–84.
10. Eskandari, M.K., Bolgos, G., Miller, C., Nguyen, D.T., DeForge, L.E., and Remick, D.G. (1992) Anti-tumor necrosis factor antibody therapy fails to prevent lethality after cecal ligation and puncture or endotoxemia. *J. Immunol.* **148,** 2724–2730.
11. Le Roy, D., Morand, P., Lengacher, S., Celio, M., Grau, G.E., Glauser, M. P., et al. (1996) Streptococcus mitis cell walls and lipopolysaccharide induce lethality in D-galactosamine-sensitized mice by a tumor necrosis factor-dependent pathway. *Infect. Immun.* **64,** 1846–1849.
12. Heumann, D., Le Roy, D., and Glauser, M. P. (1996) Contribution of TNF and of LPS in endotoxemic shock in mice. A reappraisal. *J. Endotoxin Res.* **3,** 163–168.
13. Tracey, K. J., Fong, Y., Hesse, D. G., Manogue, K. R., Lee, A. T., Kuo, G. C., et al. (1987) Anti-cachectin/TNF monoclonal antibodies prevent septic shock during lethal bacteraemia. *Nature* **330,** 662–664.
14. Schlag, G., Redl, H., Davies, J., and Haller, I. (1994) Anti-tumor necrosis factor antibody treatment of recurrent bacteremia in a baboon model. *Shock* **2,** 10–18.
15. Hinshaw, L. B., Tekamp-Olson, P., Chang, A. C. K., Lee, P. A., Taylor, F. B., Murray, C. K., et al. (1990) Survival of primates in LD100 septic shock following therapy with antibody to tumor necrosis factor (TNFα). *Circ. Shock* **30,** 279–292.
16. Silva, A.T., Bayston, K.F., and Cohen, J. (1990) Prophylactic and therapeutic effects of a monoclonal antibody to tumor necrosis factor-α in experimental gram-negative shock. *J. Infect. Dis.* **162,** 421–427.
17. Jesmok, G., Lindsey, C., Duerr, M., Fournel, M., and Emerson, T. (1992) Efficacy of monoclonal antibody against human recombinant tumor necrosis factor in E. coli- challenged swine. *Am. J. Pathol.* **141,** 1197–1207.
18. Hinshaw, L.B., Emerson, T.E., Taylor, F.B.J., Chang, A.C.K., Duerr, M., Peer, G. T., et al. (1992) Lethal Staphylococcus aureus-induced shock in primates: prevention of death with anti-TNF antibody. *J. Trauma* **33,** 568–573.
19. Hultgren, O., Eugster, H. P., Sedgwick, J. D., Körner, H., and Tarkowski, A. (1998) TNF/lymphotoxin-α double-mutant mice resist septic arthritis but display increased mortality in response to *Staphylococcus aureus*. *J. Immunol.* **161,** 5937–5942.
20. Martin, R.A., Silva, A.T., and Cohen, J. (1993) Effect of anti-TNFalpha treatment in an antibiotic treatment model of shock due to *Streptococcus pyogenes*. *FEMS Microbiol. Lett.* **110,** 175–178.
21. Opal, S.M., Cross, A.S., Sadoff, J.C., Collins, H.H., Kelly, N.M., Victor, G.H., et al. (1991) Efficacy of antilipopolysaccharide and anti-tumor necrosis factor monoclonal antibodies in a neutropenic rat model of *Pseudomonas sepsis*. *J. Clin. Invest.* **88,** 885–890.
22. Nassif, X., Mathison, J.C., Wolfson, E., Koziol, J.A., Ulevitch, R.J., and So, M. (1992) Tumour necrosis factor alpha antibody protects against lethal meningococcaemia. *Mol. Microbiol.* **6,** 591–597.

23. Teti, G., Mancuso, G., and Tomasello, F. (1993) Cytokine appearance and effects of anti-tumor necrosis factor alpha antibodies in a neonatal rat model of group B streptococcal infection. *Infect. Immun.* **61,** 227-235.

24. Echtenacher, B., Falk, W., Männel, D.N., and Krammer, P.H. (1990) Requirement of endogenous tumor necrosis factor/cachectin for recovery from experimental peritonitis. *J. Immunol.* **145,** 3762–3766.

25. Evans, G. F., Snyder, Y. M., Butler, L. D., and Zuckerman, S. H. (1989) Differential expression of interleukin-1 and tumor necrosis factor in murine septic shock models. *Circ. Shock* **29,** 279–290.

26. van der Poll, T., Keogh, CV., Buurman, W. A., and Lowry, S. F. (1997) Passive immunization against tumor necrosis factor-α impairs host defense during pneumococcal pneumonia in mice. *Am. J. Resp. Crit. Care Med.* **155,** 603–608.

27. Takashima, K., Tateda, K., Matsumoto, T., Iizawa, Y., Nakao, M., and Yamaguchi, K. (1997) Role of tumor necrosis factor alpha in pathogenesis of pneumococcal pneumonia in mice.*Infect. Immun.* **65,** 257–250.

28. Gosselin, D., DeSanctis, J., Boulé, M., Skamene, E., Matouk, C., and Radzioch, D. (1995) Role of tumor necrosis factor alpha in innate resistance to mouse pulmonary infection with Pseudomonas aeruginosa. *Infect. Immun.* **63,** 3272–3278.

29. Havell, E. A. (1989) Evidence that tumor necrosis factor has an important role in antibacterial resistance. *J. Immunol.* **143,** 2894–2899.

30. Nakane, A., Minagawa, T., and Kato, K. (1988) Endogenous tumor necrosis factor (cachectin) is essential to host resistance against *Listeria monocytogenes* infection. *Infect. Immun.* **56,** 2563–2569.

31. van Furth, R., Van Zwet, T. L., Buisman, A. M., and Van Dissel, J. T. (1994) Anti-tumor necrosis factor antibodies inhibit the influx of granulocytes and monocytes into an inflammatory exudate and enhance the growth of *Listeria monocytogenes* in various organs. *J. Infect. Dis.* **170,** 234–237.

32. Müller, M., Althaus, R., Fröhlich, D., Frei, K., and Eugster, H. P. (1999) Reduced antilisterial activity of TNF-deficient bone marrow-derived macrophages is due to impaired superoxide production. *Eur. J. Immunol.* **29,** 3089–3097.

33. Williams, D. M., Magee, D. M., Bonewald, L. F., Smith, J. G., Bleicker, C. A., Byrne, G. I.,et al. (1990) A role in vivo for tumor necrosis factor alpha in host defense against Chlamydia trachomatis. *Infect. Immun.* **58,** 1572–1576.

34. Nauciel, C. and Espinasse-Maes, F. (1992) Role of gamma interferon and tumor necrosis factor alpha in resistance to *Salmonella typhimurium* infection. *Infect. Immun.* **60,** 450–454.

35. Mastroeni, P., Skepper, J. N., and Hormaeche, C. E. (1995) Effect of anti-tumor necrosis factor alpha antibodies on histopathology of primary Salmonella infections. *Infect. Immun.* **63,** 3674–3682.

36. Louie, A., Baltch, A. L., Smith, R. P., Franke, M. A., Ritz, W. J., Singh, J. K., et al. (1994) Tumor necrosis factor alpha has a protective role in a murine model of systemic candidiasis. *Infect. Immun.* **62,** 2761–2772.

37. Netea, M. G., van Tits, L. J. H., Curfs, J. H. A., Amiot, F., Meis, J. F. G. M., Van der Meer, J. W. M., et al. (1999) Increased susceptibility of TNF-α lymphotoxin-α double knockout mice to systemic candidiasis through impaired recruitment of neutrophils and phagocytosis of *Candida albicans. J Immunol* **163,** 1498–1505.

38. Mencacci, A., Cenci, E., Del Sero, G., Fè d'Ostiani, C., Mosci, P., Montagnoli, C., et al. (1998) Defective and impaired Th1 development in tumor necrosis factor/lymphotoxin-α double-deficient mice infected with *Candida albicans. Intern. Immunol.* **10,** 37–48.

39. Rayhane, N., Lortholary, O., Fitting, C., Callebert, J., Huerre, M., Dromer, F., et al. (1999) Enhanced sensitivity of tumor necrosis factor/lymphotoxin-α-deficient mice to Cryptococcus neoformans infection despite increased levels of nitrite/nitrate, interferon-γ, and interleukin-12. *J. Infect. Dis.* **180,** 1637–1647.

40. Ashkenazi, A., Marsters, S. A., Capon, D. J., Chamow, S. M., Figari, I. S., Pennica, D., et al. (1991) Protection against endotoxin shock by a tumor necrosis factor receptor immunoadhesin. *Proc. Natl. Acad. Sci. USA* **88,** 10535–10539.

41. Loetscher, H., Angehrn, P., Schlaeger, E. J., Gentz, R., and Lesslauer, W. (1993) Efficacy of a chimeric TNFR-IgG fusion protein to inhibit TNF activity in animal models of septic shock, in *Bacterial Endotoxin: Recognition and Effector Mechanisms* (Levin, J., Alving, C. R., Munford, R. S., and Stütz, P. L., eds.), Elsevier Science, Amsterdam, pp. 455–462.

42. Lesslauer, W., Tabuchi, H., Gentz, R., Brockhaus, M., Schlaeger, E.J., Grau, G.E., et al. (1991) Recombinant soluble tumor necrosis factor receptor proteins protect mice from lipopolysaccharide-induced lethality. *Eur. J. Immunol.* **21,** 2883–2886.

43. Acton, R. D., Dahlberg, P. S., Uknis, M. E., Klaerner, H. G., Fink, G. S., Norman, J. G., et al. (1996) Differential sensitivity to Escherichia coli infection in mice lacking tumor necrosis factor p55 or interleukin-1 p80 receptors. *Arch. Surg.* **131,** 1216–1221.

44. Peschon, J.J., Torrance, D.S., Stocking, K.L., Glaccum, M.B., Otten, C., Willis, C.R., Charrier, K., et al. (1998) TNF receptor-deficient mice reveal divergent roles for p55 and p75 in several models of inflammation. *J. Immunol.* **160,** 943–952.

45. Rothe, J., Lesslauer, W., Lötscher, H., Lang, Y., Koebel, P., Köntgen, F., et al. (1993) Mice lacking the tumour necrosis factor receptor 1 are resistant to TNF-mediated toxicity but highly susceptible to infection by *Listeria monocytogenes. Nature* **364,** 798–802.

46. Evans, T.J., Moyes, D., Carpenter, A., Martin, R., Loetscher, H., Lesslauer, W., et al. (1994) Protective effect of 55- but not 75-kD soluble tumor necrosis factor receptor-immunoglobulin G fusion proteins in an animal model of gram-negative sepsis. *J. Exp. Med.* **180,** 2173–2179.

47. Van Zee, K. J., Moldawer, L. L., Oldenburg, H. S. A., Thompson, W. A., Stackpole, S. A., Montegut, W. J., et al. (1996) Protection against lethal Escherichia coli bacteremia in baboons (Papio anubis) by pretreatment with a 55-kDa TNF receptor (CD120a)—Ig fusion protein, Ro 45-2081. *J. Immunol.* **156,** 2221–2230.

48. O'Brien, D.P., Briles, D.E., Szalai, A.J., Tu, A.H., Sanz, I., and Nahm, M.H. (1999) Tumor necrosis factor alpha receptor I is important for survival from *Streptococcus pneumoniae* infections. *Infect. Immun.* **67,** 595–601.

49. Heumann, D., Le Roy, D., Zanetti, G., Eugster, H.P., Ryffel, B., Hahne, M., et al. (1996) Contribution of TNF/TNF receptor and of Fas ligand to toxicity in murine models of endotoxemia and bacterial peritonitis. *J. Inflamma.* **47,** 173–179.
50. Laichalk, L.L., Kunkel, S.L., Strieter, R.M., Danforth, J.M., Bailie, M.B., and Standiford, T.J. (1996) Tumor necrosis factor mediates lung antibacterial host defense in murine *Klebsiella pneumonia*. *Infect. Immun.* **64,** 5211–5218.
51. Erickson, S. L., de Sauvage, F. J., Kikly, K., Carver-Moore, K., Pitts-Meek, S., Gillett, N., et al. (1994) Decreased sensitivity to tumour-necrosis factor but normal T-cell development in TNF receptor-2-deficient mice. *Nature* **372,** 560–563.
52. Ohlsson, K., Björk, P., Bergenfeldt, M., Hageman, R., and Thompson, R.C. (1990) Interleukin-1 receptor antagonist reduces mortality from endotoxin shock. *Nature* **348,** 550–552.
53. Alexander, H.R., Doherty, G.M., Buresh, C.M., Venzon, D.J., and Norton, J.A. (1991) A recombinant human receptor antagonist to interleukin 1 improves survival after lethal endotoxemia in mice. *J. Exp. Med.* **173,** 1029–1032.
54. Fischer, E., Marano, M.A., Van Zee, K.J., Rock, C.S., Hawes, A.S., Thompson, W.A., et al. (1992) Interleukin-1 receptor blockade improves survival and hemodynamic performance in Escherichia coli septic shock, but fails to alter host responses to sublethal endotoxemia. *J. Clin. Invest.* **89,** 1551–1557
55. Wakabayashi, G., Gelfand, J. A., Burke, J. F., Thompson, R. C., and Dinarello, C. A. (1991) A specific receptor antagonist for interleukin 1 prevents Escherichia coli-induced shock in rabbits. *FASEB J.* **5,** 338–343.
56. Aiura, K., Gelfand, J. A., Burke, J. F., Thompson, R. C., and Dinarello, C. A. (1993) Interleukin-1 (IL-1) receptor antagonist prevents Staphylococcus epidermidis- induced hypotension and reduces circulating levels of tumor necrosis factor and IL-1 β in rabbits. *Infect. Immun.* **61,** 3342–3350.
57. Mancilla, J., Garcia, P., and Dinarello, C. A. (1993) The interleukin-1 receptor antagonist can either reduce or enhance the lethality of Klebsiella pneumoniae sepsis in newborn rats. *Infect. Immun.* **61,**926–932.
58. Bernhagen, J., Calandra, T., Mitchell, R.A., Martin, S.B., Tracey, K.J., Voelter, W., et al. (1993) MIF is a pituitary-derived cytokine that potentiates lethal endotoxaemia. *Nature* **365,** 756–759.
59. Bozza, M., Satoskar, A.R., Lin, G., Lu, B., Humbles, A.A., Gerard, C., et al. (1999) Targeted disruption of migration inhibitory factor gene reveals its critical role in sepsis. *J. Exp. Med.* **189,** 341–346.
60. Makita, H., Nishimura, M., Miyamoto, K., Nakano, T., Tanino, Y., Hirokawa, J., et al. (1998) Effect of anti-macrophage migration inhibitory factor antibody on lipopolysaccharide-induced pulmonary neutrophil accumulation. *Am. J. Resp. Crit. Care Med.* **158,** 573–579.
61. Calandra, T., Echtenacher, B., Roy, D.L., Pugin, J., Metz, C.N., Hultner, L., et al. (2000) Protection from septic shock by neutralization of macrophage migration inhibitory factor. *Nat. Med* **6,** 164–170.
62. Car, B.D., Eng, V.M., Schnyder, B., Ozmen, L., Huang, S., Gallay, P., et al. (1994) Interferon gamma receptor deficient mice are resistant to endotoxic shock. *J Exp. Med.* **179,** 1437–1444.
63. Doherty, G.M., Lange, J.R., Langstein, H.N., Alexander, H.R., Buresh, C.M., and Norton, J.A. (1992) Evidence for IFN-gamma as a mediator of the lethality of endotoxin and tumor necrosis factor-alpha. *J Immunol.* **149,** 1666–1670.
64. Heinzel, F.P. (1990) The role of IFN-gamma in the pathology of experimental endotoxemia. *J. Immunol.* **145,** 2920–2924.
65. Kamijo, R., Le, J., Shapiro, D., Havell, E. A., Huang, S., Aguet, M., Bosland, M., and Vilcek, J. (1993) Mice that lack the interferon-γ receptor have profoundly altered responses to infection with Bacillus Calmette-Guérin and subsequent challenge with lipopolysaccharide. *J. Exp. Med.* **178,** 1435–1440.
66. Matthys, P., Mitera, T., Heremans, H., Van Damme, J., and Billiau, A. (1995) Anti-gamma interferon and anti-interleukin-6 antibodies affect staphylococcal enterotoxin B-induced weight loss, hypoglycemia, and cytokine release in D-galactosamine-sensitized and unsensitized mice. *Infect. Immun.* **63,** 1158–1164.
67. Silva, A.T. and Cohen, J. (1992) Role of interferon-gamma in experimental gram-negative sepsis. *J Infect. Dis.* **166,** 331–335.
68. Kohler, J., Heumann, D., Garotta, G., LeRoy, D., Bailat, S., Barras, C., et al. (1993) IFN-gamma involvement in the severity of gram-negative infections in mice. *J. Immunol.* **151,** 916–921.
69. Zantl, N., Uebe, A., Neumann, B., Wagner, H., Siewert, J.R., Holzmann, B., et al. (1998) Essential role of gamma interferon in survival of colon ascendens stent peritonitis, a novel murine model of abdominal sepsis. *Infect. Immun.* **66,** 2300–2309.
70. Nakane, A., Minagawa, T., Kohanawa, M., Chen, Y., Sato, H., Moriyama, M., et al. (1989) Interactions between endogenous gamma interferon and tumor necrosis factor in host resistance against primary and secondary Listeria monocytogenes infections. *Infect. Immun.* **57,** 3331–3337.
71. Huang, S., Hendricks, W., Althage, A., Hemmi, S., Bluethmann, H., Kamijo, R., et al. (1993) Immune responses in mice that lack the interferon-γ receptor. *Science* **259,** 1742–1745.
72. Langermans, J. A. M., Mayanski, D. M., Hibbering, P. H., Van der Hulst, M. E. B., Van de Gevel, J. S., and van Furth, R. (1994) Effect of IFN-gamma and endogenous TNF on the histopathological changes in the liver of Listeria monocytogenes-infected mice. *Immunology* **81,** 192–197.
73. Autenrieth, I. B., Beer, M., Bohn, E., Kaufmann, S. H. E., and Heesemann, J. (1994) Immune responses to Yersinia enterocolitica in susceptible Balb/c and resistant C57BL/6 mice: an essential role for gamma interferon. *Infect. Immun.* **62,** 2590–2599.
74 Cooper, A. M., Dalton, D. K., Stewart, T. A., Griffin, J. P., Russell, D. G., and Orme, I. M. (1993) Disseminated tuberculosis in interferon-γ gene-disrupted mice. *J. Exp. Med.* **178,** 2243–2247.
75. Flynn, J. L., Chan, J., Triebold, K. J., Dalton, D. K., Stewart, T. A., and Bloom, B. R. (1993) An essential role for interferon-γ in resistance to Mycobacterium tuberculosis infection. *J. Exp. Med.* **178,**2249–2254.
76. Dalton, D. K., Pitts-Meek, S., Keshav, S., Figari, I. S., Bradley, A., and Stewart, T. A. (1993) Multiple defects of immune cell functions in mice with disrupted interferon-γ gene. *Science* **259,** 1739–1742.

77. Wysocka, M., Kubin, M., Vieira, L. Q., Ozmen, L., Garotta, G., Scott, P., et al. (1995) Interleukin-12 is required for interferon-γ production and lethality in lipopolysaccharide-induced shock in mice. *Eur. J. Immunol.* **25,** 672–676.
78. Zisman, D.A., Kunkel, S.L., Strieter, R.M., Gauldie, J., Tsai, W.C., Bramson, J., et al. (1997) Anti-interleukin-12 therapy protects mice in lethal endotoxemia but impairs bacterial clearance in murine *Escherichia coli* peritoneal sepsis. *Shock* **8,** 349–356.
79. Mancuso, G., Cusumano, V., Genovese, F., Gambuzza, M., Beninati, C., and Teti, G. (1997) Role of interleukin 12 in experimental neonatal sepsis caused by group B streptococci. *Infect. Immun.* **65,** 3731–3735.
80. Steinhauser, M. L., Hogaboam, C. M., Lukacs, N. W., Strieter, R. M., and Kunkel, S. L. (1999) Multiple roles of IL-12 in a model of acute septic peritonitis. *J. Immunol.* **162,** 5437–5443.
81. Greenberger, M. J., Kunkel, S. L., Strieter, R. M., Lukacs, N. W., Bramson, J., Gauldie, J., et al. (1996) IL-12 gene therapy protects mice from lethal Klebsiella pneumonia. *J. Immunol.* **157,** 3006–3012
82. Bohn, E. and Autenrieth, I.B. (1996) IL-12 is essential for resistance against Yersinia enterocolitica by triggering IFN-gamma production in NK cells and CD4+ T cells. *J. Immunol.* **156,** 1458–1468.
83. Cooper, A. M., Magram, J., Ferrante, J., and Orme, I. M. (1997) Interleukin12 (IL-12) is crucial to the development of protective immunity in mice intravenously infected with Mycobacterium tuberculosis. *J. Exp. Med.* **186,** 39–45.
84. Decken, K., Köhler, G., Palmer-Lehmann, K., Wunderlin, A., Mattner, F., Magram, J., et al. (1998) Interleukin-12 is essential for a protective Th1 response in mice infected with Cryptococcus neoformans. *Infect. Immun.* **66,** 4994–5000.
85. Sakao, Y., Takeda, K., Tsutsui, H., Kaisho, T., Nomura, F., Okamura, H., et al. (1999) IL-18-deficient mice are resistant to endotoxin-induced liver injury but highly susceptible to endotoxin shock. *Int. Immunol.* **11,** 471–480.
86. Tsutsui, H., Matsui, K., Kawada, N., Hyodo, Y., Hayashi, N., Okamura, H., Higashino, K., and Nakanishi, K. (1997) IL-18 accounts for both TNF-α and Fas ligand-mediated hepatotoxic pathways in endotoxin-induced liver injury in mice. *J. Immunol.* **159,** 3961–3967.
87. Netea, M. G., Fantuzzi, G., Kullberg, B. J., Stuyt, R. L., Pulido, E. J., McIntyre, R. C., et al. (2000) Neutralization of IL-18 reduces neutrophil tissue accumulation and protects against lethal Escherichia coli and Salmonella typhimurium endotoxemia. *J. Immunol.* **164,** 2644–2649.
88. Wei, X.Q., Leung, B.P., Niedbala, W., Piedrafita, D., Feng, G.J., Sweet, M., et al. (1999) Altered immune responses and susceptibility to Leishmania major and Staphylococcus aureus infection in IL-18-deficient mice. *J. Immunol.* **163,** 2821–2828.
89. Dybing, J. K., Walters, N., and Pascual, D. W. (1999) Role of endogenous interleukin-18 in resolving wild-type and attenuated Salmonella typhimurium infections. *Infect. Immun.* **67,** 6242–6248.
90. Bohn, E., Sing, A., Zumbihl, R., Bielfeldt, C., Okamura, H., Kurimoto, M., et al. (1998) IL-18 (IFN-γ-inducing factor) regulates early cytokine production in, and promotes resolution of, bacterial infection in mice. *J. Immunol.* **160,** 299–307.
91. Sugawara, I., Yamada, H., Kaneko, H., Mizuno, S., Takeda, K., and Akira, S. (1999) Role of interleukin-18 (IL-18) in mycobacterial infection in IL-18-gene-disrupted mice. *Infect. Immun.* **67,** 2585–2589.
92. Calandra, T. and Heumann, D. (2000) Inhibitory cytokines, in *Immune Response in the Critically Ill. Update in Intensive Care and Emergency Medicine* (Marshall, J.C. and Cohen, J., eds.), Springer-Verlag, Berlin, pp. 67–83.
93. Fisher, C.J., Jr., Opal, S.M., Dhainaut, J.F., Stephens, S., Zimmerman, J.L., Nightingale, P., et al. (1993) Influence of an anti-tumor necrosis factor monoclonal antibody on cytokine levels in patients with sepsis. The CB0006 Sepsis Syndrome Study Group. *Crit. Care Med.* **21,** 318–327.
94. Dhainaut, J.F., Vincent, J.L., Richard, C., Lejeune, P., Martin, C., Fierobe, L., et al. (1995) CDP571, a humanized antibody to human tumor necrosis factor-alpha: safety, pharmacokinetics, immune response, and influence of the antibody on cytokine concentrations in patients with septic shock. CPD571 Sepsis Study Group. *Crit. Care Med.* **23,** 1461–1469.
95. Abraham, E., Wunderink, R., Silverman, H., Perl, T.M., Nasraway, S., Levy, H., et al, and for the TNFα MAb Sepsis Study Group (1995) Efficacy and safety of monoclonal antibody to human tumor necrosis factor _ in patients with sepsis syndrome. A randomized, controlled, double-blind, multicenter clinical trial. *JAMA* **273,** 934–941.
96. Cohen, J., Carlet, J., and for the INTERSEPT Study Group (1996) INTERSEPT: an international, multicenter, placebo-controlled trial of monoclonal antibody to human tumor necrosis factor-α in patients with sepsis. *Crit. Care. Med.* **24,** 1431–1440.
97. Reinhart, K., Wiegand-Löhnert, C., Grimminger, F., Kaul, M., Withington, S., Treacher, D., et al., and the MAK 195F Sepsis Study Group (1996) Assessment of the safety and efficacy of the monoclonal anti-tumor necrosis factor antibody-fragment, MAK 195F, in patients with sepsis and septic shock: a multicenter, randomized, placebo-controlled, dose-ranging study. *Crit. Care Med.* **24,** 733–742.
98. Abraham, E., Anzueto, A., Gutierrez, G., Tessler, S., San Pedro, G., Wunderink, R., et al. (1998) Double-blind randomised controlled trial of monoclonal antibody to human tumour necrosis factor in treatment of septic shock. NORASEPT II Study Group. *Lancet* **351,** 929–933.
99. Reinhart, K., Menges, T., Garlund, B., Zwaveling, J.H., Smithes, M., Vincent, J.L., et al. (2001) Randomized, placebo-controlled trial of the anti-tumor necrosis factor antibody fragment afelimomab in hyperinflammatory response during severe sepsis: the RAMSES study. *Crit. Care Med.* **29,** 765–769.
100. Panacek, E.A., Marshall, J., Fischkoff, S., Barchuk, W., and Teoh, L. (2000) Neutralization of TNF by monoclonal antibody improves survival and reduces organ dysfunction in human sepsis: results of the MONARCS trial. *Chest* **118,** S88.
101. Fisher, C.J., Agosti, J.M., Opal, S.M., Lowry, S.F., Balk, R.A., Sadoff, J.C., et al., and for the Soluble TNF Receptor Sepsis Study Group (1996) Treatment of septic shock with the tumor necrosis factor receptor:Fc fusion protein. *N. Engl. J. Med.* **334,** 1697–1702.

102. Abraham, E., Glauser, M.P., Butler, T., Garbino, J., Gelmont, D., Laterre, P.F., et al., and for the Ro 45-2081 Study Group (1997) p55 tumor necrosis factor receptor fusion protein in the treatment of patients with severe sepsis and septic shock. A randomized controlled multicenter trial. *JAMA* **277**, 1531–1538.
103. Abraham, E., Laterre, P.F., Garbino, J., Pingleton, S., Butler, T., Dugernier, T., et al. (2001) Lenercept (p55 tumor necrosis factor receptor fusion protein) in severe sepsis and early septic shock: a randomized, double-blind, placebo-controlled, multicenter phase III trial with 1342 patients. *Crit. Care Med.* **29**, 503–510.
104. Fisher, C.J., Slotman, G.J., Opal, S.M., Pribble, J.P., Bone, R.C., Emmanuel, G., et al., and the IL-1 RA Sepsis Study Group (1994) Initial evaluation of human recombinant interleukin-1 receptor antagonist in the treatment of sepsis syndrome: a randomized, open-label, placebo-controlled multicenter trial. *Crit. Care Med.* **22**, 12–21.
105. Fisher, C.J., Dhainaut, J.F., Opal, S.M., et al. (1994) Recombinant human interleukin 1 receptor antagonist in the treatment of patients with sepsis syndrome: results from a randomized, double-blind, placebo-controlled trial. *JAMA* **271**, 1836–1843.
106. Opal, S.M., Fisher, C.J., Dhainaut, J.F., Vincent, J.L., Brase, R., Lowry, S.F., ET AL., and the Interleukin-1 Receptor Antagonist Sepsis Investigator Group (1997) Confirmatory interleukin-1 receptor antagonist trial in severe sepsis: a phase III, randomized, double-blind, placebo-controlled, multicenter trial. *Crit. Care. Med.* **25**, 1115–1124.
107. Glauser, M.P. and Cohen, J. (1996) Tumor necrosis factor receptor: Fc fusion protein in septic shock. *N. Engl. J. Med.* **335**, 1608–1609.
108. The International Chronic Granulomatous Disease Cooperative Study Group (1991) A controlled trial of interferon gamma to prevent infection in chronic granulomatous disease. *N. Engl. J. Med.* **324**, 509–516.
109. Dries, D.J. (1996) Interferon gamma in trauma-related infections. *Intensive Care Med.* 22 *(Suppl. 4)*, S462–S467.
110. Polk, H.C., Jr., Cheadle, W.G., Livingston, D.H., Rodriguez, J.L., Starko, K.M., Izu, A.E., et al. (1992) A randomized prospective clinical trial to determine the efficacy of interferon-gamma in severely injured patients. *Am. J Surg.* **163**, 191–196.
111. Wasserman, D., Ioannovich, J.D., Hinzmann, R.D., Deichsel, G., and Steinmann, G.G. (1998) Interferon-gamma in the prevention of severe burn-related infections: a European phase III multicenter trial. The Severe Burns Study Group. *Crit. Care Med.* **26**, 434–439.
112. David, J. (1966) Delayed hypersensitivity in vitro: its mediation by cell-free substances formed by lymphoid cell-antigen interaction. *Proc. Natl. Acad. Sci. USA* **56**, 72–77.
113. Bloom, B.R. and Bennett, B. (1966) Mechanism of a reaction in vitro associated with delayed-type hypersensitivity. *Science* **153**, 80–82.
114. Calandra, T., Bernhagen, J., Mitchell, R.A., and Bucala, R. (1994) The macrophage is an important and previously unrecognized source of macrophage migration inhibitory factor. *J Exp. Med.* **179**, 1895–1902.
115. Calandra, T., Spiegel, L.A., Metz, C.N., and Bucala, R. (1998) Macrophage migration inhibitory factor is a critical mediator of the activation of immune cells by exotoxins of Gram-positive bacteria. *Proc. Natl. Acad. Sci. USA* **95**, 11,383–11,388.
116. Bacher, M., Metz, C.N., Calandra, T., Mayer, K., Chesney, J., Lohoff, M., et al. (1996) An essential regulatory role for macrophage migration inhibitory factor in T-cell activation. *Proc. Natl. Acad. Sci. USA* **93**, 7849–7854.
117. Calandra, T., Bernhagen, J., Metz, C.N., Spiegel, L.A., Bacher, M., Donnelly, T., et al. (1995) MIF as a glucocorticoid-induced modulator of cytokine production. *Nature* **377**, 68–71.
118. Beishuizen, A., Thijs, L.G., Haanen, C., and Vermes, I. (2001) Macrophage migration inhibitory factor and hypothalamo–pituitary–adrenal function during critical illness. *J. Clin. Endocrinol. Metab.* **86**, 2811–2816.
119. Yang, H., Wang, H., and Tracey, K.J. (2001) HMG-1 rediscovered as a cytokine. *Shock* **15**, 247–253.
120. Hori, O., Brett, J., Slattery, T., Cao, R., Zhang, J., Chen, J.X., et al. (1995) The receptor for advanced glycation end products (RAGE) is a cellular binding site for amphoterin. Mediation of neurite outgrowth and co- expression of rage and amphoterin in the developing nervous system. *J. Biol. Chem.* **270**, 25,752–25,761.
121. Wang, H., Bloom, O., Zhang, M., Vishnubhakat, J.M., Ombrellino, M., Che, J., et al. (1999) HMG-1 as a late mediator of endotoxin lethality in mice. *Science* **285**, 248–251.
122. Andersson, U., Wang, H., Palmblad, K., Aveberger, A.C., Bloom, O., Erlandsson-Harris, H., et al. (2000) High mobility group 1 protein (HMG-1) stimulates proinflammatory cytokine synthesis in human monocytes. *J. Exp. Med.* **192**, 565–570.
123. Abraham, E., Arcaroli, J., Carmody, A., Wang, H., and Tracey, K.J. (2000) HMG-1 as a mediator of acute lung inflammation. *J. Immunol.* **165**, 2950–2954.
124. Howard, M., O'Garra, A., Ishida, H., de Waal Malefyt, R., and de Vries, J. (1993) Biological properties of interleukin 10. *J. Clin. Immunol.* **12**, 239.
125. Wang, P., Wu, P., Siegel, M.I., Egan, R.W., and Billah, M.M. (1995) Interleukin (IL)-10 inhibits nuclear factor kappa B (NF kappa B) activation in human monocytes. IL-10 and IL-4 suppress cytokine synthesis by different mechanisms. *J Biol. Chem.* **270**, 9558–9563.
126. Bogdan, C., Paik, J., Vodovotz, Y., and Nathan, C. (1992) Contrasting mechanisms for suppression of macrophage cytokine release by transforming growth factor-beta and interleukin-10. *J. Biol. Chem.* **267**, 23,301–23,308.
127. Dickensheets, H.L., Freeman, S.L., Smith, M.F., and Donnelly, R.P. (1997) Interleukin-10 upregulates tumor necrosis factor receptor type-II (p75) gene expression in endotoxin-stimulated human monocytes. *Blood* **90**, 4162–4171.
128. Joyce, D.A., Gibbons, D.P., Green, P., Steer, J.H., Feldmann, M., and Brennan, F.M. (1994) Two inhibitors of proinflammatory cytokine release, interleukin-10 and interleukin-4, have contrasting effects on release of soluble p75 tumor necrosis factor receptor by cultured monocytes. *Eur. J. Immunol.* **24**, 2699–2705.

129. Essner, R., Rhoades, K., McBride, W.H., Morton, D.L., and Economou, J.S. (1989) IL-4 down-regulates IL-1 and TNF gene expression in human monocytes. *J Immunol.* **142**, 3857–3861.

130. Shen, C.H. and Stavnezer, J. (1998) Interaction of stat6 and NF-kappaB: direct association and synergistic activation of interleukin-4-induced transcription. **Mol. Cell Biol. 18**, 3395–3404.

131. Barton, B.E. (1997) IL-6: insights into novel biological activities. *Clin Immunol. Immunopathol.* **85**, 16–20.

132. Standiford, T. J., Strieter, R. M., Lukacs, N. W., and Kunkel, S. L. (1998) Neutralization of IL-10 increases lethality in endotoxemia. Cooperative effects of macrophage inflammatory protein-2 and tumor necrosis factor. *J. Immunol.* **155**, 2222–2229.

133. Howard, M., Muchamuel, T., Andrade, S., and Menon, S. (1993) Interleukin 10 protects mice from lethal endotoxemia. *J. Exp. Med.* **177**, 1205–1208.

134. Marchant, A., Bruyns, C., Vandenabeele, P., Ducarme, M., Gérard, C., Delvaux, A., et al. (1994) Interleukin-10 controls interferon-γ and tumor necrosis factor production during experimental endotoxemia. *Eur. J. Immunol.* **24**, 1167–1171.

135. Gerard, C., Bruyns, C., Marchant, A., Abramowicz, D., Vandenabeele, P., Delvaux, A., et al. (1993) Interleukin 10 reduces the release of tumor necrosis factor and prevents lethality in experimental endotoxemia. *J. Exp. Med.* **177**, 547–550.

136. Bean, A. G., Freiberg, R. A., Andrade, S., Menon, S., and Zlotnik, A. (1993) Interleukin 10 protects mice against staphylococcal enterotoxin B-induced lethal shock. *Infect. Immun.* **61**, 4937–4939.

137. Florquin, S., Amraoui, Z., Abramowicz, D., and Goldman, M. (1994) Systemic release and protective role of IL-10 in staphylococcal enterotoxin B-induced shock in mice. *J. Immunol.* **153**, 2618–2623.

138. Hasko, G., Virag, L., Egnaczyk, G., Salzman, A.L., and Szabo, C. (1998) The crucial role of IL-10 in the suppression of the immunological response in mice exposed to staphylococcal enterotoxin B. *Eur. J. Immunol.* **28**, 1417–1425.

139. Cusumano, V., Genovese, F., Mancuso, G., Carbone, M., Fera, M. T., and Teti, G. (1996) Interleukin-10 protects neonatal mice from lethal Group B streptococcal infection. *Infect. Immun.* **64**, 2850–2852.

140. Sawa, T., Corry, D. B., Gropper, M. A., Ohara, M., Kurahashi, K., and Wiener-Kronish, J. P. (1997) IL-10 improves lung injury and survival in *Pseudomonas aeruginosa* pneumonia. *J Immunol.* **159**, 2858–2866.

141. van der Poll, T., Marchant, A., Buurman, W.A., Berman, L., Keogh, C.V., Lazarus, D.D., et al. (1995) Endogenous IL-10 protects mice from death during septic peritonitis. *J. Immunol.* **155**, 5397–5401.

142. Remick, D. G., Garg, S. J., Newcomb, D. E., Wollenberg, G., Huie, T. K., and Bolgos, G. L. (1998) Endogenous IL-10 fails to decrease the mortality of morbidity of sepsis. *Crit. Care Med.* **26**, 895–904.

143. Montravers, P., Maulin, L., Mohler, J., and Carbon, C. (1999) Microbiological and inflammatory effects of murine recombinant interleukin-10 in two models of polymicrobial peritonitis in rats. *Infect. Immun.* **67**, 1579–1584.

144. van der Poll, T., Marchant, A., Keogh, C.V., Goldman, M., and Lowry, S.F. (1996) Interleukin-10 impairs host defense in murine pneumococcal pneumonia. *J. Infect. Dis.* **174**, 994–1000.

145. Dai, W., Köhler, G., and Brombacher, F. (1997) Both innate and acquired immunity to Listeria monocytogenes infections are increased in IL-10-deficient mice. *J. Immunol.* **158**, 2259–2267.

146. Genovese, F., Mancuso, G., Cuzzola, M., Biondo, C., Beninati, C., Delfino, D., et al. (1999) Role of IL-10 in a neonatal mouse listeriosis model. *J. Immunol.* **163**, 2777–2782.

147. Tonnetti, L., Spaccapelo, R., Cenci, E., Mencacci, A., Puccetti, P., Coffman, R. L., et al. (1995) Interleukin-4 and -10 exacerbate candidiasis in mice. *Eur. J. Immunol.* **25**, 1559–1565.

148. Baumhofer, J.M., Beinhauer, B.G., Wang, J.E., Brandmeier, H., Geissler, K., Losert, U., et al. (1998) Gene transfer with IL-4 and IL-13 improves survival in lethal endotoxemia in the mouse and ameliorates peritoneal macrophages immune competence. *Eur. J Immunol.* **28**, 610–615.

149. Jain-Vora, S., LeVine, A. M., Chroneos, Z., Ross, G. F., Hull, W. M., and Whitsett, J. A. (1998) Interleukin-4 enhances pulmonary clearance of Pseudomonas aeruginosa. *Infect. Immun.* **66**, 4229–4236.

150. Keane-Myers, A., Maliszewski, C. R., Finkelman, F. D., and Nickell, S. P. (1996) Recombinant IL-4 augments rersistance to Borrelia burgdoreferi infections in both normal susceptible and antibody-deficient susceptible mice. *J. Immunol.* **156**, 2448–2494.

151. Hultgren, O., Kopf, M., and Tarkowski, A. (1998) Staphylococcus aureus- induced septic arthritis and septic death is decreased in IL-4-deficient mice: role of IL-4 as promoter for bacterial growth. *J. Immunol.* **160**, 5082–5087.

152. Szalay, G., Ladel, C. H., Blum, C., and Kaufmann, S. H. E. (1996) IL-4 neutralization of TNF-α treatment ameliorates disease by an intracellular pathogen in IFN-γ receptor-deficient mice. *J. Immunol.* **157**, 4746–4750.

153. Samson, J. N., Annema, A., Langermans, J. A. M., and van Furth, R. (1998) Endogenous interleukin-4 does not suppress the resistance against a primary or a secondary Listeria monocytogenes infection in mice. *Scand. J. Immunol.* **47**, 369–374.

154. Xing, Z., Gauldie, J., Cox, G., Baumann, H., Jordana, M., Lei, X. F., et al. (1998) IL-6 is an antiinflammatory cytokine required for controlling local or systemic acute inflammatory responses. *J. Clin. Invest.* **101**, 311–320.

155. Bucklin, S. E., Silverstein, R., and Morrison, D. C. (1993) An interleukin-6-induced acute-phase response does not confer protection against lipopolysaccharide lethality. *Infect. Immun.* **61**, 3184–3189.

156. Barton, B.E., Shortall, J., and Jackson, J.V. (1996) Interleukins 6 and 11 protect mice from mortality in a staphylococcal enterotoxin-induced toxic shock model. *Infect. Immun.* **64**, 714–718.

157. Dalrymple, S.A., Slattery, R., Aud, D.M., Krishna, M., Lucian, L.A., and Murray, R. (1996) Interleukin-6 is required for a protective immune response to systemic *Escherichia coli* infection. *Infect. Immun.* **64**, 3231–3235.

158. van der Poll, T., Keogh, C.V., Guirao, X., Buurman, W.A., Kopf, M., and Lowry, S.F. (1997) Interleukin-6 gene-deficient mice show impaired defense against pneumococcal pneumonia. *J. Infect. Dis.* **176**, 439–444.

159. van der Poll, T., Keogh, CV., Guirao, X., Buurman, W. A., Kopf, M., and Lowry, S. F. (1998) Interleukin-6 gene-deficient mice show impaited defense against pneumococcal pneumonia. *J. Infect. Dis.* **176**, 439–444.

160. Mancuso, G., Tomasello, F., Migliardo, M., Delfino, D., Cochran, J., Cook, J. A., et al. (1994) Beneficial effects of interleukin-6 in neonatal mouse models of Group B streptococcal disease. *Infect. Immun.* **62,** 4997–5002.

161. Liu, Z., Simpson, R. J., and Cheers, C. (1992) Recombinant interleukin-6 protects mice against experimental bacterial infection. *Infect. Immun.* **60,** 4402–4406.

162. Kopf, M., Baumann, H., Freer, G., Freudenberg, M., Lamers, M., Kishimoto, T., et al. (1994) Impaired immune and acute-phase responses in interleukin-6-deficient mice. *Nature* **368,** 339–342.

163. Dalrymple, S. A., Lucian, L. A., Slattery, R., McNeil, T., Aud, D. M., Fuchino, S., et al. (1995) Interleukin-6-deficient mice are highly susceptible to *Listeria monocytogenes* infection: correlation with inefficient neutrophilia. *Infect. Immun.* **63,** 2262–2268.

164. Ladel, C.H., Blum, C., Dreher, A., Reifenberg, K., Kopf, M., and Kaufmann, S.H. (1997) Lethal tuberculosis in interleukin-6-deficient mutant mice. *Infect. Immun.* **65,** 4843–4849.

165. Everest, P., Allen, J., Papakonstantinopoulou, A., Mastroeni, P., Roberts, M., and Dougan, G. (1997) Salmonella typhimurium infections in mice deficient in interlukin-4 production. Role of IL-4 in infection-associated pathology. *J. Immunol.* **159,** 1820–1827.

166. Kaposzta, R., Tree, P., Marodi, L., and Gordon, S. (1998) Characteristics of invasive candidiasis in gamma interferon- and interleukin-4-deficient mice: role of macrophages in host defense against *Candida albicans. Infect. Immun.* **66,** 1708–1717.

167. Nicoletti, F., Mancuso, G., Cusumano, V., Di Marco, R., Zaccone, P., Bendtzen, K., and Teti, G. (1997) Prevention of endotoxin-induced lethality in neonatal mice by interleukin-13. *Eur. J. Immunol.* **27,** 1580–1583.

168. Muchamuel, T., Menon, S., Pisacane, P., Howard, M. C., and Cockayne, D. A. (1997) IL-13 protects mice from lipopolysaccharide-induced lethal endotoxemia. Correlation with down-modulation of TNF-α, IFN-γ, and IL-12 production. *J. Immunol.* **157,** 2898–2903.

169. Matsukawa, A., Hogaboam, C. M., Lukacs, N. W., Lincoln, P. M., Evanoff, H. L., Strieter, R. M., and Kunkel, S. L. (2000) Expression and contribution of endogenous IL-13 in an experimental model of sepsis. *J. Immunol.* **164,** 2738–2744.

170. Flesch, I. E., Wandersee, A., and Kaufmann, S. H. (1997) Effects of IL-13 on murine listeriosis. *Intern. Immunol.* **9,** 467–474.

171. Gorgen, I., Hartung, T., Leist, M., Niehorster, M., Tiegs, G., Uhlig, S., et al. (1992) Granulocyte colony-stimulating factor treatment protects rodents against lipopolysaccharide-induced toxicity via suppression of systemic tumor necrosis factor-alpha. *J. Immunol.* **149,** 918–924.

172. Villa, P., Shaklee, C.L., Meazza, C., Agnello, D., Ghezzi, P., and Senaldi, G. (1998) Granulocyte colony-stimulating factor and antibiotics in the prophylaxis of a murine model of polymicrobial peritonitis and sepsis. *J Infect. Dis.* **178,** 471–477.

173. Toda, H., Murata, A., Matsuura, N., Uda, K., Oka, Y., Tanaka, N., et al. (1993) Therapeutic efficacy of granulocyte colony stimulating factor against rat cecal ligation and puncture model. *Stem Cells* **11,** 228–234.

174. Lorenz, W., Reimund, K.P., Weitzel, F., Celik, I., Kurnatowski, M., Schneider, C., et al. (1994) Granulocyte colony-stimulating factor prophylaxis before operation protects against lethal consequences of postoperative peritonitis. *Surgery* **116,** 925–934.

175. Lundblad, R., Nesland, J.M., and Giercksky, K.E. (1996) Granulocyte colony-stimulating factor improves survival rate and reduces concentrations of bacteria, endotoxin, tumor necrosis factor, and endothelin-1 in fulminant intra-abdominal sepsis in rats. *Crit. Care Med.* **24,** 820–826.

176. Eichacker, P. Q., Waisman, Y., Natanson, C., Farese, A., Hoffman, W. D., Banks, S. M., and MacVittie, T. J. (1994) Cardiopulmonary effects of granulocyte colony-stimulating factor in a canine model of bacterial sepsis. *J Appl. Physiol* **77,** 2366–2373.

177. Dunne, J.R., Dunkin, B.J., Nelson, S., and White, J.C. (1996) Effects of granulocyte colony stimulating factor in a nonneutropenic rodent model of *Escherichia coli* peritonitis. *J Surg. Res.* **61,** 348–354.

178. Barsig, J., Bundschuh, D.S., Hartung, T., Bauhofer, A., Sauer, A., and Wendel, A. (1996) Control of fecal peritoneal infection in mice by colony-stimulating factors. *J. Infect. Dis.* **174,** 790–799.

179. Karzai, W., von Specht, B.U., Parent, C., Haberstroh, J., Wollersen, K., Natanson, C., et al. (1999) G-CSF during *Escherichia coli* versus *Staphylococcus aureus* pneumonia in rats has fundamentally different and opposite effects. *Am. J. Respir. Crit. Care Med.* **159,** 1377–1382.

180. Smith, W.S., Sumnicht, G.E., Sharpe, R.W., Samuelson, D., and Millard, F.E. (1995) Granulocyte colony-stimulating factor versus placebo in addition to penicillin G in a randomized blinded study of gram-negative pneumonia sepsis: analysis of survival and multisystem organ failure. *Blood* **86,** 1301–1309.

181. Hebert, J.C. and O'Reilly, M. (1996) Granulocyte-macrophage colony-stimulating factor (GM-CSF) enhances pulmonary defenses against pneumococcal infections after splenectomy. *J Trauma* **41,** 663–666.

182. Dallaire, F., Ouellet, N., Simard, M., Bergeron, Y., and Bergeron, M.G. (2001) Efficacy of recombinant human granulocyte colony-stimulating factor in a murine model of pneumococcal pneumonia: effects of lung inflammation and timing of treatment. *J Infect. Dis.* **183,** 70–77.

183. Hebert, J.C., O'Reilly, M., and Gamelli, R.L. (1990) Protective effect of recombinant human granulocyte colony-stimulating factor against pneumococcal infections in splenectomized mice. *Arch. Surg.* **125,** 1075–1078.

184. Freeman, B.D., Quezado, Z., Zeni, F., Natanson, C., Danner, R.L., Banks, S., et al. (1997) rG-CSF reduces endotoxemia and improves survival during E. coli pneumonia. *J. Appl. Physiol.* **83,** 1467–1475.

185. Held, T.K., Mielke, M.E., Chedid, M., Unger, M., Trautmann, M., Huhn, D., et al. (1998) Granulocyte colony-stimulating factor worsens the outcome of experimental *Klebsiella pneumoniae* pneumonia through direct interaction with the bacteria. *Blood* **91,** 2525–2535.

186. Haberstroh, J., Wiese, K., Geist, A., Dursunoglu, G.B., Gippner-Steppert, C., Jochum, M., et al. (1998) Effect of delayed treatment with recombinant human granulocyte colony-stimulating factor on survival and plasma cytokine levels in a non-neutropenic porcine model of *Pseudomonas aeruginosa* sepsis. *Shock* **9**, 128–134.

187. Haberstroh, J., Breuer, H., Lucke, I., Massarrat, K., Fruh, R., Mand, U., et al. (1995) Effect of recombinant human granulocyte colony-stimulating factor on hemodynamic and cytokine response in a porcine model of *Pseudomonas* sepsis. *Shock* **4**, 216–224.

188. Greenberger, M.J., Strieter, R.M., Kunkel, S.L., Danforth, J.M., Goodman, R.E., and Standiford, T.J. (1995) Neutralization of IL-10 increases survival in a murine model of Klebsiella pneumonia. *J. Immunol.* **155**, 722–729.

189. Camargo, C.A., Jr., Madden, J.F., Gao, W., Selvan, R.S., and Clavien, P.A. (1997) Interleukin-6 protects liver against warm ischemia/reperfusion injury and promotes hepatocyte proliferation in the rodent. *Hepatology* **26**, 1513–1520.

190. Libert, C., Takahashi, N., Cauwels, A., Brouckaert, P., Bluethmann, H., and Fiers, W. (1994) Response of interleukin-6-deficient mice to tumor necrosis factor-induced metabolic changes and lethality. *Eur. J Immunol.* 24. 2237–2242.

191. Root, R.K. and Dale, D.C. (1999) Granulocyte colony-stimulating factor and granulocyte-macrophage colony- stimulating factor: comparisons and potential for use in the treatment of infections in nonneutropenic patients. *J. Infect. Dis.* **(179 Suppl. 2),** S342–S352.

192. Ozer, H., Armitage, J.O., Bennett, C.L., Crawford, J., Demetri, G.D., Pizzo, P.A., et al. (2000) 2000 update of recommendations for the use of hematopoietic colony- stimulating factors: evidence-based, clinical practice guidelines. American Society of Clinical Oncology Growth Factors Expert Panel. *J. Clin. Oncol.* **18**, 3558–3585.

193. Weiss, M., Moldawer, L.L., and Schneider, E.M. (1999) Granulocyte colony-stimulating factor to prevent the progression of systemic nonresponsiveness in systemic inflammatory response syndrome and sepsis. *Blood* **93**, 425–439.

194. Wiedermann, F.J., Mittermayr, M., Hoffmann, G., and Schobersberger, W. (2001) Recombinant granulocyte colony-stimulating factor (G-CSF) in infectious diseases: still a debate. *Wien. Klin. Wochenschr.* **113**, 90–96.

195. Heard, S.O., Fink, M.P., Gamelli, R.L., Solomkin, J.S., Joshi, M., Trask, A.L., et al. (1998) Effect of prophylactic administration of recombinant human granulocyte colony-stimulating factor (filgrastim) on the frequency of nosocomial infections in patients with acute traumatic brain injury or cerebral hemorrhage. The Filgrastim Study Group. *Crit. Care Med.* **26**, 748–754.

196. Wenisch, C., Werkgartner, T., Sailer, H., Patruta, S., Krause, R., Daxboeck, F., et al. (2000) Effect of preoperative prophylaxis with filgrastim in cancer neck dissection. *Eur. J. Clin. Invest.* **30**, 460–466.

197. Schafer, H., Hubel, K., Bohlen, H., Mansmann, G., Hegener, K., Richarz, B., et al. (2000) Perioperative treatment with filgrastim stimulates granulocyte function and reduces infectious complications after esophagectomy. *Ann. Hematol.* **79**, 143–151.

198. Winston, D.J., Foster, P.F., Somberg, K.A., Busuttil, R.W., Levy, M.F., Sheiner, P.A., et al. (1999) Randomized, placebo-controlled, double-blind, multicenter trial of efficacy and safety of granulocyte colony-stimulating factor in liver transplant recipients. *Transplantation* **68**, 1298–1304.

199. Gough, A., Clapperton, M., Rolando, N., Foster, A.V., Philpott-Howard, J., and Edmonds, M.E. (1997) Randomised placebo-controlled trial of granulocyte-colony stimulating factor in diabetic foot infection. *Lancet* **350**, 855–859.

200. Nelson, S., Belknap, S.M., Carlson, R.W., Dale, D., DeBoisblanc, B., Farkas, S., et al. (1998) A randomized controlled trial of filgrastim as an adjunct to antibiotics for treatment of hospitalized patients with community- acquired pneumonia. CAP Study Group. *J. Infect. Dis.* **178**, 1075–1080.

201. Nelson, S., Heyder, A.M., Stone, J., Bergeron, M.G., Daugherty, S., Peterson, G., et al. (2000) A randomized controlled trial of filgrastim for the treatment of hospitalized patients with multilobar pneumonia. *J Infect. Dis.* **182**, 970–973.

202. Ishikawa, K., Tanaka, H., Takaoka, M., Ogura, H., Shiozaki, T., Hosotsubo, H., et al. (1999) Granulocyte colony-stimulating factor ameliorates life-threatening infections after combined therapy with barbiturates and mild hypothermia in patients with severe head injuries. *J. Trauma* **46**, 999–1007.

203. Wunderink, R., Leeper, K., Jr., Schein, R., Nelson, S., DeBoisblanc, B., Fotheringham, N., et al. (2001) Filgrastim in patients with pneumonia and severe sepsis or septic shock. *Chest* **119**, 523–529.

204. Auphan, N., DiDonato, J.A., Rosette, C., Helmberg, A., and Karin, M. (1995) Immunosuppression by glucocorticoids: inhibition of NF-kB activity trough induction of IkB synthesis. *Science* **270**, 286–290.

205. Scheinman, R.I., Cogswell, P.C., Lofquist, A.K., and Baldwin Jr, A.S. (1995) Role of transcriptional activation of IkBα mediation of immunosuppression by glucocorticoids. *Science* **270**, 283–286.

206. Hinshaw, L.B. (1985) High-dose corticosteroids in the critically ill patient. Current concept and future developments. *Acta Chir Scand.* **526 (Suppl.),** 129–137.

207. Hinshaw, L.B., Archer, L.T., Beller-Todd, B.K., Benjamin, B., Flournoy, D.J., and Passey, R. (1981) Survival of primates in lethal septic shock following delayed treatment with steroid. *Circ. Shock* **8**, 291–300.

208. Hinshaw, L.B., Beller, B.K., Archer, L.T., Flournoy, D.J., White, G.L., and Phillips, R.W. (1979) Recovery from lethal Escherichia coli shock in dogs. *Surg. Gynecol. Obstet.* **149**, 545–553.

209. Hinshaw, L.B., Archer, L.T., Beller-Todd, B.K., Coalson, J.J., Flournoy, D.J., Passey, R., et al. (1980) Survival of primates in LD100 septic shock following steroid/antibiotic therapy. *J. Surg. Res.* **28**, 151–170.

210. Schummer, W. (1976) Steroids in the treatment of clinical septic shock. *Ann. Surg.* **184**, 333–341.

211. Thompson, W.L., Gurley, H.T., Lutz, B.A., Jackson, D.L., Kvols, L.K., and Morris, I.A. (1976) Inefficacy of glucocorticoids in shock (double-blind study). *Clin. Res.* **24**, 258A.

212. Sprung, C.L., Caralis, P.V., Marcial, E.H., Pierce, M., Gelbard, M.A., Long, W.M., et al. (1984) The effect of high-dose corticosteroids in patients with septic shock. *N. Engl. J. Med.* **311**, 1137–1143.

213. Lucas, C.E. and Ledgerwood, A.M. (1984) The cardiopulmonary response to massive doses of steroids in patients with septic shock. *Arch. Surg.* **119**, 537–541.

214. The Veterans Administration Systemic Sepsis Cooperative Study Group (1987) Effect of high-dose glucocorticoid therapy on mortality in patients with clinical signs of systemic sepsis. *N. Engl. J. Med.* **317,** 659–665.

215. Bone, R.C., Fisher, C.J., Clemmer, T.P., Slotman, G.J., Metz, G.A., Balk, R.A., and the Methylprednisolone Severe Sepsis Study Group (1987) A controlled clinical trial of high-dose methylprednisolone in the treatment of severe sepsis and septic shock. *N. Engl. J. Med.* **317,** 653–658.

216. Luce, J.M., Montgomery, A.B., Marks, J.D., Turner, J., Metz, G.A., and Murray, J.F. (1988) Ineffectiveness of high-dose methylprednisolone in preventing parenchymal lung injury and improving mortality in patients with septic shock. *Am. Rev. Respir. Dis.* **138,** 62–68.

217. Cooperative Study Group (1963) The effectiveness of hydrocortison in the management of severe infection. *JAMA* **183,** 462–465.

218. Klastersky, J., Cappel, R., and Debusscher, L. (1971) Effectiveness of betamethasone in management of severe infections. A double-blind study. *N. Engl. J. Med.* **284,** 1248–1250.

219. Bollaert, P.E., Charpentier, C., Levy, B., Debouverie, M., Audibert, G., and Larcan, A. (1998) Reversal of late septic shock with supraphysiologic doses of hydrocortisone. *Crit Care Med.* **26,** 645–650.

220. Briegel, J., Forst, H., Haller, M., Schelling, G., Kilger, E., Kuprat, G., et al. (1999) Stress doses of hydrocortisone reverse hyperdynamic septic shock: a prospective, randomized, double-blind, single-center study. *Crit. Care Med.* **27,** 723–732.

221. Annane, D. (2000) Effects of the combination of hydrocortisone-fludrocortisone on mortality in septic shock. *Crit. Care Med. 28(12 Suppl.),* A46.

222. Bone, R. C., Sibbald, W. J., and Sprung, C. L. (1992) The ACCP-SCCM consensus conference on sepsis and organ failure. *Chest* **101,** 1481–1483.

223. Lefering, R. and Neugebauer, E.A. (1995) Steroid controversy in sepsis and septic shock: a meta-analysis. *Crit. Care Med.* **23,** 1294–1303.

224. Zeni, F., Freeman, B., and Natanson, C. (1997) Anti-inflammatory therapies to treat sepsis and septic shock: a reassessment. *Crit. Care Med.* **25,** 1095–1100.

225. Cronin, L., Cook, D.J., Carlet, J., Heyland, D.K., King, D., Lansang, M.A., et al. (1995) Corticosteroid treatment for sepsis: a critical appraisal and meta- analysis of the literature. *Crit Care Med.* **23,** 1430–1439.

226. Wiegers, G.J. and Reul, J.M. (1998) Induction of cytokine receptors by glucocorticoids: functional and pathological significance. *Trends Pharmacol. Sci.* **19,** 317–321.

227. Wilckens, T. and De Rijk, R. (1997) Glucocorticoids and immune function: unknown dimensions and new frontiers. *Immunol. Today* **18,** 418–424.

228. Jurney, T.H., Cockrell, J.L., Jr., Lindberg, J.S., Lamiell, J.M., and Wade, C.E. (1987) Spectrum of serum cortisol response to ACTH in ICU patients. Correlation with degree of illness and mortality. *Chest* **92,** 292–295.

229. Moran, J.L., Chapman, M.J., O'Fathartaigh, M.S., Peisach, A.R., Pannall, P.R., and Leppard, P. (1994) Hypocortisolaemia and adrenocortical responsiveness at onset of septic shock. *Intensive Care Med.* **20,** 489–495.

230. Soni, A., Pepper, G.M., Wyrwinski, P.M., Ramirez, N.E., Simon, R., Pina, T., et al. (1995) Adrenal insufficiency occurring during septic shock: incidence, outcome, and relationship to peripheral cytokine levels. *Am. J. Med.* **98,** 266–271.

231. Rothwell, P.M., Udwadia, Z.F., and Lawler, P.G. (1991) Cortisol response to corticotropin and survival in septic shock. *Lancet* **337,** 582–583.

232. Schneider, A.J. and Voerman, H.J. (1991) Abrupt hemodynamic improvement in late septic shock with physiological doses of glucocorticoids. *Intensive Care Med.* **17,** 436–437.

233. Briegel, J., Forst, H., Hellinger, H., and Haller, M. (1991) Contribution of cortisol deficiency to septic shock. *Lancet* **338,** 507–508.

234. Zimmerman, J.J. (1999) Appraising the potential of pentoxifylline in septic premies. *Crit. Care Med.* **27,** 695–697.

235. Schade, U.F., von der, B.J., and Schonharting, M. (1989) Pentoxifylline increases survival of mice in endotoxic shock. *Prog. Clin. Biol. Res.* **301,** 223–227.

236. Schade, U.F. (1990) Pentoxifylline increases survival in murine endotoxin shock and decreases formation of tumor necrosis factor. *Circ. Shock* **31,** 171–181.

237. Badger, A.M., Olivera, D.L., and Esser, K.M. (1994) Beneficial effects of the phosphodiesterase inhibitors BRL 61063, pentoxifylline, and rolipram in a murine model of endotoxin shock. *Circ. Shock* **44,** 188–195.

238. Arrieta, O., Ortiz-Reyes, A., Rembao, D., Calvillo, M., Rivera, E., and Sotelo, J. (1999) Protective effect of pentoxifylline plus thalidomide against septic shock in mice. *Int. J. Exp. Pathol.* **80,** 11–16.

239. Fletcher, M.A., McKenna, T.M., Owens, E.H., and Nadkarni, V.M. (1992) Effects of in vivo pentoxifylline treatment on survival and ex vivo vascular contractility in a rat lipopolysaccharide shock model. *Circ. Shock* **36,** 74–80.

240. Puranapanda, V., Hinshaw, L.B., O'Rear, E.A., Chang, A.C., and Whitsett, T.L. (1987) Erythrocyte deformability in canine septic shock and the efficacy of pentoxifylline and a leukotriene antagonist. *Proc. Soc. Exp. Biol. Med.* **185,** 206–210.

241. Masouye, P., Gunning, K., Pittet, J.F., Suter, P.M., and Morel, D.R. (1992) Xanthine derivative HWA 138 attenuates hemodynamic and oxygen uptake dysfunction secondary to severe endotoxin shock in sheep. *Circ. Shock* **36,** 113–119.

242. Krakauer, T. and Stiles, B.G. (1999) Pentoxifylline inhibits superantigen-induced toxic shock and cytokine release. *Clin. Diagn. Lab. Immunol.* **6,** 594–598.

243. Lundblad, R., Ekstrom, P., and Giercksky, K.E. (1995) Pentoxifylline improves survival and reduces tumor necrosis factor, interleukin-6, and endothelin-1 in fulminant intra-abdominal sepsis in rats. *Shock* **3,** 210–215.

244. Yang, S., Zhou, M., Koo, D.J., Chaudry, I.H., and Wang, P. (1999) Pentoxifylline prevents the transition from the hyperdynamic to hypodynamic response during sepsis. *Am. J. Physiol* **277,** H1036–H1044.

245. Law, W.R., Nadkarni, V.M., Fletcher, M.A., Nevola, J.J., Eckstein, J.M., Quance, J., et al. (1992) Pentoxifylline treatment of sepsis in conscious Yucatan minipigs. *Circ. Shock* **37**, 291–300.
246. Netea, M.G., Blok, W.L., Kullberg, B.J., Bemelmans, M., Vogels, M.T., Buurman, W.A., et al. (1995) Pharmacologic inhibitors of tumor necrosis factor production exert differential effects in lethal endotoxemia and in infection with live microorganisms in mice. *J. Infect. Dis.* **171**, 393–399.
247. Lechner, A.J., Rouben, L.R., Potthoff, L.H., Tredway, T.L., and Matuschak, G.M. (1993) Effects of pentoxifylline on tumor necrosis factor production and survival during lethal *E. coli* sepsis vs. disseminated candidiasis with fungal septic shock. *Circ. Shock* **39**, 306–315.
248. Quezado, Z.M., Hoffman, W.D., Banks, S.M., Danner, R.L., Eichacker, P.Q., Susla, G.M., et al. (1999) Increasing doses of pentoxifylline as a continuous infusion in canine septic shock. *J. Pharmacol. Exp. Ther.* **288**, 107–113.
249. Hadjiminas, D. J., McMasters, K. M., Robertson, S. E., and Cheadle, W. G. (1994) Enhanced survival from cecal ligation and puncture with pentoxifylline is associated with altered neutrophil trafficking and reduced interleukin-1 beta expression but not inhibition of tumor necrosis factor synthesis. *Surgery* **116**, 348–355.
250. Nelson, J. L., Alexander, J. W., Mao, J. X., Vohs, T., and Ogle, C. K. (1999) Effect of pentoxifylline on survival and intestinal cytokine messenger RNA transcription in a rat model of ongoing peritoneal sepsis. *Crit. Care Med.* **27**, 113–119.
251. Hemmer, C. J., Hort, G., Chiwakata, C. B., Seitz, R., Egbring, R., Gaus, W., et al. (1997) Supportive pentoxifylline in falciparum malaria: no effect on tumor necrosis factor alpha levels or clinical outcome: a prospective, randomized, placebo-controlled study. *Am. J. Trop. Med. Hyg.* **56**, 397–403.
252. Bacher, A., Mayer, N., Klimscha, W., Oismuller, C., Steltzer, H., and Hammerle, A. (1997) Effects of pentoxifylline on hemodynamics and oxygenation in septic and nonseptic patients. *Crit. Care Med.* **25**, 795–800.
253. Staudinger, T., Presterl, E., Graninger, W., Locker, G. J., Knapp, S., Laczika, K., et al. (1996) Influence of pentoxifylline on cytokine levels and inflammatory parameters in septic shock. *Intensive Care Med.* **22**, 888–893.
254. Lauterbach, R. and Zembala, M. (1996) Pentoxifylline reduces plasma tumour necrosis factor-alpha concentration in premature infants with sepsis. *Eur. J. Pediatr.* **155**, 404–409.
255. Lauterbach, R., Pawlik, D., Tomaszczyk, B., and Cholewa, B. (1994) Pentoxifylline treatment of sepsis of premature infants: preliminary clinical observations. *Eur. J. Pediatr.* **153**, 672–674.
256. Zeni, F., Pain, P., Vindimian, M., Gay, J. P., Gery, P., Bertrand, M., Page, Y., et al. (1996) Effects of pentoxifylline on circulating cytokine concentrations and hemodynamics in patients with septic shock: results from a double- blind, randomized, placebo-controlled study. *Crit Care Med.* **24**, 207–214.
257. Mandi, Y., Farkas, G., Ocsovszky, I., and Nagy, Z. (1995) Inhibition of tumor necrosis factor production and ICAM-1 expression by pentoxifylline: beneficial effects in sepsis syndrome. *Res. Exp. Med. (Berl)* **195**, 297–307.
258. Staubach, K. H., Schroder, J., Stuber, F., Gehrke, K., Traumann, E., and Zabel, P. (1998) Effect of pentoxifylline in severe sepsis: results of a randomized, double-blind, placebo-controlled study. *Arch. Surg.* **133**, 94–100.
259. Lauterbach, R., Pawlik, D., Kowalczyk, D., Ksycinski, W., Helwich, E., and Zembala, M. (1999) Effect of the immunomodulating agent, pentoxifylline, in the treatment of sepsis in prematurely delivered infants: a placebo-controlled, double-blind trial. *Crit Care Med.* **27**, 807–814.
260. Jacobson, J. M. (2000) Thalidomide: a remarkable comeback. *Expert. Opin. Pharmacother.* **1**, 849–863.
261. Moreira, A. L., Wang, J., Sarno, E. N., and Kaplan, G. (1997) Thalidomide protects mice against LPS-induced shock. *Braz. J. Med. Biol. Res.* **30**, 1199–1207.
262. Schmidt, H., Rush, B., Simonian, G., Murphy, T., Hsieh, J., and Condon, M. (1996) Thalidomide inhibits TNF response and increases survival following endotoxin injection in rats. *J. Surg. Res.* **63**, 143–146.
263. Stirling, D. I. (1998) Thalidomide and its impact in dermatology. *Semin. Cutan. Med. Surg.* **17**, 231–242.
264. Calabrese, L. and Fleischer, A. B. (2000) Thalidomide: current and potential clinical applications. *Am. J. Med.* **108**, 487–495.
265. Ravot, E., Lisziewicz, J., and Lori, F. (1999) New uses for old drugs in HIV infection: the role of hydroxyurea, cyclosporin and thalidomide. *Drugs* **58**, 953–963.
266. Pollmacher, T., Haack, M., Schuld, A., Kraus, T., and Hinze-Selch, D. (2000) Effects of antipsychotic drugs on cytokine networks. *J. Psychiatr. Res.* **34**, 369–382.
267. Song, S. M., Lu, S. M., Wang, Z. G., Liu, J. C., Guo, S. Q., and Li, Z. (1999) Subcellular membrane impairment and application of phospholipase A2 inhibitors in endotoxic shock. *Injury* **30**, 9–14.
268. Vadas, P., Stefanski, E., and Pruzanski, W. (1986) Potential therapeutic efficacy of inhibitors of human phospholipase A2 in septic shock. *Agents Actions* **19**, 194–202.
269. Gadina, M., Bertini, R., Mengozzi, M., Zandalasini, M., Mantovani, A., and Ghezzi, P. (1991) Protective effect of chlorpromazine on endotoxin toxicity and TNF production in glucocorticoid-sensitive and glucocorticoid-resistant models of endotoxic shock. 2*J. Exp. Med.* **173**, *1305–1310.*
270. Ohtsuka, H., Higuchi, T., Matsuzawa, H., Sato, H., Takahashi, K., Takahashi, J., et al. (1997) Inhibitory effect on LPS-induced tumor necrosis factor in calves treated with chlorpromazine or pentoxifylline. *J. Vet. Med. Sci.* **59**, 1075–1077.
271. Ziegler, E. J., McCutchan, J. A., Fierer, J., Glauser, M. P., Sadoff, J. C., Douglas, H., et al. (1982) Treatment of gram-negative bacteremia and shock with human antiserum to a mutant *Escherichia coli. N. Engl. J Med.* **307**, 1225–1230.
272. Ziegler, E. J., Fisher, C. J., Jr., Sprung, C. L., Straube, R. C., Sadoff, J. C., Foulke, G. E., et al. (1991) Treatment of gram-negative bacteremia and septic shock with HA-1A human monoclonal antibody against endotoxin. A randomized, double-blind, placebo-controlled trial. The HA-1A Sepsis Study Group. *N. Engl. J Med.* **324**, 429–436.
273. McCloskey, R. V., Straube, R. C., Sanders, C., Smith, S. M., and Smith, C. R. (1994) Treatment of septic shock with human monoclonal antibody HA-1A. A randomized, double-blind, placebo-controlled trial. *CHESS Trial Study Group. Ann. Intern. Med.* **121**, 1–5.

274. Greenman, R. L., Schein, R. M., Martin, M. A., Wenzel, R. P., MacIntyre, N. R., Emmanuel, G., Chmel, H., Kohler, R. B., McCarthy, M., Plouffe, J., and . (1991) A controlled clinical trial of E5 murine monoclonal IgM antibody to endotoxin in the treatment of gram-negative sepsis. The XOMA Sepsis Study Group. *JAMA* **266**, 1097–1102.

275. Calandra, T., Glauser, M. P., Schellekens, J., and Verhoef, J. (1988) Treatment of gram-negative septic shock with human IgG antibody to Escherichia coli J5: a prospective, double-blind, randomized trial. *J Infect. Dis.* **158**, 312–319.

276. Bone, R. C., Balk, R. A., Fein, A. M., Perl, T. M., Wenzel, R. P., Reines, H. D., et al. (1995) A second large controlled clinical study of E5, a monoclonal antibody to endotoxin: results of a prospective, multicenter, randomized, controlled trial. The E5 Sepsis Study Group. *Crit Care Med.* **23**, 994–1006.

277. J5 study Group (1992) Treatment of severe infectious purpura in children with human plasma from donors immunized with *Escherichia coli* J5: a prospective double- blind study. *J Infect. Dis.* **165**, 695–701.

278. Avontuur, J. A., Tutein Nolthenius, R. P., van Bodegom, J. W., and Bruining, H. A. (1998) Prolonged inhibition of nitric oxide synthesis in severe septic shock: a clinical study. *Crit. Care Med.* **26**, 660–667.

279. Grover, R., Zaccardelli, D., Colice, G., Guntupalli, K., Watson, D., and Vincent, J. L. (1999) An open-label dose escalation study of the nitric oxide synthase inhibitor, N(G)-methyl-L-arginine hydrochloride (546C88), in patients with septic shock. Glaxo Wellcome International Septic Shock Study Group. *Crit. Care Med.* **27**, 913–922.

280. Nasraway, S. A., Jr. (1999) Sepsis research: we must change course. *Crit. Care Med.* **27**, 427–430.

281. Fein, A. M., Bernard, G. R., Criner, G. J., Fletcher, E. C., Good, J. T., Knaus, W. A., et al. and for the CP-0127 SIRS and Sepsis Study Group (1997) Treatment of severe systemic inflammatory response syndrome and sepsis with a novel bradykinin antagonist, Deltibant (CP-0127). *JAMA* **277**, 482–487.

282. Bernard, G. R., Reines, H. D., Halushka, P. V., Higgins, S. B., Metz, C. A., Swindell, B. B., Wright, P. E., Watts, F. L., and Vrbanac, J. J. (1991) Prostacyclin and thromboxane A2 formation is increased in human sepsis syndrome. Effects of cyclooxygenase inhibition. *Am. Rev. Respir. Dis.* **144**, 1095–1101.

283. Haupt, M. T., Jastremski, M. S., Clemmer, T. P., Metz, C. A., and Goris, G. B. (1991) Effect of ibuprofen in patients with severe sepsis: a randomized, double-blind, multicenter study. The Ibuprofen Study Group. *Crit Care Med.* **19**, 1339–1347.

284. Bernard, G. R., Wheeler, A. P., Russell, J. A., Schein, R., Summer, W. R., Steinberg, K. P., et al. and for the Ibuprofen in Sepsis Study Group (1997) The effecs of ibuprofen on the physiology and survival of patients with sepsis. *N. Engl. J. Med.* **336**, 912–918.

285. Arons, M. M., Wheeler, A. P., Bernard, G. R., Christman, B. W., Russell, J. A., Schein, R., Summer, W. R., Steinberg, K. P., Fulkerson, W., Wright, P., Dupont, W. D., and Swindell, B. B. (1999) Effects of ibuprofen on the physiology and survival of hypothermic sepsis. Ibuprofen in Sepsis Study Group. *Crit. Care Med.* **27**, 699–707.

286. Reines, H. D., Halushka, P. V., Olanoff, L. S., and Hunt, P. S. (1985) Dazoxiben in human sepsis and adult respiratory distress syndrome. *Clin. Pharmacol. Ther.* **37**, 391–395.

287. Leeman, M., Boeynaems, J. M., Degaute, J. P., Vincent, J. L., and Kahn, R. J. (1985) Administration of dazoxiben, a selective thromboxane synthetase inhibitor, in the adult respiratory distress syndrome. *Chest* **87**, 726–730.

288. Yu, M. and Tomasa, G. (1993) A double-blind, prospective, randomized trial of ketoconazole, a thromboxane synthetase inhibitor, in the prophylaxis of the adult respiratory distress syndrome. *Crit. Care Med.* **21**, 1635–1642.

289. The ARDS Network (2000) Ketoconazole for early treatment of acute lung injury and acute respiratory distress syndrome: a randomized controlled trial. *JAMA* **283**, 1995–2002.

290. Holcroft, J. W., Vassar, M. J., and Weber, C. J. (1986) Prostaglandin E1 and survival in patients with the adult respiratory distress syndrome. A prospective trial. *Ann. Surg.* **203**, 371–378.

291. Abraham, E., Baughman, R., Fletcher, E., Heard, S., Lamberti, J., Levy, H., et al. (1999) Liposomal prostaglandin E1 (TLC C-53) in acute respiratory distress syndrome: a controlled, randomized, double-blind, multicenter clinical trial. TLC C-53 ARDS Study Group. *Crit. Care Med.* **27**, 1478–1485.

292. Abraham, E., Park, Y. C., Covington, P., Conrad, S. A., and Schwartz, M. (1996) Liposomal prostaglandin E1 in acute respiratory distress syndrome: a placebo-controlled, randomized, double-blind, multicenter clinical trial. *Crit. Care Med.* **24**, 10–15.

293. Bone, R. C., Slotman, G., Maunder, R., Silverman, H., Hyers, T. M., Kerstein, M. D., et al. (1989) Randomized doubleblind, multicenter study of prostaglandin E1 in patients with the adult respiratory distress syndrome. Prostaglandin E1 Study Group. *Chest* **96**, 114–119.

294. Silverman, H. J., Slotman, G., Bone, R. C., Maunder, R., Hyers, T. M., Kerstein, M. D., et al. (1990) Effects of prostaglandin E1 on oxygen delivery and consumption in patients with the adult respiratory distress syndrome. Results from the prostaglandin E1 multicenter trial. The Prostaglandin E1 Study Group. *Chest* **98**, 405–410.

295. Dhainaut, J. F., Tenaillon, A., Le Tulzo, Y., Schlemmer, B., Solet, J. P., Wolff, M., et al. (1994) Platelet-activating factor receptor antagonist BN 52021 in the treatment of severe sepsis: a randomized, double-blind, placebo- controlled, multicenter clinical trial. BN 52021 Sepsis Study Group. *Crit Care Med.* **22**, 1720–1728.

296. Dhainaut, J. F., Tenaillon, A., Hemmer, M., Damas, P., Le Tulzo, Y., Radermacher, P., et al. (1998) Confirmatory platelet-activating factor receptor antagonist trial in patients with severe gram-negative bacterial sepsis: a phase III, randomized, double-blind, placebo-controlled, multicenter trial. BN 52021 Sepsis Investigator Group. *Crit Care Med.* **26**, 1963–1971.

297. Carlet, J. (2001) Immunological therapy in sepsis: currently available. *Intensive Care Med.* **27 Suppl 1**, S93–103.

298. Arndt, P. and Abraham, E. (2001) Immunological therapy of sepsis: experimental therapies. *Intensive Care Med.* **27 Suppl 1**, S104–S115.

299. Esmon, C. T. (1992) The protein C anticoagulant pathway. *Arterioscler. Thromb.* **12**, 135–145.

300. Lorente, J. A., Garcia-Frade, L. J., Landin, L., de Pablo, R., Torrado, C., Renes, E., et al. (1993) Time course of hemostatic abnormalities in sepsis and its relation to outcome. *Chest* **103**, 1536–1542.

301. Bernard, G. R., Vincent, J. L., Laterre, P. F., LaRosa, S. P., Dhainaut, J. F., Lopez-Rodriguez, A., et al. (2001) Efficacy and safety of recombinant human activated protein C for severe sepsis. *N. Engl. J Med.* **344,** 699–709.

302. Abraham, E. (1999) Why immunomodulatory therapies have not worked in sepsis. *Intensive Care Med.* **25,** 556–566.

303. Glauser, M. P. (2000) Pathophysiologic basis of sepsis: considerations for future strategies of intervention. *Crit. Care Med.* **28,** S4–S8.

304. Cohen, J., Guyatt, G., Bernard, G. R., Calandra, T., Cook, D., Elbourne, D., et al. (2001) New strategies for clinical trials in patients with sepsis and septic shock. *Crit. Care Med.* **29,** 880–886.

305. Kox, W. J., Volk, T., Kox, S. N., and Volk, H. D. (2000) Immunomodulatory therapies in sepsis. *Intensive Care Med.* **26 Suppl 1,** S124–S128.

306. Bouchon, A., Facchetti, F., Weigand, M. A., and Colonna, M. (2001) TREM-1 amplifies inflammation and is a crucial mediator of septic shock. *Nature* **410,** 1103–1107.

26

Intravenous Immunoglobulin Adjunctive Therapy in Patients with Streptococcal Toxic Shock Syndrome and Necrotizing Fasciitis

Anna Norrby-Teglund, Donald E. Low, and Malak Kotb

1. INTRODUCTION

Streptococcal toxic shock syndrome (STSS) and necrotizing fasciitis caused by group A streptococcus (GAS) are rapidly-progressive invasive diseases that are associated with high mortality rates, ranging from 30% to 80% despite prompt antibiotic therapy and surgical debridement (1). Intense research in the field of GAS pathogenesis has unraveled complex host–pathogen interplay and provided an impetus for the design of novel therapeutic strategies to attenuate or prevent these diseases. One of the more promising therapeutic strategies is the intravenous administration of polyspecific immunoglobulin (IVIG) to patients with severe invasive GAS infections. In this chapter, we will review the mechanistic actions and use of IVIG as adjunctive therapy for severe invasive GAS infections. In doing so, we will also highlight epidemiological and pathogenic aspects of invasive GAS infections and show how IVIG acts, in part, by attenuating the inflammatory cytokine cascade in these patients.

2. CLINICAL AND EPIDEMIOLOGICAL ASPECTS OF SEVERE INVASIVE GAS INFECTIONS

Severe GAS infections have long been recognized and the history of GAS disease has been characterized by periodic changes in severity of disease. Streptococcal infections were recognized by Greek physicians in the 5th century. Sydenham described the disease as "febris scarlatina" as early as 1664 (2). This description clearly differentiated this disease from measles and other rashes, which allowed outbreaks of scarlet fever to be documented throughout the world. The most severe forms of streptococcal disease were well known long before the discovery of the bacterium. Hippocrates recorded epidemic erysipelas and clinical descriptions of a disease that we would clinically refer to today as necrotizing fasciitis (3).

In the United States during the middle part of the last century, there was a dramatic decline in the occurrence and mortality of scarlet fever (4). This occurred without an associated decrease in pharyngitis caused by GAS and with continuing severe infections and their sequelae in developing countries (5). This decline in severity began in the 1930s, before the advent of antibiotics for the treatment of streptococcal disease, and continued up to and including the 1970s (6). The mortality declined from 72% in the preantibiotic era to 7–27% (7–9). However, in the early 1980s, reports began to appear

From: *Cytokines and Chemokines in Infectious Diseases Handbook*
Edited by: M. Kotb and T. Calandra © Humana Press Inc., Totowa, NJ

that described not only an increased mortality as a result of GAS bacteremia (35–48%) but also anecdotal reports emphasizing a rapidly fatal outcome in bacteremic patients presenting with shock *(10)*. This syndrome was designated as the streptococcal toxic shock syndrome (STSS) and was reported from several areas of the world including Europe, the United States, Canada, New Zealand, and Japan *(11–16)*.

Streptococci toxic shock syndrome was defined by criteria established by The Working Group on Severe Streptococcal Infections *(17)*. Patients were considered to have STSS if they had hypotension in combination with two or more of the following: acute renal failure, coagulation abnormalities, liver abnormalities, acute respiratory distress syndrome, generalized rash, and necrotizing fasciitis. In addition to the increase in STSS during the 1980s, there were increased reports of necrotizing fasciitis *(13,18–21)*. The hallmark of necrotizing fasciitis is infection of the subcutaneous tissue and fascia that often results in necrosis with relative sparing of the underlying muscle. The diagnosis can be made if histopathology demonstrates both necrosis of superficial fascia and polymorphonuclear infiltrate and edema of the reticular dermis, subcutaneous fat, and superficial fascia. In the absence of examined specimens, the diagnosis requires the presence of gross fascial edema and necrosis detected at surgery *(20)*.

Clinically, it appears that STSS is a separate entity from necrotizing fasciitis. The studies from Britain and Sweden, which reported an increase in severe GAS infection, did not report the concomitant presence of necrotizing fasciitis *(11,16,22)*. Martin and Høiby *(14)* in their report of an increase in incidence and severity of GAS disease in Norway, resulting primarily from M1 strains, reported only a small number of cases of necrotizing fasciitis. Hoge et al. *(12)* carried out a retrospective survey of the medical records from all 10 hospitals in Pima County, Arizona, to identify sterile site isolates of GAS between 1985 and 1990. They found significant changes in the clinical spectrum of invasive infections, with an increase in patients with clinical features of STSS during the last 3 yr of the study. Necrotizing fasciitis was not associated with shock or any of the other clinical features of STSS, suggesting that fasciitis was not a component of the syndrome. Kaul et al. *(20)* found only 36 of 77 cases of GAS necrotizing fasciitis associated with STSS.

Epidemiological studies revealed that the majority of the outbreaks of severe invasive GAS infections outbreaks, although reported from different countries and on different continents, were caused predominantly by GAS strains of M1 and M3 serotypes *(14,16,23–31)*. However, although serotypes M1 and M3 accounted for the vast majority of strains isolated from cases of STSS and necrotizing fasciitis during the recent outbreaks, many other M types, including some nontypeble strains, are known to cause these disease *(32)*.

3. VIRULENCE MECHANISMS OF GAS

Group A streptococci express several virulence factors, both cell associated and secreted, which, in various ways, interact with human cells to promote growth, dissemination, and survival of the organism. The different virulence factors interact closely in a complex network involving synergistic, additive, and inhibitory effects *(see* Fig. 1). The majority of the membrane-bound molecules, including capsule, M, and M-like proteins, and fibronectin-binding proteins, are important for evasion of phagocytosis and bacterial adherence to host cells and tissue, whereas several of the secreted proteins such as peptidases, strepolysins, superantigens, and proteases are important for the spread and growth of the bacteria and result in induction of inflammatory responses (reviewed in refs. *32–35*) *(see* Fig. 1). The biological and clinical consequences of the interplay between GAS virulence factors and host cells range from asymptomatic bacterial colonization to severe systemic effects such as inflammation, tissue destruction, multiorgan failure, and shock. Specific virulence factors and their actions are described in more detail in Chapter 6.

Superantigens are by far the most potent streptococcal factors in the induction of proinflammatory responses *(36)* and therefore have been implicated as crucial players in the pathogenesis of STSS and

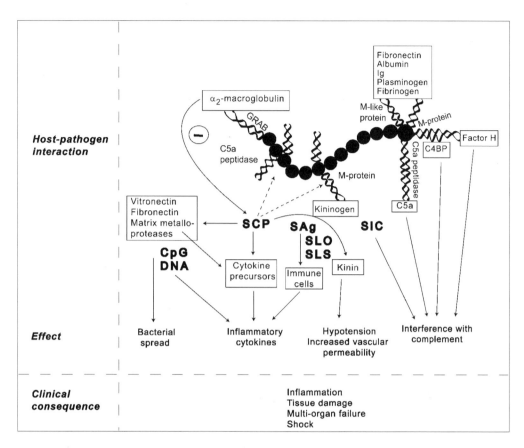

Fig. 1. Schematic model of the interaction between GAS virulence factors and human proteins and cells. Group A streptococcal cell-surface proteins, including M and M-like proteins, α_2-macroglobulin binding protein (GRAB), and C5a peptidase, interact with human plasma proteins (boxed) to promote bacterial adherence, spread, and evasion of phagocytosis. Secreted GAS factors (indicated by bold text), include streptococcal cysteine protease (SCP), unmethylated CpG DNA, streptolysin O and S (SLO,SLS), streptococcal inhibitor of complement (SIC), and superantigens (SAg). These factors strongly influence both the complement system and promote a pathologic proinflammatory response and, subsequently, the clinical symptoms of severe invasive GAS infections.

necrotizing fasciitis. There are several different superantigens produced by GAS including streptococcal pyrogenic exotoxins (Spe) A, B, C, F, G, H, J *(37,38)*, streptococcal superantigen (SSA) *(39)*, and the streptococcal mitogenic exotoxin Z and Z-2 *(38,40)*. Most GAS strains express several different superantigens, although the repertoire of genes encoding superantigens varies between GAS strains. Some of the superantigen genes are universally present in all strains regardless of serotype, whereas others are only seen in distinct lineages, such as SSA, which is only present in certain serotypes, including, among others, M3 and M4 *(41)*. It seems likely that several different superantigens can trigger invasive GAS diseases and that the bacteria during the infection produce more than one superantigen that contribute to disease pathogenesis.

4. HUMORAL IMMUNITY AGAINST GAS VIRULENCE FACTORS

It was established already in 1962 that opsonic antibodies against the M-protein conferred resistance against GAS infection; however, the protection was shown to be serotype-specific and the

Table 1

Acute-Phase Humoral Immunity Against GAS Virulence Factors in Patients with Varying Clinical Manifestations

Antibodies against	GAS serotype distribution[a]	Differences in antibody levels between patient proups	Ref.
M1-protein	>70% M1T1	Pharyngotonsillitis > bacteremia	25
	Clonal M1T1	Controls > Severe and nonsevere invasive[b]	44
SpeA	>70% M1T1	Pharyngotonsillitis = STSS = bacteremia	47
	Clonal M1T1	Controls = Severe and nonsevere invasive[b]	45
	Mixed	Controls[c] > non-STSS > STSS	46
	Mixed	Erysipelas and bacteremia > STSS	26
SpeB	>70% M1T1	Pharyngotonsillitis > STSS and bacteremia	47
	Clonal M1T1	Controls = Severe and nonsevere invasive[b]	45
	Mixed	Controls[c] and non-STSS>STSS	46
	Mixed	Erysipelas and bacteremia > STSS	26
SpeF	>70% M1T1	Pharyngotonsillitis > bacteremia and STSS	47
	Clonal M1T1	Controls = Severe and nonsevere invasive[b]	45
	Mixed	Erysipelas = bacteremia =STSS	26
M1T1 Sup[d]	Clonal M1T1	Controls > Severe and nonsevere invasive[b]	45

[a]The serotype distribution in the patient materials are indicated.

[b]Severe cases, patients with STSS, and/or necrotizing fasciitis; nonsevere cases, no signs of hypotension or multiorgan failure; controls, healthy age-matched blood donors *(44,45)*.

[c]Controls, healthy blood donors as well as preoperative orthopedic patients *(46)*.

[d]Culture supernatant (Sup) were prepared from M1T1 isolates, and each patient's plasma were tested for neutralizing activity against Sup from their own isolate *(45)*.

individual remained susceptible to infection by other GAS serotypes *(42)*. There are, to date, 93 different serotypes of GAS verified *(43)*. Analyses of the recent outbreaks in the late 1980s, which were caused predominantly by M1T1 strains, revealed that invasive cases, regardless of severe or nonsevere manifestations, had significantly lower antibody levels against the M1-protein than healthy controls or pharyngotonsillitis cases *(25,44)*, *(see* Table 1). These data suggested that low immunity to the M1-protein rendered the individuals susceptible to invasive infection by M1T1 strains, but did not influence the severity of systemic manifestation as evident by equally low antibody levels in severe or nonsevere invasive cases *(see* Table 1).

Humoral immunity against different superantigens was also assessed in patient materials collected during the recent outbreaks, and the studies revealed somewhat inconsistent results *(25,26,45–47)*, *(see* Table 1). A Swedish study reported a strong correlation between more severe invasive disease and lower levels of neutralizing antibodies against SpeB and SpeF, whereas equal antibody levels against SpeA was found in bacteremia and pharyngotonsillitis cases *(47)*. Similarly, two other studies reported higher anti-SpeB reactivity in plasma from controls than in severe invasive cases *(26,46)*; however, these two latter studies also observed a correlation between more severe cases and lower titers of anti-SpeA antibodies. The varying results obtained from the different studies may simply reflect the involvement of different superantigens in the respective study. Together, these studies show that humoral immunity toward GAS virulence factors is important for protection against infection. Basma et al. *(45)* analyzed a clinical material for neutralizing antibodies against specific toxins and against culture supernatants, containing superantigens and other extracellular virulence factors, prepared from each patient's isolate. The study showed that although there was no significant difference in neutralizing activity against specific superantigens between controls and patients with invasive infection, the patients had significantly lower immunity toward superantigens secreted by their own isolate, as compared to the controls. Equally low neutralizing activity was detected in plasma from severe or nonsevere invasive cases, indicating that low immunity to the patient's own isolate is clinically relevant and contributes to susceptibility to the superantigens. Importantly, the studies demonstrate a crucial role for antibodies against GAS virulence factors in protection against invasive infection.

5. CONVENTIONAL THERAPY OF SEVERE INVASIVE GAS INFECTIONS

Conventional therapy of invasive GAS infections has consisted of antimicrobials and, when necessary in severe invasive disease, support of vital functions for those patients with STSS and surgery for those patients with necrotizing fasciitis. Penicillin and cephalosporins are the antimicrobials most frequently used for treating GAS pharyngitis, cellulitis, and impetigo. However, concern has been raised that in more severe infections, the organism is less likely to respond to β-lactam antibiotics. Stevens et al. *(48)* showed that penicillin was ineffective in a mouse model of myositis caused by GAS if treatment was delayed ≥2 h after initiation of treatment. The targets for the β-lactams are the penicillin-binding proteins (PBPs), enzymes responsible for the formation of the peptidoglycan in the bacterial cell wall, which are expressed during the log-phase of growth. Stevens et al. *(49)* found that in addition to decreased binding of radiolabeled penicillin by all PBPs in large inocula stationary cells, PBPs 1 and 4 were undetectable at 36 h. They speculated that the loss of certain PBPs during stationary-phase growth in vitro may account for the failure of penicillin in both experimental and human cases of severe streptococcal infection. Furthermore, they found that antimicrobials that inhibit protein synthesis were able to improve survival over penicillin in a mouse model of myositis caused by GAS *(48)*. Survival of erythromycin-treated mice was greater than that of penicillin-treated mice and untreated controls, but only if treatment was begun within 24 h. Mice receiving clindamycin had survival rates of 100%, 100%, 80%, and 70%, even if the treatment was delayed 0, 2, 6, and 16.5 h, respectively.

Although GAS has remained exquisitely sensitive to penicillin, resistance to the macrolides and clindamycin has emerged worldwide. Depending of the prevalence of resistance and the mechanism of resistance, either erythromycin or clindamycin or both may not be active against the infecting GAS. Therefore, an approach for severe invasive GAS infection has been to utilize a combination of penicillin and clindamycin, since the penicillin provides coverage against 100% of *Streptococcus pyogenes* strains.

Patients with STSS require supportive therapy to manage their hypotension and multiorgan failure. However, as with severe invasive *S. pneumoniae* disease where there has been a failure of intensive care unit support to influence mortality, the mortality from STSS has not changed significantly *(50,51)*. Often, patients succumb to their infection before antimicrobials can have any beneficial effect, emphasizing the importance of research in immune modulation therapy.

The treatment of necrotizing fasciitis has emphasized the importance of early surgical intervention for diagnosis or surgical debridement and/or hyperbaric oxygen *(52)*. Early aggressive surgery has been advocated in order to reduce the systemic inflammatory response and the spread of local infection *(53)*. Hyperbaric oxygen is recommended in order to administer oxygen at greater than normal pressure so as to lead to better wound healing. Unfortunately, both procedures usually occur at a time when the patient is most unstable and therefore interferes with monitoring and treatment. In addition, there is no evidence to support the use of hyperbaric oxygen and there is new information that we may allow surgery to be delayed until the patient is stable and the degree of surgery required is better defined, thereby reducing unnecessary tissue debridement and/or amputation *(54,55)*.

6. IVIG AS ADJUNCTIVE THERAPY

The finding that low levels of protective antibodies against the M-protein and superantigens correlated with invasive GAS disease highlighted the importance of antibodies in protection against these infections and suggested that immunoglobulins might be a potential adjunctive therapy *(25,26,45–*

Table 2

Clinical Trials of the Use of IVIG Therapy in Sepsis Patients[a]

Patients	Study design[b]	Study drugs	All-cause mortality IVIG	Controls	OR (95% confidence interval)	Ref.
Preterm neonates, sepsis	SC, NB	Pentaglobin; no intervention	6/20	9/24	0.72 (0.21, 2.49)	63
Premature, early-onset sepsis	MS, DB	Standard IVIG; albumin	2/14	5/17	0.43 (0.08, 2.29)	64
Neonates, sepsis	SC	Intraglobin; saline	2/28	1/28	2.0 (0.2, 20.03)	65
Neonates, sepsis	SC, DB	Standard IVIG; dextrose	1/30	6/30	0.2 (0.04, 0.97)	66
Adults, severe sepsis	SC, NB	Sandoglobulin; no intervention	7/12	9/12	0.49 (0.09, 2.57)	67
Adults, Gram-negative septic shock	SC, NB	Pentaglobin; no intervention	1/27	9/28	0.22 (0.06, 0.81)	68
Adults, surgical sepsis	MC, DB	Sandoglobulin; albumin	11/29	22/33	0.32 (0.12, 0.87)	69
Adults, postoperative sepsis and G- endotoxemia	SC, BD	Intraglobin; no intervention	15/24	19/22	0.3 (0.08, 1.10)	70
Adults, postoperative sepsis	SC, NB	Pentaglobin; placebo	8/18	13/17	0.27 (0.07, 1.04)	71

[a]Table includes randomized controlled trials assessing the use of IVIG therapy, summarized in ref. *62*.
[b]SC; single center (SC), MC, multicenter; NB, unblinded; B, blinded; DB, double-blinded.

47). In order for an immunoglobulin therapy to be efficacious, broad antibody specificity would be required to cover all of the different serotypes of GAS and the whole spectrum of superantigens, as well as other important virulence factors. IVIG exhibits high polyspecificity generated by antibodies pooled from several thousands of donors and is a commonly used therapy in a number of neuroimmunological and primary immunodeficiency disorders, as well as in Kawasaki disease (reviewed in refs. *56–59*). The proven efficacy of IVIG in Kawasaki disease is of special interest because this disease share several common clinical features with STSS and superantigens have been proposed to be involved also in the pathogenesis of Kawasaki disease *(60)*.

There have been several studies investigating the use of IVIG for prophylaxis or adjunctive therapy of sepsis, however, large multicenter trials are lacking (reviewed in refs. *61* and *62*). The Cochrane library recently evaluated the efficacy of IVIG in the treatment of sepsis and septic shock and included randomized trials that compared polyclonal IVIG to either placebo or no intervention *(62)* (*see* Table 2). The study showed an overall reduction in mortality in patients who received polyclonal IVIG as compared to controls. However, the results of the score-based immunoglobulin treatment in sepsis (SBITS) study, which included 653 patients with a score-defined degree of sepsis (Elebute and Stoner score: 12–27) and a score-defined severity of disease (Acute Physiology and Schronic Health Evaluation score APACHE II score: 20–35) *(72)*, was not included in the Cochrane database. In the SBITS study, the patients received either IVIG (Polyglobin N) or placebo. No difference in mortality d 28 could be demonstrated. Hence, the efficacy of IVIG therapy in sepsis, in general, remains to be proven and may relate to certain sepsis subgroups. As recently reviewed by Werdan *(61)*, the most impressive reductions in mortality has been reported in specific sepsis subgroups, such as post-opera-

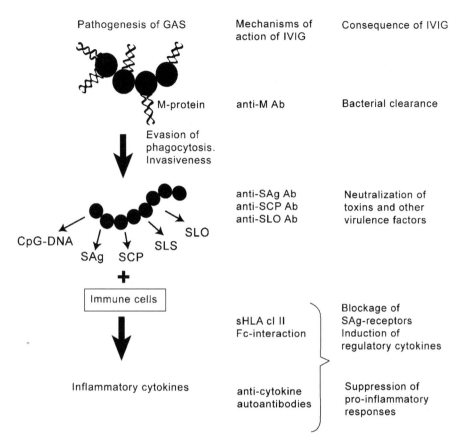

Fig. 2. Proposed mechanisms of action of intravenous immunoglobulin (IVIG) in severe invasive GAS infections. Intravenous immunoglobulin have potential to interact at different stages in the GAS pathogenesis. Ab, antibodies; SAg, superantigens; SCP, streptococcal cysteine protease (i.e., SpeB); SLO, streptolysin O; SLS, streptolysin S.

tive sepsis with a sepsis score greater than 17, septic shock with endotoxemia, neutropenic leukemia patients with sepsis syndrome, fulminant meningococcal sepsis, and STSS, the latter being discussed in detail in Subheading 6.2.

6.1. Mechanistic Actions of IVIG

Several different modes of actions that contribute to the beneficial effect in autoimmune and systemic inflammatory diseases have been described for IVIG. These include blockade of Fc receptors on reticuloendothelial cell system and phagocytic cells, modulation of Fc-receptor expression, interference with activated complement, modulation of cytokine responses, modulation of immune cell functions, interaction with idiotypic–anti-idiotypic network, antigen neutralization, and selection of immune repertoires (reviewed in refs. *56* and *57*). A crucial pathway by which IVIG exerts its anti-inflammatory activity was recently identified in a murine model of immune thrombocytopenia and involved increased expression of the Fc inhibitory receptor for IgG, Fc-γRIIB and, consequently, abrogated platelet destruction by macrophage phagocytosis (*73*). Mechanistic actions directly related to the pathogenesis of invasive GAS infections, such as antigen neutralization, bacterial opsonization, as well as cytokine modulation (*see* Fig. 2), are discussed further in Subheadings 6.1.1. and 6.1.2.

6.1.1. Antibodies Against GAS Virulence Factors

Opsonizing antibodies that promote phagocytosis and bacterial clearance of several pathogenic microorganisms, including GAS, have been demonstrated in IVIG preparations (44,74–77). Basma et al. (44) recently showed that opsonizing anti-M1 antibodies present in IVIG preparations were conferred to the patients upon IVIG therapy, as evident by elevated opsonizing titers in plasma obtained post-IVIG administration. Based on these data, it was suggested that increased bacterial clearance through opsonizing antibodies against GAS could be a potential mechanistic action of IVIG contributing to clinical efficacy of IVIG in invasive GAS infections (see Fig. 2). However, an experimental murine model of necrotizing fascitiis that compared the efficacy of clindamycin, penicillin, and IVIG, alone or in combination, failed to support this hypothesis (78). In this model, the efficacy of the various treatment regimens was assessed based on quantitative bacterial clearance, and IVIG did not enhance bacterial clearance of the M3 strain. This study does not rule out that IVIG-conferred opsonic antibodies may effect bacterial clearance in patients; however, the results emphasize the need for further studies to define the exact role of this mechanistic action in the efficacy of IVIG therapy in severe invasive GAS infections.

Intravenous immunoglobulin has also been found to contain antibodies against a wide array of GAS superantigens as well as other secreted GAS virulence factors (79–84). Specific antibodies against the superantigens SpeA, SpeB, and SpeC (80), Dnase B, and streptolysin O (83,84) have been demonstrated. The extraordinary broad specificity of IVIG was further highlighted by the finding that IVIG could completely inhibit culture supernatants, containing a mixture of superantigens and other extracellular bacterial virulence factors, from several different GAS serotypes, including M1, M3, M4, M6, and M28 (81). The inhibitory effect of IVIG was noted both on the proliferative and cytokine-inducing capacity of GAS superantigens, and the neutralizing activity was found to be transferred to the patients upon administration of IVIG with subsequent increased superantigen-neutralizing activity in patients' plasma (79,80). This inhibitory activity of IVIG is not only exclusive for superantigens expressed by GAS but also superantigens produced by S. aureus are potently inhibited by IVIG (85,86).

Analyses of different IVIG preparations containing varying concentrations of IgG, IgA, and/or IgM revealed that they varied in opsonizing and toxin-neutralizing capacity, and variation in inhibitory activity was even observed between lots of the same preparation (77,81,87). IgA and IgM were found to be potent inhibitors of GAS superantigens, and in the case of SpeA, the most efficient neutralization was achieved by a preparation containing a mixture of IgG, IgA, and IgM (87). These findings suggest that optimization of IVIG therapy may be achieved by changing the type or lot of IVIG preparation. In fact, the recent Cochrane report on IVIG therapy in sepsis demonstrated a superior reduction in mortality by IgM-enriched IVIG preparations ($n=194$; RR=0.48; 95% confidence interval [CI] 0.30–0.76) compared to standard polyclonal IVIG ($n=219$; RR=0.68; 95% CI-0.51–0.89) (62).

6.1.2. Modulation of Cytokine Responses

Intravenous immunoglobulin is a powerful modulator of cytokine production, not only via direct antigen neutralization but also through immunomodulatory activities that are mediated by pathways not yet completely defined. These pathways are believed to include Fc interactions, soluble immune components, and induction of regulatory cytokines (reviewed in 56 and 57), (see Table 3). A strong induction of interleukin (IL)-1ra has been shown in human monocytes following culture on adherent IgG (88) or coculture with IVIG (89,102). Also, IL-8 production is induced in human monocytes following coculture with IVIG (90,91). IL1-ra is well known to exert anti-inflammatory activity because of its interaction with IL-1 signaling; however, the effect of IL-8 as an anti-inflammatory agent is not as clearly defined but has been suggested to inhibit the accumulation of neutrophils to the sites of inflammation when induced systemically (103).

Table 3
Proposed Mechanistic Actions of IVIG in Cytokine Modulation

Mode of action of IVIG	Proposed mechanism	Consequence	Ref.
SAg neutralization	Anti-SAg antibodies	Inhibition of super-antigenic activity	*79, 80, 82, 86, 87*
Upregulation of interleukin (IL)-1ra	Partly Fc interaction	Anti-inflammatory	*88–90*
Upregulation of transforming growth factor (TGF)-β	Partly Fc interaction	Anti-inflammatory	*91–93*
Upregulation of IL-8	Not defined	Anti-inflammatory	*90, 91*
Cytokine neutralization	Cytokine-specific autoantibodies	Immunosuppression	*94–98*
Blockage of receptors on immune cells	Soluble HLA cl I and II, sCD4, sCD8	Immunosuppression	*99–101*

Note: SAg, superantigen.

Intravenous immunoglobulin has been shown to be a strong inhibitor of superantigen-induced lymphokine production in vitro, with the strongest suppression seen for the Th1 cytokines interferon (IFN)-γ and tumor necrosis factor (TNF)-β, as their production was almost completely abolished *(79,82,87,91)*. This inhibitory effect was seen, although to a lesser extent, even when the addition of IVIG was delayed 24 hr poststimulation with superantigen, suggesting that additional mechanisms of IVIG, aside from antigen neutralization, contribute to the inhibitory effect *(82,91)*. A differential effect of IVIG has been noted on superantigen-induced monokine production with upregulated IL-8 and decreased IL-6 production *(91)*. Studies on the effect of IVIG on superantigen-induced IL-1 production have reported conflicting results, as one study demonstrated no effect on IL-1 production *(82)*, whereas the other reported a significant reduction of IL-1 *(87)*. Thus, superantigen-induced lymphokine production is potently suppressed by IVIG, and the monokine production may also be modulated by IVIG, but further studies are required to define the effect of IVIG on superantigen-induced monokines. However, because the Th1 type of cytokines is the hallmark of a superantigen response, the powerful inhibition of these cytokines by IVIG most likely represents a major mechanistic action of IVIG contributing to clinical efficacy.

Cytokine modulation by IVIG have also been shown in vivo in several diseases, including, among others, severe invasive GAS infections where patients showed decreased levels of TNF-α and IL-6 *(23,104)*; Guillain–Barré syndrome patients who showed a selective down-regulation of pro-inflammatory cytokines *(105)*, and Kawasaki patients who demonstrated elevated IL-1ra and IL-8, as well as decreased proinflammatory cytokines following IVIG-therapy *(106)*.

6.2. Clinical Studies of IVIG Therapy in STSS and Necrotizing Fasciitis

Several case reports have demonstrated clinical improvement after IVIG therapy of patients with severe invasive GAS infections, including STSS, necrotizing fasciitis, and necrotizing myositis *(84,104,107–114)* (*see* Table 4). There have been three reports on IVIG therapy in patients with necrotizing fasciitis *(20,54,63)* (*see* Table 4). In the study by Kaul et al. *(20)*, a reduction in mortality rate (10% compared to 37%) was noted between IVIG-treated patients and nontreated controls. However, the only factors in this study that were independently associated with mortality of streptococcal necrotizing fasciitis were age, hypotension, and bacteremia. Muller et al. *(54)* described six patients with severe GAS disease and soft tissue involvement that were managed conservatively. Treatment in all cases included clindamycin, a β-lactam, and high dose IVIG. All patients were hypotensive and three patients developed STSS. One patient had limited exploratory surgery without debridement.

Table 4
Clinical Studies of the Use of IVIG as Adjunctive Therapy in Severe Invasive GAS Infections

Diagnosis of patients	No. of patients	Case patality rate (%)	GAS serotype	Ref.
NF	16 IVIG	19	No predominate serotype	*107*
	4, no IVIG	25		
NF	10 IVIG	10	35% M1, 25% M3	*20*
	67, no IVIG	37		
NF	6	0	No predominate serotype	*54*
STSS + NM	1	0	M1	*111*
STSS + NF	1	0	NA	*113*
STSS + NF	1	0	NA	*108*
STSS + NF	1	0	NA	*114*
STSS	1	0	M1	*112*
STSS	1	0	M49	*109*
STSS	1	0	M1	*104*
STSS	1	0	M74	*110*
STSS	5	20	M1	*84*
STSS	21 IVIG	7 d: 10%; 30 d: 33%[a]	48% M1, 19% M3	*23*
	32, no IVIG	7 d: 50%; 30 d: 66%	6% M1, 28% M3	

Note: NF, necrotizing fascilitis; STSS, streptococcal toxic shock syndrome; NM, necrotizing myositis.
[a]Case fatality rate was determined at 7 and 30 d after diagnosis *(23)*.

Table 5
Results of a Comparative Observational Study
of the Efficacy of IVIG Therapy in STSS

Variables	IVIG-treated cases (*n*=21)	Controls (*n*=32)	*p*-Value
Mean APACHE II score	26	25	0.99
Clindamycin therapy (%)	95	55	<0.01
Surgery (%)	67	38	0.04
Case fatality rates (%)			
All patients			
7 d	10	50	<0.01
10 d	33	66	0.02
Patients receiving clindamycin	30	53	0.06

Source: Data are adapted from *(23)*.

One patient had repeated bedside drainage of her olecranon bursa. No other patient had surgery, and all patients survived. This study, although limited in numbers, suggests that high-dose IVIG therapy may, by virtue of its effects on both bacterial and host factors, slow or limit the systemic illness in patients with severe GAS soft tissue infections, thereby allowing for nonoperative or minimally invasive approaches in these patients.

An observational cohort study designed to evaluate the efficacy of IVIG therapy in patients with STSS was conducted in Canada *(23)* *(see* Table 5). The study included 21 cases that were treated with IVIG during 1994–1995 and 32 nontreated controls identified through Ontario's Streptococcal Study Group's active surveillance during 1992–1995. Multivariate analysis revealed that IVIG therapy and a lower acute physiology and chronic health evaluation II (APACHE) score was significantly associated with survival. One confounding factor in the material was that IVIG-treated cases were more likely to have received clindamycin therapy than the controls *(see* Table 5). Therefore, a secondary multivariate analysis considering only cases and controls that had received clindamycin was performed, and the APACHE II score and IVIG therapy remained the two variables associated with survival. Further support for the use of IVIG was provided by in vitro studies of blood samples collected pre-IVIG and post-IVIG therapy *(23)*. Neutralizing activity against culture supernatant prepared from the patient's own infecting isolate increased significantly posttherapy, and the majority of patient's plasma caused 80–100% inhibition of the bacterial supernatants following IVIG-administration. The clinical studies included patients infected with GAS strains of varying serotype (*see* Table 4), which further supports the in vitro findings that IVIG has a very broad spectrum of superantigen-neutralizing antibodies *(23,79,81)*. IVIG therapy also resulted in a significantly reduced TNF-α and IL-6 production in peripheral blood mononuclear cells in four patients tested *(23)*. Thus, together these data suggest that the clinical improvement achieved by IVIG therapy is partly attributed to inhibition of the superantigens produced by the clinical isolates and a reduction in the proinflammatory response.

7. CONCLUDING REMARKS

There is much data from both in vitro and in vivo studies that support the use of IVIG as adjunctive therapy in severe invasive GAS infections. The data suggest that IVIG most likely is efficacious against GAS strains of varying serotypes with different superantigen expression profiles and that the efficacy is contributed to direct antigen neutralization, suppression of proinflammatory responses, and, potentially, bacterial opsonization (*see* Fig. 2). Although it would be desirable to have a large controlled multicenter trial to provide definite proof of clinical efficacy of IVIG in these diseases, considering the high mortality and morbidity of STSS and necrotizing fasciitis, it seems reasonable that IVIG be used in conjunction with conventional therapy and surgery.

REFERENCES

1. Low, D.E., Schwartz, B., and McGeer, A. (1998) The reemergence of severe group A streptococcal disease: an evolutionary perspective, in *Emerging Pathogens, Vol. 7*, ASM Press, Washington, DC.
2. Katz, A.R. and Morens, D.M. (1992) Severe streptococcal infections in historical perspective. *Clin. Infect. Dis.* **14**, 298–307.
3. Descamps, V., Aitken, J., and Lee, M.G. (1994) Hippocrates on necrotising fasciitis. *Lancet* **344**, 556.
4. Quinn, R.W. (1982) Epidemiology of group A streptococcal infections—their changing frequency and severity. *Yale J. Biol. Med.* **55**, 265–270.
5. Kaplan, E. (1993) Global assessment of rheumatic fever and rheumatic heart disease at the close of the century. The influences and dynamics of population and pathogens: a failure to realize prevention? (The T. Duckettt Jones Memorial Lecture). *Circulation* **88**, 1964–1972.
6. Kaplan, E.L. (1996) Recent epidemiology of group A streptococcal infections in North America and abroad: an overview. *Paediatrics* **97**, 945–948.
7. Keefer, C.S., Inglefinger, F.J., and Spink, W.W. (1937) Significance of hemolytic streptococci bacteraemia: a study of two hundred and forty six patients. *Arch. Intern. Med.* **60**, 1084–1097.
8. Hable, K.A., Horstmeirer, C., Wold, A.D., and Washington, J.A. (1973) Group A β-hemolytic streptococcemia: bacteriologic and clinical study of 44 cases. *Mayo Clin. Proc.* **48**, 336–339.
9. Duma, R.J., Weinberg, A.N., Medrek, T.F., and Kunz, L.J. (1969) Streptococcal infections: a bacteriologic and clinical study of streptococcal bacteremia. *Medicine* **48**, 87–127.
10. Goepel, J.R., Richards, D.G., Harris, D.M., and Henry, L. (1980) Fulminant Streptococcus pyogenes infection. *Br. Med. J.* **281**, 1412.
11. Gaworzewska, E. and Colman, G. (1988) Changes in the pattern of infection caused by Streptococcus pyogenes. *Epidemiol. Infect.* **100**, 257–269.
12. Hoge, C.W., Schwartz, B., Talkington, D.F., Breiman, R., MacNeill, E.M., and Englender, S.J. (1993) The changing epidemiology of invasive group A streptococcal infections and the emergence of streptococcal toxic shock-like syndrome. A retrospective population-based study. *JAMA* **269**, 384–389.
13. Cone, L.A., Woodard, D.R., Schlievert, P.M., and Tomory, G.S. (1987) Clinical and bacteriological observations of a toxic shock-like syndrome due to Streptococcus pyogenes. *N. Engl. J. Med.* **317**, 146–149.
14. Martin, P.R. and Høiby, E.A. (1990) Streptococcal serogroup A epidemic in Norway 1987–1988. *Scand. J. Infect. Dis.* **22**, 421–429.
15. Schwartz, B., Facklam, R.R., and Breiman, R.F. (1990) Changing epidemiology of group A streptococcal infection in the USA. *Lancet* **336**, 1167–1171.

16. Strömberg, A., Romanus, V., and Burman, L.G. (1991) Outbreak of group A streptococcal bacteremia in Sweden: an epidemiological and clinical study. *J. Infect. Dis.* **164**, 595–598.
17. The Working Group on Severe Streptococcal Infections (1993) Defining the group A streptococcal toxic shock syndrome. Rationale and consensus definition. *JAMA* **269**, 390–391.
18. Chelsom, J., Halstensen, A., Haga, T., and Hoiby, A. (1994) Necrotizing fasciitis due to group A streptococci in western Norway: incidence and clinical features. *Lancet* **344**, 1111–1115.
19. Demers, B., Simor, A.E., Vellend, H., Schlievert, P.M., Byrne, S., Jamieson, F., et al. (1993) Severe invasive group A streptococcal infections in Ontario, Canada: 1987–1991. *Clin. Infect. Dis.* **16**, 792–800.
20. Kaul, R., McGeer, A., Low, D.E., Green, K., Schwartz, B., Ontario group A Streptococcal Study Group, and Simor, E. (1997) Population-based surveillance for group A streptococcal necrotizing fasciitis: clinical features, prognostic indicators, and microbiologic analysis of seventy-seven cases. *Am. J. Med.* **103**, 18–24.
21. Stevens, D.L., Tanner, M.H., Winship, J., Swarts, R., Ries, K.M., Schlievert, P.M., et al. (1989) Severe group A streptococcal infections associated with a toxic shock-like syndrome and scarlet fever toxin A. *N. Engl. J. Med.* **321**, 1–7.
22. Colman, G., Tanna, A., Efstratiou, A., and Gaworzewska, E. (1993) The serotypes of Streptococcus pyogenes present in Britain during 1980-1990 and their association with disease. *J. Med. Microbiol.* **39**, 165–178.
23. Kaul, R., McGeer, A., Norrby-Teglund, A., Kotb, M., Schwartz, B., O'Rourke, K., et al., and The Canadian Streptococcal Study Group (1999) Intravenous immunoglobulin therapy for streptococcal toxic shock syndrome - a comparative observational study. *Clin. Infect. Dis.* **28**, 800–807.
24. Cockerill, F.R., 3rd., MacDonald, K.L., Thompson, R.L., Roberson, F., Kohner, P.C., Besser-Wiekm, J., et al. (1997) An outbreak of invasive group A streptococcal disease associated with high carriage rates of the invasive clone among school-aged children. *JAMA* **277**, 38–43.
25. Holm, S.E., Norrby, A., Bergholm, A.-M., and Norgren, M. (1992) Aspects of the pathogenesis in serious group A streptococcal infections in Sweden 1988–1989. *J. Infect. Dis.* **166**, 31–37.
26. Eriksson, B.K., Andersson, J., Holm, S.E., and Norgren, M. (1999) Invasive group A streptococcal infections: T1M1 isolates expressing pyrogenic exotoxins A and B in combination with selective lack of toxin-neutralizing antibodies are associated with increased risk of streptococcal toxic shock syndrome. *J. Infect. Dis.* **180**, 410–418.
27. Kiska, D.L., Thiede, B., Caracciolo, J., Jordan, M., Johnson, D., Kaplan, E.L., et al. (1997) Invasive group A streptococcal infections in North Carolina: epidemiology, clinical features, and genetic and serotype analysis of causative organisms. *J. Infect. Dis.* **176**, 992–1000.
28. Nakashima, K., Ichiyama, S., Iinuma, Y., Hasgawa, Y., Ohta, M., Ooe, K., et al. (1997) A clinical and bacteriologic investigation of invasive streptococcal infections in Japan on the basis of serotypes, toxin production, and genomic DNA fingerprints. *Clin. Infect. Dis.* **25**, 260–266.
29. Upton, M., Carter, P.E., Orange, G., and Pennington, T.H. (1996) Genetic heterogeneity of M type 3 group A streptococci causing severe infections in Tayside, Scotland. *J. Clin. Microbiol.* **34**, 196–198.
30 Svensson, N., Oberg, S., Henriques, B., Holm, S., Kallenius, G., Romanus, V. et al. (2000) Invasive group A streptococcal infections in Sweden in 1994 and 1995: epidemiology and clinical spectrum. *Scand. J. Infect. Dis.* **32**, 609–614.
31. McGeer, A., Willey, B., Schwartz, B., Green, K., Bernston, A., Trpeski, L., et al., Group A Streptococcal Study and Low D.E. (1998) Epidemiology of invasive GAS disease due to M3 serotypes in Ontario, Canada, in *Abstracts of 38th Interscience Conference on Antimicrobial Agents and Chemotherapy*, ASM, Washington, DC.
32. Cunningham, M.W. (2000) Pathogenesis of group A streptococcal infections. *Clin. Microbiol. Rev.* **13**, 470–511.
33. Boyle, M.D. (1995) Variation of multifunctional surface binding proteins—a virulence strategy for group A streptococci? *J. Theor. Biol.* **21**, 415–426.
34. Fischetti, V.A. (1989) Streptococcal M protein: molecular design and biological behavior. *Clin. Microbiol. Rev.* **2**, 285–314.
35. Norrby-Teglund, A. and Kotb, M. (2000) Host-microbe interactions in the pathogenesis of invasive group A streptococcal infections. *J. Med. Microbiol.* **49**, 849–852.
36. Kotb, M. (1998) Superantigens of gram-positive bacteria: structure–function analyses and their implications for biological activity. *Curr. Opin. Microbiol.* **1**, 56–65.
37. Kotb, M. (1995) Bacterial pyrogenic exotoxins as superantigens. *Clin. Microbiol. Rev.* **8**, 411–426.
38. Proft, T., Louise Moffatt, S., Berkahn, C.J., and Fraser, J.D. (1999) Identification and characterization of novel superantigens from Streptococcus pyogenes. *J. Exp. Med.* **189**, 89–102.
39. Mollick, J.A., Miller, G.G., Musser, J., Cook, R.G., Grossman, D., and Rich, R.R. (1993) A novel superantigen isolated from pathogenic strains of S. pyogenes with aminoterminal homology to staphylococcal enterotoxins B and C. *J. Clin. Invest.* **92**, 710–719.
40. Kamezawa, Y., Nakahara, T., Nakano, S., Abe, Y., Nozaki-Renard, J., and Isono, T. (1997) Streptococcal mitogenic exotoxin Z, a novel acidic superantigenic toxin produced by a T1 strain of *Streptococcus pyogenes*. *Infect. Immun.* **65**, 3828–3833.
41. Reda, K.B., Kapur, V., Goela, D., Lamphear, J.G., Musser, J.M., and Rich, R.R. (1996) Phylogenetic distribution of streptococcal superantigen SSA allelic variants provides evidence for horizontal transfer of ssa within *Streptococcus pyogenes*. *Infect. Immun.* **64**, 1161–1165.
42. Lancefield, R.C. (1962) Current knowledge of type-specific M antigen of group A streptococci. *J. Immunol.* **89**, 307–313.
43. Facklam, R., Beall, B., Efstratiou, A., Fischetti, V., Johnson, D., Kaplan, E., et al. (1999) emm typing and validation of provisional M types for group A streptococci. *Emerg. Infect. Dis.* **5**, 247–253.
44. Basma, H., Norrby-Teglund, A., McGeer, A., Low, D.E., El-Ahmedy, O., Dale, J.B., et al. (1998) Opsonic antibodies to the surface M protein, present in pooled normal immunoglobulins (IVIG), may contribute to its clinical efficacy in severe invasive group A streptococcal infections. *Infect. Immun.* **66**, 2279–2283.

45. Basma, H., Norrby-Teglund, A., Guedez, Y., McGeer, A., Low, D.E., El-Ahmedy, O., et al. (1999) Risk factors in the pathogenesis of invasive group A streptococcal infections: role of protective humoral immunity. *Infect. Immun* **67,** 1871–1877.
46. Mascini, E.M., Jansze, M., Schellekens, J.F., Musser, J.M., Faber, J.A., Verhoef-Verhage, L.A., et al. (2000) Invasive group A streptococcal disease in the Netherlands: evidence for a protective role of anti-exotoxin A antibodies. *J. Infect. Dis.* **181,** 631–638.
47. Norrby-Teglund, A., Pauksens, K., Holm, S.E., and Norgren, M. (1994) Relation between low capacity of human sera to inhibit streptococcal mitogens and serious manifestation of disease. *J. Infect. Dis.* **170,** 585–591.
48. Stevens, D.L., Gibbons, A.E., Bergstrom, R., and Winn, V. (1988) The Eagle effect revisited: efficacy of clindamycin, erythromycin, and penicillin in the treatment of streptococcal myositis. *J. Infect. Dis.* **158,** 23–28.
49. Stevens, D.L., Yan, S., and Bryant, A.E. (1993) Penicillin-binding protein expression at different growth stages determines penicillin efficacy in vitro and in vivo: an explanation for the inoculum effect. *J. Infect. Dis.* **167,** 1401–1405.
50. Hook, E.W., Horton, C.A., and Schaberg, D.R. (1983) Failure of intensive care unit support to influence mortality from pneumococcal bacteremia. *JAMA* **249,** 1055–1057.
51. Davies, D.H., McGeer, A., Schwartz, B., Green, K., Cann, D., Simor, A.E., et al., and The Ontario Group A Streptococcal Study Group (1996) Invasive group A streptococcal infections in Ontario, Canada. *N. Engl. J. Med.* **135,** 547–554.
52. Bisno, A.L. and Stevens, D.L. (1996) Streptococcal infections of skin and soft tissues. *N. Engl. J. Med.* **334,** 240–245.
53. Stevens, D.L. (1999) The flesh-eating bacterium: what's next? *J. Infect. Dis 179(Suppl. 2),* S366–S374.
54. Muller, M.P., McGeer, A., Low, D.E., and Ontario Group A Streptococcal Study (2001) Successful outcome in six patients treated conservatively for suspected necrotizing fasciitis (NF) due to group A streptococccus (GAS), in *Abstracts of 41st Interscience Conference on Antimicrobial Agents and Chemotherapy,* ASM, Washington, DC.
55. Brown, D.R., Davis, N.L., Lepawsky, M., Cunningham, J., and Kortbeek, J. (1994) A multicenter review of the treatment of major truncal necrotizing infections with and without hyperbaric oxygen therapy. *Am. J. Surg.* **167,** 485–489.
56. Mouthon, L., Kaveri, S.V., Spalter, S.H., Lacroix-Desmazes, S., Lefranc, C., Desai, R., et al. (1996) Mechanisms of action of intravenous immune globulin in immune-mediated diseases. *Clin. Exp. Immunol.* **104(Suppl. 1),** 3–9.
57. Ballow, M. (1997) Mechanisms of action of intravenous immune serum globulin in autoimmune and inflammatory diseases. *Allergy Clin. Immunol.* **100,** 151–157.
58. Shulman, S.R. and Bendet, M. (1997) Kawasaki disease. *Compr. Ther.* **23,** 13–18.
59. Sacher, R.A. and the IVIG Advisory Panel (2001) Intravenous immunoglobulin consensus statement. *J. Allergy Clin. Immunol.* **108,** S139–S146.
60. Leung, D.Y. (1996) Kawaski syndrome: immunomodulatory benefit and potential toxin neutralization by intravenous immune globulin. *Clin. Exp. Immunol.* **104(Suppl. 1),,** 49–54.
61. Werdan, K. (2001) Intravenous immunoglobulin for prophylaxis and therapy of sepsis. *Curr. Opin. Crit. Care* **7,** 354–361.
62. Alejandria, M.M., Lansang, M.A., Dans, L.F., and Mantaring, J.B.V. (2001) Intravenous immunoglobulin for treating sepsis and septic shock. *Cochrane Database Syst. Rev.* **2,** CD001090.
63. Erdem, G., Yurdakok, M., Tekinalp, G., and Ersoy, F. (1993) The use of IgM-enriched intravenous immunoglobulin for the treatment of neonatal sepsis in preterm infants. *Turk. J. Pediatr* **35,** 277–281.
64. Weisman, L.E., Stoll, B.J., and Kueser, T.J. (1992) Intravenous immune globulin therapy for early onset sepsis in premature neonates. *J. Pediatr.* **121,** 434–443.
65. Chen, J.Y. (1996) Intravneous immunoglobulin in the treatment of full term and premature newborns with sepsis. *J. Formos. Med. Assoc.* **24,** 733–742.
66. Haque, K.N., Zaidi, M.H., and Bahakim, H. (1988) IgM-enriched intravenous immunoglobulin therapy in neonatal sepsis. *Am. J. Dis. Child.* **142,** 1293–1296.
67. De Simone, C., Delogu, G., and Corbetta, G. (1988) Intravenous immunoglobulins in association with antibiotics: a therapeutic trial in septic intensive care unit patients. *Crit. Care Med.* **16,** 23–26.
68. Schedel, I., Dreikhausen, U., Nentwig, B., Hockenschnieder, M., Rauthmann, D., Balikcioglu, S., et al. (1991) Treatment of gram-negative septic shock with an immunoglobulin preparation: a prospective, randomized clinical trial. *Crit. Care Med* **19,** 1004–1113.
69. Dominioni, L., Dionigi, R., Zanello, M., Chiaranda, M., Dionigi, R., Acquarolo, A., et al. (1991) Effect of high-dose IgG on survival of surgical patients with sepsis scores of 20 or greater. *Arch. Surg.* **126,** 236–240.
70. Grundmann, R. and Hornung, M. (1988) Immunoglobulin therapy in patients with endotoxemia and postoperative sepsis—a prospective randomized study. *Prog. Clin. Biol. Res.* **272,** 339–349.
71. Wesloy, C., Kipping, N., and Grundmann, R. (1990) Immunoglobulin therapy of postoperative sepsis. *Z. Exp. Chir. Transplant. Kunstliche Organe* **23,** 213–216.
72. Werdan, K., Pilz, G., and and the SBITS Study Group (1997) Polyvalent immune globulins (abstract). *Shock* **7(Suppl.),** 5/1918.
73. Samuelsson, A., Towers, T.L., and Ravetch, J.V. (2001) Anti-inflammatory activity of IVIG mediated through the inhibitory Fc receptor. *Science* **291,** 484–486.
74. Weisman, L.E., Cruess, D.F., and Fisher, G.W. (1994) Opsonic activity of commercially available standard intravenous immunoglobulin preparations. *Pediatr. Infect. Dis.* **13,** 1122–1125.
75. Fisher, G.W., Cieslak, T.J., Wilson, S.R., Weisman, L.E., and Heeming, V.G. (1994) Opsonic antibodies to *Staphylococcus epidermis:* in vitro and in vivo studies using human intravenous immune globulin. *J. Infect. Dis.* **169,** 324–329.
76. Yang, K.D., Bathras, J.M., Shigeoka, A.O., James, J., Pincus, S.H., and Hill, H.R. (1989) Mechanisms of bacterial opsonization by immune globulin intravenous: correlation of complement consumption with opsonic activity and protective efficacy. *J. Infect. Dis.* **159,** 701–707.

77. Hiemstra, P.S., Brands-Tajouiti, J., and van Furth, R. (1994) Comparison of antibody activity against various microorganisms in intravenous immunoglobulin preparations determined by ELISA and opsonic assay. *J. Lab. Clin. Med.* **123,** 241–246.
78. Patel, R., Rouse, M.S., Florez, M.V., Piper, K.E., Cockerill, F.R., Wilson, W.R. et al. (2000) Lack of benefit of intravenous immune globulin in a murine model of group A streptococcal necrotizing fasciitis. *J. Infect. Dis.* **181,** 230–234.
79. Norrby-Teglund, A., Kaul, R., Low, D.E., McGeer, A., Newton, D., et al. (1996) Plasma from patients with severe invasive group A streptococcal infections treated with normal polyspecific IgG inhibits streptococcal superantigen-induced T cell proliferation and cytokine production. *J. Immunol.* **156,** 3057–3064.
80. Norrby-Teglund, A., Kaul, R., Low, D. E., McGeer, A., Andersson, J., Andersson, U., et al. (1996) Evidence for the presence of streptococcal superantigen neutralizing antibodies in normal polyspecific IgG (IVIG). *Infect. Immun.* **64,** 5395–5398.
81. Norrby-Teglund, A., Basma, H., Andersson, J., McGeer, A., Low, D. E., and Kotb, M. (1998) Varying titres of neutralizing antibodies to streptococcal superantigens in different preparations of normal polyspecific immunoglobulin G (IVIG): implications for therapeutic efficacy. *Clin. Infect. Dis.* **26,** 631–638.
82. Skansen-Saphir, U., Andersson, J., Björk, L., and Andersson, U. (1994) Lymphokine production induced by streptococcal pyrogenic exotoxin-A is selectively down-regulated by pooled human IgG. *Eur. J. Immunol.* **24,** 916–922.
83. Lissner, R., Struff, W.G., Autenrieth, I.B., Woodcock, B.G., and Karch, H. (1999) Efficacy and potential clinical applications of Pentaglobin, an IgM-enriched immunoglobulin concentrate suitable for intravenous infusion. *Eur. J. Surg.* **584 (Suppl.),** 17–25.
84. Stegmayr, B., Bjorck, S., Holm, S., Nisell, J., Rydvall, A., and Settergren, B. (1992) Septic shock induced by group A streptococcal infection: clinical and therapeutic aspects. *Scand. J. Infect. Dis.* **24,** 589–597.
85. Darville, T., Milligan, L.B., and Laffoon, K.K. (1997) Intravenous immunoglobulin inhibits staphylococcal toxin-induced human mononuclear phagocyte tumor necrosis factor alpha production. *Infect. Immun.* **65,** 366–372.
86. Takei, S., Arora, Y. K., and Walker, S. M. (1993) Intravenous immunoglobulin contains specific antibodies inhibitory to activation of T cells by staphylococcal toxin superantigens. *J. Clin. Invest.* **91,** 602–607.
87. Norrby-Teglund, A., Ihendyane, N., Kansal, R., Basma, H., Kotb, M., Andersson, J., et al. (2000) Relative neutralizing activity in polyspecific IgM, IgA, and IgG preparations against group A streptococcal superantigens. *Clin. Inf. Dis.* **31,** 1175–1182.
88. Arend, W.P., Smith, M.F.J., Janson, R.W., and Joslin, F.G. (1991) IL-1 receptor antagonist and IL-1 beta production in human monocytes are regulated differently. *J. Immunol.* **147,** 1530–1536.
89. Poutsiaka, D.D., Clark, B.D., Vannier, E., and Dinarello, C.A. (1991) Production of interleukin-1 receptor antagonist and interleukin-1 beta by peripheral blood mononuclear cells is differentially regulated. *Blood* **78,** 1275–1281.
90. Ruiz de Souza, V., Carreno, M.P., Kaveri, S.V., Ledur, A., Sadeghi, H., Cavaillon, J.M., et al. (1995) Selective induction of interleukin-1 receptor antagonist and interleukin-8 in human monocytes by normal polyspecific IgG (intravenous immunoglobulin). *Eur. J. Immunol.* **25,** 1267–1273.
91. Andersson, U., Björck, L., Skansén-Saphir, U., and Andersson, J. (1994) Pooled human IgG modulates cytokine production in lymphocytes and monocytes. *Immunol. Rev.* **139,** 21–43.
92. Schalch, L., Rordorf-Adam, C., Dasch, J., and Jungi, T.W. (1991) IgG-stimulated and LPS-stimulated monocytes elaborate transforming growth factor type beta (TGF-beta) in active form. *Biochem. Biophys. Res. Commun.* **174,** 885–891.
93. Sasaki, H., Pollard, R.B., Schmitt, D., and Suzuki, F. (1992) Transforming growth factor-beta in the regulation of the immune response. *Clin. Immunol. Immunopathol.* **65,** 1–9.
94. Svenson, M., Hansen, M.B., and Bendtzen, K. (1993) Binding of cytokines to pharmaceutically prepared human immunoglobulin. *J. Clin. Invest.* **92,** 2533–2539.
95. Svenson, M., Hansen, M.B., Ross, C., Diamant, M., Rieneck, K., Nielsen, H., et al. (1998) Antibody to granulocyte-macrophage colony-stimulating factor is a dominant anti-cytokine activity in human IgG preparations. *Blood* **91,** 2054–2061.
96. Wadhwa, M., Meager, A., Dilger, P., Bird, C., Dolman, C., Das, R.G., et al. (2000) Neutralizing antibodies to granulocyte-macrophage colony-stimulating factor, interleukin-1alpha and interferon-alpha but not other cytokines in human immunoglobulin preparations. *Immunology* **99,** 113–123.
98. Ross, C., Svenson, M., Hansen, M. B., Vejlsgaard, G. L. and Bendtzen, K. (1995) High avidity IFN-neutralizing antibodies in pharmaceutically prepared human IgG. *J. Clin. Invest.* **95,** 1974–1978.
99. Grosse-Wilde, H., Blaszczyk, R., and Westhoff, U. (1992) Soluble HLA class I and class II concentrations in commercial immunoglobulin preparations. *Tissue Antigens* **39,** 74–77.
100. Lam, L., Whitsett, C. F., McNicholl, J. M., Hodge, T. W. and Hooper, J. (1993) Immunologically active proteins in intravenous immunoglobulin. *Lancet* **342,** 678.
101. Blaszczyk, R., Westhoff, U., and Grosse-Wilde, H. (1993) Soluble CD4, CD8, and HLA molecules in commercial immunoglobulin preparations. *Lancet* **341,** 789–790.
102. Andersson, J., Skansén-Saphir, U., Sparrelid, E., and Andersson, U. (1994) Intravenous immune globulin affects cytokine production in T lymphocytes and monocytes/macrophages. *Clin. Exp. Immunol.* **104(Suppl.),** 10–20.
103. Asano, T. and Ogawa, S. (2000) Expression of IL-8 in Kawasaki disease. *Clin. Exp. Immunol.* **122,** 514–519.
104. Nadal, D., Lauener, R.P., Braegger, C.P., Kaufhold, A., Simma, B., Lutticken, R. et al. (1993) T cell activation and cytokine release in streptococcal toxic shock-like syndrome. *J. Pediatr.* **122,** 727–729.
105. Sharief, M.K., Ingram, D.A., Swash, M., and Thompson, E.J. (1999) IV immunoglobulin reduces circulating proinflammatory cytokines in Guillain–Barré syndrome. *Neurology* **52,** 1833–1838.

106. Leung, D.Y., Cotran, R.S., Kurt-Jones, E., Burns, J.C., Newburger, J.W., and Pober, J.S. (1989) Endothelial cell activation and high interleukin-1 secretion in the pathogenesis of acute Kawasaki disease. *Lancet* **2,** 1298–1302.
107. Haywood, C.T., McGeer, A., and Low, D.E. (1999) Clinical experience with 20 cases of group A streptococcus necrotizing fasciitis and myonecrosis: 1995 to 1997. *Plast. Reconstr. Surg.* **103,** 1567–1573.
108. Cawley, M.J., Briggs, M., Haith, L.R.J., Reilly, K.J., Guilday, R.E., Braxton, G.R., et al. (1999) Intravenous immunoglobulin as adjunctive treatment for streptococcal toxic shock syndrome associated with necrotizing fasciitis: case report and review. *Pharmacotherapy* **19,** 1094–1098.
109. Barry, W., Hudgins, L., Donta, S.T., and Pesanti, E.L. (1992) Intravenous immunoglobulin therapy for toxic shock syndrome. *JAMA* **267,** 3315–3316.
110. Chiu, C.H., Ou, J.T., Chang, K.S., and Lin, T.Y. (1997) Successful treatment of severe streptococcal toxic shock syndrome with a combination of intravenous immunoglobulin, dexamethasone and antibiotics. *Infection* **25,** 47–48.
111. Lamothe, F., D'Amico, P., Ghosn, P., Tremblay, C., Braidy, J., and Patenaude, J. (1995) Clinical usefulness of intravenous human immunoglobulins in invasive group A streptococcal disease: case report and review. *J. Clin. Inf. Dis.* **21,** 1469–1470.
112. Mahieu, L.M., Holm, S.E., Goossens, H.J., and Van Acker, K.J. (1995) Congenital streptococcal toxic shock syndrome with absence of antibodies against streptococcal pyrogenic exotoxins. *J. Pediatr.* **127,** 987–989.
113. Perez, C.M., Kubak, B.M., Cryer, H.G., Salemugodam, S., Vespa, P., and Farmer, D. (1997) Adjunctive treatment of streptococcal toxic shock syndrome with intravenous immunoglobulin:case report and review. *Am. J. Med.* **102,** 111–113.
114. Yong, J.M. (1994) Necrotising fasciitis. *Lancet* **343,** 1427.

Index

From: *Cytokines and Chemokines in Infectious Diseases Handbook*
Edited by: M. Kotb and T. Calandra © Humana Press Inc., Totowa, NJ